Hemisyndromes

Psychobiology, Neurology, Psychiatry

Hemisyndromes

Psychobiology, Neurology, Psychiatry

Edited by

MICHAEL S. MYSLOBODSKY

Psychobiology Research Unit
Tel Aviv University
Ramat Aviv, Israel

ACADEMIC PRESS 1983

A Subsidiary of Harcourt Brace Jovanovich, Publishers

New York London
Paris San Diego San Francisco São Paulo Sydney Tokyo Toronto

ACADEMIC PRESS, INC.
111 Fifth Avenue, New York, New York 10003

United Kingdom Edition published by
ACADEMIC PRESS, INC. (LONDON) LTD.
24/28 Oval Road, London NW1 7DX

Library of Congress Cataloging in Publication Data
Main entry under title:

Hemisyndromes: Psychobiology, neurology, psychiatry.

Includes index.
1. Brain damage--Complications and sequelae--Addresses, essays, lectures. 2. Cerebral dominance--Addresses, essays, lectures. 3. Psychobiology--Addresses, essays. lectures. 4. Neuropsychiatry--Addresses, essays, lectures. I. Myslobodsky, Michael. [DNLM: 1. Brain injuries--Complications. 2. Brain diseases--Etiology. 3. Dominance, Cerebral. WL 354 H488]
RC387.5.H45 1983 616.8 83-2823
ISBN 0-12-512460-0

PRINTED IN THE UNITED STATES OF AMERICA

83 84 85 86 9 8 7 6 5 4 3 2 1

Contents

Contributors *xi*
Preface *xiii*

1: Introduction 1
MICHAEL S. MYSLOBODSKY

2: Cerebral Lateralization in the Rat and Tentative Extrapolations to Man 7
STANLEY D. GLICK

I. Introduction 8
II. Turning in Circles in Historical Perspective 8
III. Side Preferences and Lateralized Dopamine Function 10
IV. Lateralized Effects of Unilateral Brain Lesions 11
V. Multiple Asymmetries in Rat Brain and Developmental Changes Using the Labeled 2-Deoxy-D-glucose Technique 12
VI. Lateralization of Reward Mechanisms: Relation to Drug Euphoria and Psychopathological States 13
VII. Population Bias and Cortical Modulation 17
VIII. Striatal Dopamine Receptor Asymmetries and Sex Differences 18
IX. Neurochemical Laterality in the Human Brain 21
References 23

3: Behavioral and Neural Plasticity following Unilateral Brain Lesions 27
MONIKA PRITZEL and JOSEPH P. HUSTON

I. Introduction 28
II. Interhemispheric Projections of Substantia Nigra Neurons and Cessation of Lesion-Induced Turning 28
III. Plasticity of Interhemispheric Fiber Connections 51
References 60

4: Experimental Model of Hemi-Parkinsonism 69
C. J. PYCOCK

I. Introduction 70
II. The Rotating Rodent as an Experimental Model of Parkinson's Disease 70
III. Organization and Outflows of the Basal Ganglia: Relevance to the Rotation Model 73
IV. The Rotating Rodent: A Model of Human Hemi-Parkinsonism? 77
V. The Rotating Rodent Model: Assessment of Potential Anti-Parkinsonian Drugs 80
VI. Concluding Remarks: Hemi-Parkinsonism versus the Rotating Rodent 83
References 84

5: Sex Differences in Behavioral and Brain Asymmetries 91
TERRY E. ROBINSON, JILL B. BECKER, and DIANNE M. CAMP

I. Introduction 91
II. Behavioral and Brain Asymmetries 92
III. Sex Differences in Behavioral and Brain Asymmetries 103
IV. Conclusions 115
References 122

6: Gyratory and Cursive Epilepsy 129
RUGGERO G. FARIELLO and ANAND MEHENDALE

I. Historical Note 129
II. Gyratory Epilepsy 131
III. Cursive Epilepsy 141
IV. Summary and Conclusions 145
References 146

7: Hemisyndromes of Temporal Lobe Epilepsy: Review of Evidence Relating Psychopathological Manifestations in Epilepsy to Right- and Left-Sided Epilepsy 149
PIERRE FLOR-HENRY

I. Introduction 149
II. Laterality and Psychopathology: Evidence from Epilepsy 150

III. Forced Normalization 156
IV. Endogenous Psychoses and Laterality 159
V. Mood, Motility, Visuospatial Systems, Dreams, and Erotic Arousal 164
VI. Conclusion 167
References 169

8: Laterality of Affect: The Emotional Behavior of Right- and Left-Brain-Damaged Patients 175

GUIDO GAINOTTI

I. Introduction 175
II. Clinical Aspects of Emotional Reactions Associated with Unilateral Brain Lesions 177
III. Experimental Studies of Emotional Comprehension, Emotional Appropriateness, and Emotional Expression in Right- and Left-Brain-Damaged Patients 181
IV. Meaning of the Emotional Behavior of Right- and Left-Brain-Damaged Patients 184
References 189

9: Is There Hemi-aging? 193

MARGO B. LAPIDOT

I. Introduction 193
II. Aging Cognitive Abilities: Evidence for Asymmetric Decline 194
III. Central Measures of the Aging Brain: Known and Unexplored Territory 201
IV. Concluding Remarks 206
References 208

10: Two Types of Hemisphere Imbalance in Hemi-Parkinsonism Coded by Brain Electrical Activity and Electrodermal Activity 213

MATTI MINTZ and MICHAEL S. MYSLOBODSKY

I. Introduction 213
II. Hemi-Parkinsonism 214
III. Debut of the Syndrome 215
IV. Symmetry of Sleep Electroencephalogram Abnormalities in Hemi-Parkinsonism 216
V. Visual Evoked Potentials in Hemi-Parkinsonism 219
VI. Attention-Related Visual Evoked Potentials Asymmetry Reduction 222
VII. Components of Hemisphere Interdependence 223
VIII. Asymmetrics of Electrodermal Activity 229
IX. Summary 234
References 235

11:Epileptic Laughter 239
MICHAEL S. MYSLOBODSKY

I. Introduction 239
II. Symptoms of Gelastic Epilepsy 240
III. Brain Pathology and Pathophysiology of Epileptic Laughter 251
IV. Postscript 256
References 258

12:A Critical Assessment and Integration of Lateral Asymmetries in Schizophrenia 265
JOHN H. GRUZELIER

I. Introduction 265
II. British Origins 270
III. Experimental Approaches 275
IV. Conclusions 311
References 318

13:Temporal and Spatial Dynamics Underlying Two Neuropsychobiological Hemisyndromes: Hysterical and Compulsive Personality Styles 327
ARNOLD J. MANDELL

I. Dynamic Patterns in Brain Processes 327
II. Relevant Notions from Modern Mathematical Theory 329
III. The Concepts of Dimensionality and Stability 331
IV. Additive versus Multiplicative Information Processing 335
V. Intermittency: Cluster Behavior in the Time Domain 337
VI. A Neurochemical Locus for Spatiotemporal Asymmetries and Hemispheric Disconnection 338
References 342

14:Neuroleptic Effects and the Site of Abnormality in Schizophrenia 347
MICHAEL S. MYSLOBODSKY, MATTI MINTZ, and RACHEL TOMER

I. Introduction 347
II. Lateral Eye Movements: An Index of Abnormal Hemisphere Balance in Schizophrenia or Neuroleptic Effects? 348
III. Neuroleptic-Induced Asymmetry of Visual Evoked Potentials 350
IV. Attention-Induced Changes of P_{300} 360
V. Who Is the "Nonresponder"? 364
VI. Who Is the Blinker? 368
VII. Is the Deficit in Schizophrenia Left-sided, Right-sided, or of Callosal Transfer Origin? 371
VIII. Epilogue: Diagnosis *ex Juvantibus* 377
References 379

15: Hemisphere Dysfunction in Psychopathy and Behavior Disorders 389
ISRAEL NACHSHON

I. Historical Antecedents 389
II. Performance > Verbal Pattern 390
III. Clinical Evidence 394
IV. Experimental Evidence 397
V. Summary and Conclusions 403
VI. Theoretical Speculations and Applications 404
References 406

16: Psychogenic Somatic Symptoms on the Left Side: Review and Interpretation 415
DONNEL B. STERN

I. Introduction 415
II. Evidence for Symptom Lateralization 416
III. Explanations for Symptom Lateralization 428
References 441

17: Pharmacopsychotherapy and Aberrant Brain Laterality 447
MICHAEL S. MYSLOBODSKY and MURRAY WEINER

I. Introduction 447
II. What, Where, and Why? 448
III. Personality and Situational Variables in Drug Responses 450
IV. Psychopharmacology of the "Artistic" and "Intellectual" Brain 453
V. Components of Brain Asymmetry 456
VI. Activity and Drug Disposition 460
VII. Pharmacopsychotherapy 465
VIII. Psychotherapy and Dissociative Experience 468
IX. Epilogue 472
References 473

Index *479*

Contributors

Numbers in parentheses indicate the pages on which the authors' contributions begin.

JILL B. BECKER (91), Psychology Department, The University of Michigan, Ann Arbor, Michigan 48109

DIANNE M. CAMP (91), Psychology Department, The University of Michigan, Ann Arbor, Michigan 48109

RUGGERO G. FARIELLO (129), Department of Neurology, Jefferson Medical College, Philadelphia, Pennsylvania 19107

PIERRE FLOR-HENRY (149), Alberta Hospital and Department of Psychiatry, University of Alberta, Edmonton, Alberta, Canada

GUIDO GAINOTTI (175), Institute of Neurology, Catholic University, Rome, Italy

STANLEY D. GLICK (7), Department of Pharmacology, Mount Sinai School of Medicine, City University of New York, New York, New York 10029

JOHN H. GRUZELIER (265), Department of Psychiatry, Charing Cross Hospital Medical School, London W6 8RF, England

JOSEPH P. HUSTON (27), Laboratory of Comparativc and Physiological Psychology, Institute of Psychology, University of Dusseldorf, 4000 Dusseldorf, West Germany

MARGO B. LAPIDOT (193), School of Communication Disorders, Speech and Hearing, Chaim Sheba Medical Center, Tel-Hashomer, Israel 52621

ARNOLD J. MANDELL (327), Department of Psychiatry, University of California, San Diego, La Jolla, California 92093

ANAND MEHENDALE[1] (129), Neurology Section, Audie Murphy Veterans Memorial Hospital, San Antonio, Texas 78284

MATTI MINTZ (213, 347), Psychobiology Research Unit, Department of Psychology, Tel Aviv University, Ramat Aviv 69978, Israel

MICHAEL S. MYSLOBODSKY (1, 213, 239, 347, 447), Psychobiology Research Unit, Department of Psychology, Tel Aviv University, Ramat Aviv 69978, Israel

ISRAEL NACHSHON (389), Department of Criminology, Bar-Ilan University, Ramat-Gan 52100, Israel

MONIKA PRITZEL (27), Laboratory of Comparative and Physiological Psychology, Institute of Psychology, University of Dusseldorf, 4000 Dusseldorf, West Germany

C. J. PYCOCK (69), Department of Pharmacology, Medical School, The University of Bristol, Bristol BS8 1TD, England

TERRY E. ROBINSON (91), Department of Psychology, The University of Michigan, Ann Arbor, Michigan 48109

DONNEL B. STERN (415), Department of Psychology, The City College of the City University of New York, New York, New York

RACHEL TOMER (347), Psychobiology Research Unit, Department of Psychology, Tel Aviv University, Ramat Aviv 69978, Israel

MURRAY WEINER (447), Division of Clinical Pharmacology, Department of Internal Medicine, University of Cincinnati Medical Center, Cincinnati, Ohio 45267

[1]*Present address:* Department of Neurology, Kerrville State Hospital, Kerrville, Texas 78028.

Preface

The term *hemisyndrome,* embodied in the title of this volume, is typically employed to denote a unilateral loss of brain control over the contralateral side of the body. It is most often encountered in a form of muscular weakness or paralysis, but may assume a form of extrapyramidal hemisyndrome (Hemi-Parkinsonism, hemichorea, hemiballism), cerebellar hemisyndrome (unilateral cerebellar ataxy), lateralized pain (hemicrania), inattention (hemineglect), transient ictal or postictal hemiphenomena (adversive fits, gyratory epilepsy, Todd's paralysis), and so on.

Hemisyndromes are interesting abnormalities as they permit, in a search for pathophysiology of respective brain disorders, a "comparison of the patient with himself" rather than with other patients or control individuals. Also, there is growing recognition that hemisyndromes may differ in intensity, and that they may be accompanied by various psychopathological manifestations depending upon whether the damage is predominantly in the right or the left hemisphere. Some of these disturbances are barely distinguishable from symptoms of schizophrenia or affective psychoses. Regardless of the uncertainty concerning the type and location of organic lesions conducive to certain mental abnormalities, hemisyndromes may be a convenient way to examine aberrant behaviors. Applied to psychopathological phenomena, *hemisyndrome* may be looked at as a metaphor that suggests the necessity for juxtaposition of illnesses with dissimilar clinical pictures, etiology, social consequences, and effects in order to find some commonality of pathophysiology.

This book was organized to feature the most significant manifestations implicit in the commonality of the hemisyndrome concept, and to demonstrate its limitations in psychiatry and the perspectives of its experimental analysis. Each chapter is a comprehensive "state-of-the-art" treatise chosen for its general scientific and clinical significance to highlight the hemisyndrome approach. Chapters 1–4 center on the fast-growing literature on intrinsic and experimentally produced brain asymmetries in animals. Models of asymmetric attention, emotional responsiveness, and locomotion provide answers to questions posed by concepts of aberrant laterality. In the formerly blurred area of inferences and guesswork, these answers have an exquisite sharpness and expand the epiphenomenal–descriptive level of human laterality research into the areas of biochemistry and psychopharmacology. Today much of the work with experimental hemisyndromes is motivated by their putative value in human psychopathology and neurology.

Chapters 5–9 represent the neurological section of the volume. They examine those hemisyndromes frequently encountered in clinical practice which can be juxtaposed with experimental models. A reassuring feature of this juxtaposition is that instead of thinking of hemisphere interrelations as events in a black box with a totally obscure interior, the problem develops into an area where the complexities of higher mental functions—very often examined in the course of the diagnostic and treatment routine—may be illuminated by pathological changes of neurophysiology, brain anatomy, and neurochemistry. The reader should be forewarned that some interesting clinical phenomena are not represented. Possibly because the data banks of hemiballism, hemichorea, and Todd's paralysis are practically empty, I failed to find authors ready to meet the challenge of these topics. On the other hand, such areas as hemineglect became so "overpopulated" after several recent comprehensive reviews that neither experimental nor clinical aspects needed to be represented.

Chapters 10–16 test hemisyndrome concepts in psychiatry. They provide examples of major controversies: the directionality and magnitude of aberrant laterality in psychopathology, asymmetry of conversion symptomatology, pharmacologic evidence of hemisphere imbalance, and so forth. There was no intention, of course, to cover the entire spectrum of psychiatry in this section. The area has become so vast that I had to draw the line before the section became too cumbersome to be useful. In general, however, despite some notable omissions, the coverage should provide a firm foundation of knowledge on which to build.

There are two major groups of readers to whom this volume is addressed: research neurologists and psychiatrists interested in expanding their knowledge or contemplating an independent project in the area, and clinically minded psychologists and neurobiologists concerned with clinical application of their experimental findings.

The planning and preparation of this volume was greatly aided by a gift from Mrs. Arthur J. Biederman. Rachel Tomer did a splendid job as editorial assistant; she located missing references and, with Ora Kofman, helped with extensive correspondence. Also, I take this opportunity to express my appreciation to Rachel Pardee for her readiness to lend a hand at all stages of this project. Finally, I wish to express my gratitude to the editors at Academic Press for their patient assistance in coping with many problems connected with the preparation of this volume.

1: Introduction

MICHAEL S. MYSLOBODSKY

Psychobiology Research Unit
Tel Aviv University
Ramat Aviv, Israel

Clinical neurology has provided abundant evidence that, unlike the system of locomotion (*homo faber*), other brain functions, such as perception, cognition, emotion, and verbal capacity (*homo sensi, sapience, felix,* and *loquens*), are not uniformly damaged by right and left hemisphere lesions. In many cases the various faculties of the human brain may not necessarily be deranged in the sense of a functional deficit of Jacksonian "minus symptomatology." On the contrary, perception may acquire unique sharpness. Speech may become neologistic. Behavior may become bizarre, manneristic, or impulsive and motivated by hallucinations. Rich parallel experience, normally jealously concealed from consciousness, can be retrieved from oblivion. Emotional reactions are misplaced, grotesque, inadequate. Epileptic foci in the temporal lobe are frequently associated with this drama, and temporal lobe epilepsy has long been perceived as a tempting bridge between frank psychiatric disorders and localized brain lesions. In fact, after Gowers and Jackson, numerous efforts have been made to cross this bridge.

In 1969 Flor-Henry marshaled recalcitrant facts showing that clinical patterns associated with epileptic foci in the temporal lobe of the left hemisphere may be likened to schizophrenia. Abnormalities of affect and emotions, however, have been more often associated with right temporal lobe epileptic lesions. This initial observation was taken one step farther, to hypothesize that corresponding psychoses may be related to either left or right hemisphere dysfunction. The subsequent development of this conjecture generated a flurry of research aimed at comparing measures reflecting activities of the right and left hemispheres. Despite the some-

HEMISYNDROMES:
Psychobiology, Neurology,
Psychiatry

ISBN 0-12-512460-0

what wry, yet always hopeful mood in the field, the original concept of Flor-Henry continues to serve as a provocative stimulus in psychopathology, and the present volume summarizes the "neurological step" in a search in this general direction.

The idea that psychoses are related to hemisphere imbalance of pathological proportions proved to be useful for cutting through the confusion of psychiatric theories, suggested unexpected links among various disease subcategories, and supplied a logical and coherent basis for inquiry into the rationale of psychological, physical, and pharmacological management of the mentally ill (Chapters 6–9 and 10–17).

However, the complexity of brain functions, of which laterality is probably a modest part, made Roger Sperry (1982) in his Nobel lecture warn:

> The left–right dichotomy in cognitive mode is an idea with which it is very easy to run wild. Qualitative shifts in mental control may involve up–down, front–back, or various other organizational changes as well as left–right differences. Furthermore, in the normal state, the two hemispheres appear to work closely together as a unit, rather than one being turned on while the other idles. Much yet remains to be settled in all these matters. Even the main idea of differential left and right cognitive modes is still under challenge in some quarters [p. 1225].

There is no need to recapitulate the abundant evidence that in psychopathological syndromes laterality changes cannot be detected with the same sharpness as in cases of unilateral brain lesion. The outcome of the different approaches and experimental designs is frequently disconcerting, showing that psychoses have no distinct diagnostic landmarks of lateralized pathology similar to that seen in epilepsy. Some investigators detect no laterality dysfunction in mental diseases. Some propose a more complicated schema of abnormal laterality. Still others believe that laterality is a tightly spun web, seamless so to speak along the midline and with connections between numerous circuits in both hemispheres, so that the two sides of the web change in different areas to a different extent in various disease subcategories and in different stages of a disease. In addition, there is a suspicion that we are often wrestling with medication-induced asymmetry rather than a pathophysiologically meaningful imbalance (Chapter 14). Thus, we have no clear picture of what is wrong with brain laterality in psychoses or whether anything is wrong at all.

Efforts to separate the pathogenetic mechanisms of mental diseases along the left–right dichotomy have never been entirely satisfying. As often happens with novel ideas, however, inconsistencies, inaccuracies, and contradictions are temporarily ignored, even suppressed, or, to use Lakatos's label, placed in some sort of "quarantine" in order not to inhibit "positive heuristics" of the program. Now that the "quarantine" is over, it is apparent that numerous amendments, elaborations, specifications, and parallel explanatory hypotheses have been grafted to compensate for the simplicity and insufficiency of the original scheme. These grafts, however useful, were formulated as noncontradictory ("yes. . . but") hypotheses, creating an atmosphere of conceptual and phenomenological "egalitarianism." As a result the aberrant laterality paradigm today resembles those liberal theories which, as Lakatos ironically observed, are generally admired because they fail to forbid any observable state of affairs.

There has been no shortage of explanations as to why psychopathologists and scholars continue to entertain ideas of aberrant laterality theory. However, some readers might well be wondering, "What, then, justifies this volume if the field has not yet advanced to the stage where some findings or some basic laws stay unchallenged?" Readers of Antoine de Saint-Exupery's celebrated story, *The Little Prince,* will recall a brilliant parody of this question. On a remote planet the Little Prince meets an old geographer who devotedly collects reports of traveling explorers. His belief about what deserves to be put in print is very instructive: "The recitals of explorers," he explains to the Little Prince, "are put down first in pencil. One must wait until the explorer has furnished proofs before putting them down in ink." The old scholar-pedant may have been right about some branches of geography. In neuroscience, however, very much as in physics, understanding is imprecise, and things that are true in certain situations may not be true in general. Therefore, according to Popper virtue in science lies not in caution in avoiding errors, but in ruthlessness in eliminating them. Popper's dictum, boldness in conjectures on the one hand and austerity in refutations on the other, requires that painstaking measures be taken to test a theory. The raison d'être of this book is to review some methods of testing the aberrant laterality ideas using experimental and clinical hemisyndromes as a vehicle (Chapters 2–8, 10).

Diagnosis in psychiatry remains by and large a position taken by a physician with respect to the patient's story. Neurological hemisyndromes admittedly narrow the range of symptoms and therefore are not expected to model all aspects of psychoses. Rather, they are anticipated to provide rules of thumb in psychiatric research by showing the degree of hemisphere disparity, the clarity of symptoms they generate, and the range of dissociation between the intensity of the clinical symptoms and the magnitude of psychophysiological changes, which different hemisyndromes would typically produce on the two sides. In the area of psychopathology, in which, as Garmezy (1972) noted, "our scientific efforts are often primitive, our observations too frequently imprecise, or the phenomena we observe unreliable [p. 13]," the hemisyndrome template, although somewhat restrictive, offers a neurological style, a set of rules, and in addition may make possible the capturing of the "passing moment," the freezing, so to speak, of an otherwise volatile, confusing, and frustratingly opulent psychopathological symptomatology. It abandons ambiguous, suggestive language and imposes a more committal mode of expression directly stating what is meant. Finally, the program of hemisyndromes has been enunciated as a step toward imposing a style of academic inquiry by which one may legitimately ask whether, according to the logic of Popperian falsificationalism, the imbalance produced by the unilateral hemisphere lesion would lead to expected symptoms of psychopathology—whether it would create a pattern of psychophysiological asymmetries comparable to that encountered in conceptual ("metaphoric") hemisyndromes. The methodological prize of this approach is obvious. It invites a strong corroborative statement at the cost of an easier observational hurdle. It prepares a retreat from a possible corroborative failure (the advantage of the corroborative success is clear), suggesting that the hemisyndrome, the admittedly stipulative definition of aberrant laterality, should be declared inadequate as a model for psychopathology.

In closing, it should be acknowledged that there are, of course, serious difficulties inherent in the proposed approach. Earlier contentions that unilateral brain lesions produce a static disbalance are giving way to a more dynamic picture of the multilevel (multistructural) compensatory interhemispheric "seesaw." The pattern of this complex system, securing "hemisphere interdependence," is only beginning to emerge (Chapter 10). One of its functions is restoring the unity of the brain by reducing the disparity of hemispheric reactivity caused by lateralized damage (Chapter 5). So far, the need to assess the changing anatomy, electrophysiology, and neurochemistry of this compensatory circuitry and the roles of age, gender, and activity in its organization is largely satisfied by studies of experimental hemisyndromes. Although this young area is advancing rapidly, problems typical of joint psychophysiological and neurochemical approaches continue to exist:

> Numerous difficulties are interposed between the findings of correlations and the establishment of causal relationships between chemically and electrically observed events, not the least of which is the failure of the neurobiochemist and neurophysiologist to understand anything but the most superficial aspects of the companion science. It is a rare neurophysiologist who has a good understanding of the tricarbolic acid cycle and even rarer chemist who has an appreciation of the details of neuronal structure or the meaning of an oscilloscope's recording [Roberts and Eidelberg, 1960, p. 326].

There are, however, hopeful signs that the gap between the two approaches is closing, as evidenced by the results of much recent research, partially represented in this book. As a result, experimental and clinical hemisyndromes are destined to become a more widespread paradigm in laterality research. The present volume exposes the gaps in the field that are pressing to be filled and is a prelude of that to come.

References

Flor-Henry, P. (1969). Psychosis and temporal lobe epilepsy: A controlled investigation. *Epilepsia* **10,** 363–395.

Garmezy, N. (1972). Models of etiology for the study of children who are at risk for schizophrenia. In "Life History Research in Psychopathology" (M. Roff, L. Robins, and M. M. Pollack, eds.), Vol. 2, pp. 9–23. Univ. of Minnesota Press, Minneapolis.

Roberts, E., and Eidelberg, E. (1960). Metabolic and neurophysiological roles of aminobutyric acid. *Int. Rev. Neurobiol.* **2,** 280–327.

Sperry, R. (1982). Some effects of disconnecting the cerebral hemispheres. *Science* **217,** 1223–1226.

2: Cerebral Lateralization in the Rat and Tentative Extrapolations to Man

STANLEY D. GLICK

Department of Pharmacology
Mount Sinai School of Medicine
City University of New York
New York, New York

I. Introduction 8
II. Turning in Circles in Historical Perspective 8
A. Circus Movements and the Corpus Striatum 8
B. Rotation and the Dopaminergic Nigrostriatal System 9
C. Endogenous Asymmetry in Striatal Dopamine Content 10
III. Side Preferences and Lateralized Dopamine Function 10
IV. Lateralized Effects of Unilateral Brain Lesions 11
V. Multiple Asymmetries in Rat Brain and Developmental Changes Using the Labeled 2-Deoxy-D-glucose Technique 12
A. Different Kinds of Asymmetry in Different Structures 12
B. Ontogeny of Cerebral Asymmetries 12
VI. Lateralization of Reward Mechanisms: Relation to Drug Euphoria and Psychopathological States 13
A. Asymmetries in Lateral Hypothalamic Self-stimulation Thresholds 13
B. Effects of *d*-Amphetamine and Morphine on Lateral Hypothalamic Self-stimulation Asymmetries 14
C. Asymmetries in Hippocampal Self-stimulation and Effects of D-Lysergic Acid Diethylamide and Phencyclidine 15
D. Cerebral Asymmetries and Psychopathology 16
VII. Population Bias and Cortical Modulation 17
VIII. Striatal Dopamine Receptor Asymmetries and Sex Differences 18
A. Two Sites of [^{3}H]Apomorphine Binding 18
B. Sex Differences in D3 Sites and Left–Right D3 Asymmetry in Right-Sided Rats 19
C. Left versus Right in Rat and Man 20
IX. Neurochemical Laterality in the Human Brain 21
References 23

ISBN 0-12-512460-0

I. Introduction

Functional asymmetry in the human brain has been recognized since Broca's (1861) discovery that lesions resulting in language disorders were, in most cases, located in the left hemisphere (Galaburda *et al.*, 1978). Indeed, for many years it was generally believed that lateralization of cerebral function was uniquely human and in fact "arose in response to specifically human selective pressures [Levy, 1977]." However, evidence of lateralization of function has now been documented in the brains of several animal species (e.g., LeMay and Geschwind, 1975; Webster, 1977; Nottebohm, 1977; Glick *et al.*, 1977a), and some studies (Denenberg, 1981; Glick and Ross, 1981a) have brought into question the view (Warren, 1980) that the human pattern of cerebral laterality is "species unique."

In 1885 Ernst Mach postulated a mechanism of spatial behavior that applied to both man and beast. He recounted, "The idea that the distinction between right and left depends upon an asymmetry, and possibly in the last resort upon a chemical difference, is one which has been present to me from my earliest years." It was not until about nine decades later that the implications of Mach's "idea" were investigated. The purpose of this chapter is to summarize the results of such investigations and indicate the extent to which animal and human brains share common mechanisms of asymmetry.

II. Turning in Circles in Historical Perspective

A. Circus Movements and the Corpus Striatum

As will soon become evident, the propensity of animals to turn in circles after unilateral brain damage was an important starting point of studies concerned with the characterization of cerebral asymmetry in rats. It is now a commonplace observation that rats with nigrostriatal lesions rotate, or turn in circles, in response to various drugs. Although this phenomenon has been examined intensively only in the past 15 years, the mention of a relationship between turning and striatal function or dysfunction has been in the literature for more than 100 years. In 1873 Nothnagel found that injections of chromic acid into the striatum caused a bending of the trunk to the side of the lesion (Wilson, 1914). Ferrier (1876) stated that "irritation of the corpus striatum causes general muscular contraction on the opposite side of the body. The head and body are strongly flexed to the opposite side, so that the head and tail become approximated." These results were seen in monkeys, cats, dogs, jackals, and rabbits. In 1921 Lashley described a rotation syndrome after combined unilateral destruction of the caudate nucleus and the motor cortex above it. "Circus" movements after "partial and unsymmetrical injuries to the striatum" in rats were reported by Herrick in 1926. Unilateral striatal lesions in dogs caused circus movements and a forced posture toward the side of the lesion in a study by Mettler and Mettler in 1942. After observing that striatal stimulation elicited contraversive circling in cats, Laursen concluded in 1962 that circling was the only motor response of caudate origin and that the "circling response is a complex behavioral manifestation rather than a stereotyped movement." Noting that the stimulated cats looked "as if they were searching for something," Laursen suggested that "the function of the caudate is at a high level of integration."

B. Rotation and the Dopaminergic Nigrostriatal System

Renewed interest in the phenomenon of circling, or rotation, after unilateral striatal dysfunction is attributable to findings implicating a critical role for nigrostriatal afferents containing dopamine (Andén *et al.*, 1966) and subsequent demonstrations that rats with unilateral nigrostriatal lesions can be used as a model of dopaminergic drug action (e.g., Ungerstedt, 1971; Glick *et al.*, 1976; Pycock, 1980). Initial studies indicated that damage to the nigrostriatal system was both necessary and sufficient for the appearance of drug-induced rotation. However, subsequent studies in this laboratory and others showed that normal animals also rotate, albeit at lower rates, when administered the same drugs as those administered to lesioned animals. Amphetamine, apomorphine, L-dopa, scopolamine, D-lysergic acid diethyamide (LSD), morphine, and phencyclidine (PCP) all induce rotation in naive rats (e.g., Jerussi and Glick, 1976; Morihisa and Glick, 1977; Fleisher and Glick, 1979; Glick *et al.*, 1980a) and, as with lesioned rats, the direction of rotation is consistent. Thus, when subjected to repeated testing with the same dose of a given drug, some animals rotate consistently to the left whereas others rotate to the right. It was further shown that nonlesioned, untreated rats also rotate at night (the more active half of their circadian cycle) and that this rotation is in the same direction as that induced by amphetamine (Glick and Cox, 1978). Normal dogs and cats have similarly been reported to rotate spontaneously as well as in response to drugs (Nymark, 1972; Glick *et al.*, 1981a). A possibly related observation in human beings is that people lost in fogs find that they walk in complete circles (Howard and Templeton, 1966). Mach (1885) also noted that "human beings and animals that have lost their direction move, almost without exception, nearly in circle."

C. Endogenous Asymmetry in Striatal Dopamine Content

The phenomenon of rotation in normal rats was one of the first indications that normal animals may have an intrinsic asymmetry in nigrostriatal function that is accentuated by some drugs. Such an asymmetry was eventually demonstrated directly in rats. The concentrations of dopamine in the two striata were found to differ by about 15% (Zimmerberg *et al.*, 1974). High doses of *d*-amphetamine (20 mg/kg, ip) increased this difference to approximately 25% (Glick *et al.*, 1974) while causing rats to rotate contralaterally to the side with the higher dopamine levels. The nigrostriatal asymmetry was also shown to have both pre- and post synaptic components in reciprocal relationship to each other. Thus, there was a bilateral imbalance in the metabolites of dopamine, indicative of presynaptic activity, and an oppositely directed imbalance in striatal dopamine-stimulated adenylate cyclase activity, indicative of postsynaptic receptors (Jerussi *et al.*, 1977). The implication was that the side of the brain with more active terminals had fewer, or less sensitive, postsynaptic receptors. Normally, the dominant asymmetry appeared to be presynaptic.

III. Side Preferences and Lateralized Dopamine Function

Several experiments have been concerned with the general functional significance of the nigrostriatal asymmetry revealed by the rotation studies. On the basis of earlier findings on the effects of amphetamine on side preferences in operant situations (Glick, 1973; Glick and Jerussi, 1974), it was hypothesized that this asymmetry might be related to spatial behavior. It was of interest that the normal spatial preferences of rats for the left or right lever while responding for water were correlated with the direction of amphetamine-induced rotation. Side preferences in a T maze were also correlated with amphetamine-induced rotation, and neurochemical experiments demonstrated that dopamine concentration was significantly higher in the striata contralateral to rats' side preferences in the T maze (Zimmerberg *et al.*, 1974). The asymmetry in striatal dopamine was shown not to be attributable to any learning or stress-related change induced by the testing procedure. In another experiment the effect of unilateral caudate stimulation on spatial preferences was studied. Rats were first trained to bar-press for water in a two-lever operant chamber. Electrical stimulation of the caudate nucleus ipsilateral to a rat's side preference resulted in the rat switching levers for the duration of stimulation; upon termination of the stimulation, rats would immediately return to the original lever (Zimmerberg and Glick, 1975). All of these results suggested that rotation is a stereotyped form of spatial behavior and that spatial tendencies are derived, at least in part, from a nigrostriatal asymmetry. Comparisons of rats having stronger or weaker directional biases showed that the strength of the biases was related generally to overall learning ability (Glick *et al.*, 1977b) as well as specifically to the ability to discriminate between left and right (Zimmerberg *et al.*, 1978). Rats lacking clear spatial biases were hyperactive, had difficulty learning a variety of tasks, and were unable to distinguish left from right. A persistent lateral or orienting bias appeared to function as a proprioceptive reference with alterations of proprioceptive feedback from the biased side enabling the animal to differentiate between left and right movement.

It has been proposed (Glick *et al.*, 1977a) that nonlateralized or weakly lateralized rats may represent a model of minimal brain dysfunction (MBD). Children having this disorder are characterized by hyperactivity and learning difficulties. Minimal brain dysfunction is frequently associated with poor cerebral dominance (Gazzaniga, 1973), and motor disabilities as well as electrophysiological abnormalities may appear asymmetrically (Conners, 1973; Reitan and Boll, 1973). Amphetamines and related drugs have been found to be useful in treating MBD, especially when neurological evidence of brain damage has been demonstrated (Millichap, 1973; Satterfield *et al.*, 1973). The therapeutic effects of these drugs are perhaps attributable to enhancement of nigrostriatal asymmetry and/or of cerebral dominance generally.

IV. Lateralized Effects of Unilateral Brain Lesions

That normal animals rotate and have side preferences has some interesting and important implications from an experimental viewpoint. It might be predicted, for example, that rotation following the infliction of a unilateral lesion would vary depending on whether the lesion were in the side of the brain ipsilateral or contralateral to the preoperative direction of rotation. This prediction was verified in rats administered apomorphine (Jerussi and Glick, 1975) and amphetamine (Glick, 1976) following unilateral striatal damage ipsilateral and contralateral to the preoperative direction of rotation. After surgery all rats rotated toward the side of the lesion; for both drugs, however, the intensity of rotation (full turns per hour) was twice as great in rats with lesions ipsilateral to the preoperative direction as in rats with lesions contralateral to the preoperative direction. Thus, the preoperative bias is an important determinant of the postoperative effect. Other work with unilateral striatal lesions demonstrated qualitative as well as quantitative differences in the effects of lesions of either side of the brain. In one study lesions ipsilateral to side preferences facilitated rats' timing performance, whereas contralateral lesions impaired timing performance (Glick and Cox, 1976). In another study lesions ipsilateral and contralateral to side preferences facilitated and impaired, respectively, passive avoidance learning (Rothman and Glick, 1976). These data indicate the importance of the side of the lesion in assessing the effect of the lesion. They also illustrate how faulty conclusions about the kind or magnitude of an effect produced by a lesion can sometimes be drawn when the preoperative state is not considered. Lesion sidedness is an established and ordinary facet of clinical neurology; it is clearly time for this to become an ordinary variable in lesion studies with animals.

V. Multiple Asymmetries in Rat Brain and Developmental Changes Using the Labeled 2-Deoxy-D-glucose Technique

A. Different Kinds of Asymmetry in Different Structures

The 2-deoxy-D-glucose (dGlc) technique, as originally described by Sokoloff and colleagues (1977), can be used to assess the functional state of the nervous system under a variety of experimental conditions. Reasoning that intrinsic cerebral asymmetry is in some way reflected by altered activity in the two sides of the brain, we used a modified dGlc technique (Meibach *et al.*, 1980) to evaluate potential asymmetries in several brain regions (Glick *et al.*, 1979). Data from this study indicated that hemispheric asymmetry in the rat is more prevalent and more complex than was previously envisioned. Most structures showed evidence of functional brain asymmetry. Three kinds of asymmetry were identified: (*a*) differences in activity between sides of the brain contralateral and ipsilateral to the direction of rotation (midbrain and striatum); (*b*) differences in activity between left and right sides (frontal cortex and hippocampus); and (*c*) absolute differences in activity between sides that were correlated with the rate of rotation (thalamus and hypothalamus) or with random movement (cerebellum). *d*-Amphetamine (1.0 mg/kg, ip), administered 15 min before a dGlc injection, altered asymmetries in striatum, frontal cortex, and hippocampus but not those in midbrain, thalamus, hypothalamus, and cerebellum. These data suggested that different asymmetries are organized along different dimensions in the rat; more recent data, to be reviewed later, indicate that this is probably the case in human beings as well (see Section IX).

B. Ontogeny of Cerebral Asymmetries

The labeled dGlc technique has also been used to investigate the ontogeny of cerebral laterality in rats. Animals were administered dGlc at various ages during postnatal development, and dGlc uptake was compared on the two sides of the brain in several structures (Ross *et al.*, 1981, 1982). The data clearly established that newborn rats have left–right asymmetries in dGlc uptake in many structures and that these asymmetries change during development. In females there were significant left-to-right gradients in brainstem and midbrain and right-to-left gradients in hippocampus and diencephalon (e.g., the hippocampus was right-biased in the neonate and left-biased in the adult). The only gradient observed in males was a right-to-left gradient in midbrain. In most brain regions and in both sexes, there was a significant relationship between brain activity (dGlc uptake) and brain asymmetry: the more active a structure relative to the rest of the brain, the more likely that the structure was right-biased and vice versa. There were significant differences between sexes in the slopes of these relationships in some structures (cortex, striatum).

In both sexes we also observed neonatal asymmetries in tail position that were predictive of adult turning preferences; there were significant differences between sexes in the strength of these preferences, both in the neonate (Ross *et al.*, 1981) and in the adult (Glick *et al.*, 1980b). In human beings Michel (1981) demonstrated that an asymmetry in neonatal head posture predicts handedness at 16 and 22 weeks of age. The observations of tail position and turning preference in rats and of head posture and handedness in human beings may be related.

Cerebral lateralization in the rat is clearly present at birth, changes during development, and is sexually dimorphic. Neuroanatomical (e.g., Galaburda *et al.*, 1978) and functional (e.g., Witelson, 1976) findings support the same conclusion in human beings. Corballis and Morgan (1978) suggested that the development of cerebral lateralization in the human and other species might be explicable in terms of a left–right maturational gradient; the left hemisphere presumably develops earlier and/or more rapidly than the right. This hypothesis is based largely on functional evidence concerning handedness and lateralization of language and is not based on direct measurements of brain development. The present dGlc data indicate that maturational gradients do indeed exist but that such gradients are structure specific as well as sexually dimorphic.

VI. Lateralization of Reward Mechanisms: Relation to Drug Euphoria and Psychopathological States

A. Asymmetries in Lateral Hypothalamic Self-stimulation Thresholds

Neurological findings indicating that the two sides of the human brain are specialized for affect, with one hemisphere characterized as more joyful and the other as more depressive (Gainotti, 1972; Galin, 1974; Terzian, 1964), prompted us to investigate the possibility of affectual lateralization in rats. We suggested that differences in affect might result from differences in the activity of mechanisms mediating reinforcement and then demonstrated that the two sides of the rat brain are differentially sensitive to reinforcing lateral hypothalamic stimulation (Glick *et al.*, 1980c). Bipolar stainless steel electrodes were implanted in both lateral hypothalami of naive female Sprague–Dawley rats. Rats were subsequently placed in operant chambers and allowed to self-stimulate (0.5-sec, 60-Hz sine wave, 10–150 μA), during which time rotation was also measured. All rats rotated in a preferential direction regardless of the side of the brain stimulated and, in each case, the direction was the same as that subsequently determined in response to *d*-amphetamine (1.0 mg/kg). All rats had asymmetries in self-stimulation thresholds related to the preferred direction of rotation: thresholds were lower on the contralateral side, and entire rate–intensity functions were generally higher and displaced to the left on that side. Inasmuch as sources of artifact could be excluded, the results indicated that reward processes in the rat are, to some extent, lateralized.

B. Effects of *d*-Amphetamine and Morphine on Lateral Hypothalamic Self-stimulation Asymmetries

The finding of a self-stimulation asymmetry suggested a model of affectual lateralization in which quantitative differences in neuronal firing could be translated into apparent qualitative specialization, with the two sides of the brain appearing to be specialized for high and low mood, respectively. With this in mind we hypothesized that differences in the reinforcing qualities of different drugs could conceivably be due to their differential effects on mood mechanisms in the two sides of the brain. Testing of this hypothesis has begun. Using the same experimental design, the effects of *d*-amphetamine and morphine on the lateral hypothalamic reward asymmetry were examined. Various doses of each drug were administered twice, once with the left side of the brain stimulated first and once with the right side of the brain stimulated first. The effects of the two drugs, with respect to lateralization, were quite different. Whereas *d*-amphetamine preferentially affected the low-threshold side of the brain, low doses (e.g., 2.5 mg/kg) of morphine preferentially affected the high-threshold side. The low-dose effects of both drugs were to shift the rate–intensity functions to the left. However, with *d*-amphetamine this shift occurred more for the side contralateral to the direction of rotation, whereas with morphine it occurred more for the ipsilateral side. The dose–response curve for *d*-amphetamine was an inverted-U function (Glick *et al.*, 1981b), with high doses (e.g., 2.0 mg/kg) producing a smaller increase in reward sensitivity and asymmetry than lower doses (e.g., 0.25–0.5 mg/kg). In contrast, high doses (e.g., 10.0–20.0 mg/kg) of morphine augmented reinforcement thresholds and shifted rate–intensity functions to the right. However, this depressant effect was more pronounced in the low-threshold side of the brain such that the morphine-induced reversal of reward asymmetry was fairly constant across doses (Glick *et al.*, 1982). Therefore, the facilitatory and depressant actions of morphine on lateral hypothalamic self-stimulation preferentially occurred on opposite sides of the brain.

If one side of the brain is more sensitive to reinforcement than the other, one might predict that, given a choice, rats would prefer to self-stimulate the more sensitive side provided that stimulation currents were equated in some way. This hypothesis was tested using a two-lever operant chamber in which each lever delivers stimulation to either the left or right side of the brain, respectively. All rats tested in this manner prefer to stimulate their low-threshold side. The sidedness of the stimulation supercedes any lever preferences; switching which lever affects which side of the brain quickly results in the rat switching levers. However, by increasing the current administered to the high-threshold side and/or decreasing the current administered to the low-threshold side, one can establish no-preference behavior, with rats alternately stimulating each side of the brain. The effects of *d*-amphetamine and morphine on this type of baseline have also been studied. *d*-Amphetamine induces a preference for the low-threshold side of the brain (Glick *et al.*, 1981b), whereas morphine induces a preference for the high-threshold side (Glick *et al.*, 1982); the effects of both drugs are apparent across a wide range of doses. It is of interest that the effect of a low dose of morphine is attributable to a greater increase in responding for stimulation to the high-threshold side of the brain, and the effect of a high dose is attributable to a greater decrease in stimulation of the low-threshold side. These results are entirely consistent with the rate–intensity data discussed earlier.

C. Asymmetries in Hippocampal Self-stimulation and Effects of D-Lysergic Acid Diethylamide and Phencyclidine

All of our self-stimulation work has heretofore involved the medial forebrain bundle as it courses through the lateral hypothalamus. More recently, we have begun investigating the possibility of self-stimulation asymmetries in other brain regions involving, most likely, other pathways. Some particularly interesting findings have resulted from electrode placements in the dorsal hippocampus. Rats self-stimulate the dorsal hippocampus, although rates are considerably lower than those generated from the lateral hypothalamus. An asymmetry in self-stimulation sensitivity is also evident in the dorsal hippocampus but, in contrast to the lateral hypothalamus, the hippocampal asymmetry is unrelated to the direction of rats' rotation. Instead, it appears that the hippocampal asymmetry may be organized with respect to left versus right; that is, regardless of rats' spatial biases, the left hippocampus has had a lower self-stimulation threshold than the right hippocampus in 9 of 11 rats tested so far. In our dGlc studies (Glick *et al.*, 1979), the left hippocampus was also found to be more active than the right.

Studies comparing the effects of drugs on the lateral hypothalamic and hippocampal self-stimulation asymmetries are in progress, and some preliminary findings can be noted. In contrast to their robust effects on the lateral hypothalamus, described above, *d*-amphetamine and morphine have negligible effects on hippocampal self-stimulation, hardly altering rates or thresholds in either side of the brain in any rat. However, two hallucinogens, LSD and PCP, although having little or no effect on lateral hypothalamic self-stimulation, have quite substantial effects on hippocampal self-stimulation. Optimal doses of both drugs enhance rates and lower thresholds, but the two drugs preferentially affect opposite sides of the brain. Whereas LSD (0.25 mg/kg) has larger effects on the normally more sensitive side, PCP (2.5 mg/kg) has larger effects on the normally less sensitive side. The former enhances the hippocampal asymmetry, whereas PCP reduces or reverses it. Thus, the mechanisms of action of four commonly abused drugs can be dissociated in terms of both their site of action and their side of action. Table 2.1 summarizes these data.

D. Cerebral Asymmetries and Psychopathology

Aside from helping to elucidate the mode of action of different reinforcers, the finding that reward processes are lateralized may have broad relevance to our understanding of psychopathological states. Increasing evidence has supported an association between psychosis and disorders of cerebral laterality (Gruzelier and Flor-Henry, 1979; Wexler and Heninger, 1979). Numerous observations indicate that the dominant hemisphere is overactive in schizophrenia (Flor-Henry, 1976; Gur, 1978). The latter is of particular interest in relation to other data suggesting that disturbances of reward mechanisms underlie schizophrenia (Stein and Wise, 1971; Wise *et al.*, 1978), that amphetamine potentiates or induces motor and delusional symptoms of schizophrenia (Angrist and Gershon, 1970, 1972), and that dopaminergic systems in the brain are hyperactive in schizophrenia (e.g., Snyder, 1976). These seemingly disparate findings may have a common basis: schizophrenia may be, in part, a disorder of a hyperactive dopaminergic pathway in the dominant hemisphere, and amphetamine may exacerbate or induce the disorder by selectively affecting the dominant side. The "dominance" of the dominant side may be

TABLE 2.1
Summary of Drug Effects on Self-stimulation Asymmetries

Medial forebrain bundle
d-Amphetamine
Potentiates endogenous asymmetry: preferentially increases sensitivity in dominant (lower-threshold) side
Morphine
Reverses endogenous asymmetry: Low doses preferentially increase sensitivity in nondominant (higher-threshold) side; high doses preferentially decrease sensitivity in dominant side
LSD and phencyclidine
No asymmetric effects: Low doses and high doses of both drugs increase and decrease sensitivity, respectively; effects are small and bilaterally symmetric
Dorsal hippocampus
d-amphetamine and morphine
No asymmetric effects: neither drug significantly alters sensitivity of either side
LSD
Potentiates endogenous asymmetry: preferentially increases sensitivity in dominant side
Phencyclidine
Reverses endogenous asymmetry: preferentially increases sensitivity in nondominant side

attributable to a lower threshold for excitation and, as in the self-stimulation paradigm, amphetamine may enhance "dominance" by inducing a lateralized increase in reward sensitivity.

Schizophrenic hallucinations may be mediated by abnormal activity in several brain regions, apparently including the globus pallidus, a probable site of amphetamine action, but more importantly the hippocampus and other limbic structures (e.g., Horowitz and Adams, 1970). The involvement of the hippocampus is especially intriguing in relation to our observations that LSD and PCP alter hippocampal asymmetry in reward sensitivity. LSD and PCP induce visual and auditory hallucinations, respectively (e.g., Martin, 1977), and the mechanisms of both visual and auditory hallucinations appear to be lateralized in human brain (Penfield and Perot, 1963).

VII. Population Bias and Cortical Modulation

Until recently we believed that the directional asymmetries in rotation and side preference occurred randomly in a rat population; that is, in a typical experiment it was generally observed that approximately 50% of rats rotated to the right and 50% to the left. In contrast were the findings of a left–right asymmetry in rat cortex, indicated by differences in cortical thickness (Diamond *et al.*, 1975), differences in the behavioral effects of left and right cortical lesions (e.g., Denenberg *et al.*, 1978; Robinson, 1979), and a difference in frontal cortical energy metabolism (Glick *et al.*, 1979). The results of the last study indicated that the left–right asymmetry in frontal cortex modulated or interacted with the nigrostriatal asymmetry: Rats' side preferences were higher if frontal cortex was also higher on the contralateral side. Because left frontal cortex was usually more active than right frontal cortex, the implication was that, in a large population, more rats should have right side preferences than left side preferences and right preferences should be greater than left preferences. We therefore reexamined the data we had accumulated for the past several years and determined that, in a group of 602 rats, there was a small (54.8%) but significant ($p < 0.025$) right population bias; right-sided rats were also found to be both more active and have greater side preferences than left-sided rats (Glick and Ross, 1981b). If frontal cortex is indeed lateralized and modulates spatial bias, it was reasoned further that bilateral frontal cortical lesions, by removing this modulation, should decrease side preferences and activity in right-sided rats and increase these parameters in left-sided rats. This is precisely what occurred (Ross and Glick, 1981). We speculated that the increase in population bias in human beings as compared with rodents is perhaps related to the evolution and growth of the cortex in relation to subcortical structures. The population bias would be expected to increase in parallel with phylogeny if the left–right asymmetry in cortex increased as the cortex became more convoluted in conjunction with an enhanced modulation of subcortical structures (e.g., striatum).

VIII. Striatal Dopamine Receptor Asymmetries and Sex Differences

A. Two Sites of [^{3}H]Apomorphine Binding

We conducted studies to determine whether there are cerebral asymmetries of dopamine receptor populations and, if so, whether the asymmetries can be related to the direction of rats' nocturnal and *d*-amphetamine-induced (1.0 mg/kg) rotation. It was also of interest to determine whether dopamine receptor populations differ with respect to sex. Differences between receptor populations can be quantified by the amount of binding of a selective radioligand. If separate tissue preparations are exposed to a saturating concentration of radioligand, at equilibrium a difference in the amount of binding reflects a difference in the number of receptors, the affinity of the ligand for the receptor, or both.

[^{3}H]Apomorphine was employed as a radioligand to assay for putative dopamine receptors in rat striatum. This ligand is particularly relevant because apomorphine itself elicits rotational behavior (Jerussi and Glick, 1976). Preliminary experiments confirmed the findings of others (Seeman, 1980; Sokoloff *et al.*, 1980) that [^{3}H]apomorphine labels two distinct binding sites in this tissue. Sex, directional bias, and side of the brain comprised the independent variables. The two levels of each factor were male/female, right rotator/left rotator, and right side of the brain/left side of the brain, respectively. To avoid confounding variance due to the interexperiment variation of [^{3}H]apomorphine concentration, data were blocked by single experiment, and each block included all permutations of factors and levels ($2\times2\times2$). Each experiment therefore included 4 rats, 1 from each group with respect to sex and directional bias; the left–right sides of the brain, being derived from the same animal, were obviously paired. [^{3}H]Apomorphine binding to both sites was assayed in triplicate and replicated eight times (i.e., eight blocks or $N=8$ rats per group). The concentration of [^{3}H]apomorphine varied from 2 to 3 n*M* among blocks but was constant within a block.

B. Sex Differences in D3 Sites and Left–Right D3 Asymmetry in Right-Sided Rats

Three-way analyses of variance revealed several findings (Stollak and Glick, 1982). First, the [^{3}H]apomorphine binding that is sensitive to 200 n*M* domperidone appears to be homogeneous regardless of sex, behavioral bias, or side of the brain. This binding site has been reported to be postsynaptic in rat striatum and has been classified a D4 dopamine receptor (Seeman, 1980; Sokoloff *et al.*, 1980). In contrast, the [^{3}H]apomorphine binding that occurs in the presence of 200 n*M* domperidone and is sensitive to 2 μM ADTN (2-amino-6,7-dihydroxy-1,2,3,4-tetrahydronaphthalene) is evidently heterogeneous with respect to the three variables. This binding site has been classified a D3 dopamine receptor and has been reported to be largely presynaptic in rat striatum (Seeman, 1980; Sokoloff *et al.*, 1980). Most striking was the observation of significantly more total binding to the D3 site in the striata from females than in those from males (mean difference of 20.5%, $p<0.0003$). Also observed were the following. Right rotators exhibited significantly more total binding than left rotators, the right side of the brain bound significantly more [^{3}H]apomorphine than the left side, and there was significantly more binding on the side of the brain ipsilateral to the directional bias of the animal ($p<0.05$ in each case). The last three results are accounted for by the composite finding that right rotators show a significant right–left asymmetry of binding, whereas left rotators do not. That is, there is an equivalent amount of binding on both sides of the brain in left rotators, which is equivalent to the amount of binding on the left side of the brain of right rotators, but there is significantly greater binding, an average of 21.7% more, in the right striata of right rotators ($p<0.05$) in both males and females. It is important to note that these significant differences were observed only with respect to the D3 receptor even though both D3 and D4 binding were assayed simultaneously using the same tissue preparations.

The fact that significant differences between sexes and between sides of the brain were observed only with respect to the D3 site suggests that the mechanism(s) responsible for regulating asymmetry in striatal dopaminergic activity as well as those responsible for sex differences in rotation (Glick *et al.*, 1980b; Robinson *et al.*, 1980; Brass and Glick, 1981) are, at least in the Sprague–Dawley rat, predominantly presynaptic. This conclusion is consistent with other behavioral (Glick *et al.*, 1977c) and biochemical (Jerussi *et al.*, 1977) data. Current studies are concerned with determining whether the observed differences of [^{3}H]apomorphine binding to the D3 site are due to differences in either the total number of binding sites available or the affinity of the radioligand for the site.

C. Left versus Right in Rat and Man

A final point regarding the binding results concerns the differences between left- and right-sided rats. Until recently, as noted earlier, we were unaware of any behavioral differences associated with a left versus a right bias; the possibility of any neurochemical differences indeed appeared remote. Contrary to expectation, it is now apparent that left- and right-sided rats differ behaviorally (see Section VII) as well as neurochemically (also see Valdes *et al.*, 1981). Behavioral and cerebral differences between left- and right-handed human beings are well documented (e.g., Rasmussen and Milner, 1977). Of special interest is that, whereas right-handed individuals almost always have left cerebral dominance, left-handed individuals have either right cerebral dominance, left cerebral dominance, or ambivalent dominance (e.g., Hécaen and Sauget, 1971). If one were to suppose that underlying neurochemical asymmetries mediated or at least were correlated with cerebral dominance, one might expect neurochemical data from a random population of right-handed individuals to exhibit clear left–right differences but similar data from a random population of left-handed individuals to exhibit no clear patterns of asymmetry. This result certainly appears to be the case in left- versus right-sided rats, at least with respect to the D3 striatal site that we have so far investigated. Although the similarity may be only superficial, it is likely that we may have a model of the human situation that is worthy of further research and substantiation.

IX. Neurochemical Laterality in the Human Brain

We were recently presented an opportunity to investigate directly the possibility of neurochemical asymmetries in postmortem human brain. Rossor *et al.* (1980) measured concentrations of three to five neurotransmitters in nine structures, both left and right sides, of normal brains; their primary goal was to learn whether left–right differences need consideration in comparisons of abnormal and normal brains. Because only one substance [γ-aminobutyric acid (GABA)] in one structure (substantia nigra) showed a left–right difference by a t test, it was concluded that neurochemical laterality, although still possibly a substrate for functional asymmetry, was unlikely to be an important consideration in such comparisons. Because data on handedness or cerebral dominance were not available to Rossor *et al.* (1980), it did not appear to be possible to assess the functional significance of asymmetries. However, upon reading the Rossor *et al.* (1980) paper, we were impressed with the variation in left–right ratios among the brains. The variation in many cases was huge, with standard deviations nearly as large as the means. It seemed that the absolute asymmetries, at least for some neurotransmitters in some brains, must have been quite large. If the latter were true, it seemed that there should be a strong likelihood of lateral asymmetry of neurotransmitters being related to some functional characteristic. It was reasoned further that, if different neurochemical asymmetries were related to the same function, at least in terms of lateral bias, then there should be correlations among such asymmetries. We therefore wrote to Dr. Rossor, explaining our intentions and requesting a copy of the raw data. With the generous cooperation of all authors, the original Rossor *et al.* (1980) data were eventually subjected to correlational analysis. The results showed that human brain indeed has lateral asymmetries in several structures and transmitter systems (Glick *et al.*, 1982).

The major findings were the following:

1. Correlations of left–right asymmetries between and within structures and transmitters yielded a nonrandom distribution of significant correlations.
2. Left–right asymmetries in glutamate decarboxylase (GAD) and GABA were positively correlated in all nine structures. This is especially important because GABA and GAD are indices of the same transmitter system, and the two substances were measured by different methods.
3. Correlations between left–right asymmetries of different neurotransmitters within the same structure tended to be positive, whereas correlations between different structures tended to be negative. Both trends were significant.

4. Choline acetyltransferase (ChAT) and dopamine (DA) were both significantly left-biased, as shown by chi-square tests (see Glick *et al.*, 1982, for details as to why *t* tests were inappropriate), in globus pallidus. Left–right asymmetries in ChAT and DA were positively correlated in globus pallidus as well as in caudate nucleus and putamen.
5. Left–right asymmetries in ChAT and GAD were positively correlated in all cortical areas and negatively correlated in all nigrostriatal structures.
6. In caudate, putamen, and globus pallidus there was a significant trend for brains with lower dopamine levels to be left-biased, and vice versa.
7. There was a highly significant inverse correlation of age with absolute asymmetry in globus pallidus ChAT.
8. Correlations of absolute asymmetries between the same or different transmitters in different structures were usually positive, indicating that a greater or lesser degree of asymmetry probably characterizes each brain.

There were several similarities between the human data and those previously reported in rats. Thus, even though information on cerebral dominance was lacking in human beings it was clearly demonstrated that levels of ChAT and DA were higher in the left globus pallidus than in the right globus pallidus. Since most of the patients ($N=14$) should have been right-handed, pallidal ChAT and DA levels were obviously higher on the side contralateral to hand preferences. Similarly, in rats striatal DA levels were higher on the side contralateral to side preferences (Zimmerberg *et al.*, 1974). The relationship between dopamine levels and left–right asymmetry in human basal ganglia suggests that brain asymmetry is a dynamic process, depending in part on the activity of the particular functional or neuroanatomical/neurochemical system as a whole. Using labeled dGlc as an index of neuronal activity, as discussed earlier, we made a similar finding in the rat: a correlation between activity (dGlc uptake) and left–right bias, with right bias being associated with higher activity and vice versa (Ross *et al.*, 1982). Considered together, all the results showed that chemical laterality not only is present but is an important and perhaps salient characteristic of the human brain. Moreover, the similarities between rat and human brains demonstrated that studies in the rat may reveal mechanisms and functions of brain asymmetry that are relevant to human beings.

Acknowledgments

I wish to thank the many individuals who have collaborated with me in various phases of this research. These include, especially, R. C. Meibach and D. A. Ross for their participation in the deoxyglucose studies, J. S. Stollak for conducting the [^{3}H]apomorphine-binding experiments, and L. B. Hough for his help in analyzing the human neurochemical data. The research was supported by the National Institute on Drug Abuse Grant DA 01044 and Research Scientist Development Award DA 70082 and by the National Institute on Neurological and Communicative Disorders and Stroke Grant NS 14812.

References

Andén, N. E., Dahlström, A., Fuxe, K., and Larsson, K. (1966). Functional role of the nigro-neostriatal dopamine neurons. *Acta Pharmacol. Toxicol.* **24,** 263–274.

Angrist, B. M., and Gershon, S. (1970). The phenomenology of experimentally induced amphetamine psychosis: Preliminary observations. *Biol. Psychiatry* **2,** 95–107.

Angrist, B. M., and Gershon, S. (1972). Psychiatric sequelae of amphetamine use. *In* "Psychiatric Complications of Medical Drugs" (R. I. Shader, ed.), pp. 175–199. Raven Press, New York.

Brass, C. A., and Glick, S. D. (1981). Sex differences in drug-induced rotation in two strains of rats. *Brain Res.* **223,** 229–234.

Conners, K. (1973). Psychological assessment of children with minimal brain dysfunction. *Ann. N.Y. Acad. Sci.* **205,** 283–302.

Corballis, M. C., and Morgan, M. J. (1978). On the biological basis of human laterality. I. Evidence for a maturational left-right gradient. *Behav. Brain Sci.* **1,** 261–336.

Denenberg, V. H. (1981). Hemispheric laterality in animals and the effects of early experience. *Behav. Brain Sci.* **4,** 1–49.

Denenberg, V. H., Garbanati, J., Sherman, G., Yutzey, D. A., and Kaplan, R. (1978). Infantile stimulation induces brain lateralization in rats. *Science* **201,** 1150–1152.

Diamond, M. C., Johnson, R. E., and Ingham, C. A. (1975). Morphological changes in the young, adult and aging rat cerebral cortex, hippocampus and diencephalon. *Behav. Biol.* **14,** 163–174.

Ferrier, D. (1876). "The Functions of the Brain." Dawson, London (reprinted, 1966).

Fleisher, L. N., and Glick, S. D. (1979). Hallucinogen-induced rotational behavior in rats. *Psychopharmacology* **62,** 193–200.

Flor-Henry, P. (1976). Lateralized temporal-limbic dysfunction and psychopathology. *Ann. N.Y. Acad. Sci.* **280,** 777–795.

Gainotti, G. (1972). Emotional behavior and hemispheric side of the lesion. *Cortex* **8,** 41–55.

Galaburda, A. M., Lemay, M., Kemper, T. L., and Geschwind, N. (1978). Right-left asymmetries in the brain. *Science* **199,** 852–856.

Galin, D. (1974). Implications for psychiatry of left and right cerebral specialization. *Arch. Gen. Psychiatry* **31,** 572–583.

Gazzaniga, M. S. (1973). Brain theory and minimal brain dysfunction. *Ann. N.Y. Acad. Sci.* **205,** 89–92.

Glick, S. D. (1973). Enhancement of spatial preferences by (+)-amphetamine. *Neuropharmacology* **12,** 43–47.

Glick, S. D. (1976). Behavioral effects of amphetamine in brain damaged animals: Problems in the search for sites of action. *In* "Cocaine and Other Stimulants" (E. Ellinwood, ed.), pp. 77–96. Plenum, New York.

Glick, S. D., and Cox, R. D. (1976). Differential effects of unilateral and bilateral caudate lesions on side preferences and timing behavior in rats. *J. Comp. Physiol. Psychol.* **90,** 528–535.

Glick, S. D., and Cox, R. D. (1978). Nocturnal rotation in normal rats: Correlation with amphetamine-induced rotation and effects of nigrostriatal lesions. *Brain Res.* **150,** 149–161.

Glick, S. D., and Jerussi, T. P. (1974). Spatial and paw preferences in rats: Their relationship to rate-dependent effects of d-amphetamine. *J. Pharmacol. Exp. Ther.* **188,** 714–725.

Glick, S. D., and Ross, D. A. (1981a). Lateralization of function in the rat brain: Basic mechanisms may be operative in humans. *Trends Neurosci.* **4,** 196–199.

Glick, S. D., and Ross, D. A. (1981b). Lateralized effects of bilateral frontal cortex lesions in rats. *Brain Res.* **210,** 379–382.

Glick, S. D., Jerussi, T. P., Waters, D. H., and Green, J. P. (1974). Amphetamine-induced changes in striatal dopamine and acetylcholine levels and relationship to rotation (circling behavior) in rats. *Biochem. Pharmacol.* **23,** 3223–3225.

Glick, S. D., Jerussi, T. P., and Fleisher, L. N. (1976). Turning in circles: The neuropharmacology of rotation. *Life Sci.* **18,** 889–896.

Glick, S. D., Jerussi, T. P., and Zimmerberg, B. (1977a). Behavioral and neuropharmacological correlates of nigrostriatal asymmetry in rats. *In* "Lateralization in the Nervous System" (S. Harnad, L. Goldstien, R. W. Doty, J. Jaynes, and G. Krauthamer, eds.), pp. 213–249. Academic Press, New York.

Glick, S. D., Zimmerberg, B., and Jerussi, T. P. (1977b). Adaptive significance of laterality in the rodent. *Ann. N.Y. Acad. Sci.* **299,** 180–185.

Glick, S. D., Jerussi, T. P., Cox, R. D., and Fleisher, L. N. (1977c). Pre- and post-synaptic actions of apomorphine: Differentiation by rotatory effects in normal rats. *Arch. Int. Pharmacodyn. Ther.* **225,** 303–307.

Glick, S. D., Meibach, R. C., Cox, R. D., and Maayani, S. (1979). Multiple and interrelated functional asymmetries in rat brain. *Life Sci.* **25,** 395–400.

Glick, S. D., Meibach, R. C., Cox, R. D., and Maayani, S. (1980a). Phencyclidine-induced rotation and hippocampal modulation of nigrostriatal asymmetry. *Brain Res.* **196,** 99–107.

Glick, S. D., Schonfeld, A. R., and Strumpf, A. J. (1980b). Sex differences in brain asymmetry of the rodent. *Behav. Brain Sci.* **3,** 236.

Glick, S. D., Weaver, L. M., and Meibach, R. C. (1980c). Lateralization of reward in rats: Differences in reinforcing thresholds. *Science* **207,** 1093–1095.

Glick, S. D., Weaver, L. M., and Meibach, R. C. (1981a). Amphetamine-induced rotation in normal cats. *Brain Res.* **208,** 227–229.

Glick, S. D., Weaver, L. M., and Meibach, R. C. (1981b). Amphetamine enhancement of reward asymmetry. *Psychopharmacology* **73,** 323–327.

Glick, S. D., Ross, D. A., and Hough, L. B. (1982). Lateral asymmetry of neurotransmitters in human brain. *Brain Res.* **234,** 53–63.

Glick, S. D., Weaver, L. M., and Meibach, R. C. (1982). Asymmetrical effects of morphine and naloxone on reward mechanisms. *Psychopharmacology* **78,** 219–224.

Gruzelier, J. H., and Flor-Henry, P. (1979). "Hemisphere Asymmetries and Psychopathology." Elsevier, Amsterdam.

Gur, R. E. (1978). Left hemisphere dysfunction and left hemisphere overactivation in schizophrenia. *J. Abnorm. Psychol.* **87,** 226–238.

Hécaen, H., and Sauguet, J. (1971). Cerebral dominance in left-handed subjects. *Cortex* **7,** 19–48.

Herrick, C. J. (1926). "Brains in Rats and Men." Hafner, New York (reprinted, 1963).

Horowitz, M. J., and Adams, J. E. (1970). Hallucinations on brain stimulation: Evidence for revision of the Penfield hypothesis. *In* "Origin and Mechanisms of Hallucinations" (W. Keup, ed.), pp. 13–22. Plenum, New York.

Howard, I. P., and Templeton, W. B. (1966). "Human Spatial Orientation." Wiley, New York.

Jerussi, T. P., and Glick, S. D. (1975). Apomorphine-induced rotation in normal rats and interaction with unilateral caudate lesions. *Psychopharmacologia* **40,** 329–334.

Jerussi, T. P., and Glick, S. D. (1976). Drug-induced rotation in rats without lesions: Behavioral and neurochemical indices of a normal asymmetry in nigrostriatal function. *Psychopharmacology* **47,** 249–260.

Jerussi, T. P., Glick, S. D., and Johnson, C. L. (1977). Reciprocity of pre- and post-synaptic mechanisms involved in rotation as revealed by dopamine metabolism and adenylate cyclase stimulation. *Brain Res.* **129,** 385–388.

Lashley, K. S. (1921). Studies of cerebral function in learning. No. III. Motor areas. *Brain* **44,** 255–285.

Laursen, A. M. (1962). Movements evoked from the region of the caudate nucleus in rats. *Acta Physiol. Scand.* **54,** 175–184.

LeMay, M., and Geschwind, N. (1975). Hemispheric differences in the brains of great apes. *Brain Behav. Evol.* **11,** 48–52.

Levy, J. (1977). The mammalian brain and the adaptive advantage of cerebral asymmetry. *Ann. N.Y. Acad. Sci.* **299,** 264–272.

Mach, E. (1885). "The Analysis of Sensations." Dover, New York (translated and reprinted, 1959).

Martin, W. R. (1977). *Handb. Exp. Pharmakol.* [N.S.] **45,** Part 2.

Meibach, R. C., Glick, S. D., Ross, D. A., Cox, R. D., and Maayani, S. (1980). Intraperitoneal administration and other modifications of the 2-deoxy-D-glucose technique. *Brain Res.* **195,** 167–176.

Mettler, F. A., and Mettler, C. C. (1942). The effects of striatal injury. *Brain* **65,** 242–255.

Michel, G. F. (1981). Right-handedness: A consequence of infant supine head-orientation preference. *Science* **212,** 685–687.

Millichap, G. L. (1973). Drugs in management of minimal brain dysfunction. *Ann. N.Y. Acad. Sci.* **205,** 321–334.

Morihisa, J. M., and Glick, S. D. (1977). Morphine-induced rotation (circling behavior) in rats and mice: Species differences, persistence of withdrawal-induced rotation and antagonism by naloxone. *Brain Res.* **123,** 180–187.

Nottebohm, F. (1977). Asymmetries in neural control of vocalization in the canary. *In* "Lateralization in the Nervous System" (S. Harnad, L. Goldstien, R. W. Doty, J. Jaynes, and G. Krauthamer, eds.), pp. 23–44. Academic Press, New York.

Nymark, M. (1972). Apomorphine provoked stereotypy in the dog. *Psychopharmacologia* **26,** 361–368.

Penfield, W., and Perot, P. (1963). The brain's record of auditory and visual experience—a final summary and discussion. *Brain* **86,** 596–696.

Pycock, C. J. (1980). Turning behaviour in animals. *Neuroscience* **5,** 461–514.

Rasmussen, T., and Milner, B. (1977). The role of early left-brain injury in determining lateralization of cerebral speech functions. *Ann. N.Y. Acad. Sci.* **299,** 353–369.

Reitan, R. M., and Boll, T. J. (1973). Neuropsychological correlates of minimal brain dysfunction. *Ann. N.Y. Acad. Sci.* **205,** 65–88.

Robinson, R. G. (1979). Differential behavioral and biochemical effects of right and left hemispheric cerebral infarction in the rat. *Science* **205,** 707–710.

Robinson, T. E., Becker, J. B., and Ramirez, V. D. (1980). Sex differences in amphetamine-elicited rotational behavior and the lateralization of striatal dopamine in rats. *Brain Res. Bull.* **5,** 539–545.

Ross, D. A., and Glick, S. D. (1981). Lateralized effects of bilateral frontal cortex lesions in rats. *Brain Res.* **210,** 379–382.

Ross, D. A., Glick, S. D., and Meibach, R. C. (1981). Sexually dimorphic brain and behavioral asymmetries in the neonatal rat. *Proc. Natl. Acad. Sci. U.S.A.* **78,** 1958–1961.

Ross, D. A., Glick, S. D., and Meibach, R. C. (1982). Sexually dimorphic cerebral asymmetries in 2-deoxy-D-glucose uptake during postnatal development of the rat: Correlations with age and relative brain activity. *Dev. Brain Res.* **3,** 341–347.

Rossor, M., Garrett, N., and Iversen, L. (1980). No evidence for lateral asymmetry of neurotransmitters in post-mortem human brain. *J. Neurochem.* **35,** 743–745.

Rothman, A. H., and Glick, S. D. (1976). Differential effects of unilateral and bilateral caudate lesions on side preference and passive avoidance behavior in rats. *Brain Res.* **118,** 361–369.

Satterfield, J. H., Lesser, L. L., Saul, R. E., and Cantwell, D. P. (1973). EEG aspects in the diagnosis and treatment of minimal brain dysfunction. *Ann. N.Y. Acad. Sci.* **205,** 274–282.

Seeman, P. (1980). Brain dopamine receptors. *Pharmacol. Rev.* **32,** 229–313.

Snyder, S. H. (1976). The dopamine hypothesis of schizophrenia: Focus on the dopamine receptor. *Am. J. Psychiatry* **133,** 197–202.

Sokoloff, L., Reivich, M., Kennedy, C., Des Rosiers, M. H., Patlak, C. S., Pettigrew, K. D., Sakurada, O., and Shinohara, M. (1977). The [^{14}C]deoxyglucose method for the measurement of local cerebral glucose utilization: Theory, procedure and normal values in the conscious and anesthetized albino rat. *J. Neurochem.* **28,** 897–916.

Sokoloff, P., Martres, M. P., and Schwartz, J. C. (1980). ^{3}H-Apomorphine labels both dopamine postsynaptic receptors and autoreceptors. *Nature (London)* **288,** 283–288.

Stein, L., and Wise, C. D. (1971). Possible etiology of schizophrenia: Progressive damage to the noradrenergic reward system by 6-hydroxy-dopamine. *Science* **171,** 1032–1036.

Stollak, J. S., and Glick, S. D. (1982). [^{3}H]Apomorphine binding to rat striatum reveals sexual and behavioral dimorphism. *Fed. Proc., Fed. Am. Soc. Exp. Biol.* **41,** 1326.

Terzian, T. (1964). Behavioral and EEG effects of intracarotid sodium amytal injections. *Acta Neurochir.* **12,** 230–240.

Ungerstedt, U. (1971). Striatal dopamine release after amphetamine or nerve degeneration revealed by rotational behavior. *Acta Physiol. Scand., Suppl.* **367,** 49–68.

Valdes, J. J., Mactutus, C. F., Cory, R. N., and Cameron, W. R. (1981). Lateralization of norepinephrine, serotonin and choline uptake into hippocampal synaptosomes of sinistral rats. *Physiol. Behav.* **27,** 381–383.

Warren, J. M. (1980). Handedness and laterality in humans and other animals. *Physiol. Psychol.* **8,** 351–359.

Webster, W. G. (1977). Hemispheric asymmetry in cats. *In* "Lateralization in the Nervous System" (S. Harnad, L. Goldstien, R. W. Doty, J. Jaynes, and G. Krauthamer, eds.), pp. 471–480. Academic Press, New York.

Wexler, B. F., and Heninger, G. R. (1979). Alterations in cerebral laterality during acute psychotic illness. *Arch. Gen. Psychiatry* **36,** 278–284.

Wilson, S. A. K. (1914). An experimental approach into the anatomy and physiology of the corpus striatum. *Brain* **36,** 425–492.

Wise, R. A., Spindler, J., deWit, H., and Gerber, G. J. (1978). Neuroleptic-induced "anhedonia" in rats: Pimozide blocks reward quality of food. *Science* **201,** 262–264.

Witelson, S. F. (1976). Sex and the single hemisphere: Specialization of the right hemisphere for spatial processing. *Science* **193,** 425–427.

Zimmerberg, B., and Glick, S. D. (1975). Changes in side preference during unilateral electrical stimulation of the caudate nucleus in rats. *Brain Res.* **86,** 335–338.

Zimmerberg, B., Glick, S. D., and Jerussi, T. P. (1974). Neurochemical correlate of a spatial preference in rats. *Science* **185,** 623–625.

Zimmerberg, B., Strumpf, A. J., and Glick, S. D. (1978). Cerebral asymmetry and left-right discrimination. *Brain Res.* **140,** 194–196.

3: Behavioral and Neural Plasticity following Unilateral Brain Lesions

MONIKA PRITZEL and JOSEPH P. HUSTON

Institute of Psychology III
University of Düsseldorf
Düsseldorf, Federal Republic of Germany

I. Introduction 28
II. Interhemispheric Projections of Substantia Nigra Neurons and Cessation of Lesion-Induced Turning 28
A. Unilateral Removal of the Telencephalon in Adult Rats Followed by an Injection of Horseradish Peroxidase into the Thalamus 29
B. Unilateral Removal of the Telencephalon in Newborn Rats Followed by an Injection of Horseradish Peroxidase into the Thalamus 33
C. Unilateral Substantia Nigra Lesion Followed by an Injection of Horseradish Peroxidase into the Ventromedial Thalamus One Week Later 35
D. Unilateral Substantia Nigra Lesion with Subsequent Injection of Horseradish Peroxidase or Fluorescent Tracers into the Head of the Caudate Nucleus 37
E. Sensorimotor Deprivation Following a Unilateral Substantia Nigra Lesion: Tracing Nigral Afferents to the Ventromedial Thalamus 41
F. Reorganization of Nigrothalamic Projections following Unilateral Paralysis and Unilateral Sensory Deprivation 42
G. Discussion 44
III. Plasticity of Interhemispheric Fiber Connections 51
A. Neuronal Plasticity in the Red Nucleus (Nucleus Ruber) 52
B. Neuronal Plasticity in the Superior Colliculus 55
C. Neuronal Plasticity in the Dentate Gyrus of the Hippocampal-Formation. 56
D. Conclusions 57
References 60

HEMISYNDROMES:
Psychobiology, Neurology,
Psychiatry

ISBN 0-12-512460-0

I. Introduction

In the first part of this chapter we review some of our experiments, which suggest that unilateral brain lesions are soon followed by plastic changes in interhemispheric fiber connections. Our results indicate that such changes in crossed projections may be related to recovery from behavioral asymmetries that ensue from the unilateral brain damage. They may have a role in the learning to compensate for the deficit. In Section III we present an overview of related results found by others. In summary, a considerable number of studies have shown that the destruction of some unilaterally organized fiber systems leads to an increase in the number of interhemispheric projections to the denervated target area. These projections originate preferentially from brain structures in the intact side of the brain that are homologous to the destroyed regions in the other hemisphere. For example, fiber systems that are known to connect brain structures in one side of the brain, such as the corticocollicular connections, may also be found as interhemispheric projections after a unilateral lesion is inflicted in the visual cortex.

Although such neural plasticity has been demonstrated in various neural systems, virtually no progress has been made in finding behavioral concomitants of such changes. Our results may provide some advance in this direction because they show evidence for a relationship between the temporal course of the cessation of unilateral lesion-induced turning behavior and the appearance of changes in interhemispheric projections.

II. Interhemispheric Projections of Substantia Nigra Neurons and Cessation of Lesion-Induced Turning

In this section we summarize the results of a series of our experiments in which unilateral brain lesions, or in some cases unilateral lesions in the peripheral nervous system, were inflicted in rats. The animals received an injection of a tracer (horseradish peroxidase or nuclear yellow or fast blue) into either the thalamus or nucleus caudatus after various postoperative intervals. During these postoperative intervals we recorded indices of behavioral recovery from the lesion-induced sensorimotor asymmetries, and in some cases we tried to prevent behavioral recovery.

Originally, our aim was to investigate the neuronal organization of the so-called thalamic preparation, that is, of rats in which the telencephalon is removed bilaterally. Such animals exhibit a wide range of behaviors, including operant learning (Huston and Borbély, 1973, 1974; Grill and Norgren, 1978a,b). Our purpose was to examine the anatomical properties of this preparation in relation to its functional properties. We chose to investigate the unilaterally detelencephalized rat (as one of various experimental groups) because with this preparation it was considered possible to make an intraindividual comparison of degenerative effects within the brain. We decided to study the thalamus first since it is the most dorsally situated structure in the detelencephalized preparation and is thought to be an important relay station within the diencephalon. We assumed that the injection of horseradish peroxidase (HRP) into the thalamus could give us some clues about its remaining intact afferent organization and thus provide an anatomical basis for a possible functional involvement in the control of the behaviors under investigation.

Unexpectedly, we found evidence for plastic changes in the inputs to the thalamus on the denervated side of the brain as soon as 7 days after removal of the telencephalon. The experiments were repeated in unilaterally detelencephalized newborn rats because it was assumed that plastic changes, if they had taken place in the preceding experiment, would be even more pronounced in young rats. Indeed, we found alterations in thalamic input: In adult and young rats interhemispheric projections to the denervated thalamus on the side of the brain lacking the telencephalon were identified after 1 week of postoperative survival (Pritzel and Huston, 1981a; Neumann *et al.,* 1982). During this time the spontaneous turning that follows a unilateral removal of the telencephalon had ceased to occur. Therefore, it was hypothesized that behavioral recovery, especially the cessation of lesion-induced rotation, might be accompanied by plastic changes in neuronal wiring between the two sides of the brain.

We next inflicted small unilateral lesions in the substantia nigra (SN), lesions that are known to result in rotational behavior of the animals. Horseradish peroxidase was then injected into nigral projection areas ipsilateral to the damaged SN after postoperative survival times of various intervals. Later, we tried to prevent functional recovery from SN lesions by suspending the animals in a sling for the duration of the postoperative interval during which the animals normally showed recovery from lesion-induced turning. In another experiment HRP was injected into SN projection sites after unilateral lesions were made in the peripheral nervous system; these lesions also induced turning, which ceased within 1 week after the operation.

A. Unilateral Removal of the Telencephalon in Adult Rats Followed by an Injection of Horseradish Peroxidase into the Thalamus

The series of experiments was started by unilateral removal of the telencephalon in adult rats, as illustrated in Fig. 3.1a. The results have been published by Pritzel and Huston (1981a). The subjects were 108 male rats

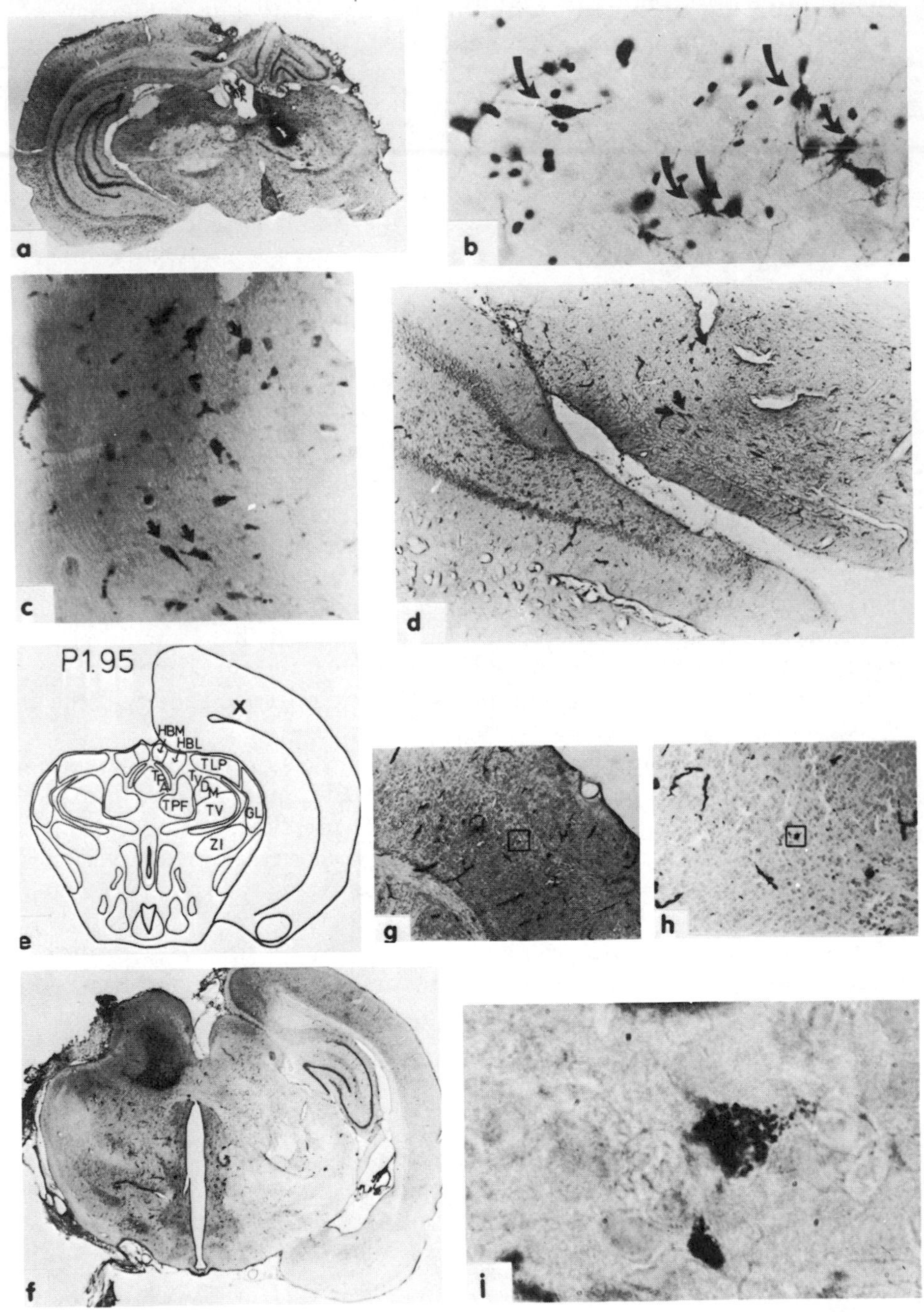
a
b
c
d
P1.95
X
HBM
HBL
TLP
TPF
TV
GL
ZI
e
g
h
f
i

(Sprague–Dawley, 200–320 g). For unilateral removal of the telencephalon, a piece of skull of the parietal bone was removed under deep anesthesia (Equithesin, 3.3 mg/kg, ip). First the cerebral cortex and striatum, and then the ventral forebrain anterior to the preoptic area and lateral to the optic tracts, were aspirated. Finally, the hippocampus was separated from the underlying thalamus.

The 7-day interval was chosen on the basis of the time course of degeneration because we wanted to trace connections that were likely to have survived the lesion. Furthermore, we had found that a 1-week interval was sufficient for the animals to cease the spontaneous rotation that they exhibit during the first postoperative days.

A similar HRP procedure was used in experiments A–D.* In experiments E and F the mode of HRP application was changed in that a crystalline implantation method was used instead of an injection method. [The HRP solution was dissolved in sterile saline (30–50%, w/v) and injected in a volume of 0.02 to 0.05 μl.] Furthermore, initially (experiments A–D) brains were processed using benzidine dihydrochloride and later (experiments E and F) were processed with tetramethylbenzidine (Mesulam, 1976; Malmgren and Olsson, 1978; Mesulam and Rosene, 1979).

In experiment A, the rats were divided into the following groups:

1. The 7-day group consisted of 15 animals in which the telencephalon was removed unilaterally and HRP was injected into the ventral or posterior part of the thalamus on the side of the brain lacking the telencephalon. In various species this part of the thalamus has been described as consistently degenerating following the infliction of massive forebrain lesions (Papez, 1938; Walker, 1938; Combs, 1949; Peacock and Combs, 1965). Four other animals received an HRP injection into the midline nuclei of the thalamus ipsilateral to the detelencephalized hemisphere.

FIG. 3.1. Unilateral removal of telencephalon in adult and newborn rats and injection of HRP into the thalamus of the denervated side of the brain 7 days later. (a) Frontal section (at about +4.2, according to the atlas of König and Klippel, 1963) showing the extent of the lesion and the locus of HRP injection into the ventromedial part of the denervated thalamus. In this example part of the hippocampal formation survived the ablation. (b) Labeled perikarya of neurons in the SN (pars reticulata) ipsilateral to the injection site. Neurons are indicated by arrows. (c, d) Labeled neurons in the SN of the intact hemisphere contralateral to the thalamus injected with HRP. Frame (c) shows the neurons presented in (d) at a higher magnification. (e) Drawing of a frontal section from a unilaterally detelencephalized neonatal rat. (The abbreviations and the A–P coordinates are adapted from the atlas of Heller *et al.*, 1979). (f) Frontal section from a unilaterally detelencephalized infant rat at the level of the superior colliculi. (g, h, i) Different magnifications of a labeled neuron in the posterior part of the intact hemisphere. In (g) and (h) the position of the neuron seen in (i) is indicated by a square.

*Experiments A–F refer to the experiments described in Sections II, A–II, F, respectively.

The midline nuclei were chosen as an injection site for this control group because they undergo only sparse degeneration following the infliction of massive lesions of the forebrain (see Walker, 1938; Combs, 1949).

2. Nine animals received an HRP injection into the ventral and posterior thalamus on the side of the brain lacking the telencephalon immediately (or at least within 24 hr) after the operation. This experiment was performed to examine whether any change in HRP-labeled neurons might be due to immediate alterations in HRP uptake in brain sites that were affected by the massive brain lesion.

3. Finally, HRP was injected into the ventral thalamus of the intact hemisphere of six unilaterally detelencephalized rats. This was done 7 days postoperatively. The purpose of this control was to test for possible differences in HRP uptake in the mainly intact part of the thalamus compared with the mainly deafferented hemithalamus. The unilateral removal of the telencephalon induced a global sensorimotor asymmetry, which led all animals to rotate spontaneously for several days.

In the following description of the results we concentrate on thalamic afferents from the SN because this structure was examined later in detail. We found labeled perikarya in the SN ipsilateral to the thalamic injection site in the detelencephalized hemisphere (see Fig. 3.1b). Unexpectedly, however, we also identified labeled neurons in the SN of the intact hemisphere contralateral to the injected hemisphere (Fig. 3.1c, d). This result led us to examine the possibility that these contralaterally organized nigrothalamic connections, which we identified all along the rostral to caudal extent of the reticular part of the SN, might have been a result of changes in HRP transport due to the massive lesion. Contralateral projections were not found in those rats in which HRP was injected into the thalamus underlying the intact telencephalon (group 3) and which, of course, exhibited the same type of sensorimotor neglect syndromes as the experimental group. However, we found many labeled cells in the ipsilateral SN of these animals, indicating that the tracing method worked in each animal tested.

The appearance of contralateral nigrothalamic projections in the experimental group was time dependent. If we injected the tracer into the thalamus of the detelencephalized side immediately or 1 day after the unilateral removal of the telencephalon (group 2), no contralateral projections from the SN were detected. The crossed projections were seen only after about 7 postoperative days.

We did not attribute this time dependency in labeling to a possible insensitivity of the HRP method applied immediately after the lesion was made since ipsilaterally situated nigrothalamic projections were clearly present then. Instead, it seemed possible that the appearance of crossed nigrothalamic connections could be related to functional consequences of the unilateral removal of the telencephalon. Specifically, we hypothesized that the crossed projections were a correlate of a compensation for the lesion-induced sensorimotor asymmetries. The cessation of spontaneous turning behavior within 7 days after infliction of the lesion seemed to provide evidence for such behavioral compensation.

The possibility that our finding of crossed nigrothalamic (and corticothalamic) projections reflected a process of sprouting of sparsely distributed crossed projections seemed to be the most parsimonious explanation of the data. The exciting prospect of the crossed connections being related to behavioral recovery from the lesion led us to continue to investigate this phenomenon with the following studies.

B. Unilateral Removal of the Telencephalon in Newborn Rats Followed by an Injection of Horseradish Peroxidase into the Thalamus

In this section we summarize experiments published by Neumann *et al.* (1982). Having obtained evidence for the development of crossed nigrothalamic projections after unilateral removal of the telencephalon in adult rats, we decided to examine the generality of this phenomenon by testing newborn animals. We believed that the crossed connections represented a morphological correlate of compensation for the lesion-induced asymmetries. If this were the case, newborn rats would be expected to exhibit even more drastic changes in postlesion neuronal organization than adults because neonatal animals are believed to show a higher degree of neuronal plasticity than adults (see Lund, 1978, for a review). We were especially interested in finding out whether there are signs of plastic changes in the brain that are correlated with the time of early functional recovery from lesion-induced rotation.

One-week-old rats were used. At that age young rats have undergone a rapid and substantial development in brain size and at the same time exhibit a repertoire of motor behavior suitable for behavioral measurements.

First, the telencephalon was removed unilaterally (Fig. 3.1e, f) by the use of a method that was in principle the same as that used with adult rats. The lesion led to gross motor asymmetries, including spontaneous turning behavior, which ceased by 6 days after the operation. The animals were then operated on for a second time, and HRP was injected unilaterally into the thalamus. The animals were divided into the following groups:

1. Nine animals were given the lesion on day 7 and received an HRP injection into the posterior part of the thalamus in the detelencephalized hemisphere at the age of 14 days.
2. In eleven 7-day-old and five 3-day-old animals HRP was successfully injected into the posterior part of the thalamus within several hours

after the telencephalic lesion was completed. Six animals of the 7-day-old group and all animals of the 3-day-old group received an injection into the thalamus of the detelencephalized hemisphere. The remaining five 7-day-old rats received HRP injections into the thalamus of the intact side of the brain.

3. To control for possible interhemispheric thalamic projections in pups with an intact brain, unilateral injections of HRP into the posterior part of the thalamus were made in 10 unoperated rats. These animals were 3, 7, or 14 days old.

Seven days after the lesion was made, the thalamus on the side of the brain lacking the telencephalon had undergone substantial degeneration; that is, it exhibited a decrease in the number of neurons. Often the neurons were pale, large, and poorly defined. There were more glia present than in the contralateral thalamus. Gross motor asymmetry following unilateral detelencephalization was observed in all animals. Spontaneous turning behavior occurred for only 3–6 days following infliction of the lesion.

We found retrogradely labeled cells in a multitude of ipsilateral diencephalic and mesencephalic structures. In addition, contralaterally situated cortical projections could be identified (Fig. 3.1e, g, h, i). The neurons were clearly stained and consistently but sparsely found in all of the injected animals of group 1. Such neurons were not found in the controls with intact brains of group 3. All the injections invaded several nuclei in the posterior part of the thalamus, which are known to have overlapping projection areas from the cortex. Therefore, we did not acquire any new information about the topographical specifity of possible "reorganization" of thalamic afferents aside from the finding that the removal of overlying cortex and other telencephalic structures led to contralateral cortical projections to the thalamus, in spite of its degenerative changes and in spite of the fact that such a crossed pathway had not been described before to our knowledge.

Some obvious artifacts were eliminated as possible explanations of these results. First, we rejected all brains in which the enzyme had spread into the contralateral part of the thalamus. Furthermore, we rejected those data in which the HRP injection included subthalamic areas and mesencephalic structures that could have crossed connections to the cortex via decussations. Second, the enzyme might have been transported into remote areas by bleeding or some other means of transport. Therefore, we repeated the experiment, injecting HRP immediately after infliction of the lesion (group 2). Since we did not find any labeled neurons in the intact cortical hemisphere when there was no delay between infliction of the lesion and HRP injection, an explanation of our data in terms of lesion artifacts seemed unwarranted.

One possible explanation of these data was that the lesion unmasked morphologically ineffective contralateral inputs of the deafferented thalamus, which then spread their terminal fields over the denervated thalamus. Because such unmasking can be shown within several days (Merrill and Wall, 1978), it could explain the appearance of contralateral projections in the present experiment with the given time span of 1 week.

Given the results of both studies with adult and young unilaterally detelencephalized rats, we decided to pursue systematically the possibility of a close relationship between changes in lesion-induced turning and the visibility of crossed projections in nigral projection systems. We next tried to minimize the extent of the lesion necessary to induce turning behavior.

This was achieved by a unilateral lesion of the SN produced with either 6-hydroxydopamine (6-OHDA) or kainic acid (KA) followed by an HRP injection into the ventrobasal thalamus (experiment C) or into the head of the caudate nucleus (NC) of the same hemisphere (experiment D). Studies C and D were planned to determine, first, whether the evidence from studies A and B of plastic changes in the nigral connections could be extended to conditions of a relatively small (SN) and selective lesion (KA or 6-OHDA) that is known to lead to an asymmetry in overt motor behavior. The neurotoxins were chosen to influence the sensorimotor asymmetry differentially with respect to the duration of lesion-induced turning behavior. Second, the HRP, an intraaxonally, retrogradely transported tracer substance, was injected into well-known ipsilateral SN projection sites that receive virtually no projections from the SN of the contralateral hemisphere (ventromedial thalamus, experiment C) and to an area that is known to receive only sparse interhemispheric projections (NC, experiment D). The fluorescent substances fast blue (FB) and nuclear yellow (NY) were used in addition to HRP to rule out HRP-specific results in labeling.

C. Unilateral Substantia Nigra Lesion Followed by an Injection of Horseradish Peroxidase into the Ventromedial Thalamus One Week Later

In this experiment (Pritzel and Huston, 1981b) (Fig. 3.2) and in the following ones the unilateral lesion of the SN was produced by injecting either 6-OHDA, which destroys catecholaminergic neurons in the SN and usually leads to spontaneous circling in a direction ipsilateral to the side with the lesion (Ungerstedt, 1971; Dray, 1979), or KA, a glutamic acid analog that has been reported to destroy mainly cell bodies (McGeer *et al.*, 1978; Mason and Fibiger, 1979) and to induce predominantly turning contralateral to the side of the unilateral lesion (DiChiara *et al.*, 1977; Papadopoulos *et al.*, 1980). Either 6-OHDA hydrochloride (Fluka AG, 8

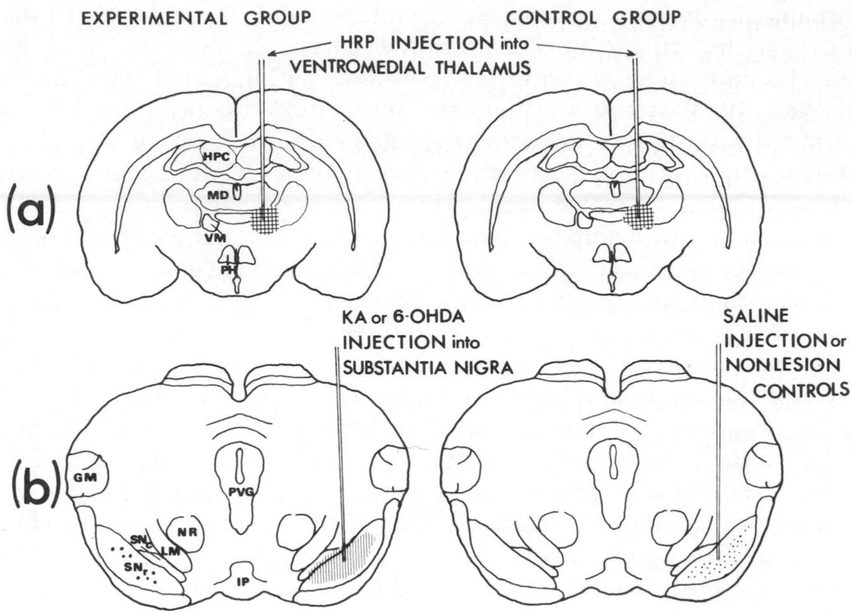

FIG. 3.2. Summary of procedure and results of (b) a KA or 6-OHDA lesion of the substantia nigra followed by (a) an HRP injection into the homolateral ventromedial thalamus 1 week later. Labeled neurons (dots) in the SN, contralateral to the injected hemisphere, appear only in the experimental group. HPC, hippocampus; LM, medical lemniscus; MD, dorsomedial nucleus of thalamus; NR, red nucleus; PH, posterior nucleus of hypothalamus; PVG, central gray substance; SN_c, substantia nigra, pars compacta; SN_r, substantia nigra pars reticulata; VM, ventromedial nucleus of thalamus; IP, interpeduncular nucleus.

μg) or KA (2 μg) was injected over a period of 5 mins. The animals were placed in the following groups:

1. Eight animals received a unilateral SN lesion by either 6-OHDA ($N=4$) or KA ($N=4$). Subsequent turning behavior lasted for several days. Seven days later the rats received an HRP injection into the medial or ventromedial part of the thalamus ipsilateral to the destroyed SN. The medioventral thalamus was chosen because it is in the center of the thalamic projection area of the reticular part of the SN (see Faull and Mehler, 1978; Bentivoglio *et al.*, 1979; Herkenham, 1979; Nauta and Domesick, 1979).

2. For control purposes, HRP was also injected into animals in whom the SN was not damaged, as well as into animals that had received unilateral injections of saline into the SN at identical coordinates, 7 days before the HRP injection into the medial and ventromedial thalamus of the same hemisphere ($N=8$).

The animals in which 6-OHDA was injected into the SN exhibited vigorous ipsiversive circling behavior immediately after awakening from anesthesia. Turning varied between 20 and 100 turns per hour for the first days after infliction of the lesion and occurred reliably for as long as 8 days after the operation.

The animals injected with KA did not exhibit a clear-cut directional preference in turning. For the first hours after the injection strong ipsiversive turning occurred in seizurelike attacks, followed sometimes by ipsiversive circling or ipsiversive torticollis. During the following days the animals developed pronounced contraversive posture and turning; however, they still exhibited intermittent phases of ipsiversive rotation. Turning ceased after about 1 week.

The injection loci of HRP extended into the dorsomedial, ventromedial, and ventrolateral nuclei of the thalamus and reached into its intralaminar group of nuclei. Several retrogradely labeled cells were identified in the medial and lateral part of the contralateral SN in each animal with an SN lesion. In the control animals, which did not receive a lesion or were injected with saline (group 2), we were unable to find labeled cells in the contralateral SN following HRP injections into the thalamus.

D. Unilateral Substantia Nigra Lesion with Subsequent Injection of Horseradish Peroxidase or Fluorescent Tracers into the Head of the Caudate Nucleus

Two experiments were performed:

1. To test for the development of crossed nigrostriatal connections after the infliction of lesions in the SN, animals received either a unilateral 6-OHDA injection ($N=30$) or a KA injection ($N=30$) into the SN (Pritzel *et al.*, 1983) (see Fig. 3.3). They were divided into three groups, with 7 ($N=20$), 21 ($N=20$), and 90 ($N=20$) days of survival time. The aim of using these intervals was to examine the time course of possible plastic changes in the nigrocaudate projections in relation to signs of behavioral recovery. By 21 days after a brain lesion is produced, neuronal plastic changes reliably take place in young and adult animals in various brain structures (see Lund, 1978, for a review). After 90 days lesion-induced plastic changes in the brain have reached their maximum according to various sources (Raisman, 1969a, b; McWilliams and Lynch, 1979). However, descriptions of behavioral recovery after the infliction of unilateral SN lesions although they vary considerably with respect to specific long-lasting deficits (Ungerstedt, 1971; Hefti *et al.*, 1980; Kozlowski and Marshall, 1980), agree in the observation that a gross behavioral compensation of sensorimotor asymmetries requires only several days of postoperative recovery.

After the different survival times, the HRP injection was centered into the head of the NC ipsilateral to the lesion. [The pars compacta of the

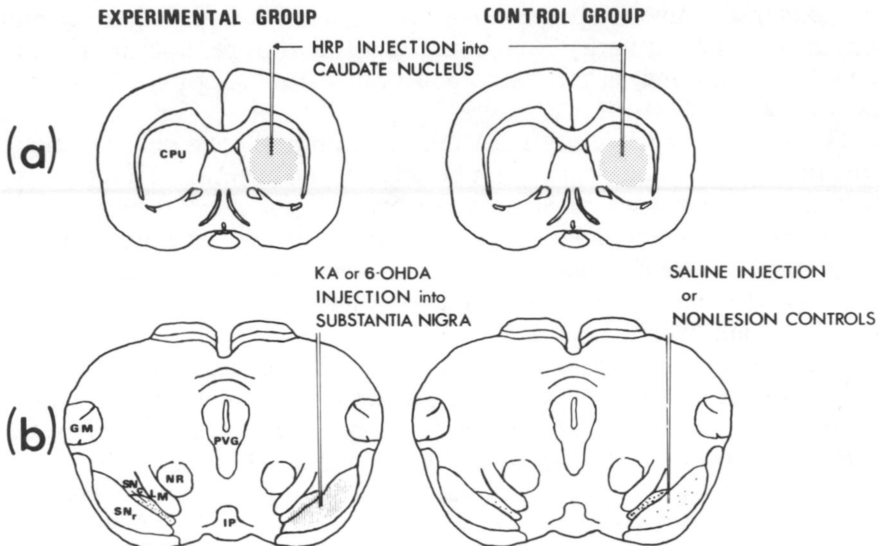

FIG. 3.3. Summary of procedure and results of (b) a KA or 6-OHDA lesion of the substantia nigra followed by (a) an HRP injection into the caudate nucleus 1–3 weeks later. An increase in the number of labeled neurons (dots) in the SN pars compacta of the contralateral hemisphere was observed only in the experimental group. CPU, caudate nucleus, potamen; GM, medial geniculate body; IP, interpeduncular nucleus; LM, medial lemniscus; NR, red nucleus, PVG, central gray substance; SN_c, substantia nigra, pars compacta; SN_r, substantia nigra, pars reticulata.

SN is one of its main afferents (for review, see Dray, 1979).]

2. Control experiments were designed to investigate, for one, whether a change in labeling of neurons might be due to a specific change in the uptake of the tracer HRP. Therefore, NY and FB were used as additional tracer substances (see Bentivoglio *et al.*, 1980a, b; Kuypers *et al.*, 1980; Bharos *et al.*, 1981; Catsman-Berrevoets and Kuypers, 1981).

Animals of this control experiment were divided into four groups. Groups a and b were injected with fluorescent, retrogradely transported tracer substance FB (group a) or NY (group b) in the head of the NC. Groups c and d were injected with FB followed by NY 1 week later. In both cases identical coordinates in the NC were used for injection. In addition, animals of group d received a 6-OHDA lesion in the SN 24 hr after FB injection. Injection of the tracers and lesion of the SN were always done in the same hemisphere. The aim of this study was to ascertain whether the tracer substance NY would show different properties in labeling of neurons, depending on whether an SN lesion (group d) preceded the NY injection or not (group c). In order to test whether FB or NY changes its properties of labeling neurons after dual injection of both tracers into the same brain locus, the tracers were also injected separately (group a and group b). The tracer substances FB and NY were selected because they have different postinjection intervals during which they can be reliably identified in the uptaking neurons (Kuypers *et al.*, 1980; Bentivoglio *et al.*, 1980a). The 7-day interval, suitable for a combined injection of FB and NY, also met the requirement of the experimental design for a postoperative survival interval of 1 week.

Between 6 and 24 hr following the NY injection (and 7 days after a single FB injection) the animals were decapitated. The fluorescent tracing of FB and NY was then coupled with histofluorescent tracing of monoamines to determine whether interhemispheric nigrocaudate projections were also mainly catecholaminergic, as is known to be the case from the unilaterally ascending nigrocaudate pathway (Ungerstedt, 1971; van der Kooy *et al.*, 1981). This was done using the sucrose–phosphate–glyoxylic method described by de la Torre (1980). Fast blue was identified (on the mounted section) as silver fluorescent grains in the cytoplasm of the uptaking neurons. Nuclear yellow was visible as golden grains that filled the nucleus of the affected neurons.

Animals of all groups were tested for rotational behavior. Turning was registered by observation or measured during 15-min periods in intervals of 2 hr by means of rotometers that counted each 360° rotation (Papadopoulos and Huston, 1980).

Twenty animals of the 21-day group and all of the animals of the 90-day group in experiment 2 received ip injections of apomorphine (8 mg/kg) and *d*-amphetamine (2 mg/kg). Rotation of the animals was measured for 2 hr after each injection. Horseradish peroxidase was then injected into the NC ipsilateral to the lesion. To characterize possible persisting unilateral deficits, the animals of the 21- and 90-day groups were administered neurological tests for sensorimotor lateralization as suggested by Marshall and Teitelbaum (1974).

A delay of 7 days between the infliction of the lesion and the injection of HRP was sufficient to reveal an increase in projections from the SN of the intact hemisphere to the NC of the contralateral hemisphere (Fig. 3.4.). This could be observed in each of the brains included in the final evaluation of data. The same was true for a 3-week interval between both operations, which yielded consistent contralateral SN–NC connections. Even small injections of HRP led to contralateral labeling of cells in the pars compacta and rostral part of the SN. All HRP injections into the NC of animals with an SN lesion on the same side of the brain led to increased labeling of cells in the SN of the other hemisphere. These projections were situated mainly within the pars compacta of the SN and corresponded macroscopically to the known organization of the ipsilateral nigrostriatal projections. We did not observe differences in the number of labeled cells between 7 and 21 days of survival. After a survival time of 90 days, however, no difference between the animals with SN

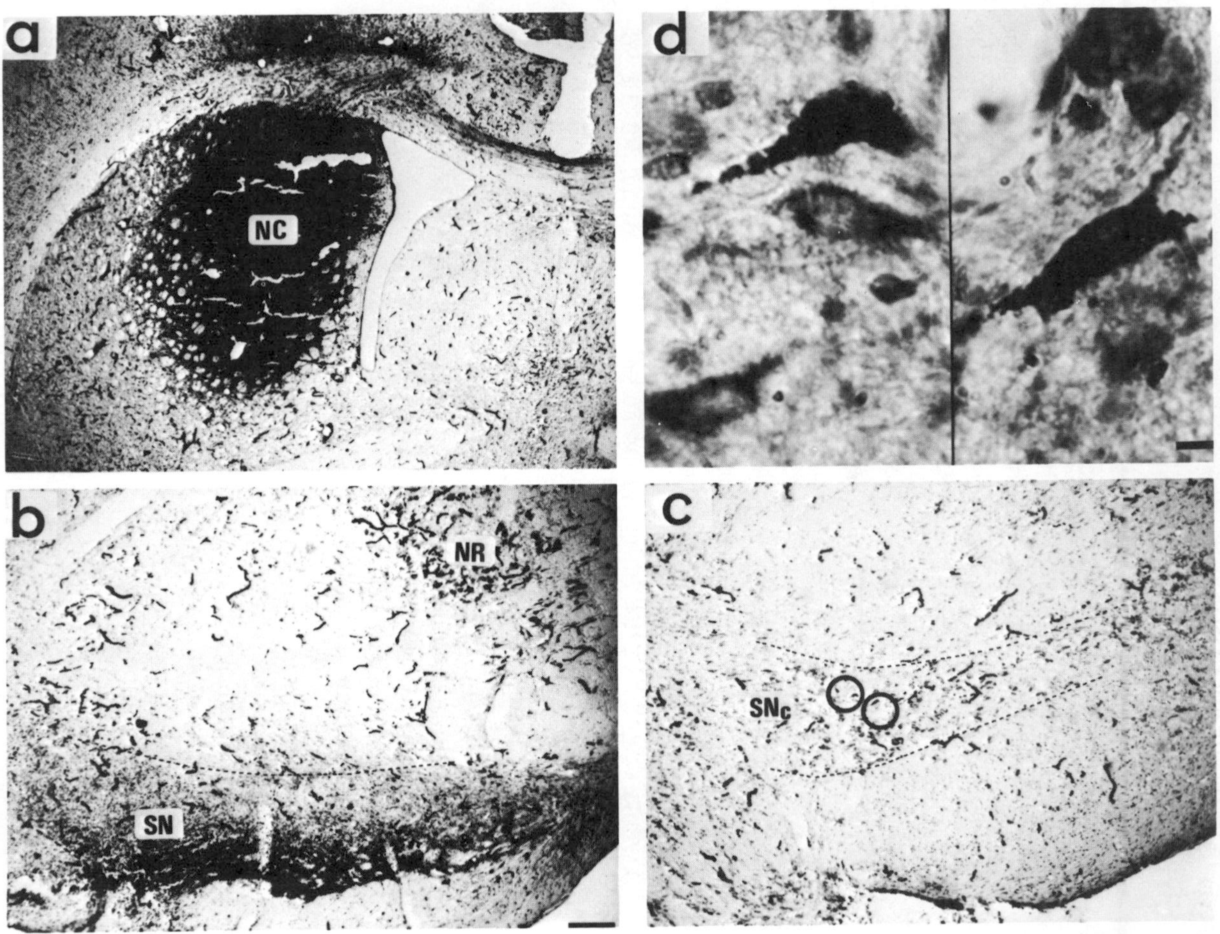
a
NC
d
b
NR
SN
c
SN_c

lesions and control animals could be found in the number of contralaterally projecting SN neurons.

The assumption that these crossed connections represent an outgrowth of already existing connections was supported by the finding of small contralateral nigrocaudate projections in the intact animals. These presumably increased in number after an insult to one of the SN. As far as can be inferred from the retrograde tracing technique, the altered contralateral organization of the SN did not increase over time; that is, the contralateral projections did not increase in number from 1 to 3 weeks after infliction of the lesion. On the contrary, a decrease was found after 90 days.

Finally, the results yielded with the HRP method could be replicated using FB or NY (group 2). If an SN lesion preceded the injections of HRP or NY by 1 week, the increase in number of contralaterally labeled neurons was in both cases significant and was about the same for HRP as for NY.

After the infliction of unilateral lesions in the SN, spontaneous turning was observed in all of the animals. Whereas rats with 6-OHDA lesions of the SN exhibited mainly ipsiversive circling, those with KA lesions did not reveal such a clear preference, either among or within subjects.

Twenty-one and 90 days after the lesion was made, the animals no longer displayed overt motor asymmetries or a specific sensorimotor lateralization. Tests of sensorimotor neglect and of deficits in reflexive reactions yielded nonsignificant results. A neurological deficit was nevertheless persistent since injection of amphetamine induced ipsiversive circling in most of the animals regardless of the type of lesion.

E. Sensorimotor Deprivation following a Unilateral Substantia Nigra Lesion: Tracing Nigral Afferents to the Ventromedial Thalamus

In the experiments described so far we accumulated evidence for the occurrence of plastic changes in interhemispheric pathways as soon as 1 week after the infliction of a unilateral brain lesion. In each case the lesion induced turning behavior that disappeared within the first week. This suggested to us that the development of the crossed connections was a concomitant of a recovery of function, that is, a morphological correlate of behavioral compensation. One way to examine the relevance of lesion-

---

FIG. 3.4. Unilateral SN lesion and HRP injection into the caudate nucleus ipsilateral to the lesion. (a) Part of a frontal section showing the HRP injection site in the head of the left caudate nucleus (NC). (b) Unilateral 6-OHDA lesion in the medially situated part of the left substantia nigra (SN) ; scale, 100 μm; NR, red nucleus. (c) Two examples of labeled neurons in the substantia nigra, pars compacta (SN_c) contralateral to the HRP injection site. (d) Magnifications of these labeled neurons; scale, 10 μm.

induced turning and its cessation to the appearance of interhemispheric projections was to prevent the turning and/or its cessation.

In a preliminary study we obtained results from five experimental and three control animals (Morgan *et al.*, 1982). As in the experiments described previously, the animals received a unilateral 6-OHDA lesion in the SN. Subsequently, they were suspended in a sling (in a sound-attenuated chamber) to prevent turning behavior. After the first postoperative week the animals received an HRP injection (via an implanted glass pipette filled with crystalline HRP) into the ventromedial (and ventrolateral) thalamus of the hemisphere ipsilateral to the lesion. During the last 24 hr of survival time, that is, between implantation of the crystalline HRP and HRP processing, the rats were kept in ordinary cages. Turning tendencies were observed. Control animals received an HRP implantation only.

All the animals of the experimental group failed to show interhemispheric nigrothalamic projections, although the HRP site was at an appropriate place in the thalamus and labeled perikarya could be identified in parts of the ipsilateral SN that were spared by the lesion.

In the nonlesion control animals between 40 and 50 neurons were counted in the SN ipsilateral to the injected thalamus. No neurons were detected in the contralateral SN.

Behavioral observations showed that the experimental animals started to turn as soon as they were released from the sling. This experiment was the first of a series in which the time of onset of behavioral recovery was varied systematically. Because in this case no interhemispheric nigrothalamic projections could be identified, it is possible that the feedback from active turning behavior or the cessation of turning behavior plays a role in their appearance.

F. Reorganization of Nigrothalamic Projections following Unilateral Paralysis and Unilateral Sensory Deprivation

In another related experiment we searched for possible plastic changes in interhemispheric nigrothalamic projections following the infliction of a peripheral lesion that also leads to a sensorimotor asymmetry (Sabel *et al.*, 1982). This asymmetry was induced in rats by unilateral paralysis (ligature of sensory and motor nerves of the forelimbs and hindlimbs) and partial sensory deprivation (vibrissae were cut and eyelid was sutured). Both paralysis and deprivation were performed on either the left or the right side of the body (Fig. 3.5a). The spontaneous turning that resulted from this operation decreased within the first 5 postoperative days. Other neurological testing for specific sensorimotor deficits revealed only minimal recovery.

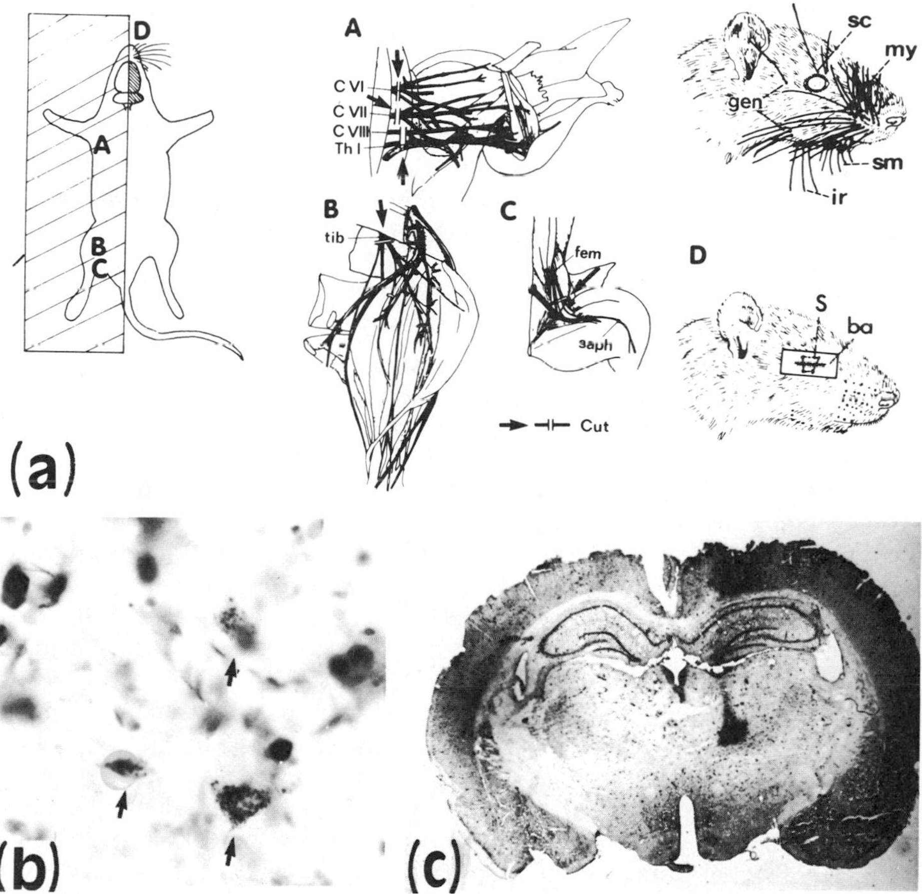

FIG. 3.5. Unilateral paralysis and unilateral partial sensory deprivation followed by an HRP injection into the ventromedial thalamus. (a) Unilateral paralysis (A, B, C) and unilateral partial sensory deprivation (D). Drawings A–C show the cuts (indicated by arrows) of the cervical (CVI, CVII, CVIII) and thoracal (Th I) spinal nerves of the forelimb (A) and the cuts of the tibial (tib) nerve (B), as well as the saphenous (saph) and femoral (fem) nerves (C) of the hindlimb. For sensory deprivation on one side of the body the superciliar (sc), mystacial (my), submental (sm), interraminal (ir), and genal (gen) vibrissae were cut and the eye was sutured (S) and covered with a Band Aid (ba) (D). (b) Examples of labeled neurons in the SN contralateral to the thalamic injection site. In this case the thalamic injection site was situated contralateral to the denervated side of the extremities. The neurons are indicated by arrows. (c) Representative microphotograph of the frontal brain section at the level of the HRP implantation site in the ventrobasal thalamus.

Sixteen days after the surgery, HRP was implanted into the ventrobasal thalamus of one hemisphere (Fig. 3.5c). This was done either ipsilateral to the denervated side of the limbs (group IDL) or contralateral to the denervated limbs (group CDL). Brains were processed according to the tetramethylbenzidine procedure. Unoperated control animals, IDL, and CDL animals were compared with respect to the number of labeled neurons found in either of the substantiae nigrae (Fig. 3.5b).

Microscopic analysis revealed that CDL animals had interhemispheric nigrothalamic projections, whereas IDL and control animals did not. At the same time there were significantly fewer labeled neurons in the substantia nigra ipsilateral to the operated side of the body. It is possible that the surgically induced behavioral asymmetry and its partial compensation may be one of the determinants of the observed neuronal plasticity.

G. Discussion

The main finding in this series of experiments was a postlesion increase in the interhemispheric organization of projection systems known to be organized primarily ipsilaterally in the intact animal (Fig. 3.6). Increases in crossed projections were found as early as 1 week after the operation, at a time when gross behavioral asymmetries (turning) were already compensated for.

Evidence for such increases in crossed projections was found for corticothalamic projections in the adult (experiment A) and in the infant rat (experiment B). Labeled neurons were found in the parieto-temporal (experiment A) and in the occipital cortex (experiment B) after HRP injection into the ventral and posterior–lateral (experiment A) and into the posterior part (experiment B) of the thalamus on the side of the ablated hemisphere (Pritzel and Huston, 1981a; Neumann *et al.*, 1982).

Similarly, in the case of nigrothalamic projections (Pritzel and Huston, 1981b) neurons were identified in the intact SN after an HRP injection into the ventromedial thalamus of the hemisphere with the SN lesion (Fig. 3.2). Furthermore, interhemispheric nigrothalamic projections were not found if the animals were prevented from turning by hanging in a sling for 1 week (experiment E). However, if a strong sensorimotor asymmetry was induced by unilateral peripheral lesions, only interhemispheric projections to the ventromedial thalamus of the deprived hemisphere (i.e., the hemisphere contralateral to the peripheral lesions) were identified (experiment F).

Microscopic inspection showed that the fiber connections to the thalamus from projection loci of the contralateral hemisphere in experiments A–D and F originate from mirror-image loci of ipsilaterally known thalamic projection sites. For example, in experiments A and B neurons were found in the deeper layers of the cerebral cortex contralateral to the

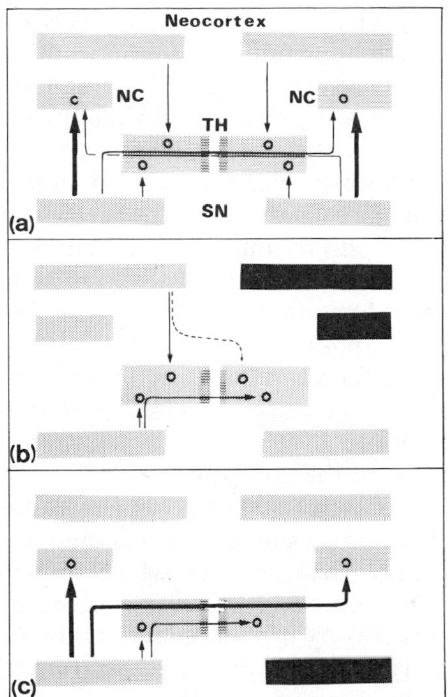

FIG. 3.6. Summary of results presented in Section II. (a) Fiber connections in the intact animal. Injections of HRP (open circles) into the head of the caudate nucleus (NC) or the thalamus (TH) reveal HRP-labeled perikarya in the substantia nigra (SN) or the neocortex homolateral to the side of injection. A sparse interhemispheric nigrocaudate projection can also be identified [which we have found to include bifurcating, monoaminergic nigrostriatal projections (Sarter *et al.*, 1982)]. (b) A unilateral lesion of telencephalic structures including neocortex and NC (blackened areas) leads to interhemispheric projections to thalamic nuclei on the side of the brain with the lesion. These crossed projections originate in both the neocortex and the SN. (c) A unilateral lesion of the SN (blackened area) leads to the identification of interhemispheric nigrothalamic projections and to an increased number of crossed projections from the intact SN to the NC.

known corticothalamic projection sites. They were situated in the pars reticulata of the intact SN following an HRP injection into the ventromedial thalamus (in experiments C and F) and in the pars compacta of the SN following an HRP injection into the head of the NC (experiment D).

The crossed projections thus originate from contralateral homotopical brain structures of ipsilaterally running corticothalamic (Colwell, 1975; Donaldson *et al.*, 1975), nigrothalamic, and nigrocaudate projection sources (Faull and Mehler, 1978; Beckstead *et al.*, 1979; Dray, 1979; Nauta and Domesick, 1979; Szabo, 1980). However, using other species and/or other methods, some investigators have also found sparse crossed corticothalamic and nigrothalamic projections in the intact animal. For example, a crossed corticothalamic projection from the prefrontal area to the mediodorsal nucleus was described in the infant and juvenile monkey (Goldman, 1979), and a sparse crossed nigrothalamic projection was found more recently in the rat, when wheat germ agglutinin-conjugated HRP (Gerfen *et al.*, 1982) was used as a tracer substance.

Our findings of increased interhemispheric projections following the infliction of unilateral brain lesions interest us primarily with respect to their possible correlation with functional recovery from lesion-induced behavior asymmetries. However, we shall first consider other possible determinants, such as a possible specificity of HRP labeling due to immediate or chronic deafferentation or peculiarities in HRP transport of regenerating neurons or an alteration in HRP labeling due to the size and locus of the brain lesion.

Injections of HRP into the thalamus of the ablated side of the brain immediately (or within 24 hr) after the operation did not reveal contralateral nigral or cortical projections. However, neurons were found in the ipsilateral SN. Therefore, the transport of HRP by transected axons (Halperin and La Vail, 1975; Geyer *et al.*, 1979; Olsson *et al.*, 1980) running through the thalamus and with their parent cell bodies in the SN can be considered an unlikely explanation of the results.

Moreover, an HRP injection into the thalamus of the intact hemisphere 1 week after unilateral detelencephalization did not give rise to labeled neurons in the contralaterally situated SN, even though in some animals relatively large injections had been made. This suggested that deafferentation of the injection locus might play some role in the appearance of interhemispheric projections in the experimental animals. However, deafferentation of thalamic and caudate injection sites was not likely to be the main reason for the appearance of crossed projections. In caudate and thalamic HRP injection sites the degree of deafferentation could be expected to differ with respect to the applied neurotoxin in the SN. For example, a KA lesion can be assumed to affect only partially the NC situated in the ipsilateral hemisphere (Weinreich and Seeman, 1980; Olianas *et al.*, 1978a), whereas a 6-OHDA lesion in the SN is reported to deafferent the NC projection area extensively (Hedreen, 1978; Heikkila *et al.*, 1981; van der Kooy *et al.*, 1981). The inverse holds for KA lesions in the SN and the destruction of nigrothalamic projections (Kilpatrick *et al.*, 1980). However, secondary lesion effects, seen as degeneration in distant areas of the brain (Schwob *et al.*, 1980; Zaczek *et al.*, 1980), are reported to result from KA lesions. Lesions produced by 6-OHDA injection reportedly do not induce such pronounced secondary lesion effects. However, in comparing the KA- and the 6-OHDA-injected animals we could not find a difference in the number of labeled neurons in the SN contralateral to the thalamic (experiment C) or caudate (experiment D) injection sites at either of the postoperative survival times. Furthermore, we found interhemispheric nigrothalamic projections emanating from the SN situated in the hemisphere contralateral to the denervated fore- and hindlimbs (experiment F). Thalamic deafferentation from thalamic inputs plays only a minor role in these preparations.

The HRP labeling of interhemispherically projecting SN neurons may also depend on the physiological activity of the affected cells (for review, see Thoenen and Kreutzberg, 1981). In fact, SN lesions considerably alter the firing rate of NC neurons (Hull *et al.*, 1974); furthermore, both amphetamine and apomorphine, which were used in this study, are known to interfere strongly with the activity of NC neurons (Fuxe *et al.*, 1975). However, we found no difference in the number of labeled neurons between animals that were given amphetamine or apomorphine and non-treated animals with lesions. Replacement of HRP by NY or FB or by a combined injection of both FB and NY did not influence the number of labeled SN neurons found contralateral to the NC injection site. Therefore, the increase in the number of labeled cells in the hemisphere contralateral to the HRP-injected thalamus and NC is not likely to be explained simply by lesion-induced peculiarities of HRP uptake. First, a unilateral lesion followed immediately by an HRP injection did not lead to the appearance of interhemispheric connections. Second, neither the size (experiments A and B versus experiments C and D) nor the type (6-OHDA versus KA) of the deafferentation seemed to influence the extent of the interhemispheric projection. Finally, the HRP results were repeated using other tracers with similar properties (NY and FB).

Common to all of the experiments was the observation of a lesion-induced behavioral asymmetry, registered as turning of the animals. Unilateral detelencephalization led to spontaneous rotation in most of the operated adult and young animals. It was often, but not consistently directed toward the side (ipsiversive) of the ablated hemisphere. Variation in the direction of turning occurred between as well as within animals. These findings correspond to those of others describing ipsiversive (Rothmann, 1923; Dresel, 1924; Kennard and Ectors, 1938) as well as contraversive circling (Langworthy and Kolb, 1935) after large unilateral cortical extirpation, including the removal of hemisphere (Rothmann, 1923; Dresel, 1924).

We also observed a rapid restoration of behavioral symmetry in all of the preparations. The spontaneous rotation usually ceased within 3 to 5 days and in all cases within 7 days. This finding is in agreement with other reports in which behavioral asymmetry due to extensive unilateral removal of the forebrain was described as having diminished within the first postoperative days in young rats (Hicks and D'Amato, 1970) and kittens (Wenzel *et al.*, 1962). Unilaterally forebrain-ablated monkeys were described as indistinguishable in their overt behavior from unoperated controls by 10 days after the operation (Karplus and Kreidl, 1914). Following the infliction of unilateral SN lesions, rotation was observed to be predominantly ipsiversive in rats with 6-OHDA lesions and predominantly contraversive in animals with KA lesions. These findings are also in line with other data; ipsiversive turning of animals with 6-OHDA lesions in the SN is a well-studied phenomenon (Ungerstedt and Arbuthnott, 1970; Ungerstedt, 1971). Kainic acid lesions have been found to induce mainly contraversive circling (DiChiara *et al.*, 1977; Papadopoulos and Huston, 1980). However, depending on the concentration of the excitotoxin and on the site of intranigral injection, rotation to either side of the body has been described (Olianas *et al.*, 1978b; DiChiara *et al.*, 1979; Porceddu *et al.*, 1979).

In summary, massive and focal lesions in one hemisphere of the brain as well as unilateral peripheral lesions led to spontaneous rotation, which ceased within the first postoperative week. Injection of HRP into the thalamus or caudate nucleus of these animals led to either the appearance of or a significant increase in the number of labeled cells in the contralateral hemisphere. This suggests an increase in interhemispheric cortical and nigral projections to the thalamus or NC after the first postoperative week(s).

The evidence for an increased number of interhemispherically projecting neurons of the nigrocaudate pathway after 7 to 21 days correlates well with electrophysiological (Hull *et al.*, 1974) and neurochemical (Nieoullon *et al.*, 1977) data of a lesion-induced increased interaction between the nigrostriatal systems of both sides of the brain. The observation of an increased number of labeled neurons (experiment D) or the new identification of neurons (experiments A–C and F) in contralateral mirror-image loci of otherwise ipsilateral thalamic and caudate projection sites can be interpreted in terms of terminal sprouting of already existing interhemispheric projections (Cotman and Lynch, 1977; Cotman and Nadler, 1978; Cotman *et al.*, 1982). For example, unilateral entorhinal lesions, which are known to induce neuronal sprouting, lead to an increase in HRP-labeled projections of commissural hippocampal connections by 8 days after the lesion (Goldschmidt and Steward, 1980; see also Bisby, 1980; Fernandez *et al.*, 1981; for review, see Thoenen and Kreutzberg, 1981).

An increased formation of synapses in denervated brain structures by already existing crossed projections (as may be the case in experiments A–D and F) has been described only recently. For example, the reinnervation of denervated fimbrial sites in the adult rat was described as occuring preferentially via axons from the contralateral fimbria (Field *et al.*, 1980), and unilateral denervation of the fascia dentata from the ipsilateral entorhinal cortex results in an increased projection from the entorhinal cortex of the other hemisphere (see Section III,c for references). Our anatomical results could thus be explained in terms of a preferential synapse formation of homotopical contralateral projections. Such an interpretation would concur with the known data about interhemispheric nigrocaudate (Fass and Butcher, 1981) and nigrothalamic (Gerfen *et al.*, 1982) projections in the rat. [Our more recent experiments (Sarter *et al.*, 1982) suggest that the so-called thalamic commissure (Rioch, 1931; Lumley, 1972) may be one of the loci of interhemispheric nigrocaudate decussations.]

The enhancement of synaptic contacts has long been considered a likely concomitant of experimentally increased general experience (Diamond *et al.*, 1964, 1975; Møllgaard *et al.*, 1971; Globus *et al.*, 1973; Greenough and Volkmar, 1973; Greenough *et al.*, 1973; Uylings *et al.*, 1978; for review, see Rosenzweig and Bennett, 1976) and of specific learning tasks (Greenough *et al.*, 1979; Spinelli and Jensen, 1979; Spinelli *et al.*, 1980; Vrensen and Cardozo, 1981). An increase in interhemispherically projecting neurons could constitute one morphological correlate of the animals' learning to compensate for the lesion-induced sensorimotor asymmetry during the first postoperative days. From a behavioral viewpoint it is known (Held, 1968; Taub, 1968) that an experimentally induced deprivation (or reversal) of sensory input can be compensated for by practice. That such learning takes place, for instance, in unilaterally detelencephalized animals is indicated by their *symmetric* behavior in the performance of learning tasks (Kellogg and Bashore, 1950) even within a few days after the infliction of a lesion (Hicks and D'Amato, 1970). It seems possible, therefore, that an increase in interhemispheric contacts is a structural correlate of the learning to compensate for sensorimotor asymmetries induced by the unilateral lesions. The fact that crossed connections were not found when the animals were prevented from engaging in turning behavior (experiment E) supports this hypothesis. One problem with the interpretation of this experiment, however, is that the stress of suspending the animals could have prevented the crossed connections from sprouting. For instance, Scheff *et al.* (1980b) have shown that hydrocortisone administration decreases sprouting. The results of experiment F suggest that a unilateral lesion in the central nervous system may not be a prerequisite for the development of crossed projections in the brain. Unilateral peripheral lesions also induced alterations in the nigrothalamic interaction between the hemispheres (see also Section III,A).

At a postoperative interval of 90 days the animals of experiment D had completely ceased turning, yet no changes in the number of contralaterally labeled neurons were found. Relevant to this result may be the findings of Goldschmidt and Steward (1980), who suggested that long-term processes in neuronal reorganization are only partially recognized by the HRP method. In their study the number of labeled neurons that had sprouted was not higher by 10 days than by 360 days after the brain lesion had been made, although neuronal reorganization went on (see also Section III). From a morphological viewpoint one might have expected that any reorganizational process in interhemispheric SN–NC projections would have reached its maximum after a 3-month period (Raisman, 1969a, b; McWilliams and Lynch, 1979) given that the "vacated synaptic space" would mainly determine the extent of plastic changes at the synaptic level. However, instead of the expected increase in number of interhemispheric nigrocaudate projections at 90 days over the 7- and 21-day results, we found a decrease in projections to the level found in the unoperated control animals.

One possible explanation for the failure to find an increase in the number of crossed projections after 90 days is that by that time the new synapses of crossed projections may have been replaced by more slowly developing regenerating ipsilateral nigrocaudate projections that survived the lesion. The principle of this phenomenon, namely, the replacement of sprouted synapses by regenerating axon terminals, has been reported after damage to the endings of sensory nerves in mammals (Wall, 1977; Devor and Gorrin-Lippmann, 1979; Devor *et al.*, 1979) and after denervation of muscle (Bennett *et al.*, 1979). We found that about 96% of the interhemispheric nigrocaudate projections were of monoaminergic origin, but only 6% of the fibers were crossed. This result is similar to that found for the ipsilaterally running nigrostriatal system, which is also thought to consist of about 95% dopaminergic fibers (van der Kooy *et al.*, 1981). Since monoaminergic neurons in the central nervous system have been reported to regenerate even in the adult rat (Björklund and Lindvall, 1979), it is possible that some ipsilaterally running monoaminergic nigrocaudate projections regenerated and replaced the sparse monoaminergic contralateral ones. This speculative interpretation is in accord with the concept of a permanent process of regeneration and degeneration within the central nervous system, as has been suggested by others (Sotelo and Palay, 1971; Chan-Palay, 1973; Buell and Coleman, 1979; Cupp and Uemura, 1980). Such plastic changes could also be fundamental to learning to compensate for lesion-induced sensorimotor asymmetries.

In summary, our series of experiments has shown the following. Within 1 week after unilateral removal of the telencephalon in young as well as adult rats, we identified interhemispheric nigrothalamic projections that originated in the nonoperated side of the brain. Within 1 week these animals also ceased to turn spontaneously, indicating that some compensation for gross sensorimotor asymmetries had occurred.

This temporal coincidence of newly identified, interhemispherically projecting nigral neurons with cessation of turning behavior was also found after the infliction of unilateral SN lesions. The short time span of 7 days between the infliction of the brain lesion and the appearance of crossed pathways supported the assumption that existing interhemispheric nigrothalamic and nigrocaudate pathways might have been activated after the unilateral lesion—for example, by the activation of "silent synapses" and/or by an increase in interneural contacts as a result of terminal sprouting.

To test further the hypothesis of an interrelationship between behavioral recovery and neuronal reorganization of interhemispherically projecting neurons, we examined the effects of partial unilateral sensory deprivation and paralysis of fore- and hindlimbs. We found that the SN of the nonaffected (or at least less affected) side of the brain (i.e., the side ipsilateral to deprivation and denervation) showed interhemispheric projections to the thalamus on the deprived side. The SN contralateral to the denervated limbs did not. Thus, depriving the thalamus of its ipsilateral nigral input by either a central or a peripheral lesion results in the appearance of interhemispheric nigrothalamic projections.

To determine the extent to which the behavioral asymmetry and its compensation are necessary determinants for plastic changes in interhemispherically projecting neurons, we tried to prevent behavioral recovery after the infliction of unilateral brain lesions. Our first results showed that rats that were suspended in a sling for the first postoperative week after the infliction of an SN lesion failed to exhibit an increase in interhemispheric projecting nigrothalamic neurons. This finding encourages further investigations of possible behavioral concomitants of postoperative sprouting phenomena.

III. Plasticity of Interhemispheric Fiber Connections

In the central nervous system of adult mammals sprouting has been investigated systematically since the work of Liu and Chambers (1958). The progress in this field has been summarized in various reviews (Chambers *et al.*, 1973; Kerr, 1975; Tsukahara, 1981; Cotman and Nieto-Sampedro, 1982) and books (Cotman, 1978; Lund, 1978; Flohr and Precht, 1981). In this section we selectively summarize some results of other researchers that support the concept of a lesion-induced compensatory neuronal reorganization. In these studies, as in ours, the asymmetry of neuronal circuits induced by the lesion (and implicitly, as our results suggest, an asymmetry in resulting behavioral deficits) is regarded as an important stimulus for the initiation of sprouting.

In a number of experiments other than our own it was found that unilateral brain lesions in mammals may be followed by the appearance of interhemispheric fiber connections of projection systems that, in the intact animal, are known to run exclusively ipsilaterally [as we reported in the case of the nigrothalamic projection, which until recently (Gerfen *et al.*, 1982) was thought to be organized strictly ipsilaterally in the rat]. In addition, an amplification of sparsely crossing interhemispheric fiber connections in response to unilateral brain lesions was also reported (as in our results with the nigrostriatal projection, which had some crossing fibers that were visible). Similarly, unilateral brain lesions may induce the appearance or the enlargement of ipsilateral fiber systems that are known to cross the hemisphere either completely or at least to a large extent in the intact brain.

The examples of this phenomenon presented in the following pages focus on the sprouting of neurons that are situated in or are closely related to the forebrain. A likely mechanism common to all of these examples seems to be a partial compensation for lesion-induced asymmetry in otherwise symmetrically (ipsilaterally or contralaterally) organized fiber connections by a mirror-image-like remodeling of those projections. The reports differ, however, with respect to the methods used to identify plastic changes in neural connections, the presumed types of plasticity, and the hypothesized determinants of the plastic changes in the central nervous system.

A. Neuronal Plasticity in the Red Nucleus [Nucleus Ruber]

The appearance of crossed connections of projection systems that are generally known to follow a unilateral course was found, for example, in the corticorubral connections in rats after neonatal lesions had been made in the sensorimotor cortex of one hemisphere (Hicks and D'Amato, 1970; Leong and Lund, 1973; Nah and Leong, 1976a,b). Sprouting of a crossed, corticorubral projection from the intact hemicortex was reported to result in mirror-image-like contacts with respect to ipsilateral connections (Nah and Leong, 1976a). The cortical projections were confined largely to the rostral parvocellular part and to the dorsolateral portion of the magnocellular part of the contralateral red nucleus, that is, to mirror-image sites of the known ipsilaterally organized corticorubral projections (Brown, 1974).

Some spurious observations, however, indicate the existence of a very sparse interhemispheric corticorubral projection in the intact newborn rat. A small contralateral projection was detected in two cases of nearly complete unilateral decortication in which degenerated fibers were identified in the nucleus ruber of both hemispheres before any possible plastic alterations (Nah and Leong, 1976a). Therefore, the lesion-induced corticorubral connections (at the level of the pyramidal decussation), which were interpreted in terms of competition of growing fibers from each side of the brain (Leong and Lund, 1973), might in part be due to sprouting of a few already established crossed corticorubral fibers.

The lesion-bound appearance of bilateral projections from otherwise ipsilaterally or contralaterally running corticofugal pathways is not restricted to the corticorubral connections. The remaining hemicortex also develops ipsilateral projections in addition to the normally crossed projections to the spinal cord and to the pons (Castro, 1975) and crossed contacts to the superior colliculus, which is normally innervated ipsilaterally (Leong and Lund, 1973; Hicks and D'Amato, 1975; Leong, 1976a). These projections might also have sparse bilateral projections in the intact animal. In the cat, for example, a bilateral cortical projection to the superior colliculus has been described (Baleydier, 1977).

The red nucleus, however, is one of the few brain loci in which the inverse type of lesion-induced neuronal reorganization can be demonstrated as well, namely, an ipsilateral sprouting of otherwise crossed cerebellorubral projections (Lim and Leong, 1975). This pathway from the dentate and interposed nuclei to the red nucleus has been described as being exclusively crossed in various species (Mehler *et al.*, 1958; Courville, 1966; Flumerfelt *et al.*, 1973), including the adult rat (Gwyn and Flumerfelt, 1974). A unilateral lesion of both of these nuclei (Lim and Leong, 1975) or a hemicerebellectomy (Castro, 1978) in the newborn rat leads to a deflection of these cerebellorubral fibers at the decussation of the superior peduncle and to their termination in the red nucleus ipsilateral to the side of the lesion of the dentate and interposed nuclei 6 weeks after the operation (Lim and Leong, 1975). A unilateral lesion of these nuclei also leads to the development of an ipsilateral projection from the cerebellum to the ventrolateral thalamus (Lim and Leong, 1975), a connection that is normally crossed.

A dynamic interaction between developing axons, arising from both nuclei in each side of the cerebellum, was suggested as an explanation for the appearance of ipsilateral cerebellorubral and cerebellothalamic fiber connections (Lim and Leong, 1975). In addition, a sparse bilateral ascending projection from these cerebellar nuclei may be present at birth (Lund, 1978). For example, ipsilateral cerebellothalamic projections have also been reported in normal rats (Chan-Palay, 1977; Kawaguchi *et al.*, 1979a).

Finally, it has been possible to demonstrate alterations in the cortical input to the red nucleus after cerebellorubral deafferentation, and vice versa. In the red nucleus of adult cats, axons arising from the cerebellar interposed nuclei make contact at somata of neurons in the red nucleus, whereas cortical afferents synapse on the dendrites of these neurons. A frontal cortical lesion made about 25 days after the cerebellorubral fibers had been severed led to degeneration of both the axosomatic and axodendritic terminals of the red nucleus (which, by then, was already chronically deafferented from cerebellorubral fibers). Since no cortical fibers are known to terminate on somata of the red nucleus (all of the animals had been perfused 2–4 days after the cortical lesions, thus reducing the possibility of another sprouting), it is possible that corticorubral axon terminals sprouted from dendritic portions to make new synaptic contacts at the soma (Nakamura *et al.*, 1974). Furthermore, other results (McAllister *et al.*, 1982) have shown that a unilateral hemispherectomy in adult cats leads to an increased cerebellar projection to those degenerated thalamic nuclei that constitute overlapping projection sites from the cerebellum and from the telencephalon (Rinvik and Grofova, 1974; Hendry *et al.*, 1979; Nakano *et al.*, 1980).

Most of the studies on the plasticity of rubral afferents were performed with newborn rats because neuroanatomical remodeling, appears more likely to occur after the infliction of neonatal lesions (Kerr, 1975; Lund, 1978; Tsukahara, 1981).

It does not seem very likely that postnatal redirected growth of developing fibers is solely responsible for a bilateral mirror-image-like neuronal reorganization. First, for cerebrorubral (Nah and Leong, 1976a) as well as for cerebellothalamic projections (Chan-Palay, 1977; Faull and Carman, 1978; Kawaguchi *et al.*, 1979a) a small bilateral fiber connection was found to exist in unoperated animals as well. Second, experiments have demonstrated the formation of functional synapses in the red nucleus in the adult cat in response to cross-innervation of forelimb flexor and extensor nerves (Tsukahara and Fujito, 1976; Fujito *et al.*, 1982; Tsukahara *et al.*, 1982). This finding supports the idea that remodeling of the rubral afferents is not confined to plastic neuronal changes during an early stage of ontogenetic development. These experiments also raise the possibility that compensatory neural changes in the brain can occur not only after unilateral brain lesions, but also after lesions have been made in the peripheral nervous system [see also our results (Sabel *et al.*, 1982), Section II,F].

Electrophysiological evidence suggests that lesion-bound, newly formed corticofugal (Murakami *et al.*, 1977) or cerebellofugal (Kawaguchi *et al.*, 1979b) contacts may have properties of synaptic transmission comparable with those of normal animals. For instance, the newly formed synapses of the corticorubral pathway that end on the somata of red nucleus neurons exhibit facilitation and posttetanic potentiation as observed in the corticorubral excitatory postsynaptic potentials (EPSP) of axodendritic connections in normal cats (Murakami *et al.*, 1977).

The effects of lesion-bound redirected corticofugal projections on the recovery of motor behavior are difficult to delineate. This holds, for instance, for the lesion-induced ipsilaterally running corticospinal projections (Hicks and D'Amato, 1970; Leong and Lund, 1973; Castro, 1975), since even a substantial bilateral transection of the pyramidal tract of up to 90% has only minimal effects on general motor behavior (Castro, 1972) and motor learning (Lashley and Ball, 1929; Ingebritsen, 1932).

B. Neuronal Plasticity in the Superior Colliculus

A considerable number of experiments have provided evidence for bilateral compensatory neuronal alterations within the visual system following the unilateral removal of one eye (Lund and Lund, 1971; Goodman *et al.*, 1973; Baisden and Shen, 1978; Rhoades and Dellacroce, 1980; Jen and Lund, 1981; Stevenson and Lund, 1982) and/or the infliction of a unilateral lesion in the superior colliculus (Schneider, 1970, 1973; Finlay *et al.*, 1979; So, 1979) or the infliction of unilateral lesions in the visual and visually associated cortex (Schneider, 1970, 1973; Leong and Lund, 1973; Leong, 1976a,b; Mustari and Lund, 1976; Rhoades, 1981a) in newborn mammals.

As briefly mentioned in the preceding section, a unilateral lesion in the sensorimotor cortex of neonatal rats led to an aberrant contralateral corticotectal projection. The fibers were organized in a mirror-image-like manner (Leong and Lund, 1973; Leong, 1976a) compared with the normal ipsilateral corticotectal projections (Nauta and Bucher, 1954; Lund, 1966). Both ended in the upper layers of the superior colliculus. The lesion-induced contralateral corticotectal connections were described as running across the midline through the deeper layers of the superior colliculus and through the intertectal commissure; that is, they seemed to be only partly included in a known commissural pathway.

To a lesser extent such crossed corticotectal projections have also been observed in adult animals with lesions (Leong, 1976a). This finding raises the possibility that remodeling of corticotectal projections is not confined to an early stage of ontogenetic development. In young animals crossed corticotectal projections, which appear after the infliction of unilateral lesions in the visual system, are thought to be due to the development of transient exuberant projections or to the competition between growing axons (Jen and Lund, 1981).

The development of a mirror-image-like organization of crossed corticotectal projections following unilateral posterior neocortical ablation (Rhoades and Chalupa, 1978; Jen *et al.*, 1978; Mustari and Lund, 1976) can be estimated to some extent because of the known retinotopic corticotectal organization of the normal ipsilaterally running projections (Lund, 1964, 1966).

A macroscopic topographic mirror-image projection of crossed fibers in the superior colliculus was reported by Mustari and Lund (1976). Unilateral lesions in the visual cortex of young rats, which caused degeneration in the ipsilateral medial superior colliculus, also induced degeneration in the medial part of the contralateral superior colliculus. The same was true for unilateral lesions in the visual cortex, which are known to lead to degeneration in the lateral part of the superior colliculus. That is, the crossed projections between the undamaged visual cortical hemisphere and the superior colliculus did not seem to be the result of a random sprouting in the superior colliculus; instead, they occurred in a topographic array, even though no natural commissure joins the appropriate laminae in the superior colliculus (Mustari and Lund, 1976). This aberrant corticotectal pathway became more pronounced when the unilateral corticotectal ablation was accompanied by the removal of one eye contralateral to the side of the brain with the lesion (Mustari and Lund, 1976).

A more detailed analysis of topographic matching of sprouted corticotectal projections was provided by Rhoades (1981a,b). In examining some ipsilateral corticotectal fiber projections of remnants that survived the unilateral cortical lesion, Rhoades (1981a) found that this small remnant cortical region sent out axons to all portions of the superior colliculus; electrophysiological data provided no indications of any topography in the expanded corticocollicular pathway (Rhoades, 1981b). That is, mirror-image-like projections in the superior colliculus are not predetermined according to a point-to-point matching in electrophysiological mapping of the visual field. Instead, the results point to an increase in redundancy of interhemispheric corticotectal communication. From a behavioral viewpoint it is interesting that mismatching of visual information that occurred in hamsters with unilateral superior colliculus lesions and subsequent redirected axon growth was compensated for behaviorally after about 12 sessions of training (Schneider, 1979).

C. Neuronal Plasticity in the Dentate Gyrus of the Hippocampal Formation

The dentate gyrus of the hippocampal formation is one of the well-studied structures of the rat's brain in which a unilateral deafferentation from the ipsilateral projection site induces an increase in the number of commissural projections (Steward *et al.*, 1973, 1976; Zimmer and Hjorth-Simonsen, 1975; Lynch, 1979; Steward, 1980) and, vice versa, severing of commissural projections leads to an enhancement of ipsilateral projection sites (O'Leary *et al.*, 1979).

Sprouting in the dentate gyrus is not restricted to the newborn rat. Although it is more prominent there (Gall *et al.*, 1980; Scheff *et al.*, 1980a; Gall and Lynch, 1981), it has also been observed in the mature animal (Steward and Vinsant, 1978).

Unilateral destruction of the pathway from the entorhinal area to the hippocampal formation induces sprouting of a normally sparse commissural pathway (Laurberg, 1979) from the contralateral entorhinal area to the fascia dentata (Steward *et al.*, 1974, 1976). This pathway from the surviving contralateral entorhinal area may proliferate approximately five- to sixfold (Steward *et al.*, 1976) to reinnervate a portion of the zone that is normally occupied by ipsilateral entorhinal afferents. Therefore, the commissural projections spread from their normal sites of termination on proximal dendrites at granular cells in the molecular layer of the dentate gyrus to the distal dendritic regions (Lynch *et al.*, 1976) extending about 50 μm into the deafferented region.

Sprouting was reported to originate from the same neurons that send collaterals ipsilaterally to the dentate granular cell (Steward and Vinsant, 1978). The topographic distribution along the granular cell dendrites was described as being similar to the ipsilateral projection system (Zimmer and Hjorth-Simonson, 1975). Furthermore, these crossed projections share many of the electrophysiological properties of the normal ipsilateral pathway (Steward *et al.*, 1973; Wilson *et al.*, 1979).

Thus, mirror-image-like remodeling of neuronal connections in the hippocampal formation seems to lead to synaptic contacts that are morphologically and electrophysiologically appropriate. Their correlation with possible behavioral changes after the infliction of unilateral entorhinal lesions, however, remains to be determined. Unilateral lesions in the hippocampal formation and related structures have not been reported to yield obvious long-term behavioral deficits.

D. Conclusions

A summary of the findings described in this section is presented in Fig. 3.7. The figure illustrates schematically the principle of neuronal plasticity that is exemplified by all of these studies, namely, the appearance of crossed (or uncrossed) projections of otherwise uncrossed (or crossed) fiber systems after the infliction of unilateral brain lesions. The crossing fibers do not always follow known decussations between the two halves of the brain (Fig. 3.7b); that is, a number of interhemispheric connections that do not run in "bundles" may exist and play a role in interhemispheric communication. The newly identified interhemispheric projections are generally organized as mirror images of the deafferented ipsilaterally (or contralaterally) running projections. However, electrophysiological (Rhoades, 1981b) and electron microscopic mapping (Nakamura *et al.*, 1974; Lynch *et al.*, 1976) has not provided evidence for a point-to-point replacement.

The literature presented in this section concentrates mainly on newborn animals in which unilateral lesions led to the appearance of interhemispherically projecting neurons. However, in most cases of lesion-induced interhemispheric projections in young animals, such projections were eventually also found in the adult unoperated animals, although only to a very small degree.

Taken together, the reviewed experiments provide considerable evidence that adult as well as young animals exhibit plasticity of interhemi-

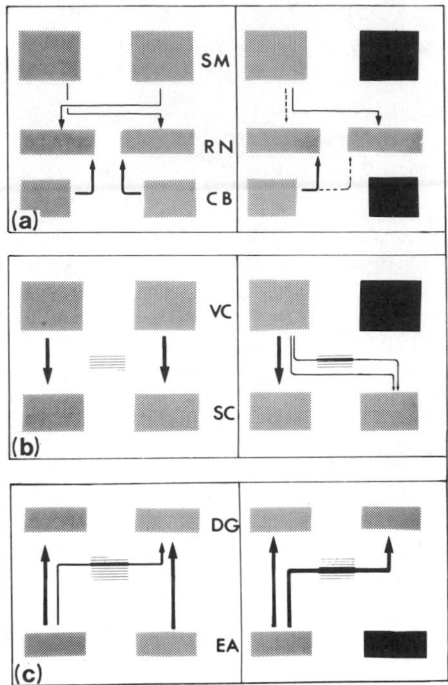

FIG. 3.7. Drawings (a), (b), and (c) refer to the data summarized in sections III, A, B, and C, respectively. Selected fiber connections in the intact animal are presented on the left side. The rearrangement of fiber connections following unilateral lesions (blackened areas) is presented on the right side. (a) Left: The red nucleus (RN) receives homolateral projections from cerebellar nuclei (CB) as well as crossed projections from the sensorimotor cortex (SM). Right: A unilateral lesion of either the SM or the CB reveals mirror-image-like projections that run ipsilateral from the SM and contralateral from the CB. (b) Left: The superior colliculus (SC) is reached by ipsilateral projections from the visual or visually associated cortex (VC). Right: A unilateral lesion within the VC reveals interhemispheric corticotectal fiber connections that run in part across the intertectal commissure. (c) Left: Projections from the entorhinal area (EA) contact granular cells of the dentate gyrus (DG) of the ipsilateral and (via the commissural system of the hippocampus) contralateral DG. Right: A unilateral lesion of the entorhinal fibers to the DG leads to an enhancement of interhemispheric projections between the entorhinal area and the dentate gyrus.

spherically projecting neurons following the infliction of a unilateral brain lesion. Such plasticity may include redirected growth of axons in young animals as well as sprouting of sparsely projecting neurons in young and adult rats. This plasticity does not seem to be associated with specific phylogenetic older or younger parts of the brain, or to certain interhemispheric connections. It has been demonstrated in the neocortex, as well as in the allocortex and in the cerebellum, with fibers traveling via known commissures or decussations or traversing the hemispheres via routes not yet defined.

It is striking that, aside from our own attempts, practically none of the studies reviewed have provided a viable link between the neural plasticity and related changes in behavior. Our evidence for a temporal relationship between recovery of function (cessation of turning) and appearance of crossed projections within 1 week after a unilateral brain lesion has been made is only a first step in the systematic functional analysis of this type of neural plasticity.

There are some reasons for our belief that an increased labeling of interhemispherically projecting neurons after the infliction of unilateral brain lesions may have behavioral relevance:

1. On the basis of the findings of others (e.g., Goldschmidt and Steward, 1980) one may assume that an increased number of labeled HRP neurons reflects plastic changes in the terminal arborization of these nerve cells.
2. An increased terminal arborization may constitute a concomitant of experience and learning. This would fit well with results of others (for review, see Rosenzweig and Bennett, 1976) describing a correlation between increased dendritic arborization and behavioral modifications.
3. An increase in such interhemispherically projecting HRP-labeled neurons within the first postoperative week also corresponds to the range of time found by others to be optimal for the identification of neural correlates of learning. Morphological changes in the brain, postulated to be related to learning processes, have been found at about 5 (Vrensen and Cardozo, 1981) days after the beginning of learning experiments.
4. In our experiments conditioning is presumably involved in the animal's compensating for the detrimental effects of the unilateral lesions. We assume that various kinds of "learning" take place to allow our unilaterally brain damaged rats to cease spontaneous turning behavior within the first postoperative week. An increase in the number of interhemispheric projections may therefore be a morphological correlate of the recovery of function after the lesion. which may or may not involve "learning."

Acknowledgments

This work was supported in part by Grant IIb5-9211.13 from the Ministry of Science of Northrhine-Westfalia and in part by Grant HU 306/1 from the Deutsche Forschungsgemeinschaft. We thank S. Morgan for a critical reading of the manuscript.

References

Baisden, R. H., and Shen, C. L. (1978). Sprouting of ipsilateral retinal projections in the optic system of the albino rat. *Exp. Neurol.* **61,** 549–560.

Baleydier, C. (1977). A bilateral cortical projection to the superior colliculus in the cat. *Neurosci. Lett.* **4,** 9–14.

Beckstead, R. M., Domesick, V. B., and Nauta, W. J. H. (1979). Efferent connections of the substantia nigra and ventral tegmental area in the rat. *Brain Res.* **175,** 191–217.

Bennett, M. R., McGrath, P. A., and Davey, D. F. (1979). The regression of synapses formed by a foreign nerve in a mature axolotl striated muscle. *Brain Res.* **173,** 451–469.

Bentivoglio, M., van der Kooy, D., and Kuypers, H. G. J. M. (1979). The organization of the efferent projections of the substantia nigra in the rat. A retrograde fluorescent double labeling study. *Brain Res.* **174,** 1–17.

Bentivoglio, M., Kuypers, H. G. J. M., and Catsman-Berrevoets, C. E. (1980a). Retrograde neuronal labeling by means of Bisbenzimide and Nuclear Yellow. Measures to prevent diffusion of the tracers out of retrogradely labeled neurons. *Neurosci. Lett.* **18,** 19–24.

Bentivoglio, M., Kuypers, H. G. J. M., Catsman-Berrevoets, C. E., Loewe, H., and Dann, O. (1980b). Two new fluorescent retrograde neuronal tracers which are transported over long distances. *Neurosci. Lett.* **18,** 25–30.

Bharos, T. B., Kuypers, H. G. J. M., Lemon, R. N., and Muir, R. B. (1981). Divergent collaterals from deep cerebellar neurons to thalamus and tectum, and to medulla oblongata and spinal cord: Retrograde fluorescent and electrophysiological studies. *Exp. Brain Res.* **42,** 399–410.

Bisby, M. A. (1980). Changes in the composition of labeled protein transported in motor axons during their regeneration. *J. Neurobiol.* **11,** 435–445.

Björklund, A., and Lindvall, O. (1979). Reformation of normal terminal innervation patterns by central noradrenergic neurons after 5, 7-dihydroxytryptamine-induced axotomy. *Brain Res.* **171,** 275–293.

Brown, L. T. (1974). Corticorubral projections in the rat. *J. Comp. Neurol.* **154,** 149–168.

Buell, S. J., and Coleman, P. D. (1979). Dendritic growth in the aged human brain and failure of growth in senile dementia. *Science* **206,** 854–856.

Castro, A. J. (1972). Motor performance in rats. The effect of pyramidal tract section. *Brain Res.* **44,** 313–323.

Castro, A. J. (1975). Ipsilateral corticospinal projections after large lesions of the cerebral hemisphere in neonatal rats. *Exp. Neurol.* **46,** 1–8.

Castro, A. J. (1978). Projections of the superior cerebellar peduncle in rats and the development of new connections in response to neonatal hemicerebellectomy. *J. Comp. Neurol.* **178,** 611–628.

Catsman-Berrevoets, C. E., and Kuypers, H. G. J. M. (1981). A search for corticospinal collaterals to thalamus and mesencephalon by means of multiple retrograde fluorescent tracers in cat and rat. *Brain Res.* **218,** 15–33.

Chambers, W. W., Liu, C. N., and McCouch, G. P. (1973). Anatomical and physiological correlates of plasticity in the central nervous system. *Brain Behav. Evol.* **8,** 5–26.

Chan-Palay, V. (1973). Neuronal plasticity in the cerebellar cortex and lateral nucleus. *Z. Anat. Entwicklungsgesch.* **142,** 23–35.

Chan-Palay, V. (1977). "Cerebellar Dentate Nucleus. Organization, Cytology, and Transmitters." Springer-Verlag, New York.

Colwell, S. A. (1975). Thalamocortical corticothalamic reciprocity: A combined anterograde-retrograde tracer technique. *Brain Res.* **92,** 443–449.

Combs, C. M. (1949). Fiber and cell degeneration in the albino rat brain after hemidecortication. *J. Comp. Neurol.* **90,** 373–402.

Cotman, C. W., ed. (1978). "Neuronal Plasticity." Raven Press, New York.

Cotman, C. W., and Lynch, G. S. (1977). Reactive synaptogenesis in the adult nervous system: The effects of partial deafferentation on new synapse formation. *In* "Neuronal Recognition" (S. H. Barondes, ed.), pp. 69–108. Chapman & Hall, London.

Cotman, C. W., and Nadler, J. V. (1978). Reactive synaptogenese in the hippocampus. *In* "Neuronal Plasticity" (C. W. Cotman, ed.), pp. 227–271. Raven Press, New York.

Cotman, C. W., and Nieto-Sampedro, M. (1982). Brain function, synapse renewal and plasticity. *Annu. Rev. Psychol.* **33,** 371–401.

Courville, J. (1966). Somatotopical organization of the projection from the nucleus interpositus anterior of the cerebellum to the red nucleus. An experimental study in the cat with silver impregnation methods. *Exp. Brain Res.* **2,** 191–215.

Cupp, C. J., and Uemura, E. (1980). Age-related changes in prefrontal cortex of *Macaca mulatta:* Quantitative analysis of dendritic branching patterns. *Exp. Neurol.* **69,** 143–163.

de la Torre, J. C. (1980). An improved approach to histofluorescence using the SPG method for tissue monoamines. *J. Neurosci. Methods* **3,** 1–5.

Devor, M., and Gorrin-Lippmann, R. (1979). Selective regeneration of sensory fibers following nerve crush injury. *Exp. Neurol.* **65,** 243–254.

Devor, M., Schonfeld, D., Seltzer, Z., and Wall, P. D. (1979). Two modes of cutaneous reinnervation following peripheral nerve injury. *J. Comp. Neurol.* **185,** 211–220.

Diamond, M. C., Krech, D., and Rosenzweig, M. R. (1964). The effects of an enriched environment on the histology of the rat cerebral cortex. *J. Comp. Neurol.* **123,** 111–119.

Diamond, M. C., Lindner, B., Johnson, R., Bennett, E. L., and Rosenzweig, M. R. (1975). Differences in occipital cortical synapses from environmentally enriched, impoverished and standard colony rats. *J. Neurosci. Res.* **1,** 109–119.

DiChiara, G., Olianas, M., Del Fiacco, M., Spano, P. F., and Tagliamonte, A. (1977). Intranigral kainic acid is evidence that nigral non-dopaminergic neurons control posture. *Nature (London)* **268,** 743.

DiChiara, G., Porceddu, M. L., Morelli, M., Mulas, M. L., and Gessa, G. L. (1979). Substantia nigra as an output station for striatal dopaminergic responses: Role of a GABA-mediated inhibition of pars reticulata neurons. *Arch. Pharm. (Weinheim, Ger.)* **306,** 153–159.

Donaldson, L., Hand, P. J., and Morrison, A. R. (1975). Corticalthalamic relationship in the rat. *Exp. Neurol.* **47,** 448–458.

Dray, A. (1979). The striatum and substantia nigra: A commentary on their relationships. *Neuroscience* **4,** 1407–1439.

Dresel, K. (1924). Die Funktionen eines grosshirn- und striatumlosen Hundes. *Klin. Wochenschr.* **3**(2), 2231–2233.

Fass, B., and Butcher, L. L. (1981). Evidence for a crossed nigrostriatal pathway in rats. *Neurosci. Lett.* **22,** 109–113.

Faull, R. L. M., and Carman, J. B. (1978). The cerebellofugal projections in the brachium conjunctivum of the rat. I. The contralateral ascending pathway. *J. Comp. Neurol.* **178,** 495–518.

Faull, R. L. M., and Mehler, W. R. (1978). The cells of origin of nigrotectal, nigrothalamic and nigrostriatal projections in the rat. *Neuroscience* **3,** 989–1002.

Fernandez, H. L., Singer, P. A., and Mehler, S. (1981). Retrograde axonal transport mediates the onset of regenerative changes in the hypoglossal nucleus. *Neurosci. Lett.* **25,** 7–11.

Field, P. M., Coldham, D. E., and Raisman, G. (1980). Synapse formation after injury in the adult rat brain: Preferential reinnervation of denervated fimbrial sites by axons of the contralateral fimbria. *Brain Res.* **189,** 103–113.

Finlay, B. L., Schneps, S. E., and Schneider, G. E. (1979). Orderly compression of the retinotectal projection following partial tectal ablation in the newborn hamster. *Nature (London)* **280,** 153–155.

Flohr, H., and Precht, W., eds. (1981). "Lesion-Induced Neuronal Plasticity in Sensorimotor Systems." Springer-Verlag, Berlin.

Flumerfelt, B. A., Otabe, S., and Courville, J. (1973). Distinct projections to the red nucleus from the dentate and interposed nuclei in the monkey. *Brain Res.* **50,** 408–414.

Fujito, Y., Tsukahara, N., Oda, Y., and Yoshida, M. (1982). Formation of functional synapses in the adult cat red nucleus from the cerebrum following cross-innervation of forelimb flexor and extensor nerves. II. Analysis of newly appeared synaptic potentials. *Exp. Brain Res.* **45,** 13–18.

Fuxe, K., Agnati, L. F., Corrodi, H., Everitt, B. J., Hökfelt, T., Löfström, A., and Ungerstedt, U. (1975). Action of dopamine receptor agonists in forebrain and hypothalamus: Rotational behavior, ovulation and dopamine turnover. *Adv. Neurol.* **9,** 223–242.

Gall, C., and Lynch, G. (1981). Fiber architecture of the dentate gyrus following ablation of the entorhinal cortex in rats of different ages: Evidence for two forms of axon sprouting in the immature brain. *Neuroscience* **6,** 903–910

Gall, C., McWilliams, R., and Lynch, G. (1980). Accelerated rates of synaptogenesis by "sprouting" afferents in the immature hippocampal formation. *J. Comp. Neurol.* **193,** 1047–1061.

Gerfen, C. R., Staines, W. A., Arbuthnott, G. W., and Fibiger, H. C. (1982). Crossed connections of the substantia nigra in the rat. *J. Comp. Neurol.* **207,** 283–303.

Geyer, G., Schmidt, H. P., and Biedermann, M. (1979). Horseradish peroxidase as a label of injured cells. *Histochem. J.* **11,** 337–344.

Globus, A., Rosenzweig, M. R., Bennett, E. L., and Diamond, M. C., (1973). Effects of differential experience on dendritic spine counts in rat cerebral cortex. *J. Comp. Physiol. Psychol.* **82,** 175–181.

Goldman, P. S. (1979). Contralateral projections to the dorsal thalamus from frontal association cortex in the rhesus monkey. *Brain Res.* **166,** 166–171.

Goldschmidt, R. B., and Steward, O. (1980). Time course of increases in retrograde labeling and increases in cell size of entorhinal cortex neurons sprouting in response to unilateral entorhinal lesions. *J. Comp. Neurol.* **189,** 359–379.

Goodman, D. C., Bogdasarian, R. S., and Horel, J. A. (1973). Axonal sprouting of ipsilateral optic tract following opposite eye removal. *Brain Behav. Evol.* **8,** 27–50.

Greenough, W. T., and Volkmar, F. R. (1973). Pattern of dendritic branching in occipital cortex of rats reared in complex environments. *Exp. Neurol.* **40,** 491–504.

Greenough, W. T., Volkmar, F. R., and Juraska, J. M. (1973). Effects of rearing complexity on dendritic branching in frontolateral and temporal cortex of the rat. *Exp. Neurol.* **41,** 371–378.

Greenough, W. T., Juraska, J. M., and Volkmar, F. R. (1979). Maze training effects on dendritic branching in occipital cortex of adult rats. *Behav. Neural Biol.* **26,** 287–297.

Grill, H. J., and Norgren, R. (1978a). The taste reactivity. II. Mimetic responses to gustatory stimuli in chronic thalamic and chronic decerebrate rats. *Brain Res.* **143,** 281–297.

Grill, H. J., and Norgren, R. (1978b). Neurological tests and behavioral deficits in chronic thalamic and chronic decerebrate rats. *Brain Res.* **143,** 299–312.

Gwyn, D. G., and Flumerfelt, B. A. (1974). A comparison of the distribution of cortical and cerebellar afferents in the red nucleus of the rat. *Brain Res.* **69,** 130–135.

Halperin, J. J., and La Vail, J. H. (1975). A study of the dynamics of retrograde transport and accumulation of horseradish peroxidase in injured neurons. *Brain Res.* **100,** 253–269.

Hedreen, J. (1978). Nondopaminergic and dopaminergic nigro-striatal pathways in rats. *Neurosci. Abstr.* **4,** 45.

Hefti, F., Melamed, E., and Wurtman, R. J. (1980). Partial lesions of the dopaminergic nigrostriatal system in rat brain: biochemical characterization. *Brain Res.* **195,** 123–137.

Heikkila, R. E., Shapiro, B. S., and Duvoisin, R. C. (1981). The relationship between loss of dopamine nerve terminals, striatal [3H] spiroperidol binding and rotational behavior in unilaterally 6-hydroxydopamine lesioned rats. *Brain Res.* **211,** 285–292.

Held, R. (1968). Plasticity in sensorimotor coordination. *In* "The Neuropsychology of Spatially Oriented Behavior" (S. J. Freedman, ed.), pp. 57–62. Dorsey Press, Homewood, Illinois.

Heller, A., Hutchens, J. O., Kirby, M. L., Karapas, F., and Fernandez, C. (1979). Stereotaxic electrode placement in the neonatal rat. *J. Neurosci. Meth.* **1,** 41–76.

Hendry, S. H. C., Jones, E. G., and Graham, J. (1979). Thalamic relay nuclei for cerebellar and certain related fiber systems in the cat. *J. Comp. Neurol.* **185,** 679–714.

Herkenham, M. (1979). The afferent and efferent connections of the ventromedial thalamic nucleus in the rat. *J. Comp. Neurol.* **183,** 487–518.

Hicks, S. P., and D'Amato, C. J. (1970). Motor-sensory and visual behavior after hemispherectomy in newborn and mature rats. *Exp. Neurol.* **29,** 416–438.

Hicks, S. P., and D'Amato, C. J. (1975). Motor-sensory cortex-corticospinal system and developing locomotion and placing in rats. *Am. J. Anat.* **143,** 1–42.

Hull, C. D., Levine, M. S., Buchwald, N. A., Heller, A., and Browning, R. A. (1974). The spontaneous firing pattern of forebrain neurons. I. The effects of dopamine and non-dopamine depleting lesions on caudate unit firing patterns. *Brain Res.* **73,** 241–262.

Huston, J. P., and Borbély, A. A. (1973). Operant conditioning in forebrain ablated rats by use of rewarding hypothalamic stimulation. *Brain Res.* **50,** 467–472.

Huston, J. P., and Borbély, A. A. (1974). The thalamic rat: General behavior, operant learning with rewarding hypothalamic stimulation and effects of amphetamine. *Physiol. Behav.* **12,** 433–448.

Ingebritsen, O. C. (1932). Maze learning after lesion in the cervical cord. *J. Comp. Psychol.* **14,** 279–294.

Jen, L. S., and Lund, R. D. (1981). Experimentally induced enlargement of the uncrossed retinotectal pathway in rats. *Brain Res.* **211,** 37–57.

Jen, L. S., Lund, R. D., and Boles, J. (1978). Further studies on the aberrant crossed visual corticotectal pathway in rats. *Exp. Brain Res.* **33,** 405–414.

Karplus, J. P., and Kreidl, A. (1914). Über Totalexstirpation einer und beider Grosshirnhemisphären an Affen (Macacus rhesus). *Arch. Anat. Physiol., Physiol. Abt.* **38,** 155–213.

Kawaguchi, S., Yamamoto, T., Samejima, A., Itoh, K., and Mizuno, N. (1979a). Morphological evidence for axonal sprouting of cerebellothalamic neurons in kittens after neonatal hemicerebellectomy. *Exp. Brain Res.* **35,** 511–518.

Kawaguchi, S., Yamamoto, T., and Samejima, A. (1979b). Electrophysiological evidence for axonal sprouting of cerebellothalamic neurons in kittens after neonatal hemicerebellectomy. *Exp. Brain Res.* **36,** 21–39.

Kellogg, W. N., and Bashore, W. D. (1950). The influence of hemidecortication upon bilateral avoidance conditioning in dogs. *J. Comp. Physiol. Psychol.* **43,** 49–62.

Kennard, M. A., and Ectors, L. (1938). Forced circling in monkeys following lesions of the frontal lobes. *J. Neurophysiol.* **1,** 45–54.

Kerr, F. W. L. (1975). Structural and functional evidence of plasticity in the central nervous system. *Exp. Neurol.* **48,** 16–31.

Kilpatrick, J. C., Starr, M. S., Fletcher, A., James, T. A., and MacLeod, N. K. (1980). Evidence for a GABA-ergic nigro-thalamic pathway in the rat. I. Behavioral and biochemical studies. *Exp. Brain Res.* **40,** 45–54.

König, J. F. R., and Klippel, R. A. (1963). "The Rat Brain: A Stereotaxic Atlas of the Forebrain and Lower Parts of the Brain Stem." R. E. Krieger, Huntington, New York.

Kozlowski, M. R., and Marshall, J. F. (1980). Plasticity of [14_C] 2-deoxy-D-glucose incorporation into neostriatum and related structures in response to dopamine neuron damage and apomorphine replacement. *Brain Res.* **197,** 167–183.

Kuypers, H. G. J. M., Bentivoglio, M., Catsman-Berrevoets, C. E., and Bharos, A. T. (1980). Double retrograde neuronal labeling through divergent axon collaterals, using two fluorescent tracers with the same excitation wavelength, which label different features of the cell. *Exp. Brain Res.* **40,** 383–392.

Langworthy, R. O., and Kolb, L. C. (1935). The experimental production in the cat of a condition simulating pseudo-bulbar palsy. *Am. J. Physiol.* **111,** 571–577.

Lashley, K. S., and Ball, J. (1929). Spinal conduction and kinesthetic sensitivity in the maze habit. *J. Comp. Psychol.* **9,** 71–105.

Laurberg, S. (1979). Commissural and intrinsic connections of the rat hippocampus. *J. Comp. Neurol.* **184,** 685–708.

Leong, S. K. (1976a). An experimental study of the corticofugal system following cerebral lesions in the albino rats. *Exp. Brain Res.* **26,** 235–247.

Leong, S. K. (1976b). A qualitative electron microscopic investigation of the anomalous corticofugal projections following neonatal lesions in the albino rats. *Brain Res.* **107,** 1–8.

Leong, S. K., and Lund, R. D. (1973). Anomalous bilateral corticofugal pathways in albino rats after neonatal lesions. *Brain Res.* **62,** 218–221.

Lim, K. H., and Leong, S. K. (1975). Aberrant bilateral projections from the dentate and interposed nuclei in albino rats after neonatal lesions. *Brain Res.* **96,** 306–309.

Liu, C.-N., and Chambers, W. W. (1958). Intraspinal sprouting of dorsal root axons. *Arch. Neurol. Psychiatry* **79,** 46–61.

Lumley, J. S. (1972). The role of the massa intermedia in motor performance in rhesus monkey. *Brain* **95,** 347–356.

Lund, R. D. (1964). Terminal distribution in the superior colliculus of fibres originating in the visual cortex. *Nature (London)* **204,** 1283–1285.

Lund, R. D. (1966). The occipitotectal pathway of the rat. *J. Anat.* **11,** 51–62.

Lund, R. D. (1978). "Development and Plasticity of the Brain." Oxford Univ. Press, New York.

Lund, R. D., and Lund, J. S. (1971). Synaptic adjustment after deafferentation of the superior colliculus of the rat. *Science* **171,** 804–807.

Lynch, G. (1979). Extrinsic influences on the development of afferent topographics in mammalian brain. *In* "The Neurosciences: Fourth Study Program" (F. O. Schmitt and F. G. Worden, eds.), pp. 957–968. MIT Press, Cambridge, Massachusetts.

Lynch G., Gall, C., and Cotman, C. (1976). Temporal parameters of axon sprouting in the adult brain. *Exp. Neurol.* **54,** 179–183.

McAllister, J. P., II, Olmstead, C. E., Villablanca, J. R., and Goméz, C. F. (1982). Residual cerebellothalamic terminal fields following hemispherectomy in the cat. *Neurosci. Lett.* **29,** 25–29.

McGeer, E. G., Olney, J. W., and McGeer, P. L. (1978). "Kainic Acid as a Tool in Neurobiology." Academic Press, New York.

McWilliams, R., and Lynch, G. (1979). Terminal proliferation in the partially deafferented dentate gyrus: Time course for the appearance and removal of degeneration and replacement of lost terminals. *J. Comp. Neurol.* **187,** 191–198.

Malmgren, L., and Olsson, Y. (1978). A sensitive method for histochemical demonstration of horseradish peroxidase in neurons following retrograde axonal transport. *Brain Res.* **148,** 279–294.

Marshall, J. F., and Teitelbaum, P. (1974). Further analysis of sensory inattention following lateral hypothalamic damage in rat. *J. Comp. Physiol. Psychol.* **86,** 375–395.

Mason, S. T., and Fibiger, H. C. (1979). On the specificity of kainic acid. *Science* **204,** 1339–1341.

Mehler, W. R., Vernier, V. G., and Nauta, W. J. H. (1958). Efferent projections from dentate and interpositus nuclei in primates. *Anat. Rec.* **130,** 430–431.

Merrill, E. G., and Wall, P. D. (1978). Plasticity of connections in the adult nervous system. *In* "Neuronal Plasticity" (C. W. Cotman, ed.), pp. 97–111. Raven Press, New York.

Mesulam, M.-M. (1976). The blue reaction product in horseradish peroxidase neurohistochemistry: incubation parameters and visibility. *J. Histochem. Cytochem.* **24,** 1273–1280.

Mesulam, M.-M., and Rosene, D. L. (1979). Sensitivity in horseradish peroxidase neurohistochemistry: A comparative and quantitative study of nine methods. *J. Histochem. Cytochem.* **27,** 763–773.

Møllgaard, K., Diamond, M. C., Bennett, E. L., Rosenzweig, M. R., and Lindner, B. (1971). Quantitative synaptic changes with differential experience in rat brain. *Int. J. Neurosci.* **2,** 113–128.

Morgan, S., Pritzel, M., Sabel, B., and Huston, J. P. (1982). Sensorimotor deprivation prevents neuronal changes induced by unilateral substantia nigra lesions. Third Meeting of Belgian, Dutch and German Physiological Psychologists, Düsseldorf (F. R. G.), May 28th.

Murakami, F., Tsukahara, N., and Fujito, Y. (1977). Analysis of unitary EPSPs mediated by the newly-formed cortico-rubral synapses after lesion of the nucleus interpositus of the cerebellum. *Exp. Brain Res.* **30,** 233–243.

Mustari, M. J., and Lund, R. O. (1976). An aberrant crossed visual corticotectal pathway in albino rats. *Brain Res.* **112,** 37–44.

Nah, S. N., and Leong, S. K. (1976a). Bilateral corticofugal projections to the red nucleus after neonatal lesions in the albino rat. *Brain Res.* **107,** 433–436.

Nah, S. N., and Leong, S. K. (1976b). An ultrastructural study of the anomalous corticorubral projection following neonatal lesions in the albino rat. *Brain Res.* **111,** 162–166.

Nakamura, Y., Mizuno, N., Konishi, A., and Sato, M. (1974). Synaptic reorganization of the red nucleus after chronic deafferentation from cerebellorubral fibers: An electron microscope study in the cat. *Brain Res.* **82,** 298–301.

Nakano, K., Takimoto, T., Kayahara, T., Takeuchi, Y., and Kobayashi, Y. (1980). Distribution of cerebellothalamic neurons projecting to the ventral nuclei of the thalamus: An HRP study in the cat. *J. Comp. Neurol.* **194,** 427–439.

Nauta, W. J. H., and Bucher, V. M. (1954). Efferent connections of the striate cortex in the albino rat. *J. Comp. Neurol.* **100,** 257–285.

Nauta, W. J. H., and Domesick, V. B. (1979). The anatomy of the extrapyramidal system. *In* "Dopaminergic Ergot Derivates and Motor Functions" (K. Fuxe and D. B. Calne, eds.), pp. 3–22. Pergamon, Oxford.

Neumann, S., Pritzel, M., and Huston, J. P. (1982). Plasticity of cortico-thalamic projections and functional recovery in the unilaterally detelencephalized infant rat. *Behav. Brain Res.* **4,** 377–388.

Nieoullon, A., Chéramy, A., and Glowinski, J. (1977). Interdependence of the nigro-striatal dopaminergic systems on the two sides of the brain. *Science* **198,** 416–418.

O'Leary, D. D. M., Fricke, R. A., Stanfield, B. B., and Cowan, W. M. (1979). Changes in the associational afferents to the dentate gyrus in the absence of its commissural input. *Anat. Embryol.* **156,** 283–299.

Olianas, M. C., De Montis, G. M., Concu, A., Tagliamonte, A., and DiChiara, G. (1978a). Intranigral kainic acid: Evidence for nigral non- dopaminergic neurons controlling posture and behavior in a manner opposite to the dopaminergic ones. *Eur. J. Pharmacol.* **49,** 223–232.

Olianas, M. C., De Montis, G. M., Mulas, G., and Tagliamonte, A. (1978b). The striatal dopaminergic function is mediated by the inhibition of a nigral, non-dopaminergic neuronal system via a strio-nigral GABAergic pathway. *Eur. J. Pharmacol.* **49,** 233–241.

Olsson, Y., and Malmgren, L. T. (1980). Axonal uptake of horseradish peroxidase isoenzymes during Wallerian degeneration. *Neurosci. Lett.* **20,** 135–140.

Papadopoulos, G., and Huston, J. P. (1980). Removal of the telencephalon spares turning induced by injection of GABA agonists and antagonists into the substantia nigra. *Behav. Brain Res.* **1,** 25–38.

Papadopoulos, G., Nef, B., and Huston, J. P. (1980). Behavioral effects of kainic acid injection into substantia nigra after ablation of the telencephalon. *Behav. Brain Res.* **1,** 331–337.

Papadopoulos, G., Huston, J. P., and Nef, B. (1981). The influence of unilateral 6-OH-dopamine lesions of the substantia nigra in the absence of the telencephalon. *Brain Res. Bull.* **6,** 165–170.

Papez, J. W. (1938). Thalamic connections in a hemidecorticate dog. *J. Comp. Neurol.* **69,** 103–120.

Peacock, J. H., and Combs, C. M. (1965). Retrograde cell degeneration in adult cats after hemidecortication. *J. Comp. Neurol.* **125,** 329–336.

Porceddu, M. L., Piacente, B., Morelli, M., and DiChiara, G. (1979). Opposite turning effects of kainic and ibotenic acid injected in the rat substantia nigra. *Neurosci. Lett.* **15,** 271–276.

Pritzel, M., and Huston, J. P. (1981a). Unilateral ablation of telencephalon induces appearance of contralateral cortical and subcortical projections to thalamic nuclei. *Behav. Brain Res.* **3,** 43–54.

Pritzel, M., and Huston, J. P. (1981b). Neural and behavioral plasticity: Crossed nigrothalamic projections following unilateral substantia nigra lesions. *Behav. Brain Res.* **3,** 393–399.

Pritzel, M., Huston, J. P., and Sarter, M. (1983). Behavioral and neuronal reorganization after unilateral substantia nigra lesions: Evidence for increased interhemispheric nigro-caudate projections. *Neuroscience* (in press).

Raisman, G. (1969a). Neuronal plasticity in the septal nuclei of the adult rat. *Brain Res.* **14,** 25–48.

Raisman, G. (1969b). A comparison of the mode of termination of the hippocampal and hypothalamic afferents to the septal nuclei as revealed by electron microscopy of degeneration. *Exp. Brain Res.* **7,** 317–343.

Rhoades, R. W. (1981a). Expansion of the ipsilateral visual corticotectal projection in hamsters subjected to partial lesions of the visual cortex during infancy: Anatomical experiments. *J. Comp. Neurol.* **197,** 425–445.

Rhoades, R. W. (1981b). Expansion of the ipsilateral visual corticotectal projection in hamsters subjected to partial lesions of the visual cortex during Infancy: Electrophysiological experiments. *J. Comp. Neurol.* **197,** 447–458.

Rhoades, R. W., and Chalupa, L. M. (1978). Functional and anatomical consequences of neonatal visual cortical damage in the superior colliculus of the golden hamster. *J. Neurophysiol.* **41,** 1466–1494.

Rhoades, R. W., and Dellacroce, D. D. (1980). Neonatal enucleation induces an asymmetric pattern of visual callosal connections in hamsters. *Brain Res.* **202,** 189–195.

Rinvik, E., and Grofová, J. (1974). Cerebellar projections to the nuclei ventralis lateralis and ventral anterior thalami: experimental electron microscopical and light microscopical studies in the cat. *Anat. Embryol.* **146,** 95–111.

Rioch, D. (1931). Studies on the diencephalon of carnivora. *J. Comp. Neurol.* **53,** 319–388.

Rosenzweig, M. R., and Bennett, E. L. (1976). "Neural Mechanisms of Learning and Memory." MIT Press, Cambridge, Massachusetts.

Rothmann, H. (1923). Zusammenfassender Bericht über den Rothmannschen grosshirnlosen Hund nach klinischer und anatomischer Untersuchung. *Z. Gesamte Neurol. Psychiatrie* **87,** 247–313.

Sabel, B., Morgan, S., Pritzel, M., and Huston, J. P. (1982). Reorganisation of nigrothalamic projections and compensation of behavioral asymmetries following unilateral paralysis and unilateral sensory deprivation. *14th Annu. Gen. Meet. Brain Behav. Soc.*, 1982 Abstract.

Sarter, M., Pritzel, M., Morgan, S., and Huston, J. P. (1982). Interhemispheric nigro-caudate projections are of mono-aminergic and of nonmono-aminergic origin, travel via interdiencephalic fiber connections and are in part due to bifurcating nigrocaudate projections to either hemisphere. *6th Eur. Neurosci. Meet. 1982* Abstract.

Scheff, S. W., Benardo, L. S., and Cotman, C. W. (1980a). Decline in reactive fiber growth in the dentate gyrus of aged rats compared to young adult rats following entorhinal cortex removal. *Brain Res.* **199,** 21–38.

Scheff, S. W., Benardo, L. S., and Cotman, C. W. (1980b). Hydrocortisone administration retards axon sprouting in the rat dentate gyrus. *Exp. Neurol.* **68,** 195–201.

Schneider, G. E. (1970). Mechanisms of functional recovery following lesions of visual cortex or superior colliculus in neonate and adult hamsters. *Brain Behav. Evol.* **3,** 295–323.

Schneider, G. E. (1973). Early lesions of superior colliculus: Factors affecting the formation of abnormal retinal projections. *Brain Behav. Evol.* **8,** 73–109.

Schneider, G. E. (1979). Is it really better to have your brain lesion early? A revision of the "Kennard principle." *Neuropsychologia* **17,** 557–583.

Schwob, J. E., Fuller, T., Price, J. L., and Olney, J. W. (1980). Widespread patterns of neuronal damage following systemic or intracerebral injections of kainic acid: A histological study. *Neuroscience* **5,** 991–1014.

So, K.-F. (1979). Development of abnormal recrossing retinotectal projections after superior colliculus lesions in newborn Syrian hamsters. *J. Comp. Neurol.* **186,** 241–257.

Sotelo, C., and Palay, S. L. (1971). Altered axons and axon terminals in the lateral vestibular nucleus of the rat. *Lab. Invest.* **25,** 653–672.

Spinelli, D. N., and Jensen, F. E. (1979). Plasticity: The mirror of experience. *Science* **203,** 75–78.

Spinelli, D. N., Jensen, F. E., and Viana di Prisco, G. (1980). Early experience effect on dendritic branching in normally reared kittens. *Exp. Neurol.* **68,** 1–11.

Stevenson, J. A., and Lund, R. D. (1982). A crossed parabigemino-lateral geniculate projection in rats blinded at birth. *Exp. Brain Res.* **45,** 95–100.

Steward, O. (1980). Trajectory of contralateral entorhinal axons, which reinnervate the fascia dentata of the rat following ipsilateral entorhinal lesions. *Brain Res.* **183,** 277–289.

Steward, O., Cotman, C. W., and Lynch, G. S. (1973). Re-establishment of electrophysiological functional entorhinal cortical input to the dentate gyrus deafferented by ipsilateral entorhinal lesions: Innervation by the contralateral entorhinal cortex. *Exp. Brain Res.* **18,** 396–414.

Steward, O., Cotman, C. W., and Lynch, G. S. (1974). Growth of a new fiber projection in the brain of adult rats: Reinnervation of the dentate gyrus by the contralateral entorhinal cortex following ipsilateral entorhinal lesions. *Exp. Brain Res.* **20,** 45–66.

Steward, O., Cotman, C. I., and Lynch, G. S. (1976). A quantitative autoradiographic and electrophysiological study of the reinnervation of the dentate gyrus by the contralateral entorhinal cortex following ipsilateral entorhinal lesions. *Brain Res.* **114,** 181–200.

Szabo, J. (1980). Distribution of striatal afferents from the mesencephalon in the cat. *Brain Res.* **188,** 3–21.

Taub, E. (1968). Prism compensation as a learning phenomenon: A phylogenetic perspective. *In* "The Neuropsychology of Spatially Oriented Behavior" (S. J. Freedman, ed.), pp. 77–106. Dorsey Press, Homewood, Illinois.

Thoenen, H., and Kreutzberg, G. W. (1981). The role of fast transport in the nervous system. *Neurosci. Res. Program Bull.* **20,** 1–138.

Tsukahara, N. (1981). Synaptic plasticity in the central nervous system. *Annu. Rev. Neurosci.* **4,** 351–379.

Tsukahara, N., and Fujito, Y. (1976). Physiological evidence of formation of new synapses from cerebrum in the red nucleus neurons following cross-union of forelimb nerves. *Brain Res.* **106,** 184–188.

Tsukahara, N., Fujito, Y., Oda, Y., and Maeda, J. (1982). Formation of functional synapses in the adult cat red nucleus from the cerebrum following cross-innervation of forelimb flexor and extensor nerves. I. Appearance of new synaptic potentials. *Exp. Brain Res.* **45,** 1–12.

Ungerstedt, U. (1971). Postsynaptic supersensitivity after 6-hydroxydopamine induced degeneration of the nigrostriatal dopamine system. *Acta Physiol. Scand.* **82,** Suppl. 367, 69–93.

Ungerstedt, U., and Arbuthnott, G. W. (1970). Quantitative recording of rotational behaviour in rats after 6-OH-dopamine lesions in the nigrostriatal dopamine system. *Brain Res.* **24,** 485–493.

Uylings, H. B. M., Kuypers, K., Diamond, M. C., and Veltman, W. A. M. (1978). Effects of differential environments on plasticity of dendrites of cortical pyramidal neurons in adult rats. *Exp. Neurol.* **62,** 658–677.

van der Kooy, D., Coscina, D. V., and Hattori, T. (1981). Is there a non-dopaminergic nigro-striatal pathway? *Neuroscience* **6,** 345–357.

Vrensen, G., and Cardozo, J. N. (1981). Changes in size and shape of synaptic connections after visual training. An ultrastructural approach of synaptic plasticity. *Brain Res.* **213,** 79–97

Walker, A. E. (1938). The thalamus of the chimpanzee. II. Its nuclear structure, normal and following hemidecortication. *J. Comp. Neurol.* **69,** 487–507.

Wall, P. D. (1977). The presence of ineffective synapses and the circumstances which unmask them. *Philos. Trans. R. Soc. London, Ser. B* **278,** 361–372.

Weinreich, P., and Seeman, P. (1980). Effect of kainic acid on striatal dopamine receptors. *Brain Res.* **198,** 491–496.

Wenzel, B. W., Tschirgi, R. D., and Taylor, J. L. (1962). Effects of early postnatal hemidecortication on spatial discrimination in cats. *Exp. Neurol.* **6,** 332–339.

Wilson, R. C., Levy, W. B., and Steward, O. (1979). Functional effects of lesion-induced plasticity: Long-term potentiation in normal and lesion-induced temporodentate connections. *Brain Res.* **176,** 65–78.

Zaczek, R., Simonton, S., and Coyle, J. T. (1980). Local and distant neuronal degeneration following intrastriatal injection of kainic acid. *J. Neuropathol. Exp. Neurol.* **39,** 245–264.

Zimmer, J., and Hjorth-Simonsen, A. (1975). Crossed pathways from the entorhinal area to the fascia dentata. II. Provokable in rats. *J. Comp. Neurol.* **161,** 71–102.

4: Experimental Model of Hemi-Parkinsonism

C. J. PYCOCK

Department of Pharmacology
University of Bristol
Bristol, United Kingdom

I. Introduction 70
II. The Rotating Rodent as an Experimental Model of Parkinson's Disease 70
A. Correlation between Striatal Dopamine Concentrations and Unilateral Motor Behavior 71
B. 6-Hydroxydopamine-Induced Nigrostriatal Lesions 72
III. Organization and Outflows of the Basal Ganglia: Relevance to the Rotation Model 73
A. Substantia Nigra as an Efferent Site 74
B. Globus Pallidus Projections 74
C. Substantia Nigra Projections 75
IV. The Rotating Rodent: A Model of Human Hemi-Parkinsonism? 77
A. Other Neurotransmitters Involved in Parkinson's Disease 78
B. Partial Nigrostriatal Lesions 79
C. Involvement of Extrastriatal Dopamine Sites: The Nucleus Accumbens 80
V. The Rotating Rodent Model: Assessment of Potential Anti-Parkinsonian Drugs 80
A. Direct and Indirect Dopamine Agonists 80
B. Uptake Blockers 81
C. Deprenyl 82
D. Presynaptic Dopamine Receptors 83
VI. Concluding Remarks: Hemi-Parkinsonism versus the Rotating Rodent 83
References 84

HEMISYNDROMES:
Psychobiology, Neurology,
Psychiatry

ISBN 0-12-512460-0

I. Introduction

The initiation and control of movement are major functions of the basal ganglia of the brain. It is hardly surprising, therefore, that many of the neurological movement disorders in man are associated with pathological lesions localized, at least in part, within the basal ganglia. Of all such disorders Parkinson's disease is the syndrome that probably has received the most physiological, biochemical, and pharmacological attention in the past 20 years. As a result Parkinsonism is perhaps the best understood basal ganglion disease (Chapter 10).

Pathologically, Parkinson's disease is associated primarily with the depletion of basal ganglion dopamine concentration, loss of this neurotransmitter being correlated with lesions of the ascending nigrostriatal pathway. Indeed, current therapeutic control of the disease is focused largely on replacement of the lost dopamine systems and stimulation of intact striatal neurons lying postsynaptically to the degenerating nigrostriatal dopamine terminals. Both the comprehensive mapping of forebrain dopamine systems (e.g., Lindvall and Björklund, 1978) and the detailed analysis of various behavioral responses observed following the manipulation of central dopamine pathways in laboratory animals (Kelly, 1977; Iversen, 1977) have enabled the behavioral pharmacologist to create valuable animal models in order to conduct research on various aspects of Parkinson's disease (Marsden *et al.*, 1975; Marsden, 1980). One such model that has been widely applied to the study of this movement disorder is the circling, or rotating, rodent.

II. The Rotating Rodent as an Experimental Model of Parkinson's Disease

In 1873 David Ferrier observed a strong contralateral pleurothotonus following unilateral stimulation of the corpus striatum in the dog, so that "the head approximated to the tail." Since that time there have been countless reports relating postural asymmetry and unilateral movement in animals (and man) after unilateral manipulation of various brain sites. Such behavior can be evoked from numerous areas within the central nervous system, ranging from caudal brainstem to rostral forebrain, and often occurs following either unilateral stimulation of selected loci or unilateral ablation of various sites. The wide variety of anatomical substrates that have been associated with the induction of postural asymmetry and circling in animals when manipulated has been reviewed (Pycock, 1980). Whereas the topics of earlier studies in this field were distributed among the enormous variety of anatomical substrates, more recent work, within the past 15 years, has concentrated mainly on the basal ganglia as the major sites associated with the induction of unilateral motor behavior. Indeed, in agreement with Ferrier's original observation, unilateral manipulation of the nigrostriatal axis routinely induces this sort of behavior in laboratory animals.

A. Correlation between Striatal Dopamine Concentrations and Unilateral Motor Behavior

The treatment of rodents with the rauwolfia alkaloid reserpine (Carlsson *et al.*, 1957; Goldstein *et al.*, 1975) or bilateral destruction of the nigrostriatal dopamine systems in the rat (Ungerstedt, 1971c) results in an akinetic Parkinsonian-like state. Temporary restoration of motor functions in both models is seen following systemic administration of L-dopa (L-3,4-dihydroxyphenylalanine). Such observations again substantiate the suggestions that, first, striatal dopamine systems are involved in the control of motor activity and, second, both preparations behave in a manner comparable to human Parkinson's disease and, as such, both may be used as an apparently reasonable model to mimic this syndrome in the laboratory. If we associate Parkinson's disease with specific lesions of the substantia nigra giant pars compacta cells with subsequent loss of melanin-containing cells and degeneration of dopamine terminals within the caudate nucleus–putamen complex, then the latter model of bilateral nigrostriatal tract destruction would appear to be a better correlate of this syndrome than the general monoamine depleting actions (with no anatomical selectivity) of reserpine. By this reasoning, therefore, the unilateral nigrostriatally lesioned rat should be a good model for hemi-Parkinsonism.

The major drawback of the bilateral nigrostriatally lesioned animal is that it becomes adipsic and aphagic and thereby fails to survive unless tube fed (Ungerstedt, 1971c; Marsden, 1980). In contrast, the unilateral nigrostriatally lesioned animal suffers no such consequences and feeds normally. Although this laboratory model is frequently used to study, for example, the assessment of putative agents for potential use in Parkinson's disease, the anatomical and pathological situation most truly represents the condition of hemi-Parkinsonism (unilateral paralysis agitans), which is characterized by unilateral damage of the nigrostriatal system (Trétiakoff, 1919; Barolin *et al.*, 1964; Hunter *et al.*, 1978).

The Swedish workers Andén and colleagues (1966) were the first to demonstrate that an electrolytic lesion of the nigrostriatal pathway at the level of the corpus mamillare in the rat produced a spontaneous curved deviation of the animal toward the side of the lesion. At times this asymmetry developed into a spontaneous turning of the animal in the direction of the lesion. Such motor activity was readily enhanced by the administration of L-dopa to the animal after pretreatment with the monoamine oxidase inhibitor nialamide, whereupon the animal actively rotated toward the operated side. These lesions caused some 60% loss of dopamine in the ipsilateral corpus striatum. Such observations were not restricted to the rat. It is known, for example, that ablation of one nigrostriatal pathway of the dog (Delmas-Marsalet, 1925) or monkey (Poirier, 1960) similarly causes the animal to turn spontaneously toward the lesioned side. In contrast, electrical stimulation of the caudate nucleus in the rat (Barnett and Goldstein, 1975; Lee *et al.*, 1980), cat (Hassler, 1956; Laursen, 1962), or monkey (Delgado *et al.*, 1975) or of the nigrostriatal pathway in the rat (Arbuthnott *et al.*, 1970; Roffman *et al.*, 1978) or cat (Skultety, 1962; York, 1973) elicits postural asymmetry, with head turning away from the stimulated side.

The experimental data considered so far suggest that an imbalance of striatal activity leads to the induction of a postural asymmetry contralateral to the dominant striatum. Pharmacological procedures have related this to striatal dopamine function. Thus, the contralateral circling component observed following electrical stimulation of the rat substantia nigra is accompanied by the release of dopamine in the ipsilateral striatum (Arbuthnott and Crow, 1971; von Voigtlander and Moore, 1971). There is much experimental evidence to support the concept of striatal dopamine-induced postural asymmetry. The administration of dopamine receptor antagonist (neuroleptic) drugs blocks electrically induced head turning observed following nigral stimulation (York, 1973; Arbuthnott and Ungerstedt, 1975). In addition, dopamine antagonists reverse the direction of spontaneous asymmetry observed following acute lesion of the nigrostriatal system (Andén *et al.*, 1966). Active circling behavior is promoted by dopamine agonists in animals with unilateral lesions of the nigrostriatal pathway (see Pycock, 1980), the effects of which are again blocked by the neuroleptic drugs (Pycock *et al.*, 1975). It is from these basic experiments that the original conclusion that circling behavior often results from "an imbalance of dopaminergic activity between the two striata" was drawn (Ungerstedt, 1971a,b).

B. 6-Hydroxydopamine-Induced Nigrostriatal Lesions

The previously mentioned experimental maneuvers employed to induce circling, namely, electrocoagulative lesions or aspiration experiments or applying electrical stimulation in the region of the ascending nigrostriatal dopamine pathways, are rather nonspecific. Because Parkinson's disease is associated primarily with dopamine loss, the application of more specific techniques to lesion the ascending midbrain–forebrain dopamine-containing projection selectively may produce a more comparable model. In this respect the neurotoxin 6-hydroxydopamine (6-OHDA) has been widely applied (Ungerstedt, 1971a). This substance, when taken up into catecholaminergic neurons, kills such cells. Hence, the injection of 6-OHDA into the region of the dopamine cell bodies within the substantia nigra leads to the specific loss of striatal dopamine concentrations, the other ascending monoamine pathways apparently remaining intact (Costall *et al.*, 1976). Animals bearing such unilateral nigrostriatal lesions, and thus modeling the situation in hemi-Parkinsonism, will circle following the administration of dopamine agonists. The action is relatively specific because, although the manipulation of other central neurotransmitter systems serves to modify such motor behavior (Pycock, 1980), only dopaminergic drugs induce reliable and vigorous circling when administered systemically in this model.

III. Organization and Outflows of the Basal Ganglia: Relevance to the Rotation Model

We accept that the basal ganglia are closely associated with the initiation and control of motor behavior, although many of the precise mechanisms involved still elude us. The basal ganglia represent a complex neuronal network and, although there has been a great deal of research on the physiology, pharmacology, and neurochemistry of these structures of the brain, the precise neuronal organization is still unknown. The results of these investigations have been reviewed (Nieuwenhuys, 1977; Graybiel and Ragsdale, 1979; Dray, 1979, 1980). Because the basic circling response is closely associated with basal ganglion function, its neuronal pathways are, of course, of interest to us in understanding our model. However, not only does manipulation of the basal ganglia itself induce this form of unilateral motor activity, but it has been noted by many groups that a similar behavior can be produced by the manipulation of proposed outflow pathways from the basal ganglia. In view of the possible relevance of understanding the actions of drugs that affect central neurotransmission other than dopamine directly, and considering the possible development of other models relevant to clinical Parkinsonism, the current knowledge regarding the status of various anatomical sites believed to receive efferent information from the basal ganglia will be summarized. For a fuller discussion see Pycock and Phillipson (1983).

The major efferent projections from the striatum are to the globus pallidus and substantia nigra (Mehler and Nauta, 1974; Carpenter, 1976). Neurochemical studies have predicted both γ-aminobutyric acid- and substance P-containing striopallidal (Fonnum *et al.*, 1978; Staines *et al.*, 1980) and strionigral pathways (Brownstein *et al.*, 1977; Jessell *et al.*,

1978). It is not surprising, therefore, that lesions or electrical stimulation of either site blocks striatally mediated circling activity or themselves induce postural asymmetries.

A. Substantia Nigra as an Efferent Site

Although the globus pallidus has received relatively little attention in this respect, the substantia nigra has been the focus of much research investigating basal ganglion outflow systems. Most interest was generated during the study of behavioral effects of manipulating nigral γ-aminobutyric acid (GABA) systems. It had originally been proposed that the strionigral GABA-mediated pathway functioned as an inhibitory feedback system that would, in accordance with striatal activity, regulate the ascending nigrostriatal dopamine pathway (Bunney and Aghajanian, 1976). Indeed, initial behavioral studies supported this contention, being illustrated by the fact that stimulation of GABA systems in the area of the nigral cell bodies of ascending axons (substantia nigra, pars compacta) produced dopamine-dependent ipsilateral rotation, whereas, conversely, blockade of GABA systems in the pars compacta induced dopamine-dependent turning away from the injected side (Arnt and Scheel-Krüger, 1979). However, GABA agonists administered in the substantia nigra, pars reticulata, initiated strong, dopamine-independent contralateral turning; GABA antagonists now evoked dopamine-independent ipsilateral circling. Thus, changing the site of injection from pars compacta to pars reticulata completely reversed the direction of rotation observed following the manipulation of GABA function within the substantia nigra and, importantly, demonstrated a motor behavior that mimicked the striatally induced phenomenon but was now completely independent of ascending dopamine function (Table 4.1). It is on the basis of these experiments, together with others using kainic acid as a lesioning tool within the nigral complex (e.g., DiChiara *et al.*, 1977, 1979a), that the substantia nigra, in addition to being the origin of the ascending dopaminergic nigrostriatal system (pars compacta), is believed to serve also as a major outflow station (pars reticulata) of the basal ganglia.

B. Globus Pallidus Projections

The globus pallidus sends projections to the subthalamus, substantia nigra, lateral habenula, nucleus tegmenti pedunculopontinus (NTPP), and ventral thalamus (Fig. 4.1). Neurochemical studies suggest that many of these pathways may be mediated by GABA, although it is probably too early to be conclusive at this stage. Again, as for the pallidum itself, relatively little work has been performed to elucidate the role of these pallidal outflows in terms of the circling model of hemi-Parkinsonism. Here,

TABLE 4.1
Motor Activity Observed after Unilateral Manipulation of Nigral GABA Systems in the Rat[a]

Nigral Site	Drug	Circling behavior	Dependence on nigrostriatal dopamine system
Pars compacta	GABA agonist	Ipsilateral	Dependent
	GABA antagonist	Contralateral	Dependent
Pars reticulata	GABA agonist	Contralateral	Not dependent
	GABA antagonist	Ipsilateral	Not dependent

[a] For references see Arnt and Scheel-Krüger (1979), James and Starr (1978), Olpe *et al.* (1977), Reavill *et al.* (1979), Scheel-Krüger *et al.* (1977), and Tarsy *et al.* (1975).

too, the reports are concerned mainly with the role of GABA at these sites. Thus, a contralateral hemiballismus in the baboon was noted by Crossman and colleagues (1980) following unilateral infusion of picrotoxin into the region of the subthalamic nucleus. In the rat a contraversive postural asymmetry was observed after unilateral injection of the GABA agonist muscimol into the latter structure (Scheel-Krüger *et al.*, 1981). However, the possible role of the subthalamic nucleus in the mechanism of basal-ganglion-mediated circling behavior has not been fully explored. Similarly, the role of the NTPP in this form of motor activity has not been fully elucidated, although preliminary studies would suggest that, at the most, its contribution is only minor (Kilpatrick and Starr, 1981; see also Section C). The possible importance of the thalamus in turning behavior is discussed in the next section.

C. Substantia Nigra Projections

The three main efferent targets of the substantia nigra are the thalamus, the superior colliculus, and the NTPP (Fig. 4.1). Since the substantia nigra is now accepted as a major output station of the basal ganglia, it is hardly surprising that subsequent work has focused on its two main efferent projections: the ventromedial thalamus and the superior colliculus. Both electrophysiological and neurochemical studies implicate the existence of inhibitory nigrotectal and nigrothalamic pathways (Deniau *et al.*, 1977, 1978; Kilpatrick *et al.*, 1980, 1982). Similarly, behavioral work supports a role of GABA in the control of certain basal-ganglion-like motor components at these sites. For example, bilateral injections of muscimol into the ventromedial nucleus of the thalamus in the rat elicit long-lasting catalepsy (DiChiara *et al.*, 1979b), a behavior most commonly associated with neuroleptic-induced blockade of striatal dopamine systems. Further work supporting a role of the thalamus in motor behavior comes from the observation that thalamic lesions significantly re-

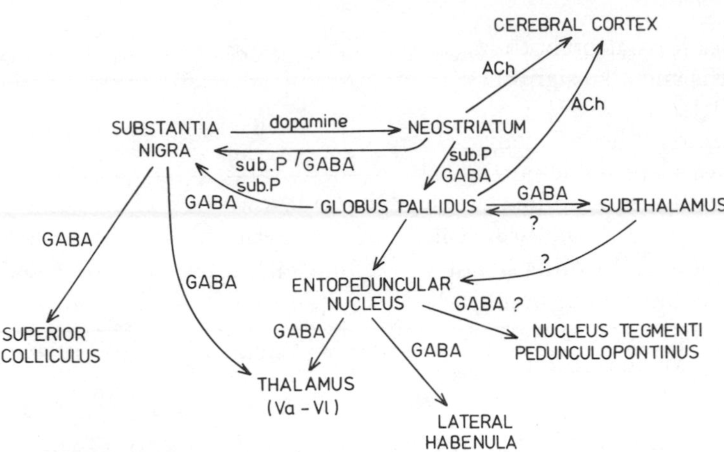

FIG. 4.1. Proposed neuroanatomical and neurochemical projections of the basal ganglia. ACh, acetylcholine; GABA, γ-aminobutyric acid; sub.P, substance P.

duce circling behavior evoked from several basal ganglion sites (Kilpatrick *et al.*, 1980), although other workers would not entirely agree with this proposal (Reavill *et al.*, 1981a).

The role of the superior colliculus in behavior mediated by the basal ganglia is similarly controversial. The superior colliculus has always been associated with the processing of visual inputs and is believed to function in visually guided behavior. However, the establishment of a strong projection from the substantia nigra to this site has prompted the suggestion that it may also contribute directly to motor behavior as a major outflow station. As with the thalamus, manipulation of GABA systems within the deep layers of this structure evokes motor activity closely comparable to basal-ganglion-mediated responses (Kilpatrick *et al.*, 1982; DiChiara *et al.*, 1981). The precise role of the superior colliculus in the circling response, however, is still far from clear. It was known originally that stimulation of the superior colliculus in cats and dogs caused turning of the head away from the stimulated side (Ferrier, 1886; Sprague and Meikle, 1965). However, with regard to the lesioning of this structure and circling behavior in rodents there is considerable disagreement among different laboratories (for further discussions, see Pycock and Phillipson, 1983). It is apparent that the site of the lesion within the superior colliculus is very important, and it would appear that the deeper and more lateral structures of the tectum, rather than the superficial and medial sites of this structure, are more consistently linked with modifications of motor behavior. However, the "colliculus controversy" has extended beyond its anatomical boundaries, and it is suggested that encroachment into the underlying mesencephalic reticular formation may be of importance in inducing these motor effects. The manipulation of dorsal mesencephalic reticular formation both induces spontaneous circling behavior (Mulas *et al.*, 1981) and also significantly modifies nigrostriatally mediated rotation (Morelli *et al.*, 1981).

Similarly, the adjacent periaqueductal gray (PAG) has also generated interest as a possible outflow site of the basal ganglia. For example, Reavill and colleagues noted that electrolytic lesions placed unilaterally in the lateral PAG drastically reduced, and in some cases abolished, apomorphine-induced circling behavior in rats with a previous 6-OHDA lesion of the ipsilateral nigrostriatal pathway (Reavill *et al.*, 1981b). Others have argued that such lesions invariably damage the adjacent mesencephalic reticular formation and thereby claim that the PAG, as such, cannot be associated with any certainty with basal-ganglion-mediated motor activity.

The third caudal site receiving nigral innervation is the NTPP. Although the neuropharmacology of this region is far from being well understood, it has been considered for some years as a possible link between the extrapyramidal motor system and the spinal outflow. However, preliminary studies of the NTPP and its possible role in motor activity are a little disappointing. It appears that unilateral lesions of the NTPP in the rat do not significantly alter striatally mediated postural asymmetry (Lee and Slater, 1981; Reavill *et al.*, 1981b). Further work is required before any definitive conclusions can be drawn regarding the role of the NTPP in motor activity.

IV. The Rotating Rodent: A Model of Human Hemi-Parkinsonism?

The rotating rodent is an animal model that has been widely used in efforts to understand human Parkinson's disease and to screen for potential anti-Parkinsonian drugs (e.g., Costall and Naylor, 1975). However, the model has some failings. For example, it is obviously based on the extreme loss of dopamine in one striatum only; the other striatum is assumed to be totally intact and functional. In Parkinson's disease loss of dopamine is usually encountered to the same degree in both striata. Similarly, the model is not a complete replica of hemi-Parkinsonism because rodents do not develop contralateral limb tremor (Marsden *et al.*, 1975; Marsden, 1980).

In the rat total loss of striatal dopamine is achieved by acute lesioning of the nigrostriatal system. The human condition is most commonly related to a chronic lesion with gradual, progressive loss of dopamine-containing neurons. Following lesioning the rat exhibits a marked postural asymmetry, the head, neck, and trunk deviating toward the side of the lesion. In the following weeks and months this asymmetry becomes much less marked, and in many cases it is not possible to differentiate between rats with a nigrostriatal lesion and those that have no such lesions. In many cases Parkinsonian patients exhibit postural asymmetries, there being a tendency to lean to one side in a scoliotic posture (Duvoisin and Marsden, 1975). The direction of this body tilt is not completely predictable; sometimes it is emphasized by the homolateral curvature of the spine, and sometimes it inclines to the opposite side as a compensatory measure. Usually, patients tend to lean contralaterally to the side exhibiting the initial and most severe Parkinsonian symptoms. Uncertainty also applies to which side patients diagnosed as having hemi-Parkinsonism will lean. Some authors predict that Parkinsonian symptoms will appear on the side opposite the reduced striatal dopamine content (Barolin *et al.*, 1964), although clinical signs of hemi-Parkinsonism have been reported as occurring on the side ipsilateral to the major lesion (Hunter *et al.*, 1978). Similarly, leaning would predominantly occur homolaterally to the dopamine loss (Duvoisin and Marsden, 1975), a result that agrees with the initial observations in animals.

A. Other Neurotransmitters Involved in Parkinson's Disease

To date, in the model of the rotating rat, as indeed in the clinical situation, the loss of striatal dopamine has been emphasized. That dopamine is a major contributory factor in both conditions cannot be denied and is reflected in the effectiveness of dopaminergic drugs in either partially reversing the symptoms of Parkinson's disease or causing active rotation in the unilaterally nigrostriatally lesioned rat. However, neurochemical surveys have provided evidence that dopamine is not necessarily the only neurotransmitter involved in these symptoms. For example, loss of the other catecholamine, norepinephrine, is reported both in human Parkinsonism (Bernheimer *et al.*, 1963; Farley and Hornykiewicz, 1977) and in the lesioned-induced animal model (Costall *et al.*, 1976). The sites at which lowered norepinephrine concentrations occur include the hypothalamus, paramedian thalamic cell groups, the nucleus accumbens, and olfactory areas of the limbic forebrain. Similarly, Hornykiewicz (1972) reported the loss of 5-hydroxytryptamine from important regions of basal ganglia such as the substantia nigra, striatum, and globus pallidus in Parkinson's disease.

A reduction of basal ganglion GABA function has also been implicated in Parkinson's disease; significant decreases in the GABA-synthesizing enzyme (glutamate decarboxylase) have been observed in many sites (Rinne *et al.*, 1974; Lloyd and Hornykiewicz, 1973; McGeer and McGeer, 1976), as has a loss of high-affinity GABA-binding sites from the substantia nigra (Lloyd *et al.*, 1977). In view of the possible existence of

GABA-mediated basal ganglion outflow pathways (see earlier), which would be directly associated with the control of locomotor activity, these postmortem observations concerning GABA function are potentially very interesting.

The state of the acetylcholinergic system remains rather uncertain. McGeer and McGeer (1976) were unable to detect a significant change in that system, save for an increase in the synthetic enzyme activity within the nucleus accumbens and a reduction of the esterase in globus pallidus. Other studies had also revealed a decrease of acetylcholinesterase activity in the caudate nucleus and putamen of Parkinsonian brains (Rinne *et al.*, 1973).

In addition to the attention focused on the monoamine neurotransmitters GABA and acetylcholine, interest in the possible role of the peptide transmitter candidates in the control of motor activity is now increasing. The basal ganglia are structures in which many such chemicals are located in high concentration, and it has been suggested that they have some neuromodulatory, if not neurotransmitter, function.

The role of peptides in neurological disorders is under investigation. For example, alterations in brain opiate receptors were noted in Parkinson's disease when a decreased number of radiolabeled naloxone-binding sites were noted in the caudate nucleus (Reisine *et al.*, 1978). Because there are few experimental data at present, it is probably too early to predict the full involvement of peptides in Parkinson's disease. However, it has been predicted, for example, that, since cholecystokinin can coexist in nerve terminals with dopamine, the levels of this peptide may be lowered in Parkinson's disease (Hökfelt *et al.*, 1980).

B. Partial Nigrostriatal Lesions

In attempting to induce circling, one usually seeks the maximal destruction of one nigrostriatal system. However, the degree of dopamine loss in man related to the first clinical signs of Parkinson's disease is not known. Some work investigating the biochemical and behavioral effects of partial unilateral lesions of the nigrostriatal tract in rats has been reported. Such partial lesions have been induced by the injection of various doses of 6-hydroxydopamine into this pathway, with a subsequent dose-related decrease in striatal dopamine and tyrosine hydroxylase activity. It has been reported that lesions destroying two-thirds or more of the nigrostriatal neurons accelerate dopamine synthesis and release in the surviving terminals of the ipsilateral striatum, as indicated by increased levels of dopamine metabolites (Hefti *et al.*, 1980b). Such an effect has been interpreted as a possible compensatory increase in activity of the surviving dopamine neurons and is in keeping with the findings showing higher homovanillic acid concentrations in postmortem Parkinsonian brains compared with control brains (Rinne *et al.*, 1971). In contrast, circling behavior in response to apomorphine or L-dopa occurred only when 90% or more of the nigrostriatal system had been destroyed, and this presumably reflects the induction of supersensitive postsynaptic dopamine receptors (Hefti *et al.*, 1980a,b). Ipsilateral rotation in response to amphetamine, however, was observed when only 50% of these neurons had been destroyed (Hefti *et al.*, 1980a).

C. Involvement of Extrastriatal Dopamine Sites: The Nucleus Accumbens

Although more difficult to identify precisely in man, the nucleus accumbens has received much attention in the rat. It is known that bilateral stimulation of dopamine receptors in this structure induces enhanced locomotor activity, although, unlike unilateral caudate injections, manipulation of one nucleus accumbens dopamine system does not induce postural asymmetry or circling behavior (see Pycock, 1980, for references). However, by the use of differential lesioning techniques directed at either striatal or mesolimbic pathways, it has been concluded that in the rodent the nucleus accumbens does significantly contribute to nigrostriatally mediated circling behavior. Whereas striatal dopamine imbalance causes postural asymmetry, the nucleus accumbens provides the locomotor component that converts the postural deviation into active turning (Kelly and Moore, 1976; Pycock and Marsden, 1978). However, the precise contribution of the nucleus accumbens or its equivalent structure to Parkinson's disease in man has yet to be fully established.

V. The Rotating Rodent Model: Assessment of Potential Anti-Parkinsonian Drugs

The most potent type of drug to induce active circling behavior in rodents with unilateral loss of nigrostriatal dopamine pathways is the dopamine agonist (see Glick *et al.*, 1976), although the number of drugs altering circling is large (Pycock, 1980, Table 1). In general, it is accepted that animals turn away (contraversively) from the side of higher striatal dopaminergic receptor stimulation.

A. Direct and Indirect Dopamine Agonists

In animals with a classic 6-OHDA lesion of the nigrostriatal pathway two forms of circling behavior are triggered by dopamine agonists, one being circling toward the lesioned side (ipsiversive). the other being circling away from the lesioned side (contraversive). It has been suggested that drugs which act presynaptically at the dopamine receptor, and are thus dependent on intact, functional dopamine terminals for their action, can act only on the unlesioned side and consequently rotate the animal toward the side of the lesion. Such drugs include the dopamine releasers, uptake blockers, and monoamine oxidase inhibitors (e.g., amphetamine, nomifensine, and deprenyl). Other dopamine agonists, which stimulate the postsynaptic dopamine receptor directly, induce circling away from the side of the lesion. It would thus appear that such drugs have a greater stimulatory effect on the lesion side, assuming that, unlike the presynaptic terminals, postsynaptic receptors would remain intact and functional on both sides of the brain after lesioning. To explain contraversive rotation it is generally accepted that the denervated postsynaptic dopamine receptors have become supersensitive (Ungerstedt, 1971b), and thus the directly acting dopamine agonists (such as apomorphine, bromocriptine, and ergometrine) have the greater pharmacological action on that side. Thus, in its basic form, the rotating rodent model is useful (*a*) for screening dopamine agonist drugs with a view to potential use in Parkinson's disease; (*b*) for predicting whether these drugs act presynaptically or postsynaptically; and (*c*) for assessing the relative potency of such drugs with respect to the well-known dopamine agonists.

B. Uptake Blockers

In addition to its use in the selection of potent dopamine agonists that may be of importance in controlling the symptoms of Parkinson's disease, the rotating model may be useful for screening other secondary agents, which, when administered with drugs such as L-dopa, greatly enhance their anti-Parkinsonian properties. Drugs that, for example, block the high-affinity uptake of monoamines into nerve terminals and are classically used as antidepressant medicines have been reported either to induce turning behavior or to enhance the effects of the dopamine agonist amphetamine in this circling model (Pycock *et al.*, 1976; Costall and Naylor, 1977; Duvoisin *et al.*, 1978). Such results indicate that these drugs inhibit the reuptake of released dopamine and thus effectively potentiate the behavioral action of amphetamine. Indeed, in other studies it has been shown that cocaine analogs, which potently block dopamine uptake systems, themselves induce intense ipsilateral rotation in rats with a unilateral 6-OHDA lesion of the substantia nigra (Heikkila *et al.*, 1979). Since this effect was attenuated by haloperidol it would suggest the primary involvement of dopamine. However, further analysis with the circling model illustrates that the interaction of uptake blocker and dopamine agonist may not be as straightforward as first proposed. Thus, in a more recent publication Fung and Uretsky (1980) showed that the concurrent use of low doses of amine uptake blockers such as nomifensine, benztropine, and mazindol in fact reduces amphetamine-induced circling behavior. The authors concluded that, in addition to inhibiting neuronal uptake, such drugs also reduced dopamine synthesis and release, and it was the effects on the latter mechanisms that caused the decreased behavioral response. Another study utilized apomorphine as the dopamine agonist, which may be of more relevance to the concept of treatment of Parkinson's disease. In agreement with the last report Delini-Stula and Vassout (1979) demonstrated that both acutely and chronically administered clomipramine and amitriptyline markedly reduced apomorphine-induced turning behavior. The authors suggested that these observations may be related to the proposed dopamine receptor-blocking properties of these drugs. From this necessarily short review of studies utilizing the rotating model, antidepressant drugs would appear to be unsuitable for supplementing dopamine agonists in the treatment of Parkinson's disease.

C. Deprenyl

A drug that has generated a great deal of interest because of its potential usefulness in Parkinson's disease is (−)-deprenyl (see Knoll, 1978). (−)-Deprenyl is a potent inhibitor of type B monoamine oxidase but lacks the characteristic "cheese effect" of many of the monoamine oxidase inhibitors. It has been studied in a number of trials for its possible anti-Parkinsonian effectiveness. It has been used to supplement (but not to replace) traditional L-dopa therapy, the general consensus being that the drug both enhances the anti-Parkinsonian effects of L-dopa and, because a smaller dose of L-dopa can then be used, may reduce some of the unwanted side effects of that drug (Lees *et al.*, 1977; Birkmayer, 1978). Others, however, are more hesitant to adopt the drug as a new treatment of Parkinson's disease and suggest that perhaps the advantages derived from using (−)-deprenyl may be related to its elevation of mood (Stern *et al.*, 1978; Eisler *et al.*, 1981). Again, this drug has been investigated in the circling model. It has been reported that by itself (−)-deprenyl causes a relatively weak ipsilateral rotation in the 6-OHDA-lesioned rat (Heikkila *et al.*, 1981). However, since another potent monoamine oxidase inhibitor, clorgyline, by itself had no motor actions in this model, it was concluded that the rotational effects of (−)-deprenyl were related to its uptake inhibition and/or dopamine-releasing properties rather than to its enzyme inhibitory effects. In conjunction with L-dopa, (−)-deprenyl enhanced the contralateral rotation evoked by this dopamine agonist, an effect that was believed, this time, to be related to its monoamine oxidase inhibitory action (Heikkila *et al.*, 1981).

D. Presynaptic Dopamine Receptors

Both in the rotational model and in the therapeutic treatment of Parkinson's disease we are dealing with postsynaptic receptor sites. The presynaptic dopamine receptors associated with the nigrostriatal terminals have presumably been lost through the process of neuronal degeneration. The rotating model therefore may be of little use for detecting potential presynaptic dopamine agonists, although some interesting observations have been documented. Experimentally, apomorphine is taken as the classic dopamine agonist that, in general, enhances motor behavior. However, in rodents it has been noted that subcutaneous administration of lower doses of apomorphine decreases locomotor activity (DiChiara *et al.*, 1976; Costall *et al.*, 1980), and this is believed to reflect a preferential action on presynaptic dopamine receptors (Van Ree and Wolterink, 1981). Similarly, in the turning model low doses of apomorphine markedly depressed the contralateral turning response seen during unilateral electrical stimulation of the nigrostriatal pathway (Barghon and Costentin, 1980). Hence, although the model described here may be useful for screening dopamine agonists, interpretations of indirect pre- or postsynaptic effects should be treated warily.

VI. Concluding Remarks: Hemi-Parkinsonism versus the Rotating Rodent

Among the extrapyramidal movement disorders, Parkinson's disease occurs most frequently and is the one about which we know the most. However, the disease appears to develop insidiously in human beings, with advancing years, whereas animals of old age very rarely exhibit comparable symptoms (Stern, 1980). Thus, because Parkinson's disease is not naturally occurring in laboratory animals and very often is of unknown etiology, it is difficult to produce experimentally an accurate model of this movement disorder (Marsden, 1980). It is only by understanding, or at least thinking that we understand, the pathophysiology underlying the disease that we are able to make a crude attempt to produce a replica in the laboratory. The unilateral nigrostriatally lesioned rodent described in this chapter has been widely used to mimic the symptoms of unilateral paralysis agitans—hemi-Parkinsonism. However, taken literally, the model displays very few of the clinical signs of hemi-Parkinsonism, such as unilateral tremor and rigidity. The most positive pathophysiological aspect of this model is the unilateral deficit in striatal dopamine concentration.

Despite the fact that the rotating rodent is a widely employed model and that very often drugs evoking strong circling behavior after systemic administration are useful in the treatment of Parkinson's disease, the precise workings of the model are still poorly understood. It has been suggested, for example, that rats with unilateral lesion of the ascending dopamine pathways exhibit a contralateral sensory deficit, and it is this lack of sensory information that is related to circling activity (Marshall and Teitelbaum, 1974; Ljungberg and Ungerstedt, 1976). The relevance of this hypothesis to circling behavior and to hemi-Parkinsonian states requires further investigation.

A further deficit in our knowledge concerning the rotating rodent, as indeed with any movement disorder related to the basal ganglia, focuses on the basal ganglion outflow pathways as discussed previously. The somewhat surprising lack of effect of large ablations of single established basal ganglion outflow sites in modifying circling behavior might suggest that more than one outflow pathway is involved in the expression of this form of motor activity or that the brain must be sufficiently plastic that, in the event of loss of one major outflow channel, information can be diverted through other efferent pathways without significant alteration in the resulting motor pattern. Clearly, such a hypothesis must be clarified, although the use of drugs modifying synapses on these outflow systems as potential anti-Parkinsonian agents is indeed an intriguing suggestion that may hold considerable hope for the future.

Additional optimism may hinge on the transplantation of cells into the central nervous system. Even with this new line of research the rotating rodent has not been neglected. Grafts of embryonic substantia nigral tissue have been transplanted into the lateral ventricle adjacent to the denervated striatum of adult rats that had previously received a unilateral 6-OHDA nigrostriatal lesion. Axons from these grafts grow into the striatum, partially reinnervating the area, and, by decreasing the dopaminergic imbalance between the two striata, reduce the rotation intensity previously recorded in this rotating rat model (Dunnett *et al.*, 1981; Freed *et al.*, 1981). The future for this type of experimentation is very exciting.

In conclusion, despite its drawbacks the rotating rodent provides a relatively inexpensive and reliable laboratory model for screening potential anti-Parkinsonian agents. It appears to have potential use for determining the basal outflow pathways expressing striatally mediated behavior and will also presumably play a part in the assessment of the roles of the new generation of peptide transmitters in this brain region.

References

Andén, N. -E., Dahlström, A., Fuxe, K., and Larsson, K. (1966). Functional role of the nigro-neostriatal dopamine neurons. *Acta Pharmacol. Toxicol.* **24,** 263–274.

Arbuthnott, G. W., and Crow, T. J. (1971). Relation of contraversive turning to unilateral release of dopamine from the nigrostriatal pathway in rats. *Exp. Neurol.* **30,** 484–491.

Arbuthnott, G. W., and Ungerstedt, U. (1975). Turning behaviour induced by electrical stimulation of the nigro-neostriatal system of the rat. *Exp. Neurol.* **47,** 162–172.

Arbuthnott, G. W., Crow, T. J., Fuxe, K., and Ungerstedt, U. (1970). Behavioural effects of stimulation in the region of the substantia nigra. *J. Physiol. (London)* **210,** 61P–62P.

Arnt, J., and Scheel-Krüger, J. (1979). Behavioural differences induced by muscimol selectively injected into pars compacta and pars reticulata of substantia nigra. *Naunyn-Schmiedeberg's Arch. Pharmacol.* **310,** 43–51.

Barghon, R., and Costentin, J. H. (1980). Rotational behaviour induced by unilateral electrical stimulations of nigro-striatal dopamine neurons: Modification by low doses of apomorphine. *Eur. J. Pharmacol.* **64,** 39–46.

Barnett, A., and Goldstein, J. (1975). Head turning induced by electrical stimulation of the caudate nucleus and its antagonism by anti-Parkinson drugs. *J. Pharmacol. Exp. Ther.* **194,** 296–302.

Barolin, G. S., Bernheimer, H., and Hornykiewicz, O. (1964). Seitenverschiedenes verhalten des dopamins (3-hydroxytryptamin) in gehirn eines falles von hemiparkinsonismus. *Arch. Neurol. Neurochir. Psychiatrie* **94,** 241–248.

Bernheimer, H., Birkmayer, W., and Hornykiewicz, O. (1963). Zur biochemie des Parkinson-syndroms des menschen. *Klin. Wochenschr.* **41,** 465–469.

Birkmayer, W. (1978). Long term treatment with L-deprenyl. *J. Neural Transm.* **43,** 239–244.

Brownstein, M. J., Mroz, E. A., Tappaz, M. L., and Leeman, S. E. (1977). On the origin of substance P and glutamic acid decarboxylase (GAD) in the substantia nigra. *Brain Res.* **135,** 315–323.

Bunney, B. S., and Aghajanian, G. K. (1976). Dopaminergic influence in the basal ganglia: Evidence for striatonigral feedback regulation. *In* "The Basal Ganglia" (M. D. Yahr, ed.), pp. 249–267. Raven Press, New York.

Carlsson, A., Lindqvist, M., and Magnusson, T. (1957). 3,4-Dihdroxyphenylalanine and 5-hydroxytryptophan as reserpine antagonists. *Nature (London)* **180,** 1200.

Carpenter, M. B. (1976). Anatomical organization of the corpus striatum and related nuclei. *In* "The Basal Ganglia" (M. D. Yahr, ed.), pp. 1–36. Raven Press, New York.

Costall, B., and Naylor, R. J. (1975). A comparison of circling models for the detection of antiparkinson activity. *Psychopharmacologia* **41,** 57–64.

Costall, B., and Naylor, R. J. (1977). Further aspects of nomifensine pharmacology. *Br. J. Clin. Pharmacol.* **4,** 89–99.

Costall, B., Marsden, C. D., Naylor, R. G., and Pycock, C. J. (1976). The relationship between striatal and mesolimbic dopamine dysfunction and the nature of circling responses following 6-hydroxydopamine and electrolytic lesions of the ascending dopamine systems of rat brain. *Brain Res.* **118,** 87–113.

Costall, B., Hui, S.-C. G., and Naylor, R. J. (1980). Denervation in the dopaminergic mesolimbic system: Functional changes followed using (−)-*N*-*n*-propylnorapomorphine depend on the basal activity levels of rats. *Neuropharmacology* **19,** 1039–1040.

Crossman, A. R., Sambrook, M. A., and Jackson, A. (1980). Experimental hemiballismus in the baboon produced by injection of a gamma-aminobutyric acid antagonist into the basal ganglia. *Neurosci. Lett.* **20,** 369–372.

Delgado, J. M. R., Delgado-García, J. M., Amérigo, J. A., and Grau, C. (1975). Behavioural inhibition induced by pallidal stimulation in monkeys. *Exp. Neurol.* **49,** 580–591.

Delini-Stula, A., and Vassout, A. (1979). Modulation of dopamine-mediated behavioural responses by antidepressants: Effects of single and repeated treatment. *Eur. J. Pharmacol.* **58,** 443–451.

Delmas-Marsalet, V. A. P. (1925). Contribution expérimentale à l'étude des fonctions du noyau caudé. Thèse de l'Université de Bordeaux.

Deniau, J. M., Hammond-Le Guyader, C., Feger, J., and McKenzie, J. S. (1977). Bilateral projection of nigro-collicular neurones: An electrophysiological study in the rat. *Neurosci. Lett.* **5,** 45–50.

Deniau, J. M., Hammond, C., Riszk, A., and Feger, J. (1978). Electrophysiological properties of identified output neurons of the rat substantia nigra (pars compacta and pars reticulata): Evidence for the existence of branched neurons. *Exp. Brain Res.* **32,** 409–422.

DiChiara, G., Porceddu, M. L., Vargiu, L., Argiolas, A., and Gessa, G. L. (1976). Evidence for dopamine receptors mediating sedation in the mouse brain. *Nature (London)* **264,** 564–566.

DiChiara, G., Olianas, M., Del Fiacco, M., Spano, P. F., and Tagliamonte, A. (1977). Intranigral kainic acid is evidence that nigral non-dopaminergic neurones control posture. *Nature (London)* **268,** 743–745.

DiChiara, G., Porceddu, M. L., Morelli, M., Mulas, M. L., and Gessa, G. L. (1979a). Substantia nigra as an output station for striatal dopaminergic responses: Role of GABA-mediated inhibition of pars reticulata neurons. *Naunyn-Schmiedebergs Arch. Pharmacol.* **306,** 153–159.

DiChiara, G., Morelli, M., Porceddu, M. L., and Gessa, G. L. (1979b). Role of thalamic γ-aminobutyrate in motor functions: Catalepsy and ipsiversive turning after intrathalamic muscimol. *Neuroscience* **4,** 1453–1465.

DiChiara, G., Porceddu, M. L., Imperato, A., and Morelli, M. (1981). Role of GABA neurons in the expression of striatal motor functions. *In* "GABA and the Basal Ganglia" (G. DiChiara and G. L. Gessa, eds.), pp. 129–163. Raven Press, New York.

Dray, A. (1979). The striatum and the substantia nigra: A commentary on their relationships. *Neuroscience* **4,** 1407–1439.

Dray, A. (1980). The physiology and pharmacology of mammalian basal ganglia. *Prog. Neurobiol.* **14,** 221–335.

Dunnett, S. B., Björklund, A., Stenevi, U., and Iversen, S. D. (1981). Behavioural recovery following transplantation of substantia nigra in rats subjected to 6-OHDA lesions of the nigrostriated pathway. I. Unilateral lesions. *Brain Res.* **215,** 147–161.

Duvoisin, R. C., and Marsden, C. D. (1975). Note on the scoliosis of Parkinsonism. *J. Neurol. Neurosurg. Psychiatry* **8,** 787–793.

Duvoisin, R. C., Heikkila, R. E., and Manzino, L. (1978). Circling induced by dopamine uptake inhibitors. *J. Pharm. Pharmacol.* **30,** 714–716.

Eisler, T., Teräväinen, H., Nelson, R., Krebs, H., Weise, V., Lake, C. R., Ebert, M. H., Whetzel, N., Murphy, D. L., Kopin, I. J., and Calne, D. B. (1981). Deprenyl in Parkinson disease. *Neurology* **31,** 19–23.

Farley, I. J., and Hornykiewicz, O. (1977). Noradrenaline distribution in subcortical areas of the human brain. *Brain Res.* **126,** 53–62.

Ferrier, D. (1873). Experimental researches in cerebral physiology and pathology. *In* "West Riding Lunatic Asylum Medical Report" (J. Crichton Browne, ed.), Vol. III, pp. 30–96.

Ferrier, D. (1886). "The Functions of the Brain." Smith, Elder & Co., London.

Fonnum, F., Gottesfeld, Z., and Grofová, I. (1978). Distribution of glutamate decarboxylase, choline acetyl transferase and aromatic amino acid decarboxylase in the basal ganglia of normal and operated rats. Evidence for striato-pallidal, striatoentopeduncular and striatonigral GABAergic fibres. *Brain Res.* **143,** 125–138.

Freed, W. J., Morihisa, J. M., Spoor, E., Hoffer, B. J., Olson, L., Seiger, A., and Wyatt, R. J. (1981). Transplanted adrenal chromaffin cells in rat brain reduce lesion-induced rotational behaviour. *Nature (London)* **292,** 351–352.

Fung, Y. K., and Uretsky, N. J. (1980). The effect of dopamine uptake blocking agents on the amphetamine-induced circling behaviour in mice with unilateral nigrostriatal lesions. *J. Pharmacol. Exp. Ther.* **214,** 651–656.

Glick, S. D., Jerussi, T. P., and Fleisher, L. N. (1976). Turning in circles: The neuropharmacology of rotation. *Life Sci.* **18,** 889–896.

Goldstein, J. M., Barnett, A., and Malick, J. B. (1975). The evaluation of anti-Parkinson drugs on reserpine-induced rigidity in rats. *Eur. J. Pharmacol.* **33,** 183–188.

Graybiel, A. M., and Ragsdale, C. W. (1979). Fiber connections of the basal ganglia. *In* "Development and Chemical Specificity of Neurons" (M. Cuénod, G. W. Kreutzberg, and F. E. Bloom, eds.), pp. 239–283. Elsevier, Amsterdam.

Hassler, R. (1956). Die Zentralen Apparate der Wendebewegungen: Ipsiverswe Wendungen durch Reizung Liner direkten Vestibulo-Thalamischen bahn im Hirnstamm der Katze. Parts I and II. *Arch. Psychiat. Nervenkr.* **194,** 456–480, 481–516.

Hefti, F., Melamed, E., Sahakian, B. J., and Wurtman, R. J. (1980a). Circling behaviour in rats with partial, unilateral nigro-striatal lesions: Effect of amphetamine, apomorphine, and DOPA. *Pharmacol., Biochem. Behav.* **12,** 185–188.

Hefti, F., Melamed, E., and Wurtman, R. J. (1980b). Partial lesions of the dopaminergic nigrostriatal system in rat brain: Biochemical characterization. *Brain Res.* **195,** 123–137.

Heikkila, R. E., Cabbat, F. S., Manzino, L., and Duvoisin, R. C. (1979). Rotational behaviour induced by cocaine analogs in rats with unilateral 6-hydroxydopamine lesions of the substantia nigra: Dependence upon dopamine uptake inhibition. *J. Pharmacol. Exp. Ther.* **211,** 189–194.

Heikkila, R. E., Cabbat, F. S., Manzino, L., and Duvoisin, R. C. (1981). Potentiation by deprenil of *l*-dopa induced circling in nigral-lesioned rats. *Pharmacol., Biochem. Behav.* **15,** 75–80.

Hökfelt, T., Rehfeld, J. F., Skirboll, L., Ivemark, B., Goldstein, M., and Markey, K. (1980). Evidence for coexistence of dopamine acid CCK in mesolimbic neurons. *Nature (London)* **285,** 476–478.

Hornykiewicz, O. (1972). Neurochemistry of Parkinson's disease. *In* "Handbook of Neurochemistry" (A. Lajtha, ed.), Vol. 7, pp. 465–501. Plenum, New York.

Hunter, R., Smith, J., Thomson, T., and Dayan, A. D. (1978). Hemiparkinsonism with infarction of the ipsilateral substantia nigra. *Neuropathol. Appl. Neurobiol.* **4,** 297–301.

Iversen, S. D. (1977). Brain dopamine systems and behaviour. *In* "Handbook of Psychopharmacology" (L. L. Iversen, S. D. Iversen, S. H. Snyder, eds.), Vol. 8, pp. 333–384. Plenum, New York.

James, T. A., and Starr, M. S. (1978). The role of GABA in the substantia nigra. *Nature (London)* **275,** 229–230.

Jessell, T. M., Emson, P. C., Paxinos, G., and Cuello, A. C. (1978). Topographic projections of substance P and GABA pathways in the striato- and pallidonigral system: A biochemical and immunohistochemical study. *Brain Res.* **152,** 487–498.

Kelly, P. H. (1977). Drug-induced motor behaviour. *In* "Handbook of Psychopharmacology" (L. L. Iversen, S. D. Iversen, and S. H. Snyder, eds.), Vol. 8, pp. 295–331. Plenum, New York.

Kelly, P. H., and Moore, K. E. (1976). Mesolimbic dopaminergic neurones in the rotational model of nigrostriatal function. *Nature (London)* **263,** 695–696.

Kilpatrick, I. C., and Starr, M. S. (1981). The nucleus tegmenti pedunculopontinus and circling behavior in the rat. *Neurosci. Lett.* **26,** 11–16.

Kilpatrick, I. C., Starr, M. S., Fletcher, A., James, T. A., and MacLeod, N. K. (1980). Evidence for a GABAergic nigrothalamic pathway in the rat. I. Behavioural and biochemical studies. *Exp. Brain Res.* **40,** 45–54.

Kilpatrick, I. C., Collingridge, G. L., and Starr, M. S. (1982). Evidence for the participation of nigrotectal GABA-containing neurones in striatal and nigral-derived circling in the rat. *Neuroscience* **7,** 207–222.

Knoll, J. (1978). The possible mechanisms of action of (−)-deprenyl in Parkinson's disease. *J. Neural Transm.* **43,** 177–198.

Laursen, A. M. (1962). Movements evoked from the region of the caudate nucleus in cats. *Acta Physiol. Scand.* **54,** 175–184.

Lee, L. A., and Slater, P. (1981). Role of globus pallidus and substantia nigra efferent pathways in striatally-evoked head turning in the rat. *Exp. Brain Res.* **44,** 170–176.

Lee, L. A., Crossman, A. R., and Slater, P. (1980). The neurological basis of striatally induced head-turning in the rat: The effects of lesions in putative output pathways. *Neuroscience* **5,** 73–79.

Lees, A. J., Shaw, K. M., Kohout, L. J., Stern, G. M., Elsworth, J. D., Sandler, M., and Youdim, M. B. H. (1977). Deprenyl in Parkinson's disease. *Lancet* **2,** 791–795.

Lindvall, O., and Björklund, A. (1978). Organization of catecholamine neurons in the rat central nervous system. *In* "Handbook of Psychopharmology" (L. L. Iversen, S. D. Iversen, and S. H. Snyder, eds.), Vol. 9, pp. 139–231. Plenum, New York.

Ljungberg, T., and Ungerstedt, U. (1976). Sensory inattention produced by 6-hydroxydopamine-induced degeneration of ascending dopamine neurons in the brain. *Exp. Neurol.* **53,** 585–600.

Lloyd, K. G., and Hornykiewicz, O. (1973). L-Glutamic acid decarboxylase in Parkinson's disease: Effect of L-Dopa therapy. *Nature (London)* **243,** 521–523.

Lloyd, K. G., Shemen, L., and Hornykiewicz, O. (1977). Distribution of high affinity sodium-independent [^{3}H]GABA binding in the human brain: Alterations in Parkinson's disease. *Brain Res.* **127,** 269–278.

McGeer, P. L., and McGeer, E. G. (1976). Enzymes associated with the metabolism of catecholamines, acetylcholine and GABA in human controls and patients with Parkinson's disease and Huntington's chorea. *J. Neurochem.* **26,** 65–76.

Marsden, C. D. (1980). Animal models of extrapyramidal diseases. *In* "Animal Models of Neurological Disease" (F. Clifford Rose and P. O. Behan, eds.), pp. 269–277. Pitman Medical, Tunbridge Wells.

Marsden, C. D., Duvoisin, R. C., Jenner, P., Parkes, J. D., Pycock, C., and Tarsy, D. (1975). Relationship between animal models and clinical Parkinsonism. *Adv. Neurol.* **9,** 165–175.

Marshall, J. F., and Teitelbaun, P. (1974). Further analysis of sensory inattention following lateral hypothalamie damage in rats. *J. Comp. Physiol. Psychol.* **86,** 375–395.

Mehler, W. R., and Nauta, W. J. H. (1974). Connections of the basal ganglia and of the cerebellum. *Confin. Neurol.* **36,** 205–222.

Morelli, M., Imperato, A., Porceddu, M. L., and DiChiara, G. (1981). Role of dorsal mesencephalic reticular formation and deep layers of superior colliculus in turning behaviour elicited from the striatum. *Brain Res.* **215,** 337–341.

Mulas, A., Longoni, R., Spina, L., Del Fiacco, M., and DiChiara, G. (1981). Ipsiversive turning behaviour after discrete unilateral lesion of the dorsal mesencephalic reticular formation by kainic acid. *Brain Res.* **208,** 468–472.

Nieuwenhuys, R. (1977). Aspects of the morphology of the striatum. *In* "Psychobiology of the Striatum" (A. R. Cools, A. H. M. Lohman, and J. H. L. van den Burken, eds.), pp. 1–19. Elsevier/North-Holland Biomedical Press, Amsterdam.

Olpe, H.-R., Schellenberg, H., and Koella, W. P. (1977). Rotational behaviour induced in rats by intranigral application of GABA-related drugs and GABA antagonists. *Eur. J. Pharmacol.* **45,** 291–294.

Poirier, L. J. (1960). Experimental and histological study of midbrain dyskinesias. *J. Neurophysiol.* **23,** 534–551.

Pycock, C. J. (1980). Turning behaviour in animals. *Neuroscience* **5,** 461–514.

Pycock, C. J., and Marsden, C. D. (1978). The rotating rodent: A two component system? *Eur. J. Pharmacol.* **47,** 167–175.

Pycock, C. J., and Phillipson, O. T. (1983). A neuroanatomical and neuropharmacological analysis of basal ganglia output. *In* "Handbook of Psychopharmacology" (L. L. Iversen, S. D. Iversen, and S. H. Snyder, eds.), Vol. 18. Plenum, New York (in press).

Pycock, C. J., Tarsy, D., and Marsden, C. D. (1975). Inhibition of circling behaviour by neuroleptic drugs in mice with unilateral 6-hydroxydopamine lesions of the striatum. *Psychopharmacologia* **45,** 211–219.

Pycock, C. J., Milson, J. A., Tarsy, D., and Marsden, C. D. (1976). The effects of blocking catecholamine uptake on amphetamine-induced circling behaviour in mice with unilateral destruction of striatal dopaminergic terminals. *J. Pharm. Pharmacol.* **28,** 530–532.

Reavill, C., Jenner, P., Leigh, N., and Marsden, C. D. (1979). Turning behaviour induced by injection of muscimol or picrotoxin into the substantia nigra demonstrates dual GABA components. *Neurosci. Lett.* **12,** 323–328.

Reavill, C., Jenner, P., Leigh, N., and Marsden, C. D. (1981a). The role of nigral projections to the thalamus in drug-induced circling behaviour in the rat. *Life Sci.* **28,** 1457–1466.

Reavill, C., Leigh, N., Jenner, P., and Marsden, C. D. (1981b). Nigrothalamic GABA pathway and nigro-reticular pathways in the expression of dopamine mediated circling behaviour. *In* "GABA and the Basal Ganglia" (G. DiChiara and G. L. Gessa, eds.), pp. 187–204. Raven Press, New York.

Reisine, T. D., Rossor, M., Spokes, E., Iversen, L. L., and Yamamura, H. I. (1978). Alterations in brain opiate receptors in Parkinson's disease. *Brain Res.* **173,** 378–382.

Rinne, U. K., Sonninen, V., and Hyyppä, M. (1971). Effect of L-DOPA on brain monoamines and their metabolites in Parkinson's disease. *Life Sci.* **10,** 549–557.

Rinne, U. K., Riekkinen, P., Sonninen, V., and Laaksonen, H. (1973). Brain acetylcholinesterase in Parkinson's disease. *Acta Neurol. Scand.* **49,** 215–226.

Rinne, U. K., Laaksonen, H., Riekkinen, P., and Sonninen, V. (1974). Brain glutamic acid decarboxylase activity in Parkinson's disease. *Eur. Neurol.* **12,** 13–19.

Roffman, M., Bernard, P. S., Dawson, K. M., Sobiski, R. E., and Saelens, J. K. (1978). The effects of haloperidol and clozapine on circling induced by electrical stimulation of the substatia nigra and the ventromedial tegmentum. *Neuropharmacology* **17,** 943–946.

Scheel-Krüger, J., Arnt, J., and Magelund, G. (1977). Behavioural stimulation induced by muscimol and other GABA agonists injected into the substantia nigra. *Neurosci. Lett.* **4,** 351–356.

Scheel-Krüger, J., Magelund, G., and Olianas, M. C. (1981). Role of GABA in the striatal output system: Globus pallidus, nucleus entopeduncularis, substantia nigra and nucleus subthalamicus. *In* "GABA and the Basal Ganglia" (G. DiChiara and G. L. Gessa, eds.), pp. 165–186. Raven Press, New York.

Skultety, F. M. (1962). Circus movements in cats following midbrain stimulation through chronically implanted electrodes. *J. Neurophysiol.* **25,** 152–164.

Sprague, J. M., and Meikle, J. M., Jr. (1965). The role of the superior colliculus in visually guided behaviour. *Exp. Neurol.* **11,** 115–146.

Staines, W. A., Nagy, J. I., Vincent, S. R., and Fibiger, H. C. (1980). Neurotransmitters contained in the efferents of the striatum. *Brain Res.* **194,** 391–402.

Stern, G. (1980). Parkinsonism in animals. *In* "Animal Models of Neurological Disease" (F. Clifford Rose and P. O. Behan, eds.), pp. 278–280. Pitman Medical, Tunbridge Wells.

Stern, G. M., Lees, A. J., and Sandler, M. (1978). Recent observations on the clinical pharmacology of (−)-deprenyl. *J. Neural Transm.* **43,** 245–251.

Tarsy, D., Pycock, C., Meldrum, B., and Marsden, C. D. (1975). Rotational behaviour induced in rats by intranigral picrotoxin. *Brain Res.* **89,** 160–165.

Trétiakoff, C. (1919). Contribution à l'étude de l'anatomie pathologique du locus niger de Soemmering. Thèse de Paris, No. 293.

Ungerstedt, U. (1971a). Striatal dopamine release after amphetamine or nerve degeneration revealed by rotational behaviour. *Acta Physiol. Scand.* **82,** Suppl. 367, 49–68.

Ungerstedt, U. (1971b). Post-synaptic supersensitivity after 6-hydroxydopamine induced degeneration of the nigro-striatal dopamine system in the rat brain. *Acta Physiol. Scand.* **82,** Suppl. 367, 69–93.

Ungerstedt, U. (1971c). Adipsia and aphagia after 6-hydroxydopamine induced degeneration of the nigro-striatal dopamine system. *Acta Physiol. Scand.* **82,** Suppl. 367, 95–122.
Van Ree, J. M., and Wolterink, G. (1981). Injection of low doses of apomorphine into the nucleus accumbens of rats reduces locomotor activity. *Eur. J. Pharmacol.* **72,** 107–111.
von Voigtlander, P. F., and Moore, K. E. (1971). The release of ^{3}H-dopamine from cat brain following electrical stimulation of the substantia nigra and caudate nucleus. *Neuropharmacology* **10,** 133–141.
York, D. H. (1973). Motor responses induced by stimulation of the substantia nigra. *Exp. Neurol.* **41,** 323–330.

5: Sex Differences in Behavioral and Brain Asymmetries

TERRY E. ROBINSON, JILL B. BECKER, and DIANNE M. CAMP

Department of Psychology
and Neuroscience Laboratory
The University of Michigan
Ann Arbor, Michigan

I. Introduction ... 91
II. Behavioral and Brain Asymmetries ... 92
A. Human Beings ... 92
B. Nonhuman Animals ... 95
III. Sex Differences in Behavioral and Brain Asymmetries ... 103
A. Human Beings ... 103
B. Nonhuman Animals ... 106
IV. Conclusions ... 115
A. Are Human Beings Unique in Having Lateralized Brains? ... 115
B. Are There Sex Differences in Lateralization? ... 115
C. Relationship between Asymmetries in Human Beings and Nonhuman Animals ... 119
References ... 122

I. Introduction

There is some debate as to who should be credited with first suggesting that the human brain is functionally lateralized. Paul Broca is usually cited as the first to observe that left hemisphere damage is associated with language disturbances, although Dax supposedly made this suggestion approximately 25 years earlier than Broca (cited in Kolb and Whishaw, 1980). Regardless of priority, since the late nineteenth century there has been a vigorous and enduring interest in the idea that the brain is asymmetrically organized.

Although research on nonhuman animals has provided a great deal of insight into human brain function, nonhuman animals have not been

HEMISYNDROMES:
Psychobiology, Neurology,
Psychiatry

ISBN 0-12-512460-0

used very much to study the factors involved in brain asymmetry. This is because for many years it was thought that an asymmetric organization was unique to the human brain. However, there is now considerable evidence that asymmetries exist in the nervous system of many different species (for reviews, see Nottebohm, 1979; Walker, 1980; Denenberg, 1981). In this chapter we review evidence for cerebral asymmetries in both human and nonhuman animals. The emphasis is on asymmetries in nonhuman animals, and therefore the literature on lateralization in human beings is only briefly summarized to facilitate comparison with the literature on nonhuman animals. After this we address the major topic of this chapter, the idea that gender may influence the patterns of behavioral and brain asymmetries observed in both human and nonhuman animals.

II. Behavioral and Brain Asymmetries

A. Human Beings

For many years there were only a few scattered and not well-substantiated reports of anatomical asymmetries in human brain. However, in more recent years a number of well-documented examples of morphological asymmetries have been reported (for reviews, see Witelson, 1977; Galaburda *et al.*, 1978). The best known asymmetry is in the size of the planum temporale (Geschwind and Levitsky, 1968), but asymmetries have also been described in the length of the Sylvian fissure, the length of the frontal pole, the length of the occipital horn of the lateral ventricle, the extent of the anterior speech region, and the distribution of gray and white matter (Gur *et al.*, 1980; Falzi *et al.*, 1982; see also previously mentioned reviews). Anatomical asymmetries may not be confined to neocortical regions. An asymmetry in the volume of the lateral posterior nucleus of the thalamus has also been described (Eidelberg and Galaburda, 1982).

In addition to these morphological asymmetries it has long been thought that there are probably subtle asymmetries in specific neurotransmitter systems within some brain regions. However, there have been very few systematic studies of neurochemical asymmetries in human brain. Glick *et al.* (1982) reanalyzed data collected by Rossor *et al.* (1980) and reported that asymmetries exist in the concentrations of several neurochemicals in several brain structures. For example, the levels of choline acetyltransferase and dopamine are higher in the left globus pallidus than in the right globus pallidus. Amaducci *et al.* (1981) reported that choline acetyltransferase activity is higher in the left superior temporal lobe than in the right. This difference is maximal in cortical layers II and IV. An asymmetry has also been described in the distribution of norepinephrine in the thalamus (Oke *et al.*, 1978). Others have inferred from pharmacological evidence that asymmetries may exist in human brain neurotransmitter systems (Mandell and Knapp, 1979; Waziri, 1980; Frumkin and Grim, 1981). How these anatomical and neurochemical asymmetries are related to brain function is not known.

Much of what we know about cerebral asymmetry in humans is derived from studies of the functional asymmetries observed in people who have received lateralized brain injuries through accident, stroke, or surgery. This topic has been reviewed in many articles and books and is only briefly summarized here (for reviews, see Geschwind, 1972; Kimura, 1973a; Milner, 1974; Sperry, 1974; Hécaen and Albert, 1978; Heilman and Valenstein, 1979; Kolb and Whishaw, 1980). The initial clinical–anatomical observations of Broca have been replicated and extended many times. Left hemisphere lesions have a relatively selective effect on language abilities, although, despite Broca's emphasis on frontal cortex, it is now known that aphasia may result from more posterior lesions as well (i.e., Wernicke's or fluent aphasia). However, left hemisphere lesions fail to disrupt performance on many nonverbal tasks. In contrast, right hemisphere lesions in humans produce deficits on nonverbal tasks without impairing language abilities to any great extent. For example, people with restricted right hemisphere lesions have been reported to be impaired at spatial tasks, recognition of faces, tactile recognition of patterns, and memory for visual location, melodies, geometric patterns, nonsense patterns, and abstract paintings.

The results from studies of people with unilateral lesions are complemented by numerous experiments with normal and commissurotomized humans. A variety of techniques have been used to present stimuli preferentially to one hemisphere or the other (e.g., dichotic listening, tachistoscopic tasks) to determine if there are hemispheric advantages in processing different kinds of stimuli. It is generally found in these kinds of experimental situations that the left hemisphere has an advantage over the right hemisphere in processing verbal stimuli (e.g., letters, words, digits), whereas the right hemisphere has an advantage in processing stimuli that are not easily verbalized (e.g., faces, nonsense patterns, melodies, geometric shapes).

A major feature of the lateralization of higher cognitive functions (e.g., language and spatial abilities) in humans is complementary specialization (Milner, 1974). The homologous right and left halves of the brain, in fact, perform similar functions but are specialized for processing particular kinds of stimuli or for generating particular patterns of motor output (Efron, 1963a,b; Kimura and Archibald, 1974; Milner, 1974; Mateer and Kimura, 1977; Schwartz and Tallal, 1980). For example, both the left and right medial temporal regions are important for normal learning and memory. After left medial temporal lobe damage the ability to learn and retain verbal material is impaired. After right medial temporal lobe damage there is an impairment in the learning and retention of material that is not easily labeled verbally. A similar complementary specialization has been described for the frontal lobe. Both the left and right frontal lobes appear to be important for the ability to order events in time (Milner, 1974). The left frontal lobe is selectively involved in the temporal ordering of verbal material, whereas the right frontal lobe is necessary for the temporal ordering of nonverbal material.

In addition to the lateralization of cognitive functions there are well-known behavioral asymmetries in humans. The most pronounced and best known asymmetry is, of course, handedness. The majority of humans preferentially use their right hand for the performance of a variety of unimanual acts. However, there are also other, less studied lateral preferences. Most humans have a preferred foot, eye, and ear as well. Newborn infants show a lateralized head posture; that is, they turn their head to the right more frequently than to the left, both spontaneously and in response to unilateral sensory stimulation (Gesell, 1938; Turkewitz, 1977). This asymmetry in head posture seen in infancy is predictive of hand preference for reaching later in life (Gesell and Ames, 1947; Liederman and Coryell, 1981; Michel, 1981). People also walk, swim, or drive in spirals when blindfolded (Schaeffer, 1928). The topic of postural–motor asymmetries in humans has been reviewed (e.g., Herron,1980; Porac and Coren, 1981).

Despite the massive literature on lateralization in the human brain that has accumulated over the past 75 years, there is still little agreement among neuropsychologists as to the basis of hemispheric asymmetry. What is special about the left hemisphere that confers on it an advantage for verbal stimuli? Why does the right hemisphere outperform the left hemisphere in processing nonverbal information? The lack of any consensual answer to these questions is reflected in the variety of ways in which left and right hemisphere specialization has been characterized. The left hemisphere has been described by such terms as verbal, sequential, temporal, digital, logical, analytical, rational, deductive, propositional, and Western. The right hemisphere has been described by the terms nonverbal, visuospatial, simultaneous, spatial, analogical, Gestalt, synthetic, holistic, intuitive, imaginative, appositional, and Eastern. This multitude of dichotomies has done little to further our knowledge of the basic differences between left and right hemisphere organization.

A major reason why progress has been slow in answering questions about the nature of hemispheric specialization in humans is probably due to the numerous constraints on research with humans. It is simply not possible with humans to design the kind of rigorously controlled studies on brain–behavior relations that are done in other species. Much of our knowledge of human brain function is actually inferred from studies in other species, in which a greater variety of experimental techniques are used. Obviously, this approach is most successful for understanding brain regions that have common functions in most mammals (e.g., many subcortical structures) but is more tenuous for understanding brain regions that may have functions that are uniquely human (e.g., association cortical areas). Nevertheless, studies on the cortex of nonhuman animals involving unit recording, neurochemical manipulations, developmental paradigms, and lesions have greatly enhanced our knowledge of the ways in which homologous human cortical regions function (e.g., see Kolb and Whishaw, 1983). However, animal models have not been widely used to study basic questions concerning hemispheric asymmetries. If nonhuman animals also had lateralized brain regions, it might be possible to ask experimentally many questions concerning brain asymmetry that are otherwise impossible to ask in humans.

B. Nonhuman Animals

In this section we review some of the evidence for behavioral and brain asymmetries in nonhumans. It should become obvious from this review that brain lateralization is not a uniquely human situation, even though the relationship between cerebral asymmetry in humans and asymmetries in nonhuman animals is not at all clear. Nevertheless, the presence of asymmetries in both humans and nonhumans makes it possible to study the factors that contribute to the development of lateralization and could provide animal models useful for testing hypotheses about the functional significance of lateralization.

1. ANATOMICAL ASYMMETRIES

There are a number of reports of anatomical asymmetries in the brains of nonhuman animals, some of which are surprisingly similar to those observed in humans. In chimpanzees the left Sylvian fissure is usually longer than the right, in orangutans and chimpanzees the right Sylvian fissure angles up higher than the left, and in baboons the right frontal pole is longer than the left (LeMay and Geschwind, 1975; LeMay, 1976; Yeni-Komshian and Benson, 1976; Cain and Wada, 1979). All of these patterns have been found in humans as well. Right–left asymmetries have been found in the skulls of some subspecies of gorilla (Groves and Humphrey, 1973), although it is not known if this is related to an anatomical asymmetry in the cerebral hemispheres. The neocortex of rats, mice, rabbits, and cats is reported to be thicker on the right than on the left (Diamond *et al.*, 1975; Kolb and Whishaw, 1981; Kolb *et al.*, 1982a), and the pattern of sulci in cats often differs between the two cerebral hemispheres (Webster and Webster, 1975). A right–left asymmetry in the thickness of the dorsal hippocampus has also been reported (Diamond *et al.*, 1982). Finally, lower vertebrates such as lampreys, eels, newts, and frogs have an asymmetry in the size of the habenular nuclei, which has been known for many years (see Nottebohm, 1979, for references).

2. NEUROCHEMICAL ASYMMETRIES

In addition to morphological asymmetries, neurochemical asymmetries have been found in a number of regions of the rat brain. Depending on the exact anterior–posterior position, thalamic norepinephrine (NE) concentrations may be higher on the left or right. In the anterior portion of the thalamus NE concentrations are higher on the left, whereas farther caudally there is a transition to higher NE levels on the right (Oke *et al.*, 1980). Asymmetries were also reported in a study in which γ-aminobutyric acid (GABA) turnover was estimated by measuring the elevation of GABA levels in discrete brain regions following inhibition of GABA catabolism (Starr and Kilpatrick, 1981). Concentrations of GABA were higher in the right substantia nigra, superior colliculus, and nucleus accumbens relative to the left and were higher in the left caudate nucleus, ventromedial thalamus, and ventral tegmentum relative to the right.

The uptake of some neurotransmitters into hippocampal synaptosomes has been reported to be lateralized in rats that turn preferentially to the left in a T maze (Valdes *et al.*, 1981). In rats with a left turn preference the uptake of [^{3}H]serotonin, [^{3}H]NE, and [^{3}H]choline is greater into synaptosomes prepared from the left than from the right hippocampus. Valdes *et al.* (1982) also reported a relationship between asymmetries in the distribution of zinc in the hippocampus and spatial preference in a T maze. In addition, these authors reported that the left hippocampus weighs significantly more than the right, but others have failed to find such a difference (Kolb *et al.*, 1982a; S. D. Glick, personal communication; T. E. Robinson and J. B. Becker, unpublished observations, 1982). Using deoxy-D-[1,2-^{3}H] glucose (2-DG) Glick *et al.* (1979) found a left–right asymmetry in hippocampal metabolic activity, the left hippocampus showing greater uptake of 2-DG (also see Stokes and McIntyre, 1981).

3. FUNCTIONAL ASYMMETRIES

There are a number of examples of functional asymmetries in nonhuman animals. Probably the best known example is the asymmetry in the neural control of bird song so elegantly demonstrated by Nottebohm (for reviews, see Nottebohm, 1979, 1980). Nottebohm found that the chaffinch and canary have "left hypoglossal dominance" for song. That is, section of the left but not right hypoglossal nerve disrupts singing in these species. Additional studies have shown that the forebrain nuclei that control the syrinx are also functionally lateralized. Damage to the left hyperstriatum ventrale, pars caudale, or robust nucleus of the archistriatum disrupts song to a greater extent than lesions to the same structures in the right hemisphere.

It is intriguing that even though there is a striking functional asymmetry for bird song no left–right morphological differences have been found in the canary forebrain (Nottebohm, 1981). Nottebohm (1981) has suggested that perhaps the lack of a left–right anatomical asymmetry reflects the equipotentiality of either hemisphere to acquire control over song. After section of the left hypoglossal nerve adult canaries can eventually learn a new song of normal complexity, and this new song is under control of the right hypoglossal nerve.

One other example of lateralization in birds comes from studies by Rogers and co-workers (Rogers and Anson, 1979; Howard *et al.*, 1980). These authors have reported that visual discrimination learning, and auditory habituation are more dependent on the left than on the right hemisphere. The direction of this asymmetry may be due to an asymmetric orientation of the chick in the egg, which results in one eye receiving more input than the other before hatching (Rogers, 1981).

In rats there have been reports of asymmetries in the effects of neocortical lesions on behavior and neurotransmitter levels. Robinson found that damage to the right frontal cortex by ligation of the right middle cerebral artery, or a suction lesion, produces a postoperative period of hyperactivity not seen after left neocortical damage (Robinson, 1979; Robinson and Coyle, 1980; Pearlson and Robinson, 1981). More hyperactivity is seen after the application of 6-hydroxydopamine (6-OHDA) or kainic acid to the right than to the left frontal cortex as well (Kubos *et al.*, 1982; Robinson and Stitt, 1981). Neurochemically, right hemisphere lesions cause a bilateral decline in cortical and locus coeruleus NE levels, whereas left neocortex lesions do not. Denenberg and co-workers (1978, 1980; Sherman *et al.*, 1980; see Denenberg, 1981, for review) reported lateralized effects of cortical lesions in rats with different developmental experiences. For example, rats handled in infancy (before weaning) that had the right neocortex ablated in adulthood were hyperactive in an open field if they had been raised in laboratory cages, but were hypoactive if raised in an enriched environment (Denenberg *et al.*, 1978). Lesions to the left neocortex did not produce significant changes in activity in handled rats raised in either environment. In nonhandled rats there was no evidence for a lateralized effect regardless of the side of the lesion. For a detailed discussion of the interactions between brain lateralization and early experience, see Denenberg (1981).

An obvious indication of an asymmetry in brain activity is the presence of persistent postural or motor asymmetries in the absence of peripheral structural asymmetries. For example, many animals other than humans show "handedness" (or "pawedness"), in that they consistently perform specific unimanual tasks with a preferred paw (e.g., Peterson, 1934; Warren, 1958; Collins, 1968). One infers from this that there is something different about the organization of the two hemispheres that leads to the predominant use of one paw over the other. Indeed, a small frontal cortex lesion, or the injection of 6-OHDA into the lateral hypothalamus, contralateral to the preferred paw, results in a reversal of paw preference (Peterson and Fracarol, 1938; Peterson and Devine, 1963; Uguru-Okorie and Arbuthnott, 1981). Damage ipsilateral to the preferred paw has no effect on paw preference. Unfortunately, little more is known about the nature of brain asymmetry that contributes to the preferred use of one paw.

Much more is known about the neural basis of postural asymmetries that result in rotational (circling) behavior in a variety of species. It has been known for many years that a unilateral lesion of ascending nigrostriatal fibers results in motor asymmetries (Andén *et al.*, 1966), as does the application of dopamine (DA) directly into the striatum (Ungerstedt *et al.*, 1969). When the nigrostriatal DA system is destroyed unilaterally with 6-OHDA, a well-documented and highly replicable behavioral syndrome ensues. In rats and mice this syndrome consists of persistent circling toward the side of the lesion (ipsiversive). The spontaneous circling following unilateral destruction of the nigrostriatal DA system usually diminishes over time but can be reinstated by an injection of a variety of drugs, particularly drugs that activate DA systems (Ungerstedt and Arbuthnott, 1970; Christie and Crow, 1971; Ungerstedt, 1971a,b). For example, amphetamine (AMPH) typically produces vigorous ipsiversive turning, whereas apomorphine produces contraversive turning. These studies on rotational behavior established that animals typically turn in the direction contralateral to the nigrostriatal DA system having the greatest activity. Thus, after a unilateral injection of 6-OHDA into the substantia nigra the DA terminals in the striatum on that side degenerate, and AMPH releases more DA on the intact side. Activity in the intact striatum induces turning toward the damaged side. However, DA receptors in both striata are intact following the infliction of a unilateral substantia nigra lesion. The fact that apomorphine elicits contraversive turning is thought to indicate that the unilaterally denervated receptors have become hypersensitive, and therefore since the more active side is ipsilateral to the lesion the animal rotates toward its intact side (Ungerstedt, 1971b).

Other brain areas probably interact with the nigrostriatal DA system to produce circling behavior. A model that is gaining acceptance is that asymmetries in the DA projections to the striata are responsible for producing postural asymmetries, and the projections to the nucleus accumbens are involved in producing locomotion (Kelly and Moore, 1977; Moore and Kelly, 1978; Pycock and Marsden, 1978). Asymmetric nigrostriatal DA activity plus an active nucleus accumbens DA system results in circling. Other neurotransmitter systems (e.g., serotonergic, cholinergic) that influence nigrostriatal DA activity also modulate rotational behavior (see Pycock, 1980, for review).

Thus, the induction of an asymmetry in the nigrostriatal DA system results in an asymmetry in behavior. However, Glick and colleagues have reported that unilateral lesions of the nigrostriatal system are not necessary to produce rotational behavior (for reviews, see Glick *et al.,* 1976, 1977a). After an injection of AMPH intact rats rotate in a dominant direction when placed in a spherical rotometer (Jerussi and Glick, 1974; Greenstein and Glick, 1975). The dominant direction of rotation elicited by AMPH is constant for individual animals when they are tested weeks apart, although approximately 50% of rats rotate predominantly to the left and 50% predominantly to the right. More recent reports suggest a slight population bias to the right (Denenberg, 1981; Glick and Ross, 1981a; see later).

Since earlier studies in unilaterally lesioned animals (see above) showed that rats rotate contralateral to the striatum with the greatest activity, the observation of rotation in unlesioned rats suggested an endogenous asymmetry in nigrostriatal DA activity. Indeed, analysis of DA levels in the striata of intact rats showed that the striatum with the highest DA content was found contralateral to the dominant direction of rotation elicited by AMPH (Glick *et al.,* 1974; Jerussi and Glick, 1976; Robinson *et al.,* 1980). Rats that rotate predominantly left after AMPH injection usually have higher DA levels in their right striatum, and vice versa. No relationship has been found between the levels of striatal acetylcholine, (ACh), telendiencephalic NE or ACh, striatal NE, or medial frontal cortex NE or DA and rotational behavior. A similar relationship between unilateral striatal activity and direction of rotation has been reported with the 2-DG technique (Glick *et al.,* 1979). The striatum showing the greatest glucose utilization after an AMPH injection was found to be contralateral to the dominant direction of rotation elicited by AMPH. In fact, drugs are not necessary to demonstrate lateralized motor tendencies. During the night, when rats are quite active, they also tend to turn in a dominant direction, and this direction is the same as the dominant direction of rotation elicited by AMPH during the day (Glick and Cox, 1978). Thus, Glick and colleagues have suggested that there is an endogenous asymmetry in nigrostriatal activity that is manifested in lateralized behavior.

We have obtained evidence supporting the idea that there is an endogenous asymmetry in the nigrostriatal DA system. In one experiment we studied the AMPH-stimulated release of DA from striatal tissue using an *in vitro* perifusion system (for a description of the technique see Becker and Ramirez, 1980, 1981). Before DA release was measured, all rats were tested for AMPH-induced rotational behavior on at least two separate occasions. On the basis of this screening one hemisphere was operationally defined as being "dominant" for rotational behavior (the side contralateral to the dominant direction of rotation), and the other side as "nondominant." At least 1 week after the last behavioral test the animals were killed, and the left and right striata were removed and placed individually in a perifusion chamber. After a 45-min equilibration period AMPH was added to the perifusion medium. The amount of AMPH-stimulated DA release from the dominant striatum was significantly greater than that from the nondominant striatum (Fig. 5.1).

If there is an asymmetry in the nigrostriatal DA system, one would predict that the effects of unilateral damage to the striata might differ, depending on which side was damaged. Indeed, Glick and co-workers (Jerussi and Glick, 1975; Glick and Cox, 1976; Rothman and Glick, 1976; Glick *et al.*, 1977a) have shown that the effects of electrolytic lesions of the caudate contralateral to an animal's dominant direction of rotation differ from the effects of ipsilateral lesions. We have also found that the direction (contraversive versus ipsiversive) of AMPH-induced rotational behavior seen after the infliction of a unilateral 6-OHDA lesion of the substantia nigra depends to a large extent on whether the substantia nigra on the dominant or nondominant side (as defined earlier) is lesioned (Robinson and Becker, 1983). In this experiment intact rats were first screened for AMPH-induced rotational behavior to identify which hemisphere was intrinsically dominant for rotational behavior (as described above). The animals were then pretreated with desipramine hydrochloride, and 6-OHDA was injected into either the dominant or the nondominant substantia nigra. After at least 2 weeks of recovery all rats were again tested for AMPH-induced rotational behavior.

The direction of rotational behavior observed after the 6-OHDA lesion depended on at least two factors: (*a*) the extent of the striatal DA

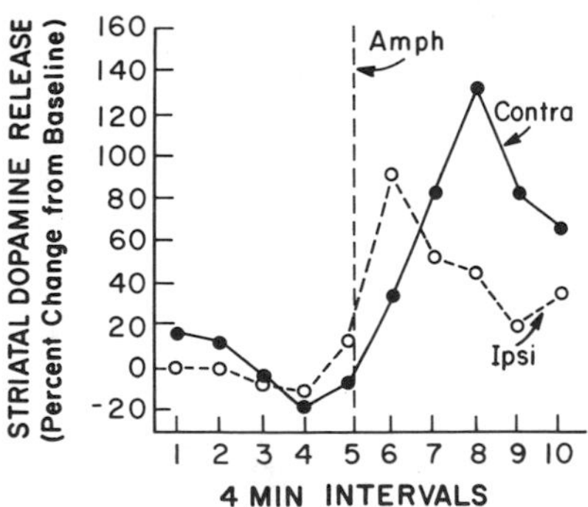

FIG. 5.1. *In vitro* dopamine release from the striatum located contralateral (Contra) versus ipsilateral (Ipsi) to the dominant direction of rotation. Amphetamine was added to the perifusion medium at the vertical dashed line. Dopamine release is plotted as a percent change from the average baseline release (intervals 1–5). The percent increase in amphetamine-stimulated dopamine release from the Contra striatum is significantly greater than that from the Ipsi striatum ($F = 4.2$, $p < 0.004$; $N = 9$).

depletion and (*b*) the side of the lesion (Table 5.1). In animals with a >90% striatal DA depletion ($\bar{x}$=98.5%) lesions of either the dominant or nondominant side had the same effect. Of rats with a nondominant-sided lesion, 9 of 9 rotated ipsilateral to the lesion. All (100%) of their total rotations (one rotation equals four consecutive 90° turns in the same direction) were ipsiversive. Of rats with a dominant-sided lesion, 9 of 10 rotated preferentially to the ipsilateral side. Almost all (93.7%) of their total rotations were ipsiversive. In contrast, if the striatal DA depletion was <90% ($\bar{x}$=67.0%), the side of the lesion had a dramatic effect. The majority of these rats (9 of 11) with dominant-sided lesions rotated in the contraversive direction (i.e., in the opposite direction of all other groups), although some of these animals had 80–90% DA depletions. These animals made only 24% of their total rotations ipsilateral to the lesion. However, animals with a <90% DA depletion on the nondominant side were like animals with a nearly total DA depletion. All of them (N= 8) showed ipsiversive rotation, making 96.5% of their total rotations in that direction. The unique effect of dominant-sided lesions was most evident when rats were tested with a low dose (1.2 mg/kg) rather than a high dose (3–5 mg/kg) of AMPH. These data suggest that functionally the endogenous asymmetry in the nigrostriatal system must be very robust. When only 10–20% of the DA input to the dominant hemisphere was left intact, most animals still turned away from that side.

Finally, the endogenous asymmetry in striatal DA reported by Glick and colleagues (1977b) may be related to broader categories of behavior than simply rotation. The asymmetry in DA content and the direction of AMPH-elicited rotation have also been related to side preferences and learning rates in a T maze, paw use in two-lever operant tasks, and response rates yielding the greatest number of reinforcements on FR 30, FI 15, and DRL 16 schedules of reinforcement (see Glick *et al.*, 1977a, for review). We have found that the rate of learning a spatial task is faster in rats that are lateralized than in nonlateralized rats (Camp *et al.*, 1981). Glick *et al.* (1977a) have suggested that "a moderate degree of striatal asymmetry may be optimal for maximal overall learning ability and side preferences may have some adaptive significance in terms of how the organism can most effectively cope with or strategically explore its environment [p. 245]."

This section is not an exhaustive review of all the literature on brain and behavioral asymmetries in nonhuman animals. For example, functional asymmetries have been reported in cats (Webster, 1972) and nonhuman primates as well (Dewson, 1977, 1978; Petersen *et al.*, 1978; for other references, see Nottebohm, 1979; Walker, 1980; Denenberg, 1981). The purpose of this section is to show that there is considerable evidence that nonhuman animals have lateralized brains. Most of this evidence has been acquired recently, and we still know relatively little about brain asymmetries in nonhuman animals.

TABLE 5.1

Effects of "Dominant" versus "Nondominant"-Sided 6-OHDA Lesions of the Substantia Nigra on Amphetamine-Induced Rotational Behavior[a]

Lesion group	N	Number of Ipsi turners (%)	DA depletion (%)	Net rotations	Total rotations		Total one-quarter turns		% Dominance
					Ipsi (%)	Contra (%)	Ipsi (%)	Contra (%)	
1. "Nondominant" (>90%)	9	9 (100)	98.6 ± 0.5	213 ± 62	213 ± 62 (100)	0 (0)	898 ± 259 (98 ± 1)	22 ± 17 (2 ± 1)	100
2. "Dominant" (>90%)	10	9 (90)	98.3 ± 0.8	152 ± 47	154 ± 46 (94 ± 6)	6 ± 6 (6 ± 6)	665 ± 183 (89 ± 5)[b]	56 ± 28[c] (11 ± 5)[b]	95.6 ± 4.0
3. "Nondominant" (<90%)	8	8 (100)	64.1 ± 4.6	172 ± 30	175 ± 29 (97 ± 3)	3 ± 3 (3 ± 3)	766 ± 109 (91 ± 3)	56 ± 16 (9 ± 3)	96.5 ± 3.2
4. "Dominant" (<90%)	11	2 (18)	69.9 ± 6.1	61 ± 12[d]	11 ± 6[e] (24 ± 11)	68 ± 15[e] (76 ± 11)	136 ± 51[e] (26 ± 8)	394 ± 82[e] (74 ± 8)	92.4 ± 3.0

[a] The "dominant" and "nondominant" hemispheres were operationally defined on the basis of screening tests for AMPH-induced rotational behavior conducted before surgery (see text). The groups are subdivided as to whether the unilateral depletion in striatal dopamine (DA) was greater or less than 90% (relative to the unlesioned side). Animals with less than a 20% DA depletion were not included. The results are for male rats tested with 1.2 mg/kg AMPH, ip. Statistical analyses consisted of Kruskal–Wallis nonparametric analyses of variance, followed by two-tailed Mann–Whitney U tests where appropriate.

[b] Differs from group 1, $p < 0.02$, tests conducted on percent scores.

[c] Differs from group 1, $p < 0.05$.

[d] Differs from groups 1 and 3, $p < 0.02$.

[e] Differs from all other groups, $H = 17.2–22.1$, $p < 0.001$; Mann–Whitney U values from $p < 0.02$ to 0.001.

Many questions concerning brain asymmetry in both humans and nonhumans are unanswered. We know very little about the factors that determine whether a particular neural system will become lateralized. What factors influence the development of different patterns of lateralization? Of what importance is lateralization for normal brain function? We do not even have a complete catalog of which neural regions have asymmetries. For example, most work with humans has concentrated on asymmetries in cortical structures, even though many nonneocortical regions may also be lateralized (Ojemann and Ward, 1971; Oke *et al.*, 1978; Glick *et al.*, 1982).

One factor that is known to influence brain organization is gender (Raisman and Field, 1973; Greenough *et al.*, 1977; Gorski *et al.*, 1978). It has also been suggested that there are sex differences in cerebral lateralization in humans (Lansdell, 1962; McGlone, 1980). Therefore, it may be profitable to investigate sex differences in brain asymmetries in nonhuman animals. The study of sex differences in brain asymmetry not only may contribute to our knowledge of sex differences in brain organization in general, but may also provide insights into those factors (genetic, hormonal, and/or experiential) that influence the development of cerebral asymmetries and into the functional significance of lateralization. In the next section we discuss the evidence for sex differences in behavioral and brain asymmetries in both human and nonhuman animals. As before, evidence on humans is only briefly summarized because it has been extensively reviewed (McGlone, 1980).

III. Sex Differences in Behavioral and Brain Asymmetries

A. Human Beings

1. LATERALIZATION OF COGNITIVE FUNCTIONS

The idea that there are sex differences in human brain organization should not be surprising. There is no question that such sex differences exist. Those that are best documented and understood are differences in the organization of the hypothalamopituitary system (Goy and McEwen, 1980; Krieger and Hughes, 1980). Sex differences in the organization of parts of the hypothalamus certainly play a prominent role in sex differences in reproductive function and related hormonal control systems. A more recent and highly controversial suggestion is that "higher" neural regions are also sexually dimorphic in humans. Most attention has focused on the idea that there are sex differences in the lateralization of cognitive (verbal and spatial) abilities. This issue has been reviewed extensively, with peer commentary (McGlone, 1980). Some of this evidence is briefly summarized here.

The evidence that there are sex differences in human cerebral asymmetry is derived primarily from three types of studies: (*a*) anatomical observations; (*b*) clinical studies; and (*c*) normative studies (see McGlone, 1980, for a comprehensive list of references). The anatomical evidence for sex differences in brain laterality is limited. In their study of morphological asymmetries in the planum temporale and frontal operculum, Wada *et al.* (1975) commented on a number of trends in sex differences that did not quite reach statistical significance. However, they did find that significantly more women than men had a reversed asymmetry of the planum (i.e., larger right than left). Sex differences have been reported in the morphology of the corpus callosum (de Lacoste-Utamsing and Holloway, 1982). In women the splenium is larger and more bulbous than in men. These authors speculated that this sex difference in the organization of interhemispheric fibers may be related to sex differences in hemispheric specialization.

The most convincing evidence for sex differences in human cerebral asymmetry comes from studies of sex differences in the effects of lateralized brain damage (Lansdell, 1961, 1962; McGlone, 1977, 1978, 1980). Generally, left hemisphere lesions are more disruptive of language abilities in men than in women, and right hemisphere lesions are more disruptive of visuospatial abilities in men than women. On most verbal and nonverbal tasks there is a difference in the effects of right versus left hemisphere lesions in men, whereas lesions of either the right or left hemisphere often have the same effect on the performance of these tasks in women (also see Inglis and Lawson, 1981, 1982). For example, McGlone (McGlone and Fox, 1981, cited in McGlone, 1982) has found that, although there is a significant difference in the effects of a sodium amytal injection into left versus right internal carotid on oral fluency in men (a left-sided injection impairs oral fluency, whereas a right-sided injection does not), there is no difference between a left- and right-sided injection in women. In women both left and right injections mildly impair oral fluency to an equal extent.

The evidence for sex differences in cerebral asymmetry from normative studies is more tentative. Some authors report sex differences, and others do not (see McGlone, 1980, for references). For example, there are some reports that in a dichotic listening task men show a greater right ear advantage for verbal stimuli than do women. Men may also show a greater right visual field advantage for verbal material and greater left field advantage for nonverbal material in tachistoscopic tasks than do women.

Although the evidence for sex differences in human cerebral asymmetry is far from overwhelming, when sex differences have been found the direction of the difference has been remarkably consistent over a variety of experimental approaches. In summarizing this literature McGlone (1980) has hypothesized that in humans the male brain is more strongly lateralized than the female brain, at least for language and visuospatial abilities. Obviously, more research is required to resolve some of the controversies raised by opponents of this view (see peer commentaries on McGlone, 1980, 1982). Merely objecting to the idea will not promote advances in our understanding of human brain organization.

A new and positive development in the study of sex differences in human brain organization has come from a finding of Kimura (1980, 1981). Kimura (1981) found that, after a left anterior cortical lesion (presumably including Broca's area), the incidence of aphasia is similar in men and women. However, after a left posterior lesion (presumably involving Wernicke's area), there is a striking sex difference in the incidence of aphasia. Men show a significantly greater incidence of aphasia after posterior lesions than do women. In fact, women aphasics with restricted left posterior damage were only rarely found. Kimura (1981) concluded that, "while it is too early to reject the idea that there are sex differences in the lateral organization of speech, it is appropriate to consider alternative and adjunct hypotheses. One of these must be that the intra-hemispheric organization of speech differs between males and females [p. 8]." This hypothesis is supported by Mateer *et al.* (1982), who found sex differences in the disruptive effects of anterior versus posterior cortical stimulation on a naming task.

2. POSTURAL AND MOTOR ASYMMETRIES

Of particular relevance to this chapter are studies on sex differences in lateral preferences, particularly lateral preferences involving postural or motor asymmetries. This topic has been thoroughly reviewed by Porac and Coren (1981), who have also provided a considerable amount of new data on the subject. Most of the following discussion on sex differences in lateral preferences is derived from Porac and Coren's (1981) book.

A number of authors have noted that there are sex differences in the incidence of left- and right-handedness (for references, see Porac and Coren, 1981, p. 36). Typically, it is reported that a higher percentage of women than men are right-handed (i.e., there are more left-handed men). Porac and Coren (1981) have discussed some of the methodological problems of previous studies and have conducted a large study of lateral preferences in a heterogeneous population of 5147 people, in which they examined the incidence and strength of handedness, footedness, eyedness, and earedness. As some previous studies suggested, they found significant sex differences in all four indices of lateral preference (see Table 3.3, Porac and Coren, 1981, p. 36). Women as a group were more right-sided than men by approximately 9.3%. Specifically, women were more right-sided for handedness (90.1% of the female population were right-handed versus 86.5% of the male population), footedness (86.0 versus 76.7%), and earedness (64.6 versus 54.8%). It is interesting that there was a small sex difference in eyedness, which was reversed in direction.

More men than women were right-eyed (72.9% of men versus 69.1% of women).

In addition to simply scoring the incidence of right and left preferences Porac and Coren (1981) used an index to calculate the strength or consistency of lateral preferences. On all four indices women showed more strength or consistency in lateral preferences than men. Not only were women more strongly lateralized than men within each of the four indices of lateral preference (hand, foot, eye, ear), but they were also more "congruent" across the indices. A person is considered "congruent" when the direction of lateral preference (left or right) is the same on two different indices of lateral preference. Porac and Coren (1981, p. 44) found

> significant gender differences in five of six possible pairwise comparisons; females are more congruent for the pairings of hand–foot, hand–ear, foot–ear, and eye–ear, while males display greater congruency in the hand–eye pairing. The female group also shows a significantly higher incidence of total congruency in sidedness when all four indexes are considered together. Thus, females are not only more consistent in their within-index response patterns, but they are also more totally congruent in their across-index patterns than are males.

To summarize, there are reliable sex differences on a variety of measures of lateral preference in humans. Annett (1980) has commented that "the greater dextrality of females than males in manual skill is one of the few facts about sex differences in laterality that I regard as firmly established [p. 227]." The direction of the sex difference in lateral preferences stands in obvious contrast to the results of studies on sex differences in cognitive (language and spatial) abilities. In studies of cognitive abilities it has been suggested that women are less lateralized than men. However, using indices of motor asymmetries one would conclude that women are more lateralized than men. This observation is most interesting in light of the studies on sex differences in neural asymmetries and in postural and motor asymmetries in nonhuman animals. These studies are discussed in the following section.

B. Nonhuman Animals

In this section we review evidence for sex differences in behavioral and brain asymmetries in nonhuman animals. This may be rather foolhardy (or at least premature), since so little is generally known about asymmetries in animals and even less about sex differences in lateralization. Nevertheless, there is enough evidence to argue that gender is an important variable in studies of lateralization. When both male and female animals are examined, sex differences in laterality are frequently found. Evidence from studies using neurochemical, neuroanatomical, and behavioral indices are discussed in turn.

1. NEURAL ASYMMETRIES

a. Neurochemical Indices. We have already reviewed evidence for neurochemical and functional asymmetries in the mesostriatal DA system of rats. Most of this evidence comes from studies by Glick and coworkers (see Glick *et al.*, 1976, 1977a, for reviews). In reading this literature we were impressed by the fact that in all of Glick's experiments of which we were aware, female rats had been used. Because other studies (e.g., Becker and Ramirez, 1981) suggested sex differences in striatal DA activity we decided to compare AMPH-induced rotational behavior and the lateralization of striatal DA in male versus female rats (Robinson *et al.*, 1980). We found sex differences in both rotational behavior and the lateralization of striatal DA. As Glick *et al.* (1974) previously reported we found that in female rats striatal DA content was higher in the striatum located contralateral to the dominant direction of rotation. However, in male rats there was no statistically significant relationship between the dominant direction of rotational behavior and the lateralization of striatal DA content. Glick *et al.* (1980) also commented that in C57BL/6J mice the striatal DA asymmetry appears to be greater in females than in males. These studies suggest that there are sex differences in the lateralization of striatal DA, and a simplistic interpretation is that females are more lateralized than males. However, the exact nature of the difference between males and females is not known and requires further study. Many variables influence striatal DA content, major ones being the dose of AMPH used and the time after AMPH injection that an animal is killed. Whether these and other variables influence the distribution of striatal DA differently in males and females is not known.

Ross *et al.* (1981) used the 2-DG technique to study asymmetries in metabolic activity in various brain regions of male and female neonatal rats. They found striking sex differences in the uptake of 2-DG. Significant left–right asymmetries were found only in brain regions dissected from female rats. Females showed greater uptake of 2-DG into the right hippocampus, right diencephalon, left cortex, and left medulla–pons. Males showed no significant left–right differences. The sex differences in the left–right distribution of 2-DG were significant in all the brain regions studied, including the previously mentioned areas as well as the cerebellum and caudate–putamen. In addition, these left–right asymmetries in 2-DG uptake appear to change with age and to be related to whether a structure is left-biased or right-biased in a sexually dimorphic manner (Ross *et al.*, 1982).

b. Neuroanatomical Indices. We know of two reports of sex differences in a morphological asymmetry. In the first Diamond *et al.* (1981) reported that in young adult male rats the right posterior neocortex is thicker than the same region on the left. However, in females an opposite, but not statistically significant trend was found, with the left neocortex tending to be thicker than the right. More recently, Diamond *et al.* (1982) reported a sex difference in the direction of a morphological hippocampal asymmetry. In male rats the right hippocampus is thicker than the left, although this asymmetry is statistically significant at some ages and not others. In contrast, female rats have a significantly thicker left hippocampus than right hippocampus. The existence of sex differences in hippocampal anatomical asymmetries may be related to sex differences in the effects of lateralized hippocampal lesions on a place–navigation learning task (Therrien *et al.*, 1982).

2. POSTURAL AND MOTOR ASYMMETRIES

The majority of studies on lateralization in nonhuman animals have involved measures of postural or motor asymmetries. For example, the work of Glick and colleagues (1977a) relating rotational behavior to an asymmetry in the nigrostriatal DA system is briefly reviewed above. Most experimenters who measure lateral preferences in behavior are usually not interested primarily in the lateral preference per se but in what the lateral preference indicates about underlying neural activity. The assumption in these studies is that postural–motor asymmetries reflect an asymmetry in neural activity. If there are not peripheral structural asymmetries that cause a postural–motor asymmetry, then one can safely assume the postural–motor asymmetry is due to an asymmetry in neural activity. Of course, in studies of lateralization one must distinguish between transient asymmetries in motor output, which, for example, may occur in response to transient changes in the sensory environment, and more stable, enduring lateral preferences in behavior. Only these latter asymmetries are of relevance to studies of cerebral asymmetry. Stable lateral preferences in behavior may occur as left–right asymmetries in which the majority of a population prefers the left or right (e.g., human handedness), or the preference for left versus right may be more equally distributed in the population (e.g., handedness in mice; Collins, 1975).

Since lateral preferences in behavior are used as an index of neural asymmetry, it is desirable to know what neural system(s) produces the lateral preference in question. For some postural–motor asymmetries we know a great deal about the underlying neural asymmetry, as is the case for AMPH-induced rotational behavior (Pycock, 1980). Unfortunately, we know little about the underlying neural asymmetry for most lateral preferences in behavior, as is the case for handedness or turn preferences in an open field (Denenberg *et al.*, 1978).

In reviewing the literature we found that seven different types of postural–motor asymmetries have been used in studies of lateralization in nonhuman animals. These are (*a*) rotational behavior; (*b*) turn preference in an open field; (*c*) turn preference when the tail is pinched; (*d*) turn preference in a T maze; (*e*) side preference in a two-lever operant situa-

TABLE 5.2
Direction of Postural–Motor Asymmetries in Male and Female Rats as Indicated by a Variety of Indices

Test	Females		Males		Reference
	Left	Right	Left	Right	
1. Rotational behavior	(a) 272/602 (45%)	330/602 (55%)[a]	—	—	Glick and Ross (1981)
	(b) 170/344 (49%)	174/344 (51%)	158/265 (60%)	107/265 (40%)[a]	This chapter
2. Turn preference in open field	(a) —	—	−0.3862(H)[b]	—	Sherman *et al.* (1980)
	(b) −0.508(NH)[b]	—	—	—	Sherman *et al.* (1982)
	(c) −0.510(NH)[b]	—	−0.3768(H)[b]	—	This chapter
3. Side preference: tail pinch	(a) 2/20 (10%)	18/20 (90%)[a]	10/20 (50%)	10/20 (50%)	This chapter
4. Turn preference: T maze	(a) —	—	3/14 (21%)	11/14 (79%)	Cowey and Bozek (1974)
	(b) 8/14 (57)	6/14 (43%)	5/15 (33%)	10/15 (67%)	Robinson and Becker (1981)
	(c) 16/20 (80%)	4/20 (20%)[a]	14/20 (70%)	6/20 (30%)	This chapter
5. Side preference: two-lever bar press	(a)124/292 (42.5%)	168/292 (57.5%)[a]	—	—	Glick and Ross (1981a)
6. Tail deviation	(a) 45/117 (38%)	72/117 (62%)[a]	65/114 (57%)	49/114 (43%)	Ross *et al.* (1981)
	(b) 626/1084 (57.7%)	395/1084 (36.4%)[a]	591/1139 (51.9%)	418/1139 (36.7%)[a]	Denenberg *et al.* (1982)
7. Handedness (mice)	(50%)	(50%)	(50%)	(50%)	Collins (1968)

[a] Left differs from right, $p < 0.05$ (χ^2 test).
[b] Differs from zero ($p < 0.05$).

tion; (*f*) tail deviation in newborn rat pups; and (*g*) handedness (see Table 5.2). In nearly all of the cases where both males and females have been tested for these postural–motor asymmetries sex differences have been reported. There are two major questions concerning sex differences in these postural–motor asymmetries. One is whether there are consistent left or right asymmetries at the population level. For example, Denenberg (1981) has argued that there is a population bias to the right for motor asymmetries such as rotational behavior, whereas we have suggested that there may be many different patterns of lateralization within a population (Robinson and Becker, 1981). The second question concerns the strength of behavioral asymmetries. We discuss each of these questions in turn for each of the measures of lateral preference listed in Table 5.2.

a. Rotational Behavior. In their studies of AMPH-induced rotational behavior Glick and co-workers originally reported that there was no right–left population bias for the preferred direction of rotation. Although the direction an individual animal turned was consistent across different test sessions, approximately 50% turned predominantly left and 50% predominantly right. However, a more recent analysis of data accumulated over a number of years resulted in a report of a small, but statistically significant population bias to the right (Glick and Ross, 1981a; see Table 5.2). Nearly all of Glick's experiments have been performed with female rats only, and therefore this population bias is reported only for females.

In the past 2 to 3 years we have also tested quite a few rats for AMPH-induced rotational behavior. As shown in Table 5.2 (line 1b) we did not find a significant right-sided bias in female rats. However, the right bias in females reported by Glick and Ross (1981a) did not reach statistical significance until N exceeded 420 (S. D. Glick, personal communication), and we tested only 344 female rats. It is interesting that we did find a significant population bias in male rats: 60% turned preferentially to the left ($p < 0.05$).

In addition to questions concerning the directionality of behavioral asymmetries, another factor to consider is the strength or magnitude of asymmetries. For example, in humans the majority of both men and women are right-handed, but women appear to be more strongly right-handed than men (see Section II). There have now been a number of reports that intact (unlesioned) female rats show significantly more AMPH-induced rotational behavior than do male rats (Brass and Glick, 1981; Robinson *et al.*, 1980; Becker *et al.*, 1982). This sex difference in rotational behavior has been found in three independently raised rat populations [Fisher and Sprague–Dawley from Perfection Laboratories (Brass and Glick, 1981) and Sprague–Dawley-derived Holtzman rats (Robinson *et al.*, 1980; Becker *et al.*, 1982] and with a number of different doses of AMPH. However, there are also sex differences in the metabolism of

AMPH, so that when males and females are injected systemically with the same dose of AMPH the brain levels of AMPH are significantly lower in males than in females (Meyer and Lytle, 1978; Becker *et al.*, 1982). To control for this variable Becker *et al.* (1982) measured the whole-brain or striatal levels of AMPH in male and female rats after an ip injection of AMPH in doses ranging from 0.625 to 10 mg/kg. From this information they calculated doses that resulted in equal brain levels of AMPH in males and females at 5, 30, and 60 min after injection. Even when the brain levels of AMPH were equivalent, females showed significantly more net rotations than males.

However, the stage of the estrous cycle in female rats was also an important consideration because the amount of AMPH-induced rotational behavior varied across the estrous cycle. Female rats made more net rotations on the day of estrus than on diestrus 1. Males made significantly fewer net rotations than estrous, diestrous 2, or proestrous females but did not differ from diestrous 1 females. Therefore, if female rats are tested randomly with regard to the estrous cycle, there will usually be a smaller sex difference than seen between estrous females and males, and the amount of variation in the female group will probably be greater.

The preceding studies were all conducted with intact rats. We also tested male and female rats that had a unilateral 6-OHDA lesion of the substantia nigra for AMPH-induced rotational behavior. In all of these rats striatal DA levels were depleted by at least 70% on the lesioned side. The males were tested for 60 min on two different occasions, once with 1.2 mg/kg and once with 1.85 mg/kg of AMPH. The females were treated similarly, but were given 0.85 mg/kg of AMPH on one occasion and 1.5 mg/kg on the other. We know from the Becker *et al.* (1982) study that, when males are injected ip with 1.2 mg/kg, they have the same brain levels of AMPH as females given 0.85 mg/kg. Males and females given 1.85 and 1.5 mg/kg of AMPH, respectively, also have equivalent brain levels of AMPH. In this study no record was kept of the stage of the estrous cycle in the female rats. After being injected with 1.2 mg/kg of AMPH, male rats ($N = 12$) made an average of 223.1 ± 46.2 (SEM) net rotations, whereas females ($N = 14$) given 0.85 mg/kg made an average of 343.8 ± 40.1 net rotations ($t = 1.98$, $df = 24$, $p < 0.03$, one-tail; $p < 0.059$, two-tail). After being injected with 1.85 mg/kg of AMPH, male rats ($N = 12$) made an average of 229.2 ± 36.8 net rotations and, after receiving 1.5 mg/kg, females ($N = 11$) made an average of 395.5 ± 43.1 net rotations ($t = 2.95$, $df = 21$, $p < 0.01$, two-tail). Therefore, the sex difference in AMPH-induced rotational behavior is also seen in rats with unilateral damage to the mesostriatal DA system.

Brass and Glick (1981) reported an interesting reversal of the normal sex difference in rotational behavior seen with AMPH. They found that Sprague–Dawley (but not Fisher) male rats given a very large dose of apomorphine (10 mg/kg, ip) made more net rotations than females. Although the significance of this finding is not clear, Brass and Glick (1981) suggested that there may be a sex difference in the predominance of a pre- versus postsynaptic asymmetry.

Finally, the greater lateralization of females in AMPH-induced rotational behavior is not confined to rats. Female gerbils also show more rotational behavior than males (Glick *et al.*, 1977b).

b. Turn Preferences in an Open Field. Sherman *et al.* (1980) first reported that under certain conditions rats turn preferentially to the left or right in an open-field situation. In this experiment Sherman *et al.* (1980) placed a rat in the starting corner of an open-field apparatus. The corner was closed off from the rest of the field by an L-shaped barrier. When the barrier was removed, an observer simply recorded whether the rat first moved along the left- or right-hand wall. In the Sherman *et al.* (1980) study all the rats were male, some had been handled early in infancy and some had not, and some had cortical lesions and some had not. Directionality bias was calculated by a directionality score (DS); $DS = (R-L)/(R+L)^{1/2}$, where R and L represent the number of responses along the right and left walls, respectively. A positive number indicates a right bias and a negative number a left bias. Of interest here are the results obtained with control (unlesioned) animals. Nonhandled control rats showed no directionality bias. However, handled control rats showed a significant left-going bias in the open field (DS = −0.3862; see Table 5.2, line 2a).

In a more recent study Sherman *et al.* (1982) tested female rats in a similar experiment. In this experiment nonhandled females raised in standard laboratory cages were compared with handled females raised in an enriched environment. In contrast to the males, only the nonhandled females showed a significant left-going bias ($DS = -0.508$; see Table 5.2 line 2b).

We have completed an experiment in which handled and nonhandled males ($N=39$) and females ($N=40$) raised in standard laboratory cages were tested in an open-field situation similar to that described by Sherman *et al.* (1980). The directionality scores obtained (Table 5.2, line 2c) were very close to those reported by Sherman *et al.* (1980, 1982). Only handled males and nonhandled females showed a significant left-going bias. The nonhandled males and handled females did not have significant directionality scores.

It is difficult to quantify the strength of the turn preference in the open-field situation because each animal was given only four trials. From the directionality scores shown in Table 5.2 it can be seen that both Sherman *et al.* (1980, 1982) and our group (Table 5.2 line 2c) reported a directionality score that is larger for nonhandled females than for handled males. However, we did not find a statistically significant difference between the two scores. The males and females were run in two different studies by Sherman *et al.* (1980, 1982) and were therefore not directly compared.

c. Side Preferences When a Rat's Tail Is Pinched. We examined the direction and strength of the postural asymmetry produced when a paper clip is attached to a rat's tail (also see Myslobodsky and Braun, 1981). After a clip is attached to its tail a rat initially deviates to one side or the other and tries to remove the clip. We simply recorded the total number of seconds each animal deviated to the right or left in a 5-min test period. Both male and female rats were tested. Table 5.2 (line 3a) shows the number of males and females that spent more time turned either to the left or right. There was no right–left bias in the male population. Exactly 50% of the males were right-biased and 50% left-biased. However, the females showed a strong right-sided bias. Of the female rats (18 of 20), 90% spent more time deviated to the right than to the left (Table 5.2).

Further analysis also revealed a sex difference in the strength of the postural asymmetry induced by tail pinch when turning direction is disregarded. The percentage of the total test period (5 min) during which each animal was in a lateralized posture (i.e., turned either to the left or right) was calculated. We found that females spent significantly more time in a lateralized posture ($46.8 \pm 2.8\%$ of the test period) than did males ($27.3 \pm 3.2\%$; $t = 4.6$, $p < 0.0001$). Animals spent the remainder of the test period (53.2% for females and 72.7% for males) walking directly ahead, rearing, or standing still without deviating to either side.

d. Turn Preferences in a T Maze. In his review of asymmetries in rodents Denenberg (1981, p. 9) noted that Cowey and Bozek (1974) found that 11 of 14 male rats chose the right arm in a Y maze (Table 5.2, line 4a). Denenberg (1981) related this right bias to the right population bias reported by Glick and Ross (1981a) in AMPH-induced rotational behavior. We also looked at the distribution of right and left turns in a T maze in two separate experiments in which both male and female rats were tested. In the first (Robinson and Becker, 1981) we found no significant side preference, but we tested only 14 males and 15 females (Table 5.2, line 4b). In a second, independent experiment we did not find a significant left–right bias in males, although 70% of the males turned preferentially to the left. The female rats did show a significant leftward-turning bias in the T maze (Table 5.2, line 4c). If the results from the experiments shown on lines 4b and 4c of Table 5.2 are combined, we see that 24 of 34 female rats showed a left turn bias ($\chi^2 = 5.8$, $p < 0.05$), whereas only 19 of 35 male rats showed a leftward bias ($\chi^2 = 0.3$). These data do not support the idea that there is a right turn bias at the population level in a T maze.

We attempted to estimate the strength of the turn preference in the T maze (Table 5.2, line 4c) by calculating the percentage of total turns made in the dominant direction for each animal, regardless of preferred direction. There were no differences between males and females on this measure.

e. Side Preferences in a Two-Lever Operant Situation. Glick and colleagues have reported that, when given a choice of two levers to press in an operant learning situation, rats usually choose the lever on the same side as their dominant direction for rotational behavior. In individual studies the side preference in the operant chamber initially appeared to be approximately 50% left and 50% right (Glick *et al.*, 1977a). However, after accumulating data for a number of years Glick and Ross (1981a) reported a right bias in this task, corresponding to the right bias found in rotational behavior (Table 5.2, line 5). All of the rats reported by Glick and Ross (1981a) were females, and unfortunately we know of no data on males involving side preferences in a two-lever operant task.

f. Tail Deviation. Ross *et al.* (1981) reported that, when newborn rat pups are removed from the nest and placed on a flat, open surface, they adopt an asymmetric posture. Specifically, the tail is usually turned strongly to either the right or left. Ross *et al.* (1981) recorded this asymmetry in tail posture and found that it is positively correlated with the dominant direction of AMPH-induced rotation seen when the rats are tested as adults. It is interesting that they also found a significant sex difference in tail posture. Significantly more female rat pups had a rightward than a leftward bias in tail position (Table 5.2, line 6a). There was no significant right–left difference in tail posture in male rats.

This study was repeated by Denenberg *et al.* (1982). However, Denenberg *et al.* (1982) used Purdue–Wistar rats rather than the Sprague–Dawley rats used by Ross *et al.* (1981). Since they had earlier found a left bias in adult Purdue–Wistar rats in an open field (Sherman *et al.*, 1980), they thought that they might see a left bias in tail posture as well. Indeed, they found that both male and female rat pups had a significant left bias in tail posture (Table 5.2, line 6b). Therefore, Denenberg *et al.* (1982) suggested that there is a strain difference in the direction of the asymmetry in tail posture.

In their study Ross *et al.* (1981) found that females were more lateralized than males in the sense that there was a significant left–right asymmetry in females but not males. However, this does not directly address the question as to the strength of the asymmetry, regardless of left–right bias. Denenberg *et al.* (1982) did address this question and reported that females are significantly more lateralized than males on this measure. They found that both males and females had a leftward bias (Table 5.2, line 6b) but that females made a greater percentage of left responses than males. This was due to the male group having significantly more animals that did not show any behavioral asymmetry.

g. Handedness. Finally, there have been a number of studies of handedness (or pawedness) in a variety of species. For example, Collins (1977, for review) has extensively studied handedness in mice. Although species other than man have a preferred "hand" that is consistently used for a specific unimanual task, we do not know of any report of a significant left–right bias at the population level. In a large study of inbred mice Collins (1968, 1975, 1977) found that 50% of males and females preferred the left paw and 50% the right paw (Table 5.2, line 7).

Even though 50% of both male and female mice are left-handed and 50% right-handed there are striking sex differences in the degree of lateralization. By a variety of measures females are shown to be more strongly lateralized than males, whether they are left-handed or right-handed. Collins (1977) concluded, "Genetic differences giving rise to sex differences are associated with variation in the strength of expressed laterality. Female mice harbor a genetic complement associated with stronger expressed laterality. Male mice harbor a genetic complement associated with weaker expressed laterally [p. 147]."

IV. Conclusions

In this chapter we have reviewed evidence addressing two major questions. One question asks whether humans are unique in having lateralized brains, and the other whether there are sex differences in behavioral and brain asymmetries. After discussing these two questions, we close with a few comments about the possible relationships between asymmetries in humans and nonhumans.

A. Are Human Beings Unique in Having Lateralized Brains?

The answer to this question is obviously no. There are now many examples of lateralization in nonhuman animals. We reviewed evidence for (*a*) behavioral (postural–motor) asymmetries, from which an asymmetry in brain activity can be inferred; (*b*) functional asymmetries, for example, different behavioral effects depending on the side of the lesion; (*c*) neurochemical asymmetries; and (*d*) neuroanatomical asymmetries. Evidence of lateralization has been found in a variety of species, including birds, rats, cats, and great apes (for reviews, see Nottebohm, 1979; Walker, 1980; Denenberg, 1981). Even though there are many examples of lateralization in nonhuman animals we are still very ignorant about the topic. We have no idea how prevalent asymmetry is. Most research in this area is still at a stage of merely documenting the neural systems that are lateralized and determining which tests might be reliable indicators of lateralization.

B. Are There Sex Differences in Lateralization?

1. HUMAN BEINGS

For human beings the answer to this question must be somewhat tentative, particularly concerning the lateralization of cognitive (language and spatial) abilities. McGlone and others (see McGlone, 1980, for review) have suggested that males are more lateralized than females for verbal and spatial abilities, but this is still a controversial idea. It is obvious from the peer commentaries of the McGlone (1980) article that there is no unanimous agreement as to whether meaningful sex differences exist in human cerebral asymmetry. Whether sex differences in the effects of unilateral brain damage can be explained by sex differences in cerebral asymmetry or whether other sexually dimorphic patterns of cerebral organization are involved (e.g., Kimura, 1980, 1981) remains a topic for future research. Certainly, McGlone (1980) has compiled enough evidence that the idea of sex differences in human cerebral asymmetry must be taken seriously and investigated further.

The evidence for sex differences in brain morphology, physiology, and function in nonhuman animals is now irrefutable (Goy and McEwen, 1980). It is also evident that circulating gonadal hormones modulate extrahypothalamic neural activity in a sexually dimorphic manner (e.g., Becker and Ramirez, 1981) and may influence neuroplasticity (Loy and Milner, 1980; Yu, 1982). This would lead one to suspect that research on sex differences in human brain organization might be profitable. Traditionally, studies on human brain function have been performed with men. This is due partly to the fact that many early studies were carried out on war veterans with head injuries. The textbook picture of human brain organization is therefore one of the male brain and thus accounts for less than 50% of the population. Obviously, we need to understand the brain of the other 50% of the population as well. Research on sex differences in brain organization not only is of basic interest, but has clinical implications. To understand the various patterns of deficits seen following brain damage, to predict recovery of function, and to design therapeutic protocols we must understand the contribution of such variables as gender. The degree to which sex differences in the effects of brain damage are due to differences in the vascular system, the response to injury, interhemispheric differences or intrahemispheric differences, etc., remains to be determined.

A comparison of the direction of the sex difference in the lateralization of cognitive abilities versus postural–motor asymmetries is interesting. For cognitive abilities the evidence would suggest that men are more lateralized than women, whereas for postural–motor asymmetries men appear to be less lateralized than women. This raises the possibility that asymmetries in cognitive abilities and lateral preferences in behavior are due to asymmetries in different neural systems. Such a suggestion runs counter to the prevailing view that right-handedness is associated with left hemisphere specialization for language (e.g., Kimura, 1973b, 1976). However, one must keep in mind that the relationship between handedness and left hemisphere specialization for language is only correlative. We do not know the neural basis of handedness or left hemisphere specialization for language. There is still even considerable debate as to the relative influence of biological and environmental factors in handedness (see Morgan and Corballis, 1978, and associated peer commentaries). In addition, like right-handed individuals, the majority of left-handed individuals have left hemisphere dominance for verbal abilities, and a few right-handed individuals have right hemisphere speech (Milner, 1974). Therefore, the correlation between hemispheric specialization for language and handedness is far from perfect. We should consider the possibility that postural–motor asymmetries in humans are due to unknown asymmetries in subcortical brain regions rather than to the asymmetries in the neocortical structures implicated in language-related functions.

2. NONHUMAN ANIMALS

In nonhuman animals many of the studies on sex differences in lateralization have involved measures of postural–motor asymmetries. One question about postural–motor asymmetries concerns directionality: Is there a consistent right–left bias, and if so is it in the same direction in males and females? Denenberg (1981) previously suggested that there is a right-sided population bias for some postural–motor asymmetries. However, Table 5.2 shows that we found very little evidence for a consistent right-sided bias. Female rats had a statistically significant right bias on four different measures: (*a*) rotational behavior (Glick and Ross, 1981a); (*b*) side preference when tail is pinched (Section III, B, 2, c); (*c*) side preference in a two-lever operant situation (Glick and Ross, 1981a); and (*d*) tail deviation (Ross *et al.*, 1981). It should be noted that in an independent study of rotational behavior we did not find a significant right bias in the rotational behavior of female rats (Table 5.2, line 1b), although we tested fewer rats than Glick and Ross (1981a). On three measures a statistically significant left-sided population bias has been reported in female rats: (*a*) turn preference in an open field (Sherman *et al.*, 1982; Section III, B, 2, b); (*b*) turn preference in a T maze (section III,B,2,b); and (*c*) tail deviation (Denenberg *et al.*, 1982). It should be noted that the left bias in the T maze was not found in all experiments and that the left bias in tail deviation reported by Denenberg *et al.* (1982) is in the opposite direction of that reported by Ross *et al.* (1981). Denenberg *et al.* (1982) suggested that the reason for the difference between their study and that of Ross *et al.* (1981) is that different strains of rats were used. Since Purdue–Wistar rats show a left-going bias in the open field and Sprague–Dawley rats a right-going bias for rotational behavior, Denenberg *et al.* (1982) predicted that the two strains would show an opposite asymmetry in tail deviation. However, following this logic one would predict that Sprague–Dawley female rats would show a right-going bias in the open field, whereas we found a significant left-going bias (Table 5.2, line 2c).

In male rats the pattern of lateralization is slightly more consistent than that in females. Male rats had a statistically significant population bias to the left on three different measures: (*a*) rotational behavior (Section III, B, 2, a; S. D. Glick, personal communication), (*b*) turn preference in an open field (Sherman *et al.*, 1980; Section III, B, 2, b), and (*c*) tail deviation (Denenberg *et al.*, 1982). There was no significant right–left bias in a T maze or following tail pinch and, although Denenberg *et al.* (1982) found a left-going bias for tail deviation in males, Ross *et al.* (1981) did not. Measures of handedness have not shown a right–left population bias in either males or females. To summarize, females do not consistently show a right or left bias across different measures of postural–motor asymmetries and, if anything, males show a left-going bias, at least with some measures.

The lack of a reliable left–right difference at the population level across different measures of lateral preferences in behavior (especially in females) strikes a chord that is familiar in research on handedness in nonhuman primates. There are many studies which show that monkeys consistently use the same hand when performing a specific unimanual task. However, when faced with a different unimanual task monkeys are nearly as likely to use a different hand as the one used in the initial task (Lehman, 1980; Warren, 1977), although there may be a weak tendency to prefer the same hand (Lehman, 1980). The important point here is that different measures of postural–motor asymmetries, even if they attempt to measure the same asymmetry, may give very different answers concerning sidedness. In our present state of ignorance we often do not know which measures are meaningful and which are not. The reliability of many of the measures listed in Table 5.2 has not yet been established. In most cases we do not know the neural basis of lateral preferences in behavior. Finally, that different measures for lateral preferences often yield asymmetries in different directions suggests either that the neural asymmetries underlying different behavioral asymmetries are different or that in some studies the direction of lateral preferences is influenced by asymmetries in the testing environment. The latter possibility must be carefully avoided in studies of lateral preferences in behavior. In summary, we would stress caution in drawing any conclusions concerning left–right asymmetries. The available evidence certainly does not provide strong support for a consistent left or right bias at the population level.

Regardless of what the measures of lateral preference in behavior reflect about neural asymmetries, it is interesting that in the majority of cases in which both males and females have been tested sex differences were found. Often the direction of the lateral preference was in the opposite direction for males and females, or a significant asymmetry was found in only one sex. This is also true for some neurochemical asymmetries. For example, in their study on the uptake of 2-DG into brain Ross *et al.* (1981) found significant left–right asymmetries in female rats but not in males. Sex differences have also been reported in a right–left asymmetry in response to visual stimuli in chicks (Andrew *et al.*, 1982).

In addition to sex differences in the direction of behavioral and brain asymmetries we noticed consistent sex differences on the strength of lateral preferences in behavior. On nearly all measures of lateral preference, if there was a sex difference, it was in the direction of females being more lateralized than males. Of the seven different measures of postural–motor asymmetries listed in Table 5.2 females are significantly more lateralized than males on four measures (rotational behavior, side preferences when the tail is pinched, tail deviation, and handedness). On two of the measures (turn preference in open field and T maze) there is no statistical difference between males and females, although the directionality scores from the open field are in the direction of greater lateralization in females (Table 5.2, lines 2a, b, and c). There are no data available for making a comparison on a two-lever operant task. On none of the measures were males found to be more lateralized than females, with the single exception of apomorphine-induced rotational behavior in one strain of rats (Glick and Ross, 1981a).

On the basis of the available evidence we think that we can conclude with some confidence that there are sex differences in behavioral and brain asymmetries in nonhuman animals. The evidence certainly implicates gender as an important variable in studies of cerebral lateralization. The factors that account for these sex differences are not known. The existence of sexually dimorphic patterns of behavioral and brain asymmetries raises the possibility that genetic differences between males and females either directly influence the pattern of behavioral and brain asymmetries or indirectly influence lateralization, perhaps via sex differences in the hormonal environment. There are a few cases in which hormonal manipulations have altered the pattern of asymmetries (e.g., Diamond *et al.*, 1981; Myslobodsky and Braun, 1981). Of course, the contribution of experiential factors must also be considered.

C. Relationship between Asymmetries in Human Beings and Nonhuman Animals

It would be of great interest to relate findings on behavioral and brain asymmetries in nonhuman animals to the lateralization of cognitive abilities in humans. In fact, a number of authors have attempted to do just that. For example, in his review of hemispheric lateralization Denenberg (1981) concluded that, for all animals, "asymmetry is an initial condition of brains. The left hemisphere is preferentially biased to receive and transmit communication; the right is selectively set to deal with spatial and affective matters [p. 20]." Robinson and Coyle (1980) have suggested that their studies on the effects of right versus left cortical lesions on motor activity and cortical catecholamine concentrations may be related to "the catastrophic reactions associated with left hemisphere lesions and apathy, irritability and depression associated with right hemisphere lesions [in humans; p. 76]." Partly from experiments on asymmetries in the nigrostriatal DA system of rats, Glick *et al.* (1981) have speculated that "schizophrenia may be a disorder of a hyperactive dopaminergic reward pathway in the dominant hemisphere [p. 327]."

However, we must remember that the kinds of measures used in studies with humans are very different from those used in most studies of nonhumans. In humans the greatest emphasis by far has been on the well-known asymmetries in cognitive (language and spatial) abilities. Although there has been a considerable amount of work on postural–motor asymmetries, and sex differences in postural–motor asymmetries are well documented, these asymmetries are not usually stressed in the literature on cerebral asymmetry in humans. In contrast, most of the examples of lateralization in nonhuman animals rely on measures of motor performance of some kind. This includes measures not only of lateral preferences, but of open-field activity, running-wheel activity, performance in learning studies, etc.

Although it would be desirable to relate postural–motor asymmetries in nonhumans to cognitive asymmetries in humans, this may be inappropriate. One must consider the hypothesis that postural–motor asymmetries in nonhumans are related not to cognitive asymmetries in humans, but to postural–motor asymmetries in humans. The evidence for sex differences in behavioral and brain asymmetries supports this idea. The direction of the sex difference in lateralization is consistent when the comparison between humans and nonhumans concerns measures of postural–motor asymmetries in both. In both humans and nonhumans, females appear to be more strongly lateralized than males. However, for cognitive asymmetries in humans the weight of the evidence is that women are less lateralized than men (McGlone, 1980). Thus, the direction of the sex difference is in opposite directions when cognitive asymmetries in humans are compared with postural–motor asymmetries in nonhumans.

Unfortunately, we know very little about the neural basis of postural–motor asymmetries in any species. As mentioned earlier, right-handedness is often related to left hemisphere dominance of speech, but this is far from an obligatory relationship. Subcortical neural systems may also be very much involved in postural–motor asymmetries in humans, and the basal ganglia are obvious suspects. It is known that there are asymmetries in subcortical regions in humans (Ojemann and Ward, 1971; Oke *et al.*, 1978; Eidelberg and Galaburda, 1982). If we knew more about the neural basis of postural–motor asymmetries, we would be in a better position to speculate about the relationship between such asymmetries across species.

It is possible that in most animals there is nothing analogous to left hemisphere specialization in humans. The neural organization of the left hemisphere in humans may, in fact, be relatively unique or at least confined to primates (e.g., Petersen *et al.*, 1978). Whether this is true or whether neocortical specialization in humans represents an elaboration of the same functions found in homologous cortical regions in other animals remains to be determined. With the exception of Nottebohm's work with birds, the only study we are aware of in which anything akin to the complementary specialization of humans is reported for nonprimates is that of the Russian researcher Bianki (1981). Since experimenters in the West (e.g., Webster, 1972; Robinson and Voneida, 1973; Hamilton, 1977; Overmann and Doty, 1978; Kolb *et al.*, 1982b; although also see Dewson, 1977) have failed to reveal functional asymmetries comparable to those described by Bianki (1981), it is difficult to evaluate this report.

In conclusion, with a few exceptions (e.g., bird song) we know next to nothing about the factors that influence the development of lateralization, the functional significance of lateralization, or the consequences of disordered lateralization. However, this area of research holds much promise for furthering our understanding of brain organization and function. To understand the organization of specific neural systems it is obviously imperative to know whether the system is lateralized. Studies on lateralization may also contribute to our understanding of the function of neural systems in ways that are not possible by studying either side independently. For example, although the topic is very speculative at this point, it has been suggested that disorders in the pattern of asymmetries may contribute to a variety of behavioral and psychiatric problems (Gruzelier and Flor-Henry, 1979; Mandell and Knapp, 1979). Particular patterns of lateralization in specific neural systems may be required for optimal function (Glick *et al.*, 1977a). Finally, studies on lateralization in nonhuman animals should lead to the development of animal models of lateralization in humans. It is hoped that this will result in a better understanding of the variables that influence the development of lateralization. One variable that has been explored by Denenberg and coworkers (Denenberg, 1981) is early experience. The factor that we have primarily addressed here is gender. How these and other variables (e.g., age, hormones, experience) interact to produce the patterns of behavioral and brain asymmetries seen in adult animals is a topic for future research.

Acknowledgments

We thank E. S. Valenstein, B. Kolb, and I. Q. Whishaw for their helpful comments on an earlier draft of this chapter and Marilyn Hoy for typing the manuscript. Some of the research reported here was supported by Grant 16437 from the NINCDS. The work contributed by Jill B. Becker was supported by a postdoctoral fellowship from the NICHHD.

References

Amaducci, L., Sorbi, S., Albanese, A., and Gainotti, G. (1981). Choline acetyltransferase (ChAT) activity differs in the right and left human temporal lobes. *Neurology* **31,** 799–805.

Andén, N. E., Dahlström, A., Fuxe, K., and Larsson, K. (1966). Functional role of the nigro-neostriatal dopamine neurons. *Acta Pharmacol. Toxicol.* **24,** 263–274.

Andrew, R. J., Mench, J., and Rainey, C. (1982). Right–left asymmetry of response to visual stimuli in the domestic chick. *In* "Analysis of Visual Behavior" (D. J. Ingle, M. A. Goodale, and R. J. W. Mansfield, eds.), pp. 197–209. MIT Press, Cambridge, Massachusetts.

Annett, M. (1980). Sex differences in laterality-meaningfulness versus reliability. *Behav. Brain Sci.* **3,** 227–228.

Becker, J. B., and Ramirez, V. D. (1980). Dynamics of endogenous catecholamine release from brain fragments of male and female rats. *Neuroendocrinology* **31,** 18–25.

Becker, J. B., and Ramirez, V. D. (1981). Sex differences in the amphetamine-stimulated release of catecholamines from rat striatal tissue in vitro. *Brain Res.* **204,** 361–372.

Becker, J. B., Robinson, T. E., and Lorenz, K. A. (1982). Sex differences and estrous cycle variations in amphetamine-elicited rotational behavior. *Eur. J. Pharmacol.* **80,** 65–72.

Bianki, V. L. (1981). Lateralization of functions in the animal brain. *Int. J. Neurosci.* **15,** 37–47.

Brass, C. A., and Glick, S. D. (1981). Sex differences in drug-induced rotation in two strains of rats. *Brain Res.* **223,** 229–234.

Cain, D. P., and Wada, J. A. (1979). An anatomical asymmetry in the baboon brain. *Brain Behav. Evol.* **16,** 222–226.

Camp, D. M., Therrien, B. A., and Robinson, T. E. (1981). Spatial learning ability is related to an endogenous asymmetry in the nigrostriatal dopamine system in rats. *Soc. Neurosci. Abstr.* **7,** 455.

Christie, J. E., and Crow, T. J. (1971). Turning behavior as an index of the action of amphetamines and ephedrines on central dopamine-containing neurons. *Br. J. Pharmacol.* **43,** 658–667.

Collins, R. L. (1968). On the inheritance of handedness. I. Laterality in inbred mice. *J. Hered.* **59,** 9–12.

Collins, R. L. (1975). When left-handed mice live in right-handed worlds. *Science* **187,** 181–184.

Collins, R. L. (1977). Toward an admissible genetic model for the inheritance of the degree and direction of asymmetry. *In* "Lateralization in the Nervous System" (S. Harnad, L. Goldstein, R. W. Doty, J. Jaynes, and G. Krauthamer, eds.), pp. 137–150. Academic Press, New York.

Cowey, A., and Bozek, T. (1974). Contralateral "neglect" after unilateral dorsomedial prefrontal lesions in rats. *Brain Res.* **72,** 53–63.

de Lacoste-Utamsing, C., and Holloway, R. L. (1982). Sexual dimorphism in the human corpus callosum. *Science* **216,** 1431–1432.

Denenberg, V. H. (1981). Hemispheric laterality in animals and the effects of early experience. *Behav. Brain Sci.* **4,** 1–49.

Denenberg, V. H., Garbanati, J., Sherman, G., Yutzey, D. A., and Kaplan, R. (1978). Infantile stimulation induces brain lateralization in rats. *Science* **201,** 1150–1152.

Denenberg, V. H., Hofmann, M., Garbanati, J. A., Sherman, G. F., Rosen, G. D., and Yutzey, D. A. (1980). Handling in infancy, taste aversion, and brain laterality in rats. *Brain Res.* **200,** 123–133.

Denenberg, V. H., Rosen, G. D., Hofmann, M., Gall, J., Stockler, J., and Yutzey, D. A. (1982). Neonatal postural asymmetry and sex differences in the rat. *Dev. Brain Res.* **2,** 417–419.

Dewson, J. H. (1977). Preliminary evidence of hemispheric asymmetry of auditory function in monkeys. *In* "Lateralization in the Nervous System" (S. Harnad, L. Goldstein, R. W. Doty, J. Jaynes, and G. Krauthamer, eds.), pp. 63–71. Academic Press, New York.

Dewson, J. H. (1978). Some behavioral effects of removal of superior temporal cortex in the monkey. *In* "Recent Advances in Primatology" (D. Chivers and J. Herbert, eds.), Vol. 1, pp. 763–768. Academic Press, New York.

Diamond, M. C., Johnson, R. E., and Ingham, C. A. (1975). Morphological changes in the young, adult and aging rat cerebral cortex, hippocampus and diencephalon. *Behav. Biol.* **14,** 163–174.

Diamond, M. C., Dowling, G. A., and Johnson, R. E. (1981). Morphologic cerebral cortical asymmetry in male and female rats. *Exp. Neurol.* **71,** 261–268.

Diamond, M. C., Murphy, G. M., Jr., Akiyama, K., and Johnson, R. E. (1982). Morphologic hippocampal asymmetry in male and female rats. *Exp. Neurol.* **76,** 553–565.

Efron, R. (1963a). The effect of handedness on the perception of simultaneity and temporal order. *Brain* **86,** 261–294.

Efron, R. (1963b). Temporal perception, aphasia and déja vu. *Brain* **86,** 403–424.

Eidelberg, D., and Galaburda, A. M. (1982). Symmetry and asymmetry in the human posterior thalamus. I. Cytoarchitectonic analysis in normal persons. *Arch. Neurol. (Chicago)* **39,** 325–332.

Falzi, G., Perrone, P., and Vignolo, L. A. (1982). Right–left asymmetry in anterior speech region. *Arch. Neurol. (Chicago)* **39,** 239–240.

Frumkin, L. R., and Grim, P. (1981). Is there pharmacological asymmetry in the human brain? An hypothesis for the differential hemispheric action of barbiturates. *Int. J. Neurosci.* **13,** 187–197.

Galaburda, A. M., LeMay, M., Kemper, T. L., and Geschwind, N. (1978). Right–left asymmetries in brain. *Science* **199,** 852–856.

Geschwind, N. (1972). Language and the brain. *Sci. Am.* **226,** 76–83.

Geschwind, N., and Levitsky, W. (1968). Human brain: Left–right asymmetries in temporal speech region. *Science* **161,** 186–187.

Gesell, A. (1938). The tonic neck reflex in the human infant. *Pediatrics* **13,** 455–464.

Gesell, A., and Ames, L. B. (1947). The development of handedness. *Genet. Psychol.* **70,** 155–175.

Glick, S. D., and Cox, R. D. (1976). Differential effects of unilateral and bilateral caudate lesions on side preferences and timing behavior in rats. *J. Comp. Physiol. Psychol.* **90,** 528–535.

Glick, S. D., and Cox, R. D. (1978). Nocturnal rotation in normal rats: Correlation with amphetamine-induced rotation and effects of nigro-striatal lesions. *Brain Res.* **150,** 149–161.

Glick, S. D., and Ross, D. A. (1981a). Right-sided population bias and lateralization of activity in normal rats. *Brain Res.* **205,** 222–225.

Glick, S. D., and Ross, D. A. (1981b). Lateralization of function in the rat brain. Basic mechanisms may be operative in humans. *Trends in Neurosci.* **4,** 196–199.

Glick, S. D., Jerussi, T. P., Waters, D. H., and Green, J. P. (1974). Amphetamine-induced changes in striatal dopamine and acetylcholine levels and relationship to rotation (circling behavior) in rats. *Biochem. Pharmacol.* **23,** 3223–3225.

Glick, S. D., Jerussi, T. P., and Fleisher, L. N. (1976). Turning in circles: The neuropharmacology of rotation. *Life Sci.* **18,** 889–896.

Glick, S. D., Jerussi, T. P., and Zimmerberg, B. (1977a). Behavioral and neuropharmacological correlates of nigrostriatal asymmetry in rats. *In* "Lateralization in the Nervous System" (S. Harnad, L. Goldstein, R. W. Doty, J. Jaynes, and G. Krauthamer, eds.), pp. 213–249. Academic Press, New York.

Glick, S. D., Zimmerberg, B., and Jerussi, T. P. (1977b). Adaptive significance of laterality in the rodent. *Ann. N. Y. Acad, Sci.* **299,** 180–185.

Glick, S. D., Meibach, R. C., Cox, R. D., and Maayani, S. (1979). Multiple and interrelated functional asymmetries in rat brain. *Life Sci.* **25,** 395–400.

Glick, S. D., Schonfeld, A. R., and Strumpf, A. J. (1980). Sex differences in brain asymmetry of the rodent. *Behav. Brain Sci.* **3,** 236.

Glick, S. D., Weaver, L. M., and Meibach, R. C. (1981). Amphetamine enhancement of reward asymmetry. *Psychopharmacology (Berlin)* **73,** 323–327.

Glick, S. D., Ross, D. A., and Hough, L. B. (1982). Lateral asymmetry of neurotransmitters in human brain. *Brain Res.* **234,** 53–64.

Gorski, R. A., Gordon, J. H., Shryne, J. E., and Southham, A. M. (1978). Evidence for a morphological sex difference within the medial preoptic area of the rat brain. *Brain Res.* **148,** 333–346.

Goy, R. W., and McEwen, B. S. (1980). "Sexual Differentiation of the Brain." MIT Press, Cambridge, Mass.

Greenough, W., Carter, C. S., Steerman, C., and DeVoogd, T. (1977). Sex differences in dendritic patterns in hamster preoptic area. *Brain Res.* **126,** 63–72.

Greenstein, S., and Glick, S. D. (1975). Improved automated apparatus for recording rotation (circling behavior) in rats or mice. *Pharmacol., Biochem. Behav.* **3,** 507–510.

Groves, C. P., and Humphrey, N. K. (1973). Asymmetry in gorilla skulls: Evidence of lateralized brain function? *Nature (London)* **244,** 53–54.

Gruzelier, J., and Flor-Henry, P. (1979). "Hemispheric Asymmetries of Function in Psychopathology." Elsevier, Amsterdam.

Gur, R. C., Packer, I. K., Hungerbuhler, J. P., Reivich, M., Obrist, W. D., Amarnek, W. S., and Sackheim, H. A. (1980). Differences in the distribution of gray and white matter in human cerebral hemispheres. *Science* **207,** 1226–1228.

Hamilton, C. R. (1977). Investigations of perceptual and mnemonic lateralization in monkeys. *In* "Lateralization in the Nervous System" (S. Harnad, L. Goldstein, R. W. Doty, J. Jaynes, and G. Krauthamer, eds.), pp. 45–62. Academic Press, New York.

Hecaen, H., and Albert, M. L. (1978). "Human Neuropsychology." Wiley, New York.

Heilman, K. M., and Valenstein, E. (1979). "Clinical Neuropsychology." Oxford Univ. Press, New York.

Herron, J., ed. (1980). "Neuropsychology of Left-Handedness." Academic Press, New York.

Howard, K. J., Rogers, L. J., and Boura, A. L. A. (1980). Functional lateralization of the chicken forebrain revealed by use of intracranial glutamate. *Brain Res.* **188,** 369–382.

Inglis, J., and Lawson, J. S. (1981). Sex differences in the effects of unilateral brain damage on intelligence. *Science* **212,** 693–695.

Inglis, J., and Lawson, J. S. (1982). Sex differences in the functional asymmetry of the damaged brain. *Behav. Brain Sci.* **5,** 307–310.

Jerussi, T. P., and Glick, S. D. (1974). Amphetamine-induced rotation in rats without lesions. *Neuropharmacology* **13,** 283–286.

Jerussi, T. P., and Glick, S. D. (1975). Apomorphine-induced rotation in normal rats and interaction with unilateral caudate lesions. *Psychopharmacologia* **40,** 329–334.

Jerussi, T. P., and Glick, S. D. (1976). Drug-induced rotation in rats without lesions: Behavioral and neurochemical indices of a normal asymmetry in nigro-striatal function. *Psychopharmacology (Berlin)* **47,** 249–260.

Kelly, P. H., and Moore, K. E. (1977). Mesolimbic dopamine neurons: Effects of 6-hydroxydopamine induced destruction and receptor blockade on drug-induced rotation of rats. *Psychopharmacology (Berlin)* **55,** 35–41.

Kimura, D. (1973a). The asymmetry of the human brain. *Sci. Am.* **228,** 70–78.

Kimura, D. (1973b). Manual activity during speaking. I. Right handers. *Neuropsychologia* **11,** 45–50.

Kimura, D. (1976). The neural basis of language qua gesture. *In* "Studies in Neurolinguistics" (H. Avakian-Whitaker and H. A. Whitaker, eds.), Vol. 2, pp. 145–156. Academic Press, New York.

Kimura, D. (1980). Sex differences in intrahemispheric organization of speech. *Behav. Brain Sci.* **3,** 240–241.
Kimura, D. (1981). "A Sex Difference in Speech Organization within the Left Hemisphere," Res. Bull. No. 548. University of Western Ontario, London, Ontario.
Kimura, D., and Archibald, Y. (1974). Motor functions of the left hemisphere. *Brain* **97,** 337–350.
Kolb, B., and Whishaw, I. Q. (1980). "Fundamentals of Human Neuropsychology." Freeman, San Francisco, California.
Kolb, B., and Whishaw, I. Q. (1981). Neonatal frontal lesions in the rat: Sparing of learned but not species-typical behaviors in the presence of reduced brain weight and cortical thickness. *J. Comp. Physiol. Psychol.* **95,** 863–879.
Kolb, B., and Whishaw, I. Q. (1983). Problems and principles underlying inter-species comparisons. *In* "Behavioral Approaches to Brain Research" (T. E. Robinson, ed.), pp. 141–211. Oxford Univ. Press, London and New York.
Kolb, B., Sutherland, R. J., Nonneman, A. J., and Whishaw, I. Q. (1982a). Asymmetry in the cerebral hemispheres of the rat, mouse, rabbit and cat: The right hemisphere is larger. *Exp. Neurol.* **78,** 348–359.
Kolb, B., Sutherland, R. J., and Whishaw, I. Q. (1982b). A comparison of the contributions of the frontal and parietal association cortex to spatial localization in rats. *J. Comp. Physiol. Psychol.* (in press).
Krieger, D. T., and Hughes, J. C. (1980). "Neuroendocrinology." Sinauer Assoc., Sunderland, Massachusetts.
Kubos, K. L., Pearlson, G. D., and Robinson, R. G. (1982). Intracortical kainic acid induces an asymmetrical behavioral response in the rat. *Brain Res.* **239,** 303–309.
Lansdell, H. (1961). The effect of neurosurgery on a test of proverbs. *Am. Psychol.* **16,** 448.
Lansdell, H. (1962). A sex difference in effect of temporal lobe neurosurgery on design preference. *Nature (London)* **194,** 852–854.
Lehman, R. A. W. (1980). The handedness of rhesus monkeys. III. Consistency within and across activities. *Cortex* **16,** 197–204.
LeMay, M. (1976). Morphological cerebral asymmetries of modern man, fossil man and nonhuman primates. *Ann. N. Y. Acad. Sci.* **280,** 349–366.
LeMay, M., and Geschwind, N. (1975). Hemispheric differences in the brains of great apes. *Brain Behav. Evol.* **11,** 48–52.
Liederman, J., and Coryell, J. (1981). Right-hand preference facilitated by rightward turning biases during infancy. *Dev. Psychobiol.* **14,** 439–450.
Loy, R., and Milner, T. A. (1980). Sexual dimorphism in extent of axonal sprouting in rat hippocampus. *Science* **208,** 1282–1284.
McGlone, J. (1977). Sex differences in the cerebral organization of verbal functions in patients with unilateral brain lesions. *Brain* **100,** 775–793.
McGlone, J. (1978). Sex differences in functional brain asymmetry. *Cortex* **14,** 122–128.
McGlone, J. (1980). Sex differences in human brain asymmetry: A critical survey. *Behav. Brain Sci.* **3,** 215–263.
McGlone, J. (1982). Faulty logic fuels controversy. *Behav. Brain Sci.* **5,** 312–315.
Mandell, A. J., and Knapp, S. (1979). Asymmetry and mood, emergent properties of serotonin regulation. *Arch. Gen. Psychiatry* **36,** 909–916.
Mateer, C., and Kimura, D. (1977). Impairment of nonverbal oral movements in aphasia. *Brain Lang.* **4,** 262–276.
Mateer, C., Polen, S. B., and Ojemann, G. A. (1982). Sexual variation in cortical localization of naming as determined by stimulation mapping. *Behav. Brain Sci.* **5,** 310–311.
Meyer, E. M., Jr., and Lytle, L. D. (1978). Sex related differences in the physiological disposition of amphetamine and its metabolites in the rat. *Proc. West. Pharmacol. Soc.* **21,** 313–316.

Michel, G. F. (1981). Right handedness: A consequence of infant supine head-orientation preference? *Science* **212,** 685–687.
Milner, B. (1974). Hemispheric specialization: Scope and limits. *In* "The Neurosciences: Third Study Program" (F. O. Schmitt and F. G. Worden, eds.), pp. 75–89. MIT Press, Cambridge, Massachusetts.
Moore, K. E., and Kelly, P. H. (1978). Biochemical pharmacology of mesolimbic and mesocortical dopaminergic neurons. *In* "Psychopharmacology: A Generation of Progress" (M. A. Lipton, A. DiMascio, and K. F. Killam, eds.), pp. 221–234. Raven Press, New York.
Morgan, M. J., and Corballis, M. C. (1978). On the biological basis of human laterality. II. The mechanisms of inheritance. *Behav. Brain Sci.* **1,** 270–336.
Myslobodsky, M. S., and Braun, H. (1981). Does postural asymmetry indicate directionality of rotation in rats: Role of sex and handling. *Behav. Brain Res.* **2,** 113–117.
Nottebohm, F. (1979). Origins and mechanisms in the establishment of cerebral dominance. *In* "Handbook of Behavioral Neurobiology" (M. S. Gazzaniga, ed.), pp. 295–344. Plenum, New York.
Nottebohm, F. (1980). Brain pathways for vocal learning in birds: A review of the first 10 years. *Prog. Psychobiol. Physiol. Psychol.* **9,** 85–124.
Nottebohm, F. (1981). Laterality, seasons and space govern the learning of a motor skill. *Trends Neurosci.* **4,** 104–106.
Ojemann, G. A., and Ward, A. A. (1971). Speech representation in ventrolateral thalamus. *Brain* **94,** 669–680.
Oke, A., Keller, R., Mefford, I., and Adams, R. N. (1978). Lateralization of norepinephrine in human thalamus. *Science* **200,** 1411–1413.
Oke, A., Lewis, R., and Adams, R. N. (1980). Hemispheric asymmetry of norepinephrine distribution in rat thalamus. *Brain Res.* **188,** 269–272.
Overman, W. H., Jr., and Doty, R. W. (1978). Hemispheric specialization of facial recognition in man but not in macaque. *Soc. Neurosci. Abstr.* **4,** 78.
Pearlson, G. D., and Robinson, R. G. (1981). Suction lesions of the frontal cerebral cortex in the rat induce asymmetrical behavioral and catecholaminergic responses. *Brain Res.* **218,** 233–242.
Petersen, M. R., Beecher, M. D., Zoloth, S. R., Moody, D. B., and Stebbins, W. C. (1978). Neural lateralization of species-specific vocalizations by Japanese macaques (*Macaca fuscata*). *Science* **202,** 324–327.
Peterson, G. M. (1934). Mechanisms of handedness in the rat. *Comp. Psychol. Monogr.* **9,** 1–67.
Peterson, G. M., and Devine, J. V. (1963). Transfers in handedness in the rat resulting from small cortical lesions after limited forced practice. *J. Comp. Physiol. Psychol.* **56,** 752–756.
Peterson, G. M., and Fracarol, La C. (1938). The relative influence of the locus and mass of destruction upon the control of handedness by the cerebral cortex. *J. Comp. Neurol.* **68,** 173–190.
Porac, C., and Coren, S. (1981). "Lateral Preferences and Human Behavior." Springer-Verlag, New York.
Pycock, C. J. (1980). Turning behavior in animals. *Neuroscience* **5,** 461–514.
Pycock, C. J., and Marsden, C. D. (1978). The rotating rodent: A two component system? *Eur. J. Pharmacol.* **47,** 167–175.
Raisman, G., and Field, P. M. (1973). Sexual dimorphism in the neuropil of the preoptic area of the rat and its dependence on neonatal androgen. *Brain Res.* **54,** 1–29.
Robinson, J. S., and Voneida, T. J. (1973). Hemisphere differences in cognitive capacity in the split-brain cat. *Exp. Neurol.* **38,** 123–134.
Robinson, R. G. (1979). Differential behavioral and biochemical effects of right and left hemispheric cerebral infarction in the rat. *Science* **205,** 707–710.
Robinson, R. G., and Coyle, J. T. (1980). The differential effect of right versus left hemi-

spheric cerebral infarction on catecholamines and behavior in the rat. *Brain Res.* **188,** 63–78.

Robinson, R. G., and Stitt, T. G. (1981). Intracortical 6-hydroxydopamine induces an asymmetrical behavioral response in the rat. *Brain Res.* **213,** 387–388.

Robinson, T. E., and Becker, J. B. (1981). Variation in lateralization: Selected samples do not a population make. *Behav. Brain Sci.* **4,** 34–35.

Robinson, T. E., and Becker, J. B. (1983). The rotational behavior model: Asymmetry in the effects of unilateral 6-OHDA lesions of the substantia nigra in rats. *Brain Res.* **264,** 127–131.

Robinson, T. E., Becker, J. B., and Ramirez, V. D. (1980). Sex differences in amphetamine-elicited rotational behavior and the lateralization of striatal dopamine in rats. *Brain Res. Bull.* **5,** 539–545.

Rogers, L. J. (1981). Environmental influences on brain lateralization. *Behav. Brain Sci.* **4,** 35–36.

Rogers, L. J., and Anson, J. M. (1979). Lateralization of function in the chicken fore-brain. *Pharmacol., Biochem. Behav.* **10,** 679–686.

Ross, D. A., Glick, S. D., and Meibach, R. C. (1981). Sexually dimorphic brain and behavioral asymmetries in the neonatal rat. *Proc. Nat. Acad. Sci. U.S.A.* **78,** 1958–1960.

Ross, D. A., Glick, S. D., and Meibach, R. C. (1982). Sexually dimorphic cerebral asymmetries in 2-deoxy-d-glucose uptake during post-natal development of the rat: Correlations with age and relative brain activity. *Brain Res.* **3,** 341–347.

Rossor, M., Garrett, N., and Iversen, L. (1980). No evidence for lateral asymmetry of neurotransmitters in post-mortem human brain. *J. Neurochem.* **35,** 743–745.

Rothman, A. H., and Glick, S. D. (1976). Differential effects of unilateral and bilateral caudate lesions on side preference and passive avoidance behavior in rats. *Brain Res.* **118,** 361–369.

Schaeffer, A. A. (1928). Spiral movements in man. *J. Morphol. Physiol.* **45,** 293–398.

Schwartz, J., and Tallal, P. (1980). Rate of acoustic change may underlie hemispheric specialization for speech perception. *Science* **207,** 1380–1381.

Sherman, G. F., Garbanati, J. A., Rosen, G. D., Yutzey, D. A., and Denenberg, V. H. (1980). Brain and behavioral asymmetries for spatial preference in rats. *Brain Res.* **192,** 61–67.

Sherman, G. F., Garbanati, J. A., Rosen, G. D., Hofmann, M., Yutzey, D. A., and Denenberg, V. H. (1983). Lateralization of spatial preference in the female rat. *Life Sci.* (in press).

Sperry, R. W. (1974). Lateral specialization in the surgically separated hemispheres. *In* "The Neurosciences: Third Study Program" (F. O. Schmitt and F. G. Worden, eds.), pp. 5–19. MIT Press, Cambridge, Massachusetts.

Starr, M. S., and Kilpatrick, I. C. (1981). Bilateral asymmetry in brain GABA function? *Neurosci. Lett.* **25,** 167–172.

Stokes, K. A., and McIntyre, D. C. (1981). Lateralized asymmetrical state-dependent learning produced by kindled convulsions from the rat hippocampus. *Physiol. Behav.* **26,** 163–169.

Therrien, B. A., Camp, D. M., and Robinson, T. E. (1982). Sex differences in the effects of unilateral hippocampal lesions on spatial learning. *Soc. Neurosci. Abstr.* **8,** 312.

Turkewitz, G. (1977). The development of lateral differentiation in the human infant. *Ann. N. Y. Acad. Sci.* **299,** 309–318.

Uguru-Okorie, D. C., and Arbuthnott, G. W. (1981). Altered paw preference after unilateral 6-hydroxydopamine injections into lateral hypothalamus. *Neuropsychologia* **19,** 463–467.

Ungerstedt, U. (1971a). Striatal dopamine release after amphetamine or nerve degeneration revealed by rotational behavior. *Acta Physiol. Scand.* **82,** Suppl. 367, 49–68.

Ungerstedt, U. (1971b). Postsynaptic supersensitivity after 6-hydroxydopamine induced degeneration of the nigrostriatal dopamine system. *Acta Physiol. Scand.* **82,** Suppl. 367, 69–92.

Ungerstedt, U., and Arbuthnott, G. W. (1970). Quantitative recording of rotational behavior in rats after 6-hydroxydopamine lesions of the nigrostriatal dopamine system. *Brain Res.* **24,** 485–493.

Ungerstedt, U., Butcher, L. L., Butcher, S. G., Andén, N. E., and Fuxe, K. (1969). Direct chemical stimulation of dopaminergic mechanisms in the neostriatum of the rat. *Brain Res.* **14,** 461–471.

Valdes, J. J., Mactutus, C. F., Cory, R. N., and Cameron, W. R. (1981). Lateralization of norepinephrine, serotonin and choline uptake into hippocampal synaptosomes of sinistral rats. *Physiol. Behav.* **27,** 381–383.

Valdes, J. J., Hartwell, S. W., Sato, S. M., and Frazier, J. M. (1982). Lateralization of zinc in rat brain and its relationship to a spatial behavior. *Pharmacol., Biochem. Behav.* **16,** 915–917.

Wada, J. A., Clarke, R., and Hamm, A. (1975). Cerebral hemispheric asymmetry in humans. *Arch. Neurol.* (*Chicago*) **32,** 239–246.

Walker, S. F. (1980). Lateralization of functions in the vertebrate brain: A review. *Br. J. Psychol.* **71,** 329–367.

Warren, J. M. (1958). The development of paw preferences in cats and monkeys. *J. Genet. Psychol.* **93,** 229–236.

Warren, J. M. (1977). Handedness and cerebral dominance in monkeys. *In* "Lateralization in the Nervous System" (S. Harnad, L. Goldstein, R. W. Doty, J. Jaynes, and G. Krauthamer, eds.), pp. 151–172. Academic Press, New York.

Waziri, R. (1980). Lateralization of neuroleptic-induced dyskinesia indicates pharmacologic asymmetry in the brain. *Psychopharmacology* (*Berlin*) **68,** 51–53.

Webster, W. G. (1972). Functional asymmetry between the cerebral hemispheres of the cat. *Neuropsychologia* **10,** 75–87.

Webster, W. G., and Webster, I. H. (1975). Anatomical asymmetry of the cerebral hemispheres of the cat brain. *Physiol. Behav.* **14,** 867–869.

Witelson, S. F. (1977). Anatomic asymmetry in the temporal lobes: its documentation, phylogenesis and relationship to functional asymmetry. *Ann. N. Y. Acad. Sci.* **299,** 328–354.

Yeni-Komshian, G. H., and Benson, D. A. (1976). Anatomical study of cerebral asymmetry in the temporal lobe of humans, chimpanzees and rhesus monkeys. *Science* **192,** 387–389.

Yu, W.-H. A. (1982). Sex difference in the regeneration of the hypoglossal nerve in rats. *Brain Res.* **238,** 404–406.

6: Gyratory and Cursive Epilepsy

RUGGERO G. FARIELLO and ANAND MEHENDALE

Department of Neurology
Jefferson Medical College
Philadelphia, Pennsylvania

Neurology Section
Audie Murphy Veterans
Memorial Hospital
San Antonio, Texas

I. Historical Note 129
II. Gyratory Epilepsy 131
A. Clinical Features 131
B. Electroencephalographic Correlates 136
C. Treatment 136
D. Summary of Clinical and Electrographic Features 137
E. Experimental Data on Sustained Turning Behavior 137
F. Extrapolation of Experimental Data to the Clinical Syndrome of Gyratory Epilepsy 139
III. Cursive Epilepsy 141
A. Clinical Features 141
B. Electroencephalographic Abnormalities 143
C. Psychiatric Aspects 143
D. Differential Diagnosis 144
E. Experimental Data on Running 145
IV. Summary and Conclusions 145
References 146

I. Historical Note

In the language of Western civilization the word *epilepsy* is derived from the Greek επὶ λάμβανω/ληπτός meaning "to be seized upon." In Sanskrit the word *mirghi* means "seizure disorder" or "being possessed by a spirit." No pathological condition more than epilepsy has been the object of human fantasy since the dawning of civilization. The repetitive occurrence of trancelike and convulsive episodes in an otherwise normal individual has kindled the imagination of observers and has been taken

HEMISYNDROMES:
Psychobiology, Neurology,
Psychiatry

ISBN 0-12-512460-0

as irrefutable proof of the dual (material and immaterial) nature of humankind. Thus, for millennia, people affected with epilepsy have been considered to be souls bridging the gap between human being and deity of either good or evil nature. Throughout the period of prelogical cultures and well into the premodern era, the concept of a supernatural origin of epileptic attacks seemed to be substantiated by people in whom, during a spell, odd and complex motor activity occurred, at times requiring fine muscle coordination and even unusual skills. When these nonconvulsive phenomena were associated not with a total loss of consciousness but, on the contrary, with verbalization, hallucinatory experiences, and mild cognitive disturbances, it is quite understandable that they were mistaken for signs of privileged communication with spirits. After all, the traditional definition of epilepsy was based on two cardinal signs: convulsions of the whole body and loss of consciousness. Thus, it is not surprising that such episodes of partial seizures were confused, even by the most scientifically oriented minds, with psychiatric disturbances, evil possession, or religious experiences. Given this historical background, it is quite remarkable that as early as 1581 Thomas Erastus clearly recognized the epileptic nature of these partial complex spells. Indeed, in his work, "Comitiis Montani Vicentini", published in Basel, he firmly established the concept of partial epilepsy, which he called the imperfect form, as distinguished from the classical, traditional, or perfect form of the grand mal type. Among the first examples of the imperfect form, the following singular case is of interest: "Superiore anno adolescentem curavi egregium, qui ex alto loco decidit, et tempus sinistrum laesit, ex quo in epilepsiam in epilepsiam incidit, qui paroxismi tempore ter, quater, saepius in gyrum se vertebat, impetuque facto, si non prohiberetur, versus locum aliquem procurrebat, priusquam prorsus caderet (plerumque non cadebat, sed manibus magna vi faciem confricabat) nec ad se reversus quicquid eorum, quae evenissent, sciebat [p. 195]." "Last year I treated a peculiar case of a lad who had fallen from a high place and injured the left side of his head, from which he derived epilepsy. At the time of his spell he was turning in circles, three, four, and even more times. Right after this, if not prevented, he would start running in some direction before falling (usually, though, he did not fall but forcefully rubbed his face with his hands). He did not have any knowledge of anything that had happened during the attack (p. 195 translated by R. F.)."

This is not only one of the first accounts of cursive epilepsy but, in addition, the first account of gyratory epilepsy (from the Greek γυρόω, "turning"). It is amazing that the two forms coexisted in the same patient. The histories of these two forms of epilepsy have developed rather differently. Cursive epilepsy (from the Latin *currere,* "to run") has consistently been the object of study by English neurologists, whereas gyratory epilepsy has been notably neglected by Anglo-Saxon authors, having been described in great detail, particularly by French, Italian, and, rarely, German authors.

II. Gyratory Epilepsy

In 1957 Inghirami reviewed the literature and cited fewer than 80 published cases of gyratory epilepsy. Cotte-Rittaud and Courjon (1962) revised their experience with 300 cases of adversive epilepsy, which they had observed over a 10-year period. Of their patients, 26 (8.6%) had gyratory epilepsy, that is, fits with complete rotation of the patient around the vertical axis, whereas only 6 (5%) showed the classical presentation of the adversive seizure as masterly described by Penfield and Jasper (1954) as the marker of a lesion located in the supplementary motor area. From their data it appears that gyratory epilepsy, although rare, is by no means exceptional in regard to frequency of occurrence. We have reviewed all the cases in the literature available to us and have summarized in Table 6.1 salient features of those reported in non-English journals, so that a comprehensive account of those cases will be available in the English language as well.

A. Clinical Features

Adversive movements are frequent during epileptic attacks. A clear definition of gyratory epilepsy must distinguish simple adversive fits from a true rotatory phenomenon. Adversive fits selectively involve eye and head turning, with occasional extension to the neck, upper trunk, and upper extremities. They may be accompanied by primitive vocalization and may herald a generalized convulsive attack, usually of the grand mal type. The localizing value of these adversive attacks has been suggested by Penfield and Jasper (1954) and confirmed by other authors (Guidetti *et al.*, 1959; Cotte-Rittaud and Courjon, 1962).

In gyratory, or rotatory, epilepsy the turning behavior is not limited to the upper part of the body but involves all of the body, which turns along its vertical axis for at least 180° but at times for an entire 360° one or more times in a pirouetting fashion. This ballet-like motion is usually seen only when the patient is in the standing position at the beginning of the attack. If the patient is lying down, turning is generally limited to a 180° rotation. Exceptions to this rule have been reported (Guidetti *et al.*, 1959), demonstrating that the incompleteness of the turning may not be exclusively related to the physical impossibility of revolving the body while lying down. The complex rotatory behavior may represent the entire attack, but more frequently it is either preceded or followed by other epileptic manifestations. The most common of these is a generalized

TABLE 6.1
Summary of Cases Described in the Non-English Literature

Sex and age (years) of patient	Loss of consciousness	Direction[a]	EEG	Pathology	Remarks	Reference
F, 8	After turning	←	Right central θ	?	—	Morocutti and Vizioli (1957)
F, 10	?	→	Left frontocentral focus	?	Followed by falling to the ground	
M, 7	Partial	←	Diffuse right-sided slowing and sharp waves	?	—	
M, 9	Yes	→	Right temporal slowings on hyperventilation	?	—	
M, 13	Yes	→	Bilaterally synchronous spike–wave discharges	?	Associated grand mal	
M, 23	No	←	?	Right frontal meningioma	Associated upper extremities dyskinesias	Riser *et al.* (1951)
F, 19	After turning	←	?	Right temporal scar	Associated with vestibular symptoms	
F, 16	No	→	Right parietal focus	?	Postictal amnesia for 3–4 hr	
F, 18	No	←	Multifocal spikes, Right–Left	?	Followed by grand mal	
M, 5	No	←	"Diffuse abnormalities"	?	—	
M, ?	No	←	?	?	Followed by grand mal	
F, 50	No	←	Left posterior spikes	?	—	
M, 14	Yes	→	Bilaterally synchronous spike–wave discharges at 3 Hz	?	Mentally retarded	

M, 22	Yes	←	Bilaterally synchronous spike–wave discharges after pentylenetetrazol	?	—	
F, 30	Yes	→	Bisynchronous spikes	?	—	
M, 30	Yes	←	Bisynchronous, asymmetric discharges	?	Followed by grand mal	
M, 12	Yes	← →	Bitemporal focus	?	Followed by grand mal	
M, 12	Yes	—	Right frontal focus	—	Followed by upper extremities and facial myocloni	
M, 14	Yes	→	Left temporal focus	—	—	
M, 47	No	←	No disturbances	?	Associated with visual hallucination	Inghirami (1957)
M, 13	Yes	←	Bilaterally synchronous spike–wave discharges at 2.5–3 Hz	?	Born while mother was standing and hit head on the ground; "cured" with trimethadione	
F, 8	Yes	←	Bilaterally synchronous spike–wave discharges at 3 Hz	?	Associated with absences; "cured" with trimethadione	
F, 17	Yes	←	Photoconvulsive response	?	Improved with trimethadione	
F, 33	Yes	→	Nonspecific	?	Associated absences	Gauthier and Berlanger (1953)
M, 12	Yes	→	Right frontal focus	?	Bout of grand mal seizures	
Four cases	—	—	All bilaterally synchronous spike–wave discharges at 3 Hz with focal onset	—	One with peduncular hallucinosis	Dell and Hécaen (1951)
M, 43	After turning	→	?	Left frontal glioblastoma	—	Guidetti *et al.* (1959)

(*Continued*)

TABLE 6.1 (*Continued*)

Sex and age (years) of patient	Loss of consciousness	Direction[a]	EEG	Pathology	Remarks	Reference
M, 61	No	↷	Diffuse θ	Bilateral subdural hematoma	Pirouetting while kneeling	
M, 39	After turning	↶	?	Left, hemispheral atrophy	Postictal nystagmus	
M, 41	After turning	↷	—	Left parieto-temporal fibrillary astrocytoma	Associated with flying-like movements of of the arms	
M, 58	Partial	↶	Ictal recruiting discharge with left parieto-occipital onset	Occlusion of right internal carotid artery	Hemianopia hallucinations (left-sided)	Vasconetto *et al.* (1969)
F, 9	Partial	↶	No disturbances	?	Associated with visual hallucinations	Kotowicz and Scherpereel (1968)
M, 14	Yes	—	3 Hz generalized spike–wave discharges	?	Associated with typical absences	Alajouanine and Nelhil (1957)
F, 22	?	↷	?	Optochiasmatic cyst	Associated vertigo followed by grand mal	Delay *et al.* (1948)

[a] ↷ denotes clockwise turning; ↶ denotes counterclockwise turning.

grand mal attack. Clonic, partial motor jerks of the upper extremities, masticatory movements and other automatisms, dystonic posturing of the upper extremities, vertiginous experiences, buzzing or ringing sounds, and complex hallucinatory visual experiences including peduncular hallucinosis have all been described in various combinations with the gyratory attack. In a peculiar case described by Mingazzini (1894), gyratory attacks were seen alternatively in a clockwise and counterclockwise direction. When turning was directed toward the left, hallucinatory experiences were perceived by the left eye and, when turning occurred toward the right, hallucinatory experiences were located in the right eye. Others (Hartenberg, 1946) have reported hallucinations limited to half of the visual field. Even cursive epilepsy may follow a gyratory fit, as in the case of the young boy described by Erastus. We could not find any other description of such an association.

A great number of patients have other types of seizure intercurrent with the one presenting the gyratory components; others have gyratory seizures only during a limited period of their epileptic condition.

As far as the direction of the gyratory phenomena is concerned, in most patients it remains constant from one attack to another, but exceptions have been reported, as mentioned earlier and in the case of a patient of Riser *et al.* (1951), who had alternating attacks of clockwise and counterclockwise turning behavior. Garcin and Kipfer (1941) suggested that, when a focal or hemispheric cerebral lesion underlies the epileptic condition, the direction of turning is away from the lesion site (contraversive turning), although exceptions to this rule have been frequently described in the literature (ipsiversive turning). Thus, as a general rule, clockwise turning is to be expected to accompany a left hemispheric lesion, whereas counterclockwise turning is commonly associated with right hemispheric pathology.

The state of consciousness may be variously compromised during the attack. Riser *et al.* (1951) analyzed 14 cases of gyratory epilepsy and divided them in two groups, one with loss of consciousness at the time of turning behavior and the other with retained consciousness and memory of the event during and after the turning. They did not comment, however, on the reasons for such a distinction and, from the analysis of their data, no other distinguishing features between the two groups can be found. These authors seem to imply that in patients with preserved consciousness there are no localizing electroencephalographic (EEG) signs or, if present, they show a tendency to spread bilaterally and diffusely. However, they fail to substantiate this impression since the same type of abnormality was found in patients with loss of consciousness. Cotte-Rittaud and Courjon (1962), who studied a comprehensive sample of adversive epilepsy, found that it was more useful to differentiate between seizures with a conscious and unconscious onset than between simple and complex (i.e., gyratory) adversive seizures. Thus, their analysis suggested that the adversive seizures with preserved consciousness at the onset appeared to have a "net presumptive value as being of frontal involvement at the level of the premotor zone [p. 6]," whereas they tend to relate the origin of the unconscious adversive seizures to any cortical area (with, however, a predilection for the temporal and occipital regions) or subcortical structures. In between the two states of consciousness there are various degrees of twilight states, memory defects and verbal unresponsiveness during the turning part of the attack.

B. Electroencephalographic Correlates

The great majority of patients reported in the literature that we reviewed exhibited various degrees of EEG abnormalities. These can be divided into three major categories:

1. *Focal epileptogenic discharges.* Spike foci have been noted in virtually all brain areas including frontal, parietal, temporal, and occipital lobes. Frank epileptiform activity was occasionally associated with different types of background slowings.
2. *Multifocal epileptogenic discharges.* These, too, did not show any selective predilection for a given cerebral localization and were both unilateral and bilateral with synchronous and/or asynchronous interhemispheric discharge pattern.
3. *Generalized seizure discharges in the form of bilateral synchronous spike–waves.* In some cases these were quite well organized at 3 cycles per second, with generalized onset as classically seen in petit mal. In other patients there were various atypical features, such as slower frequency of the spike–wave complexes, focal or lateralized onset of the bursts, asymmetry of the discharge, and interictal abnormalities. One patient was reported as having a photoconvulsive response (Inghirami, 1957).

C. Treatment

All the major anticonvulsants that were in vogue in the 1960s have been used to treat gyratory epilepsy with variable results. Inghirami (1957) advocated the use of trimetadione, which he reported to be highly effective in all of his cases associated with generalized spike–wave on EEG. On the contrary, Dell and Hécaen (1951), who administered, trimetadione to six patients exhibiting gyratory seizures and generalized spike–wave on the EEG, reported little effect in two and no effect in four of the patients. These patients, however, showed atypical and asymmetric bursts on the EEG. It seems, therefore, that there is no treatment of choice for gyratory epilepsy and that the choice of anticonvulsant must be guided by clinical and electrographic criteria in each case, as for many other forms of epilepsy.

D. Summary of Clinical and Electrographic Features

Electrical stimulation studies have shown that contraversive eye, head, and neck turning followed by gyratory movements of the whole body can be induced by delivering stimuli to a great number of cerebral structures. According to Foerster (1936) turning attacks were evoked in human subjects by electrical stimulation of various cortical areas of the frontal, parietal, temporal, and occipital lobes. Stimulation of the basis of F1 and F2 (area 6 of Broca), the posterior part of P1 (area 5 and the superior part of the interparietal sulcus), area 22, and area 19 of the occipital lobe with current intensity much higher than those used by Penfield resulted in turning (Penfield and Jasper, 1954).

Among subcortical structures, it is of interest that paroxysmal turning behavior was induced by stimulation of the amygdala (Gastaut *et al.*, 1951, 1952). By stimulating the phylogenetically older part of the amygdala in cats (the anteromedial division) Kaada *et al.* (1954) induced contralateral eye, head, and neck turning at times followed by body twists until the animal fell. Up to three or four complete turns of the body were obtained by increasing the stimulus intensity. Hess (1949) noted turning behavior upon stimulation of hypothalamic and suprathalamic nuclei. Considering that adversive components have been noted even in the course of petit mal attack, accompanied by supposedly bilaterally synchronous wave–spike discharges (Cotte-Rittaud and Courjon, 1962), the experiments of Hunter and Jasper (1969) are of particular clinical interest. These writers induced turning in cats by stimulating the same thalamic area in which electrical stimulation evoked spike–wave discharges on the EEG. They found that tonic elevation of one forepaw with turning of the head and eyes or involvement of the entire body in a circling movement was produced when the stimulating point was near or within the central median or subthalamic region or when other nuclei adjacent to the intralaminar region were stimulated. The turning movement was usually obtained with a stimulation intensity higher than that required to produce an arrest reaction, suggesting some spread to nearby structures. Further slight increases in stimulus intensity elicited forced turning of the head. Turning was at times ipsilateral but more commonly contralateral to the stimulus, which is in line with clinical observations of the relative rarity of ipsiversive seizures (Cotte-Rittaud and Courjon, 1962).

E. Experimental Data on Sustained Turning Behavior

The experimental work of Ungerstedt (1971) demonstrated that sustained turning behavior results from lesions of the substantia nigra in rodents. The original explanation of this phenomenon implied that a balance between the activity of the two dopaminergic nigrostriatal extrapyramidal systems is necessary for the maintenance of straight posture and gait. Whenever an imbalance occurs, turning behavior results, with circling movements directed away from the neostriatal system showing dopamine (DA) hyperactivity. Thus, if a toxin relatively selective for DA neurons such as 6-hydroxydopamine (6-OHDA) is injected unilaterally in the substantia nigra (SN), destroying the cells of origin of the DA-releasing dendrites in the caudate–putamen complex, the contralateral spared nigrostriatal system will become predominant and induce rotatory behavior directed away from the normal side, that is, ipsilateral to the destroying lesion. If a chronic irritating agent such as cobalt is injected in the SN, presumably inducing a temporary tonic hyperfunction of that structure, then circling will be contralateral to the side of the lesion (Shibuya *et al.*, 1978). However, in the cobalt implantation experiments the neostriatal DA content on the side of implantation increased remarkably during the first 24 hr but decreased rapidly thereafter, reaching minimal values (10% of the contralateral normal site) at 4 days. The neostriatal content of DA metabolites (homovanillic acid and dihydroxyphenylacetic acid) remained slightly higher, indicating that the remaining DA terminals might have been in a hyperfunctioning state. Since rotatory direction did not change according to the change in neostriatal DA content but remained directed contralaterally to the cobalt implantation throughout the experiments, the experiments suggested that factors other than an imbalance between the two dopaminergic systems might play a role in the genesis of turning behavior. Indeed, there is a substantial amount of experimental evidence demonstrating the role of another neurotransmitter substance, γ-aminobutyric acid (GABA), in circling behavior.

In fact, after unilateral intranigral injection of muscimol (a direct GABA receptor agonist) contralateral circling activity is noted (Oberlander *et al.*, 1977; Arnt and Scheel-Krüger, 1979). The rate of turning is dose dependent. Lesion experiments have suggested that the activation of DA neurons antagonizes this GABA function in the SN, and conversely their inactivation or destruction enhances GABA-mediated circling (Gale and Casu, 1981).

It has been recognized that the anatomical connections of the SN are much more widespread and intricate than originally thought. Among nigral afferents, in addition to the long-established nigrostriatal dopaminergic ascending pathway, other connections projecting to the thalamus, superior colliculi, and pontomesencephalic tegment have been demonstrated. A contingent of fibers from the nigra also project to the periaqueductal central gray, and another pathway ends in the pedunculopontine nucleus. Structures that project to the SN include the globus pallidus, the caudate–putamen complex, and some of the raphae nuclei. Between the pars compacta (more dorsal) and the pars reticulata (more ventral) of the SN there are abundant reciprocal connections. There seem to exist caudal projections of the SN that end at levels in the spinal cord (Commissiong and Neff, 1979).

The anatomical complexity of the SN is paralleled by the complexity of the neurochemical regulation involved, the picture of which is only beginning to emerge. Some of the highest concentrations of GABA, DA, substance P, and serotonin are found in the SN. Relatively recent experiments (Iadarola and Gale, 1981) have revived older suggestions that the SN may play an important role in the regulation of forebrain excitability. Fariello and Hornykiewicz (1979) observed that lesions of the SN are initially associated with a decrease in pentylenetetrazol (PMZ) convulsive threshold in rats and subsequently followed by an increase in the PMZ threshold. The time course of the changes in the PMZ threshold is inversely proportional to the neostriatal DA content. This was initially raised and subsequently progressively lowered, suggesting that the SN is an important locus of modulation of brain excitability (Iadarola and Gale, 1982).

In summary, the SN is now recognized as a major crossroad of pathways from the extrapyramidal motor system and a center where many neurochemical systems converge from telencephalic and rhombomesencephalic structures. Turning and circling behavior can therefore be induced by activation or deactivation not only of the SN but also of many of the other nuclei that are in strict functional connection with it. In keeping with this postulate are the findings of turning behavior induced by unilateral lesions of central vestibular nuclei (Shima and Hassler, 1982), the superior colliculi (Geula and Asdourian, 1981) and possibly also the locus coeruleus (Pycock *et al.*, 1975). According to Hassler (1956a,b) turning movements result from dysfunction of two main central systems: the ascending vestibuloreticulothalamic pathway, which is in connection with the striatum, and the descending pallidoreticulospinal pathway, which crosses the midline caudal to the central periaqueductal gray. Both the ascending and descending systems join the fasciculus tegmenti dorsolateralis at the pontine tegmental level. Experimental and clinical data point to the SN as a crucial, but not a unique structure for the genesis of turning behavior in these systems.

F. Extrapolation of Experimental Data to the Clinical Syndrome of Gyratory Epilepsy

On the basis of the experimental data described in the preceding section, it seems logical to speculate that turning behavior in human beings is caused by activation of the extrapyramidal system or at least by a part of that which is connected to the nigra. Both cortical and subcortical foci may spread during the organization of an ictal epileptic event to involve any one of the numerous structures that have been shown to connect with the nigral system. As long as a lateralization of the discharge exists, a paroxysmal imbalance between the function of the two extrapyramidal systems will result, being manifested in asymmetric motor function, with turning directed away from the side of higher level of DA receptor activity (Ungerstedt, 1971). Since it is assumed that epileptiform discharges cause paroxysmal hyperactivity of the structure in which they are generated, it is not surprising that most of the circling activity in epileptic patients is directed away from the site of predominant epileptic pathology. It is known that, in cases of multifocal discharges distributed over the two hemispheres, a focus located on one side may alternate with another focus on the other side of the brain in triggering the ictal events. This fact may explain those patients who had diffuse cerebral pathology and turning in different directions during various attacks (Riser *et al.*, 1951). Semerano *et al.* (1968) postulated, as convincingly as can be done on mere clinical and electrographic grounds, that their two patients had amygdaloid foci. As previously mentioned (Kaada *et al.*, 1954), turning behavior can be elicited by electrical stimulation of the amygdala. Gloor (1957) investigated the pattern of conduction of amygdaloid seizure discharge. Although no direct connections with the SN were explored or considered, seizures were seen to spread to the thalamus, hypothalamus, and tegmental area, which in turn might have influenced the nigral system, thus causing turning behavior. Similarly, vestibular lesions, which have been implicated in a number of patients with gyratory fits on the basis of clinical signs of vestibular dysfunction occurring as part of the seizure, may cause turning because of interference with the ascending vestibuloreticulothalamic pathways.

That gyratory epilepsy in humans is often followed by a secondary generalized grand mal attack suggests that the postulated regulatory role of the SN toward the susceptibility of the forebrain to generalized convulsions (Fariello and Hornykiewicz, 1979) may be a clinically relevant fact. Indeed, it is believed that seizure discharges are associated with impaired GABA-mediated function (Ayala *et al.*, 1973; Meldrum, 1978; Fariello and Golden, 1981). When a seizure discharge involves the SN, the excitability of the whole brain might increase, predisposing an epileptic brain to secondary generalization of the discharges.

Finally, to explain rotatory seizures in patients with generalized spike–wave discharges, one should postulate that an epileptogenic lesion exists within or in close proximity to those thalamic nuclei the stimulation of which is capable of inducing bilaterally synchronous spike–wave discharges (Hunter and Jasper, 1949) in an epilepsy-prone brain.

Three of the major thalamic nuclei (the centromedian, the ventralis anterior, and the ventrolateral) have well-established motor function and connections with many other extrapyramidal centers, including the SN. In those cases in which an asymmetry of the generalized spike–wave discharge was noted, it seems that the initially lateralized discharge sets off a predominant activation of either the right or the left extrapyramidal system, causing turning contralateral to the more stimulated side. Turning toward one side in those patients in whom a definite lateralization of the discharge was not seen in the EEG tracings may be explained by assuming that, despite the seemingly symmetric electrical activity, an asymmetry existed which did not surface to the cortical areas explored by conventional EEG. Alternatively, a genuine bilateral paroxysm may bring out asymmetric motor behavior related to cerebral dominance. A confirmation of this hypothesis should be sought through studies relating direction of turning to cerebral dominance in patients with turning and without any lateralization of their primary generalized EEG discharge.

III. Cursive Epilepsy

Another unusual and complex form of bodily movements is caused by electrical activation induced by paroxysmal epileptiform discharges. Such movement is running, and the seizure disorder that it characterizes is termed *cursive epilepsy.* Gyratory epilepsy and cursive epilepsy have no common electrophysiological correlates, as explained in Section IV, but it seems appropriate to discuss cursive epilepsy because it is also manifested by activation of an apparently specific and peculiar motor system caused by epileptogenic activity that almost always originates in the temporal lobe, irrespective of its laterality. It seems relevant to emphasize the dissimilarities between these two epileptic syndromes because they might involve two different motor systems, one definitely lateralized and having to do with posture, slow dystonic movement, and turning, the other being concerned with a more complex and specifically directed type of motion, such as running, which seems to be triggered regardless of the brain laterality and which is clinically expressed by bilateral locomotive movements without preferential lateralization.

A. Clinical Features

Cursive epilepsy is a definite clinical entity. *Epilepsia cursiva, cursive epilepsy, epilepsia cursora, epilepsia procursiva,* and the French *epilepsie retropulsive* are all terms that were used in the past to denote running fits. Nonne (1923) used the term *epilepsia procursiva.* The prefix *pro* denoted the forward direction of running, whereas other authors (see Nonne, 1923), referred to patients with backward running movement as suffering from *epilepsie retropulsive.*

Descriptions of running fits date back to the time of Hippocrates, who spoke of men "jumping up and fleeing out of doors." Erastus (1581) examined a girl who for half an hour ran back and forth across a room while people in the room tried to stop her. When asked afterward whether she had seen or heard anything, she said that she had not. "But it was a fact," wrote Erastus, "that when she saw the wall, she did not proceed further but turned back [from Lennox, 1960, p. 280]." Since then sporadic reports of cursive epilepsy have appeared in the medical literature. The two largest series are that of Sisler *et al.* (1953) and that of Chen and Forster (1973).

The others are generally single case reports mixed with quiritarian (from the Latin *quiritor,* literally meaning "call the quirites [Romans] for help" and extended to mean "crying for help and yelling with fright") and gelastic features (see Chapter 11 for review).

Although difficult to estimate, the incidence of cursive epilepsy in the general population is relatively low. It is possible to get some idea of its prevalence from the series published by Chen and Forster (1973). The University of Wisconsin Epilepsy Center studied 5000 consecutive cases of epilepsy. Of these, 6 had cursive epilepsy, and 2 had both cursive and gelastic features. In addition, these patients usually had more common seizure patterns, such as grand mal, akinetic, or partial complex spells.

Sisler *et al.* (1953) proposed that cursive epilepsy be defined as episodic alteration of awareness associated with running. According to these authors consciousness may be clouded to a variable degree. The activity is coordinated but is inappropriate to the reality situation. They consider it a type of automatism, and it is included in the ill-defined groups of psychomotor epilepsy. The cases described in the literature generally fit into this framework of description. Hans Strauss (1960) wrote about a 12-year-old boy whose developmental milestones were normal. He experienced attacks in which he would be sitting and then would rise and run. He would remember everything that he had done. At one time while at school, he had an attack but was afraid to run around the classroom for fear of appearing ridiculous. Therefore, instead of running he started making the shuffling movements that children often make to imitate a locomotive, accompanying his motion with corresponding noises. He felt that he should run but suppressed the urge to do so. Neurological findings were unremarkable. The reported EEG abnormalities in this case were 0.7–3 cycles per second activity, with spikes at the right frontal electrode extending to the right anterior temporal electrode. There were also some spikes at the left frontal electrode. The patient was reported to respond well to diphenylhydantoin therapy. This case differs from all other cases in the literature in that the boy had complete awareness of what he was doing and at one time volitionally suppressed the running, being totally conscious at the time of the spell. The EEG abnormalities in this case are questionable, at least as judged by the illustration in the article, thus, it is very difficult to presume that the diagnosis in this patient was correct, and other psychobehavioral problems such as compulsive behavior or even catatonic impulsive action had not been convincingly ruled out. It is therefore reasonable to assume that alteration of awareness occurs with cursive epilepsy and that the subject experiences complete or nearly complete amnesia for the event.

In many patients with cursive epilepsy there is no progression of the seizure toward generalized tonic clonic convulsion. In some patients running may occur as a preconvulsive phenomenon. In these patients running is followed by major motor convulsions. This type of preconvulsive running is quite rare. A more common presentation is a dreamlike state followed by running for a few minutes and then by exhaustion and complete amnesia for the episode. This may be regarded as an automatism not different from those commonly seen with partial complex seizures. Running can also occur after a major convulsion in the postictal twilight state, but this type of running is quite unusual in a patient suffering from cursive epilepsy.

Patients with cursive epilepsy invariably have additional types of seizures, and rarely is cursive epilepsy the only ictal manifestation. These seizure types include grand mal, psychomotor, adversive, petit mal, gelastic, atonic, quiritarian, and focal motor.

A lack of sophisticated diagnostic techniques was a major handicap in determining the etiology of cursive epilepsy in the past.

B. Electroencephalographic Abnormalities

The EEG abnormalities in patients with cursive epilepsy are striking. All the patients reported in the literature had abnormal interictal EEGs. The most consistent abnormality in all patients is either slowing or spike or sharp waves over the temporal region. These abnormalities do not show left or right preponderance, occurring approximately equally on both sides. This indicates that a temporal lobe focus is essential for the production of cursive epilepsy independently from its laterality. We have observed two patients with cursive epilepsy associated with other types of seizures. A 34-year-old man with partial complex seizures of the temporal lobe type and rare cursive fits had a left temporal sharp wave. A 17-year-old boy with partial motor, partial complex, generalized tonic seizures and four running seizures had widespread spike–wave discharges over the right frontal and temporal lobes, often followed by generalization.

C. Psychiatric Aspects

A significant number of patients with cursive epilepsy have psychobehavioral problems. These include low normal intelligent quotients, hyperactivity, significant psychosocial stresses, and abnormal personality traits. On a broad spectrum these patients vary from introspective, dependent, and shy individuals to rebellious and extroverted people. Few patients have been thought to be unemotional and rigid, according to Sisler *et al.* (1953). These patients have serious conflicts in their relationships with other members of their family. Acute trauma seemed to have increased the conflict immediately before the onset of running fits in most instances in this series.

We have already stated that all patients with cursive epilepsy have a temporal focus on their EEGs. Sisler *et al.* (1953) pointed to the fact that, in their series of nine patients, an acute trauma might have played a role immediately before the onset of running fits and speculated on the neuropsychological personality changes produced by the trauma.

In Penfield's series (Penfield and Perot, 1963) electrical stimulation of the temporal lobes produced pleasurable sensations or fear. It has been suggested that, in patients with cursive epilepsy, a temporal lobe electrical discharge produces an ictal experiential hallucination of unpleasant connotation because of the conflicts in the patients' interpersonal relationships. The subjects' response to such hallucinations is to run toward or away from anxiety-provoking conflicts. Thus, running epilepsy might be an outward manifestation of an internal state of fear brought about by temporal lobe electrical discharges, and it can be considered to be a form of automatism within the broad category of partial complex seizures.

D. Differential Diagnosis

A variety of neuropsychiatric conditions involve paroxysmal episodic motor dysfunction and should be ruled out before the diagnosis of cursive epilepsy is made.

1. *Compulsive behavior manifested by running.* The subject usually has an urge to carry out an act and is unable to suppress it. This urge might be running and, in that case, simulates cursive epilepsy. The main points of differentiation are that these subjects rarely have a history of other seizure types, there is usually an abnormal premorbid personality, computed tomographic (CT) scan is always normal, and EEG abnormalities are either absent or nonspecific.
2. *Panic reaction of phobic anxiety.* Panic reaction of phobic anxiety is characterized by abdominal symptoms, a choking sensation, and occasionally running with terrified facies. These attacks, however, last much longer. There is vivid recollection of the episode, and usually during a psychiatric interview the underlying phobia can be identified. The CT scan and EEG are normal or nonspecifically abnormal, and there is no history of other seizure disorders.
3. *Impulsive actions of catatonic patients.* Sometimes catatonic patients perform actions on impulse in which running is included. With a good psychiatric history and EEG, differentiation does not offer a problem.
4. *Hypnogenic paroxysmal dystonia.* In this case there are violent movements of the extremities and tonic phases of variable duration. The EEG is abnormal, but clinically running is rare and the episodes always occur at night (Lugaresi and Cirignotta, 1981).
5. *Fugue states.* In this case patients walk in a dazed state and have complete amnesia for the event. In contrast to cursive epilepsy, running is very rare. The EEG is normal or nonspecifically abnormal.
6. *Paroxysmal dyskinesias.* Paroxysmal dyskinesias may at times be confused with cursive epilepsy. Particularly in the kinesigenic form, running may trigger an attack of generalized choreoathetosis (Goodenough *et al.*, 1978). On the basis of a careful observation of the temporal se-

quence of events, the distinction should be clear. In paroxysmal kinesigenic choreoathetosis, running is started voluntarily and suddenly interrupted by afinalistic dystonic movements; in cursive epilepsy, running is unconscious but performed with correct coordination. Automatic, at times dystonic, movements occur before the act of running. Many kinesigenic dyskinesias are familial, whereas others are acquired and associated with such neurological diseases as multiple sclerosis, idiopathic hypoparathyroidism, and cerebral palsy.

E. Experimental Data on Running

Walking, trotting, and running can be produced in cats deprived of forebrain motor control by the stimulation of two brainstem regions (Orlovsky and Shik, 1976; Eidelberg *et al.*, 1981). A subthalamic locomotor region has been identified which lies laterally to the posterior hypothalamus, medial to the cerebral pedunculus, caudal to the posterior thalamus, rostral to the red nucleus, dorsal to the mamillary body, and ventral to the inferior borders of the posterior thalamus. The mesencephalic locomotor region lies in the ventral part of the inferior colliculus and extends ventrally past the aqueduct to the dorsolateral part of the brachium conjunctivum. The stimulus intensity is the determinant factor in producing various speeds of locomotion, with higher current inducing running and threshold stimulation inducing slow stepping.

In the late 1940s interest in the field of cursive epilepsy arose when Newell *et al.* (1947) reported the production of running fits in dogs maintained on a diet of flour bleached with a combination of nitrogen, tetrachloride, and benzoyl peroxide. Fits were not observed in dogs fed untreated flour or flour treated with benzoyl peroxide alone, chlorine dioxide, chlorine, nitrogen dioxide, or methyldichloramine. Monkeys fed "agenized" flour, that is, flour treated with carbon tetrachloride and benzoyl peroxide, showed some EEG abnormalities. Cats fed agenized flour displayed running fits. Human subjects who had been fed agenized flour showed no clinical seizures or EEG abnormalities. Unfortunately, these findings have not been investigated further, and the pathophysiology of those fits remains the object of speculation. A modern investigation with sophisticated electrophysiological and pharmacological techniques might help to establish whether the previously mentioned nature and sites of origin (locomotor regions) are involved in running fits.

IV. Summary and Conclusions

We have presented two forms of epilepsy characterized by complex motor activity as the integral part of the ictal event. In addition to this basic similarity and the exceptional coexistence of the forms in the same patient (Erastus, 1581) these two epileptic manifestations differ substantially, particularly with regard to lateralization of motor activity. This, in fact, is an intrinsic characteristic of gyratory epilepsy whereas, to our knowledge, it has never been observed as a feature of cursive epilepsy, at least in the cases reported in the literature and in the two patients that we have observed. This is even more remarkable when one considers that, in cursive seizures, the epileptiform discharge is almost always unilateral, whereas cases of gyratory attacks were seen in patients with bilaterally symmetric discharges. Experimental work in animals (for review see Eidelberg *et al.*, 1981) has shown that stimulation of locomotor regions in the subthalamic and mesencephalic areas induces stepping and, with progressively increasing stimulation intensity, also trotting and galloping without lateralization. We speculate that this motor system is activated by temporal discharges in cases of cursive epilepsy and has a clinical midline expression without the possibility of lateralization. The anatomically different and definitely lateralized extrapyramidal system, when activated by paroxysmal epileptiform discharges, seems to be responsible for the clinical manifestation of gyratory epilepsy.

References

Alajouanine, T., and Nelhil, J. (1957). A propos de certaines variétés particulières de petit mal: Forme salutante, la forme avec reject de la tête en arrière, la forme giratoire. *Rev. Neurol.* May, 528.

Arnt, J., and Scheel-Kruger, J. (1979). GABAergic and glycinergic mechanisms within the substantia nigra: Pharmacological specificity of dopamine independent contralateral turning behavior and interacts with other neurotransmitters. *Psychopharmacology (Berlin)* **62,** 267–277.

Ayala, G. F., Dichter, M., Gumnit, R. J., Matsumoto, H., and Spencer, A. (1973). The genesis of the epileptic spike: New knowledge of cortical feedback system suggests a neurophysiological explanation of the brief paroxysms. *Brain Res.* **52,** 1–17.

Chen, R., and Forster, M. (1973). Cursive epilepsy and gelastic epilepsy. *Neurology* **23,** 1019–1029.

Commissiong, J. H., and Neff, N. (1979). Commentary: Current status of dopamine in mammalian spinal cord. *Biochem. Pharmacol.* **28,** 1569–1573.

Cotte-Rittaud, M., and Courjon, J. (1962). Semiological value of adversive epilepsy. *Epilepsia* **3,** 151–166.

Delay, M. M. J., Puech, P., Desclaux, R., and Digo, P. (1948). Guérison de graves troubles caractériels et de crises comitiales après ouverture de la lame sus-optique et d'un kyste cysternal. *Rev. Neurol.* **13,** 375–376.

Dell, M. B., and Hécaen, H. (1951). Complex pointe-ondes a debut unilateral et épilepsie giratoire. *Rev. Neurol.* **84,** 656–659.

Eidelberg, E., Walden, J. G., and Nguyen, L. H. (1981). Locomotor control in macaque monkeys. *Brain* **104,** 647–663.

Erastus, T. (1581). Comitiis montani vicentink novi medicorum censoris quinque librorum de morbis nuper editorum viva anatome. *Basileae.*

Fariello, R., and Golden, G. (1981). Homotaurine a GABA agonist with anticonvulsant effects. *Brain Res. Bull.* **5,** Suppl. 2, 691–699.

Fariello, R., and Hornykiewicz, O. (1979). Substantia nigra and pentylenetetrazol threshold in rats: Correlation with striatal dopamine mechanism. *Exp. Neurol.* **65,** 202–208.

Foerster, F. (1936). The motor cortex in man in the light of Hughlings Jackson's doctrine. *Brain* **52,** 135.

Gale, K., and Casu, M. (1981). Dynamic utilization of GABA in substantia nigra: Regulation by dopamine and GABA in the striatum, and its clinical and behavioral implications. *Mol. Cell. Biochem.* **39,** 369–405.

Garcin, R., and Kipfer, M. (1941). L'épilepsie giratoire. *Paris Med.* **119,** 29–34.

Gastaut, H., Vigouroux, R., Corriol, J., and Badier, M. (1951). Effect de la stimulation électrique (par electrodes à demeure) du complèxe amygdalien chez le chat non narcosé. *J. Physiol. (Paris)* **43,** 740.

Gastaut, H., Naquet, R., Vigouroux, R., and Corrieol, J. (1952). Provocation de comportements émotionnels divers par stimulation rhinencéphalique chez le chat avec électrodes à demeure. *Rev. Neurol.* **86,** 319.

Gauthier, C., and Belanger, C. (1953). Contribution á l'étude de l'ěpilepsie giratoire. *Laval Med.* **18,** 12–21.

Geula, C., and Asdourian, D. (1981). Circling induced by injection of GABA into the superior colliculus. *Soc. Neurosci. Abstr.* **7,** 690.

Gloor, P. (1957). The pattern of conduction of amygdaloid seizure discharge—an experimental study in the cat. *AMA Arch. Neurol. Psychiatry* 77, 247–258.

Goodenough, D., Fariello, R., Annis, B. L., and Chun, R. W. M. (1978). Familial and acquired paroxysmal dyskinesias. *Arch. Neurol. (Chicago)* **35,** 827–831.

Guidetti, B., Fortuna, A., and Moscatelli, G. (1959). Sul valore localizzatorio delle crisi avversative e giratorie. *Riv. Patol. Nerv. Ment.* **80,** 1153–1185.

Hartenberg, P. (1946). L' epilepsie chronique. Paris: Masson.

Hassler, R. (1956a). Die Zentralen Apparate der WendebeWegungen. I. Ipsiversive Wendungen durch Reizung einer directen vestibulo-thalamischen Bahn im Hirnstamm der Katze. *Arch. Psychiatr. Z. Neurol.* **194,** 456–480.

Hassler, R. (1956b). Die zentralen Apparate der WendebeWegungen. II. Die neuronalen Apparate der vestibularen Korrecturwendungen und der Adversivbewegungen. *Arch. Psychiatr. Z. Neurol.* **194,** 481–516.

Hess, W. (1949). "Das Zwischenhirn Syndrome, Localizationen Functionen," p. 187. Schwabbe, Switzerland.

Hunter, J., and Jasper, H. (1949). Effects of thalamic stimulation in unanesthetized animals. *Electroencephalog. Clin. Neurophysiol.* **1,** 305–321.

Iadarola, M. J., and Gale, K. (1981). The substantia nigra: Site of GABA mediated anticonvulsant activity in rats. *Soc. Neurosci. Abst.* **188,**(16), 591.

Iadarola, M. D., and Gale, K. (1982). Attempts to identify the midbrain site associated with GABA mediated anticonvulsant activity. *Science* **218,** 1237–1240.

Inghirami, L. (1957). L'epilessia giratoria. *Riv. Neurobiol.* **3,** 673–702.

Kaada, B. R., Andersen, P., and Jansen, J., Jr. (1954). Stimulation of amygdaloid nuclear complex in unanesthetized cat. *Neurology* **4,** 48–64.

Kotowicz, A., and Scherpereel, P. (1968). L'épilepsie gyratoire: A propos d'un nouveau cas. *Maroc Med.* **48,** 141–143.

Lai, M., and Chen, R. (1980). Gelastic epilepsy and cursive epilepsy. *J. Formosan Med. Assoc.* **79,** 433–490.

Lennox, W. G. (1960). "Epilepsy and Related Disorders," Vol. 1, p. 280. Little, Brown, Boston, Massachusetts.

Lugaresi, E., and Cirignotta, F. (1981). Hypnogenic paroxysmal dystonia: Epileptic seizure or a new syndrome? *Sleep* **4,** 129–138.

Meldrum, B. S. (1978). Gamma-aminobutyric acid and the search for new anticonvulsant drugs. *Lancet* **2,** 304–306.

Mingazzini, G. (1894). Editorial note. *Riv. Sper. Freniatr. Med. Leg. Alienazioni Ment.* **20,** 361–378.

Morocutti, C., and Vizioli, R. (1957). L'epilessia giratoria. *Riv. Neurol.* **27,** 412–418.
Newell, G., Erickson, T., Gilson, W., Gershoff, S., and Elvehjem, C. (1947). Role of "agenized" flour in the production of running fits. *JAMA, J. Am. Med. Assoc.* **135,** 760–763.
Nonne, M. (1923). Die Neurosen. *In* "Lehrbuch der Nervnkrankheiten" (H. Oppenheim, ed.), Springer-Verlag, Berlin.
Oberlander, C., Dumont, C., and Bossier, J. R. (1977). Rotational behavior after unilateral injection of muscimol in rats. *Eur. J. Pharmacol.* **43,** 389–390.
Orlovsky, G. N., and Shik, M. L. (1976). Control of locomotion: A neurophysiological analysis of the cat locomotor system. *Neurophysiology (Engl. Transl.) II* **10,** 281–317.
Penfield, W., and Jasper, H. H. (1954). "Epilepsy and Functional Anatomy of Human Brain." Little, Brown, Boston, Massachusetts.
Penfield, W., and Perot, P. (1963). The brain's record of auditory and visual experiences. *Brain* **86,** 597–697.
Pycock, C. J., Donaldson, I. G., and Marsden, C. D. (1975). Circling behavior produced by unilateral lesions in the region of the locus ceruleus in rats. *Brain Res.* **97,** 317–329.
Riser, M., Geraud, J., Grezes-Rueff, C., Lavitary, M., and Rascol, M. (1951). A propos de 14 cas d'épilepsie giratoire. *Rev. Neurol.* **84**(4), 245–253.
Semerano, A., Testa, G. F., and Denes, F. (1968). Observazioni cliniche ed elettroencefalografiche in due casi di crisi amigdaloidea. *Riv. Patol. Nerv. Ment.* **89,** 108–118.
Shibuya, M. R., Fariello, R., Farley, K., Price, K., Lloyd, K. G., and Hornykiewicz, O. (1978). Cobalt injections into the substantia nigra of the rat: Effects of behavior and dopamine metabolism in the striatum. *Exp. Neurol.* **58,** 486–499.
Shima, F., and Hassler, R. (1982). Circling behavior produced by unilateral lesions of the central vestibular system. *Appl. Neurophysiol.* **45,** 255–260.
Sisler, G., Levy, L., and Roseman, E. (1953). Epilepsia cursiva. *Arch. Neurol. Psychiatry* **69,** 73–79.
Strauss, H. (1960). Paroxysmal compulsive running and concept of epilepsia cursiva. *Neurology* **10,** 341–344.
Ungerstedt, U. (1971). Striatal dopamine release after amphetamine or nerve degeneration revealed by rotational behavior. *Acta Physiol. Scand.* **82,** Suppl. 48–49.
Vasconetto, C., Smith, J. A. S., and Morocutti, C. (1969). Osservazioni cliniche edelectroencefalografiche a proposito di un caso di epilessia giratoria. *Riv. Neurol.* **37,** 219–230.

7: Hemisyndromes of Temporal Lobe Epilepsy: Review of Evidence Relating Psychopathological Manifestations in Epilepsy to Right- and Left-Sided Epilepsy

PIERRE FLOR-HENRY

Alberta Hospital
and Department of Psychiatry
University of Alberta
Edmonton, Alberta, Canada

I. Introduction 149
II. Laterality and Psychopathology: Evidence from Epilepsy 150
III. Forced Normalization 156
IV. Endogenous Psychoses and Laterality 159
V. Mood, Motility, Visuospatial Systems, Dreams, and Erotic Arousal 164
VI. Conclusion 167
References 169

I. Introduction

Between 1964 and 1966 I became interested in the possible lateralization of psychopathological syndromes. This was because Terzian and Cecotto (1957; Terzian, 1964) had reported a striking differential emotional reactivity of the two hemispheres to carotid barbiturization, and Lishman (1966) had shown in a study of the sequellae of penetrating war wounds that, whereas psychiatric disabilities in general were associated with left hemisphere lesions, affective disturbances were significantly correlated with right hemisphere wounds, notably right frontal and right temporal localization. Because at that time I was a registrar at the Maudsley Hospital, London, England, and had access to the well-documented and complete archives of that hospital, I was able to carry out the first controlled investigation of epileptic psychoses, comparing systematically 50 temporal lobe epileptics who had exhibited definite psychotic episodes with 50 temporal lobe epileptics who had never shown psychotic distur-

HEMISYNDROMES:
Psychobiology, Neurology,
Psychiatry

ISBN 0-12-512460-0

bances (Flor-Henry, 1966, 1969a,b). The findings are now well known, and therefore they are briefly summarized here:

1. In temporal lobe epilepsy, psychosis was significantly associated with epilepsy implicating the dominant hemisphere.
2. There was a significant trend whereby left temporal lobe epilepsy was associated with schizophrenic and right temporal lobe epilepsy with manic-depressive symptoms, schizoaffective syndromes falling in an intermediate position with respect to focus of lateralization.
3. Since in the total population (psychotic plus control) there was an equal frequency of unilateral epilepsies, right and left, and since the psychotics had an excess of left-sided epilepsies, it followed that in the controls there was a relative excess of right hemisphere epilepsies. This was because the majority of the controls, who had been referred to a unit specialized in the psychiatric aspects of epilepsy, suffered from neurotic-type depression and/or anxiety.
4. "Forced normalization" was an important parameter of psychosis. The schizophrenic syndrome was inversely correlated with the frequency of temporal–limbic seizures but independent of the frequency of generalized seizures, whereas there was a trend showing that the manic-depressive syndrome was inversely correlated with the frequency of (secondarily) generalized seizures.
5. Structural brain damage was unrelated to the emergence of psychosis but, when present in psychosis, was related to chronicity.

II. Laterality and Psychopathology: Evidence from Epilepsy

In this chapter I review the evidence, derived from studies of epilepsy, that between 1965 and 1982 confirmed and amplified the relationships delineated in the preceding section. I then integrate the cerebral correlates of psychopathology as they emerge in epilepsy into the more general question of the cerebral localization of psychopathology in the endogenous syndromes, of which epilepsy is, in a certain sense, a special but paradigmatic example.

Let us begin by examining the evidence concerning the cerebral lateralization of mood provided by epileptic studies. Mnoukhine and Dinabourg (1965) described 139 children with cerebral palsy, hemiparesis, and epilepsy. Of these, 55 had permanent hemiplegia, 28 showed postictal hemiparesis, and 56 had focal, unilateral Jacksonian sensory or motor seizures alone. Cerebral insults lateralized to the dominant hemisphere produced profound intellectual retardation (in 80% of cases) and blunting of affect. Epilepsy lateralized to the nondominant hemisphere was associated with "distinct intensification of emotional manifestations, abrupt excitability, melancholic depressions [p. 1074]" in 45% of cases in the experience of these Russian authors. Examining 100 temporal lobe epileptics who had undergone temporal resection, Falconer and Taylor (1970) found that psychopathic personality deviation (present in 48 patients) was associated with left hemisphere resections in two-thirds of cases, whereas neurosis (present in 30 patients) was related to right hemisphere epilepsy, again in two-thirds of cases. Of the 52 psychotic epileptics considered by Gregoriadis *et al.* (1971) in Athens, 9 were manic-depressive, and all 9 had right hemisphere lateralization on both electroencephalographic (EEG) and air-encephalographic indices. In Boston Bear and Fedio (1977) studied the interictal personality characteristics of unilateral temporal lobe epileptics who had never had psychotic episodes. There were 12 left and 15 right temporal lobe cases. The patients with right temporal focus were significantly different from those with left temporal focus (and from controls matched for age, sex, and socioeconomic status) and were characterized by emotionality, depression, and mood lability. In India Shukla and Katiyar (1980) in a series of 62 temporal lobe epileptics found a significant association between right temporal foci and neurosis, essentially anxiety, depression, and neurasthenic forms. In Japan Onuma *et al.* (1980) noted in a series of 51 epileptic psychoses a preponderance of right frontal foci and stated that "two out of three cases associated with manic and depressive symptoms had the right temporal lobe foci [p. 338]." A similar lateralization was described by another Japanese group, also from Tokyo. Hara *et al.* (1980) described 40 psychotic episodes occurring in 32 epileptics. The group with dysphoric or depressive mood swings exhibited "generalized epilepsy or right lateralization."

The association between left hemisphere epilepsy and schizophrenic symptoms has also been confirmed by several investigations in the past 12 years. The 43 patients with schizophrenic and paranoid psychoses in the series of Gregoriadis *et al.* (1971) all had left hemisphere lateralization on both EEG and air-encephalographic indices. Taylor (1975) at Oxford studied 88 patients who had undergone temporal lobectomy for drug-resistant temporal epilepsy. Neuropathologically, 41 had mesial–temporal sclerosis alone, and 47 exhibited "alien tissue," or hamartomas, focal dysplasias, or small benign tumors. The right and left hemisphere lesions were found to differ in both verbal and performance discrepancies preoperatively and postoperatively as a function of the nature of the neuropathological lesion. Preoperatively, the verbal–performance discrepancy was significant for right-, but not for left-sided lesions, whereas it became significant for both sides postoperatively. This was particularly true for the alien tissue group. Thus, alien tissue pathology, arising early during embryogenesis, in contrast to mesial–temporal sclerosis, which is a postnatal insult, produces a less specific dysfunction in the left hemisphere.

In addition, 13 of the 88 patients had a schizophrenic psychosis. Of the alien tissue group, 23% had psychosis compared with 5% of the mesial–temporal sclerosis patients. There was a considerable excess of sinistrality in the alien tissue group compared with mesial–temporal sclerosis, although the total sinistral group remained left hemisphere dominant as a whole. There was a significant interaction between sinistrality and psychosis. The interaction correlating with the highest probability for psychosis was the presence of alien tissue in the left hemisphere of sinistral female patients. A psychotic evolution was least probable with mesial–temporal sclerosis in the right hemisphere of dextral male patients.

Lindsay *et al.* (1979) followed prospectively for 15 years 100 children with limbic epilepsy who had been identified from a larger, unselected population of over 1000 children with epilepsy (all types) at Oxford in 1964. By 1979 the series consisted of 87 patients, as a result of deaths, but 100% follow-up was achieved. Nine patients (or 10.3%) had developed overt, schizophrenic psychosis. None of these had a right-sided focus, 7 had a left-sided focus, and 2 had bilateral foci. Of the psychotics, 8 were male and only 1 female. Although 26 patients had "grossly disordered childhood homes," this factor was not related to the emergence of adult psychiatric disorder. In the series of Hara *et al.* (1980) 10 patients had exhibited a total of 15 "schizophrenic-like" episodes. In the majority of these cases the focus was left temporal.

Sherwin (1981) carried out a retrospective analysis of 63 patients with temporal lobe epilepsy who had been subjected to unilateral temporal lobectomy in Los Angeles. There were significantly more right hemisphere epilepsies ($N=46$) than left hemisphere epilepsies in this series because an attempt had been made to exclude active psychosis. [In an earlier study of patients selected for concordance of intractable epilepsy and behavior disorder, Sherwin (1977) reported the emergence of schizophrenic episodes in 15% of the patients and stated that all the psychotic patients had left temporal lobe epileptogenic lesions on pneumoencephalographic and EEG findings.] In a 5-year follow-up period 7 patients became psychotic, 6 with paranoid–schizophrenic symptoms and 1 with a depressive psychotic syndrome. Of these, 5 had undergone left temporal and 1, a right temporal lobectomy. The relative frequencies of left hemisphere epilepsy in the psychotic and of right hemisphere epilepsy in the nonpsychotic groups were highly significant. It is also noteworthy that the patient with depressive psychosis was the one psychotic who had been subjected to right temporal lobectomy. In addition, 6 of the 7 psychotics had become seizure free postoperatively. Sherwin also demonstrated a similar and significant segregation of left temporal epilepsy in patients who became schizophrenic after unilateral temporal resections performed at Sainte Anne Hospital in Paris (Sherwin *et al.*, 1982).

Perez and Trimble (1980), working in London, compared the mental state of 23 epileptic psychotic patients with that of 10 endogenous schizophrenics using the Present State Examination. Of the 23 epileptics, 11 satisfied the CATEGO criteria for the nuclear syndrome of schizophrenia. All had temporal lobe epilepsy, revealing a significant association between temporal lobe epilepsy and schizophrenia, as opposed to other psychotic forms randomly distributed between the temporal and generalized epilepsies. Moreover, the phenomenology of the schizophrenic syndrome in the detailed description provided by the Present State Examination was essentially identical in the epileptic and in the endogenous schizophrenias, thus settling once and for all the futile discussion of the supposed special clinical features by which schizophrenic psychoses in epilepsy were alleged to differ from schizophrenia. (The only differences were that the endogenous schizophrenics had a higher incidence of visual hallucinations and more religious delusions than the epileptic psychotics; this, of course, is the opposite side of the traditional views.)

Later, Trimble and Perez (1982) further examined their material, now consisting of data for 24 consecutive patients with epilepsy and active psychosis referred to the National Hospital, Queen Square. They commented that, whereas the nuclear syndrome is seen exclusively with temporal lobe epilepsy, the depressive syndrome of endogenous type is associated with generalized epilepsy. Of the 11 temporal lobe epileptics with nuclear schizophrenia, 9 had left temporal epilepsy. It is remarkable that the 2 patients with right temporal epilepsy were both sinistrals!

Shukla and associates (1979; Shukla and Katiyar, 1980), who, as we have seen, had found a right hemisphere association with neurotic-type depressive states in epilepsy, did not find any particular lateralization for schizophrenia; neither did Kristiansen and Sindrup (1978a,b) in Denmark. In both instances this was the result of the psychiatric criteria used, which were not sufficiently discriminating. Shukla defined schizophrenia according to DSM II criteria, which would incorporate a number of thought-disordered hallucinatory depressive psychoses. Kristiansen and Sindrup excluded all affective psychoses and considered "paranoid–hallucinatory" syndromes. However, paranoid–hallucinatory syndromes are not specific to schizophrenia and occur in affective psychoses (where they may dominate the clinical presentation and obscure the affective infrastructure) and are also found in the atypical varieties of mood psychoses. If one does not rigorously define the schizophrenic syndrome, it is not surprising that the laterality dimension does not emerge. Notwithstanding these methodological considerations there is, in fact, a dominant hemisphere implication in the Kristiansen and Sindrup survey. Their psychotic group had a great excess of bilateral foci compared with the nonpsychotic controls (31 versus 7, respectively), and in addition the psychotic group had a significantly higher incidence of sinistrality.

Toone and Driver (1980) also noted a striking excess of sinistrality (17%) in 57 patients with a combined diagnosis of epilepsy and psychosis whose records they retrieved from the Maudsley Hospital for the years 1967–1980. Analyzing a subsample of 41 patients they found a majority of schizophrenic psychoses (*N*=24), affective psychoses (*N*=15), and two postictal psychotic episodes. Examining the laterality of foci in the dextral schizophrenics (*N*=12), a strong dominant temporal lateralization emerges again. Although only 2 patients showed an asymmetric pattern right > left, and no patients exhibited a unilateral right focus, 10 of the 12 had unilateral left (*N*=4) or asymmetric left > right (*N*=6). In a later report on the CAT scan findings in the 57 psychotic epileptics Toone *et al.* (1982) described a nonsignificant excess of left hemisphere abnormality. This is not particularly informative since it resulted from a comparison with epileptics who suffered from psychiatric illnesses other than psychosis or neurotic depression, which were not otherwise defined but which in principle would also demonstrate lateralized abnormalities. Much more interesting is that, when these authors segregated CAT scans showing unilateral abnormality in their psychotic group, all 5 patients with unilateral left-sided changes were schizophrenic or paranoid and the 2 with unilateral right-sided abnormality were affective!

Taylor (1969) reviewed the evidence derived from a study of aggressive psychopathy in temporal lobe epilepsy which suggested that epilepsy of very early onset in the male, and involving the dominant hemisphere, was the cerebral determinant of aggressive psychopathic behavior. Sherwin (1977) found a similar lateralization for aggressive behavior in temporal lobe epilepsy. He examined the EEG and air-encephalographic abnormalities in 35 patients with temporal lobe epilepsy coupled with aggressive or "paranoid psychotic" behavior and found that 17 had EEG localizing features: left-sided in 11, bilateral in 3, and right-sided in 3. The pneumoencephalogram was abnormal in 18 patients, with evidence of temporal horn dilatation in 14. The temporal horn dilatation was left-sided in 13 of these 14 patients. A striking confirmation was provided by the Oxford series of Lindsay *et al.* (1979). Twelve of 87 surviving patients with limbic epilepsy had exhibited severe antisocial and aggressive behavior. In all of the 12 the focus was contralateral to the preferred hand, a very significant lateralization. Of the 12, 10 were males. Catastrophic rage reactions were significantly associated with onset of epilepsy before the age of 1 year and with a significant decrement of verbal IQ for both sexes, again demonstrating disorganization of dominant hemispheric systems.

Sackeim *et al.* (1982) reviewed the international literature for all published cases in which laughing or crying was a component of the aura or of the seizure in an analysis of ictal emotional outbursts. There were 103 cases, with a preponderance of males (where sex was specified: males, 67; females, 31), and gelastic epilepsy was very much more frequent than dacrystic epilepsy (91 versus 6 cases, respectively). The incidence of laughing, or gelastic, epilepsies was twice as high in males as in females, whereas crying, or dacrystic, epilepsies were more common in females than in males. Gelastic epilepsy was significantly associated with left hemisphere epilepsy for both sexes, a lateralization effect that was more pronounced for males than females. In the male, gelastic epilepsy and its relation to unilateral left-sided focus was three times more likely than in association with a unilateral right-sided focus.

Thus, we see that strong evidence accumulated from many independent investigations in several countries shows that in epilepsy schizophrenic, paranoid, and aggressive psychopathic personality deviation is associated with epileptic disorganization of the dominant hemisphere, whereas depressive manifestations, both psychotic and neurotic forms, are related to epilepsy lateralized to the nondominant hemisphere. It is important to note not only that psychopathological syndrome complexes emerge as manifestations of altered, lateralized hemispheric shifts but that these also, as Bear and Fedio (1977) demonstrated, determine patterns of personality organization.

Studying personality characteristics of 47 patients with alien tissue tumors after unilateral temporal lobectomy, Taylor and Marsh (1979) found that right-operated males were significantly more extroverted than left-operated males and that left-operated females had a significant elevation of the Lie Scale on the Eysenck Personality Questionnaire, a result not of deliberate mendacity but of schizoid fantasy. A related observation was made by Mignone *et al.* (1970), who found that social introversion scores on the Minnesota Multiphasic Personality Inventory (MMPI) were significantly higher in patients with dominant temporal lobe lesions than in patients with nondominant lesions. In an investigation of psychological differences in right- and left-sided temporal lobe epilepsy, McIntyre *et al.* (1976) administered tests of cognitive style and affect communication to 11 right and 11 left unilateral temporal epileptics of normal intelligence selected from a neurological outpatient population. Compared with matched controls, the left temporal epileptics were more reflective and the right epileptics more impulsive. Left-lateralized patients were unusual in the assignation of affective labels to emotionally evocative stimuli, whereas the right temporal epileptics were similar to normal subjects. Nielsen and Kristensen (1981) considered 42 patients with unilateral temporal lobe epilepsy "without regard to psychiatric history." Utilizing the Bear and Fedio questionnaire they found that subjects with a left-sided focus were more aggressive and emotionally labile than patients with an exclusively right-sided EEG focus who had "obviously the most benign psychological prognosis [p. 289]."

That hemispheric balance is a determinant of personality is also suggested by some intriguing observations of so-called multiple personality in patients with temporal lobe epilepsy. In the two patients described by Schenk and Bear (1981) the switch in personality was accompanied by a switch in handedness. These authors cited five literature reports demonstrating the same phenomenon.

Particularly fascinating in this context are the two cases reported by Ischlondsky (1955). The first patient was a young woman who exhibited diametrically opposed personality types: one mischievous, impulsive, aggressive, and crude; the other shy, submissive, obedient, and affectionate. The opposed mental states were associated with opposite sensorimotor neurological lateralization. During the aggressive phase the sensory threshold on the right side of the body was high, and that on the left side was low. There was olfactory hypersensitivity in the right nostril and anosmia in the left. The pupil was small on the right and dilated on the left. Similarly, there was a unilateral absence of sweating on the right side of the body and abundant sweating on the left side. When the personality shifted to the opposite pole, the patient became friendly and shy, the lateralized sensorimotor neurological asymmetries also shifted for all the modalities described.

In the second case the neurological lateralization for aggressive and depressed personality shifts was a mirror image of the first. The depressed personality phase was associated with excitatory signs on the left side of the body and hyposensitivity on the right side, the opposite asymmetry being found in the aggressive phase. Ischlondsky remarked that no consistency was observed in the relationship between one or the other personality expression and the specific neurological manifestations and that hyposensitivity on one side was never associated with normal sensitivity on the other, but was always combined with contralateral hypersensitivity. Thus, it is suggested that there is an alteration of the relative balance between the two hemispheres involving a process of active contralateral inhibition, which is presumably responsible for the amnesia always exhibited in such patients during one personality state for the alternative one. The interesting point is that the second patient was dextral and the first sinistral.

III. Forced Normalization

The considerable body of evidence showing that in both epileptic psychoses and endogenous psychoses there is a common and fundamental alteration in neural excitability has been reviewed elsewhere (Flor-Henry, 1976a). In general, this is expressed as a reduction of neural excitability, or increased seizure threshold, accompanied by EEG normalization when the EEG was previously abnormal and correlated with psychopathological manifestations. Kristensen and Sindrup (1978b), in their controlled investigation of 96 patients with complex partial seizures and paranoid hallucinatory psychosis compared with 96 similar patients with psychosis (median duration of epilepsy 24 years), confirmed the inverse relationship between temporal–limbic seizures and psychosis and its independence of the frequency of generalized seizures first reported in 1969 (Flor-Henry, 1969a).

Reports substantiating the importance of forced normalization in psychoses continue to appear. Ishiguro (1981) studied the "periodic psychoses of puberty" in 20 young women compared with 20 age-matched controls. The psychoses were in fact brief manic–depressive episodes associated with menstruation. The patients alone exhibited 4–5 cycle per second spike–wave discharges and temporal spikes. They had a lower seizure threshold than the controls. The EEG abnormalities decreased premenstrually and disappeared altogether during the menstrual phase and the psychotic episode.

Koukkou *et al.* (1979) investigated the paroxysmal EEG activity induced by clozapine in 20 schizophrenics and by haloperidol in another 19. The EEG was monitored on days 0, 3, 10, 20, and 30 after the initiation of medication, and changes were related to baseline incidence on day 0. The EEG indices were correlated with psychopathological syndrome scores: apathetic, hallucinatory, hostile, manic, somatic–depressive, paranoid, catatonic, and retarded–depressive. Clozapine patients with paroxysmal EEG changes received significantly less clozapine than the patients who did not show EEG changes, and the former showed more noticeable alleviation of the retarded depressive syndrome than the latter. There was a negative correlation between frequency of EEG paroxysms and relief of this depressive syndrome. Moreover, the frequency of the EEG activity induced by clozapine was greater in the right than in the left temporal region, and the inverse relationship between EEG paroxysms and intensity of depression was also significantly higher in the right hemisphere than in the left. Clozapine is a neuroleptic that is structurally close to the tricyclic antidepressants, and it has an antidepressant rather than an antischizophrenic action, as was demonstrated in this trial. This study is of considerable importance, for it is probably the first that formally fuses the interaction of the two fundamental parameters of psychosis: laterality of cerebral dysfunction and forced normalization. Forced normalization can also be expressed as a consequence of the successful treatment of temporal lobe epilepsy by temporal lobectomy. In the Danish series reported by Jensen and Larsen (1979), of 74 patients who underwent temporal lobectomy, 11 were psychotic preoperatively. In 6 of the 9 who became psychotic postoperatively, the psychosis emerged after the cessation of their seizures.

In endogenous psychoses the classical, typical syndrome of schizophrenia appears to be associated with an absolute increase in seizure threshold. In the case of catatonic, phasic manic–depressive and "epileptoid" psychoses with depressive, manic, or schizoform presentations there is a background of lowered seizure threshold, the psychotic episodes supervening during transitory states of diminished neural excitability. Remarkably, there is evidence that interictal psychotic episodes during withdrawal of anticonvulsant medication (and consequent increase in clinical seizures) are also associated with forced normalization. Sironi *et al.* (1979) described two patients in Milan who were subjected to depth EEG studies and withdrawn from anticonvulsants before temporal lobectomy because of poorly controlled temporal lobe epilepsy. In the steady state, with anticonvulsant plasma levels in the therapeutic range, they had no seizures and their mental state was unremarkable. During the first 4–5 days of withdrawal they experienced a number of partial, complex seizures and secondarily generalized seizures. These were accompanied by increasing high-voltage spike discharges in the amygdaloid, temporal cortex, and frontal–orbital regions. On the fifth day a sudden dysphoric, delusional hallucinatory episode supervened, with cessation of the clinical seizures and a marked reduction in the depth EEG abnormalities in the first patient and a complete disappearance of the irritative EEG elements in the second patient. Without the information provided by the depth EEG this situation would have been considered characteristic of ictal psychotic episodes; yet, in fact, the emergence of psychosis after withdrawal from anticonvulsants and increased frequency of clinical seizures are, even then, superimposed on a sudden shift toward seizure refractoriness, diminished neural excitability, and normalization of the EEG.

Thus, the evidence from the study of psychopathological associations in epilepsy shows that schizophrenic, paranoid, and psychopathic–aggressive syndromes are correlated with epileptic disorganization of the dominant hemisphere, notably of the dominant temporal–limbic structures, whereas depressive symptoms, both psychotic and neurotic types, are related to epilepsy of the nondominant hemisphere. In the genesis of psychotic as opposed to personality or neurotic forms of mental disturbances, however, the emergence of psychosis hinges on the interaction between the (lateralized) locus of cerebral disorganization and a state of reduced neural excitability in critical cerebral regions in such a manner that there is an inverse correlation between schizophrenic symptoms and the seizure system activated during temporal–limbic seizures (partial complex seizures), as well as an inverse relationship between manic-depressive symptoms and activation of the generalized seizure system.

Furthermore, structural brain damage, measured as the proportion of patients with cerebral atrophy among psychotic epileptics and among epileptics without psychosis, is similar in both groups, suggesting that structural brain damage cannot play a part in the genesis of psychosis. However, when epileptic psychosis develops against the background of brain damage, it is correlated with chronicity of the psychotic process.

IV. Endogenous Psychoses and Laterality

The evidence, increasingly abundant and from increasingly varied sources, showing that the endogenous syndrome of schizophrenia is associated with dominant hemisphere disorganization has been reviewed by the author (Flor-Henry, 1974, 1976b, 1978, 1979a). Several other critical reviews of the question have led to the same conclusion (Gruzelier and Hammond, 1976; Wexler, 1980; Newlin *et al.*, 1981; Gruzelier, 1981b). It should be noted that the specific involvement of dominant frontal and dominant temporal cerebral regions in schizophrenia is suggested by such different approaches as the direction of electrodermal asymmetry, the statistical directionality of saccadic eye movements, accoustic threshold studies, evoked potential characteristics, and tachistoscopic analysis. Even so distant a reflection of cortical laterality and asymmetry as the recovery curve of the Hoffman reflex soleus muscle (right and left) reflects left hemisphere effects in schizophrenia and right hemisphere effects in depression (Goode *et al.*, 1981). Those computed tomographic scan investigations of chronic schizophrenia that have looked for localized points of maximal involvement within the broader context of generalized ventricular dilation–frontotemporal cortical atrophy typically found in approximately 80% of the deteriorating schizophrenias reveal once again a dominant frontal (Golden *et al.*, 1981) or dominant temporal localization (Takahashi *et al.*, 1981). In their review of psychopathology and hemispheric dysfunction, Marin and Tucker (1981) concluded that "some studies seem to indicate left hemisphere dysfunction in schizophrenia [but] a comparable number do not support this hypothesis [p. 550]." This is not surprising if one recalls the heterogeneous character of schizophrenia, the fundamental distinction between the chronic and remitting forms, the not infrequent transformation of schizophrenia into depression or mania (Sheldrick *et al.*, 1977), and the fact that the nuclear syndrome itself is nonhomogeneous since it includes a subgroup with electrodermal asymmetry (left hand responses greater than right hand responses) correlated with hypomania, delusions of grandeur, pressure of speech, depressive delusions, and hallucinations and a subgroup with the opposite pattern of electrodermal asymmetry (right hand responses greater than left hand responses) correlated with emotional withdrawal, blunted affect, apathy, and motor retardation (Gruzelier, 1981a).

The cerebral localization and lateralization of the neural systems that determine mood and its regulation constitute a more complex problem than that of the pattern of cerebral disturbance that psychopathologically is translated as schizophrenia. Although the area has been reviewed (Flor-Henry, 1979b), let us examine the question again, incorporating new information in a slightly different perspective, since evidence derived from epilepsy is crucial in unraveling otherwise perplexing but only apparent contradictions in the data.

Lishman (1968) undertook a detailed and meticulous survey of psychiatric disabilities in British soldiers who had sustained penetrating head injuries. From an initial cohort of 1024, 670 were retained for statistical analysis. Of these, 144 had severe psychiatric disability, which was affective in 113. For the affective disorders the localization was significantly right frontotemporal. Shaffer *et al.* (cited in Rutter 1981) studied the relationship between localized cortical injuries and psychiatric symptoms in childhood in 118 children with depressed unilateral skull fractures identified from 17 neurosurgical units in the United Kingdom and followed up 2 years later. Depression was found in 9%, and there was a significant association between a depressive symptom cluster and right frontal injury. A similar relationship between right hemisphere damage and depressive symptom complex in adults was observed by Folstein *et al.* (1977). In this study 10 patients with left hemisphere strokes (and right hemiplegia) and 10 patients with right hemisphere strokes (and left hemiplegia) were investigated. Of the right hemisphere group, 70% exhibited a depressive syndrome of sadness, irritability, apathy, and impaired concentration, which proved responsive to imipramine. None of the patients with left hemisphere strokes showed a depressive syndrome, although some, understandably, were unhappy with their disability, which of course included, to various degrees, dysphasic difficulties. An American group, as early as 1933, had reported on the mental symptoms accompanying right and left unilateral cerebrovascular accidents. Alford (1933) found that the "emotional–catastrophic" reaction was present in 3 of 33 right hemisphere vascular lesions but occurred in 50% of 55 cases of left hemisphere cerebrovascular lesions. In Rome Gainotti (1972; see also Chapter 8) confirmed these observations in a study of 80 left and 80 right unilateral cerebrovascular accidents. The emotional–catastrophic reaction was significantly correlated with left hemisphere insults and the presence of Broca-type aphasia. The right hemisphere lesion group showed the abnormal reaction of euphoric indifference.

In the analysis of lateralized hemispheric pathology and corresponding mood interactions it is important to differentiate the emergent emotions carefully. The evidence reviewed so far shows that the depressive syndrome complex is derivative of right hemisphere lesions, whereas the emotional–catastrophic reaction accompanies insults of the dominant hemisphere. These are quite distinct categories of mood pathology. In the emotional–catastrophic reaction a trivial stimulus triggers a sudden explosive affective storm, either of heart-rending weeping or of disinhibited hilarity or anger, which a few moments later subsides as suddenly and as unexpectedly as it arose. It implies a disturbance in the regulation or control of emotion, which thus would appear to hinge on dominant hemispheric systems. Thus, it is not surprising that the evidence shows that blunting of affect is associated with dominant hemisphere lesions (Bingley, 1958; Abrams and Taylor, 1980) or that in autism the degree of emotional rapport is correlated with verbal, but not performance IQ (DeMyer *et al.*, 1974).

Whereas the evidence from lateralized cerebral lesional studies reveals that the depressive syndrome complex is associated with nondominant hemisphere pathology, dysphoric mood, depression, or irritability, more isolated expressions of mood disturbance are statistically related to destructive lesions of the dominant hemisphere. An impressive accumulation of inquiries verifies this association. Dobrokhotova and Braghina (1975) summarized the experience from the Soviet Union. Lesions of the left hemisphere lead to depressive states, whereas lesions of the right hemisphere evoke inadequate emotional responses such as euphoria or nonchalance. Gasparini *et al.* (1978) studied 24 consecutive patients with lateralized hemispheric lesions, 16 to the left and 8 to the right hemisphere, the majority of whom had temporal lesions. Aphasics or dysphasics were excluded. Almost 50% of the left hemisphere group and 0% of the right hemisphere group had a depression score over 70 (1 SD) on the MMPI. Sackeim *et al.* (1982) reviewed the international literature for pathological laughter and pathological crying associated with lateralized cerebral lesions. Excluding epilepsy they were able to compile 119 cases (64 males and 55 females). Crying was significantly associated with left-sided lesions, and laughter with right-sided lesions. It is interesting that patients who exhibited both crying and laughter were characterized by a relative excess of bilateral lesions (compared with the other groups). Males are significantly more susceptible to pathological laughter (left hemisphere) and females to pathological crying (right hemisphere).

Thus, observations of epileptic patients indicate that abnormal activation of the right hemisphere induces crying (i.e., sadness), whereas abnormal activation of the left hemisphere evokes euphoria. The manic–depressive syndrome, when it occurs in epilepsy, is associated with right hemisphere epilepsy, as are neurotic forms of depression. The data from (nonepileptic) unilateral cerebral lesions imply that, on the one hand, the depressive syndrome complex is related to right hemisphere lesions whereas, on the other hand, dysphoric emotionality follows left hemisphere pathology and euphoric responses follow right hemisphere inactivation. Denenberg (1980) has shown, in a formal sense, that three fundamental principles are necessary and sufficient to account for the characteristics of a linked double brain system: (*a*) intrahemispheric activation; (*b*) contralateral inhibition; and (*c*) interhemispheric coupling. In this perspective a parsimonious hypothesis to account for the preceding body of evidence is apparent. Sadness is a function of right brain systems, and euphoria of left brain systems. These emotions can be generated by ipsilateral intrahemispheric activation. At the same time, as argued before for different reasons (Flor-Henry, 1979b; Flor-Henry and Koles, 1980), in the normal brain mood stability depends in part on reciprocal transcallosal neural inhibition. Thus, under certain circumstances after a lateralized insult (notably if it is nonirritative and large, as in hemispherectomies or cerebral tumors) the induced emotion reflects the abnormal activation of the contralateral hemisphere through the loss of contralateral inhibition. It would also follow from this representation that mania, although in its most fundamental origin related to right brain mechanisms, is the result of an abnormal activation of the left hemisphere as outlined earlier when it occurs in bipolar psychoses. It is obvious that the central symptoms of mania, verbal disinhibition and euphoria, immediately suggest excessive left hemisphere activation. It is of interest in this context that all cases of secondary mania that have been published in recent years have been associated with lesions, often cerebral tumors, of the nondominant hemisphere. Cohen and Niska (1980) have summarized this evidence, contributing a personal case.

It is remarkable that pharmacological inactivation of the right or left hemisphere with intracarotid barbiturization or transient neurophysiological inactivation with unilateral electroconvulsive therapy (ECT)* produces a pattern of differential emotional responses identical with those accompanying lateralized nonirritative cerebral lesions (Deglin and Nikolaenko, 1975; Rossi and Rosadini, 1967).

A number of approaches (lateral asymmetry of the electrodermal response amplitude, the direction of lateral saccadic eye movements, patterns of EEG desynchronization during mentation, and induced emotions) have verified and amplified the preceding relationships in normal and pathological subjects. For example, both Gruzelier and Venables (1974) and Myslobodsky and Horesh (1978) found in depressed patients that the electrodermal response amplitude (to an orienting stimulus) is reduced

*After unilateral ECT: transient contralateral hemiparesis, deep tendon reflex asymmetry, tactile and visual inattention, homonymous hemianopia, left visuospatial neglect after nondominant ECT and transient dysphasia after dominant ECT, elevation of the accoustic threshold to short tones in the contralateral ear, and reduction of the amplitude of the visual evoked response on the stimulated side. Duration of neurological signs, 20 min (Kriss *et al.*, 1978).

on the right and increased on the left, a right hemisphere implication. Schwartz *et al.* (1975) found evidence of right hemisphere activation in normal subjects during visuospatial and emotional–mental representations reflected by a significant excess of lateral saccadic eye movements to the left. Davidson *et al.* (1979) showed in normal subjects that positive emotions (euphoria) are associated with left frontal activation (lateral saccades to the right) and negative emotions (sadness) with right frontal activation (lateral saccades to the left). Myslobodsky and Horesh (1978) found that in both psychotic and neurotic forms of depression there was an excess of left saccades, that is, right hemisphere activation. Tucker (1981) and Tucker *et al.* (1981) induced depressive and euphoric moods in university students. During each mood condition the subjects carried out verbal and visual imagery tasks, and they were also exposed to an auditory attentional bias task. The left hemispheric tasks (verbal) were invariant in either euphoria or depression. During depression there was a highly significant decrement in visual imagery, and a right ear attention bias emerged (i.e., engagement of the left hemisphere because of right hemisphere interference during induced depression). Frontal α power was significantly reduced on the right side during depression and was symmetric, right and left, during euphoria.

Investigations of depression, both psychotic and neurotic, in which the right–left hemispheric variance ratios during depression and after recovery were analyzed with mean integrated amplitude analysis of the EEG signal, showed without exception a relative increase in right hemisphere variance during depression (right–left = 2,3/1), which returns to near unity after recovery (d'Elia and Perris, 1973; Goldstein, 1979; Rochford *et al.*, 1981; Hoffman and Goldstein, 1981). We had found a significant reduction of right parietal α power in both depressed and manic patients compared with normal subjects (Flor-Henry and Koles, 1980). Matousek *et al.* (1981) found a similar reduction in the absolute values of right parietal α power in 63 patients with endogenous depression compared with 317 controls, and a related finding was described by Kemali *et al.* (1981), who noted in 22 depressed patients a significant reduction of α mean power relative activity in the parietal regions (right < left), an effect not found in schizophrenia or controls. The distribution of the EEG amplitudes over the right and left hemispheres in normal subjects is unimodal and gaussian, 70% of the time for the right and 80% of the time for the left hemisphere. Von Knorring and Goldstein (1982) found that this distribution was abnormal and polymodal over the right hemisphere in 72% of cases of depression but not significantly different from normal subjects for the left hemisphere.

Moreover, von Knorring (1982) found that the tricyclic antidepressant imipramine administered to normal subjects produces EEG changes, with significant increases in left frontal α power—hence a state of relative right hemisphere activation. Paul (1973) had observed a similar effect in depressed patients treated with the monoamine oxidase inhibitor Nardil. We found (Flor-Henry and Koles, 1981) that lithium given for 1 week to normal subjects led to a significant increase in right parietal power and variance and also that right posterior temporal power interacted significantly with the visuospatial cognitive activation condition. Sal-Halasz *et al.* (1958) reported with astonishment that dimethyltryptamine, a euphoriant hallucinogen* structurally related to serotonin, when injected intravenously to 30 healthy physicians, induced abnormal neurological signs on the left side, demonstrating a transient abnormal activation of the right hemisphere. The asymmetric organization of neurotransmitter systems in the brain is increasingly being recognized. It is the inevitable corollary of a central nervous system organization in which structural and functional asymmetries are fundamental elements.

V. Mood, Motility, Visuospatial Systems, Dreams, and Erotic Arousal

A large body of neuropsychological investigations in the past few years, together with psychometric observations accumulated over the past 30 years, show that pathological depression is correlated with a diminished efficiency of visuospatial cognitive skills and that this phenomenon is state dependent, visuospatial abilities returning to normal with recovery from depression. This was confirmed by Fromm-Auch (1982), who reviewed about 20 studies on the effects of unilateral dominant and nondominant and bilateral ECT, which reported quantified neuropsychological measurements before and after ECT. Nondominant ECT, after the fifth treatment and coinciding with recovery from depression, was associated with a significant improvement in right hemisphere neuropsychological functions, whereas there was no systematic change in left hemisphere variables. Dominant ECT produced a decrement in verbal scores, whereas bilateral ECT was associated inconsistently with a tendency toward improvement in visuospatial measures. Brumback and Staton (1980) documented in children with endogenous depression the presence of neuropsychological dysfunction of the nondominant hemisphere, together with performance IQ deficits that significantly improved after treatment with tricyclic antidepressants and recovery. Staton *et al.* (1981) further reported on two children with endogenous depression, mild left hemiparesis, and left Babinski, all of which were resolved after treat-

*Inducing essentially mood changes (euphoria), spatial illusions, disturbance of body scheme, and contraction of subjective time.

ment with tricyclics. Described in the literature is the case of a man who exhibited a right hemiparesis and nonfluent aphasia after the removal of a left frontal convexity meningioma. Five years later during a manic episode the aphasia and right hemiparesis disappeared, returning, however, after the successful treatment of the manic episode with chlorpromazine (Robinson, 1976).

These exceptional cases illustrate the fundamental intricacy of the cerebral systems determining motility and mood. Happiness leads to movement, skipping, and hopping; sadness is linked to immobility or agitation. This intimate interdependence of mood and movement reaches its most extreme forms in the hypermotility of mania and of excited catatonias or in the mutism of melancholia with psychomotor retardation or stupor. It is not a coincidence that the cerebral mood systems (orbital and mesial frontolimbic) are coextensive and overlapping with the frontal systems, which determine volitional motility. The cerebral systems that generate mood states are fundamentally related to the brain systems that determine volitional motility and visuospatial processes. In an evolutionary perspective mood is the subjective epiphenomenon of space and motion; a biological organism must be determined by its motility in relation to visual cues. In this perspective the emotions derivative of left frontal activation, euphoria and anger, can be viewed as corresponding to approach behavior; those derived from right frontal activation, dysphoric states and sadness, correspond to withdrawal. The shift of cerebral mood systems to the nondominant hemisphere is the result of the lateralization in the left hemisphere of neural systems mediating verbal–linguistic processes. There exists, in fact, a remarkable correspondence between the two hemispheres in this respect. Ross and Rush (1981) showed that an inability to understand the emotional inflections of language follows the appearance of lesions of the posterior regions of the right hemisphere; an inability to express emotional modulations of language accompanies lesions of the anterior regions of the right hemisphere. These are the exact analogs of sensory and motor aphasias resulting from posterior and anterior lesions of the left hemisphere, respectively.

Dreams are essentially emotionally charged spatial subjective states with no, or very low, verbal connotations. The loss or reduction of dreaming accompanies unilateral lesions of the right hemisphere (Humphrey and Zangwill, 1951; Nielsen, 1955). Studies of EEG phase relationships during the waking state and sleep have shown than in the waking state the dominant hemisphere leads, whereas during sleep the nondominant hemisphere leads (Giannitrapani *et al.*, 1966). Investigations of the mean integrated amplitude of the EEG during slow-wave sleep and REM sleep indicate an activation of the right hemisphere during REM sleep and of the left hemisphere during slow-wave sleep (Goldstein *et al.*, 1972). Myslobodsky *et al.* (1977) noted reversals of right and left electrodermal response amplitude relationships during the waking state and sleep, suggesting opposite patterns of hemispheric activation in these two states. There is extensive evidence from animal studies that sleep in general is associated with right hemisphere activation and partial hemispheric disconnection, transcallosal neural activity virtually ceasing during REM sleep (Bakan, 1975).

In depression there is reduced latency of REM sleep onset. Antidepressants and ECT suppress REM sleep; withdrawal from antidepressants is associated with rebound, excessive dreaming, and unpleasant erotic stimulation. Sleep deprivation after 24 hr induces euphoria in depressed patients. Furthermore, it is well known that REM sleep is associated with penile erections in the male and with vaginal secretory changes of sexual excitement in the female. Thus, the subjective phenomenology of dreams—spatial, affective, and sexual—with its essential anatomical substrate in the nondominant hemisphere correlated with evidence of corresponding neurophysiological activation in that hemisphere, again reveals the importance of right hemisphere systems in the genesis of affective responses. Moreover, it also suggests that erotic arousal is dependent on right brain processes.

There is independent evidence that this is the case. The author compiled, through a bibliographic search, all the cases of orgasmic epilepsy published in the international literature (Flor-Henry, 1976a). Orgasmic epilepsy is a rare form of epilepsy in which the epileptic seizure is an orgasm, almost always perceived as unpleasant and often with unusual distribution; for example, it may be experienced in the left side of the body. All of the cases were of epilepsy of the nondominant hemisphere. Cohen *et al.* (1976) found that in normal male and female subjects masturbating to orgasm under EEG monitoring, orgasm was associated with a prominent increase in right parietal EEG power. Tucker (1982) found an increase in right parietal EEG coherence and a reduction in power in that region in normal subjects during erotic stimulation. It is not surprising that the orgasmic response, which, in a sense, is paradigmatic of a nonverbalizable subjective experience, should be a function of right hemisphere systems. Orgasmic epilepsy hinges on abnormal activation of right hemisphere systems. Sexual deviation in epilepsy, notably fetishistic, is related to epilepsy of the dominant hemisphere. In nonepileptic populations aggressive psychopathy and sexual deviation occur almost exclusively in the male, whose dominant hemisphere functions are more unstable, more precarious, and more vulnerable than are those of the female. A considerable number of investigations, both in epileptics and in nonepileptics, have shown (using neuropsychological indices, EEG lateralization, or even pneumoencephalographic or CAT scan surveys) that aggressive psychopathy is related to dominant frontotemporal dysfunction. These various relationships lead to a neurophysiological model for sexual deviation, the first that is justified by empirical evidence (Flor-Henry, 1980).

Normal sexuality is determined by the presence of normal verbal ideational sexual representations, which depend essentially on intact dominant hemispheric systems, and on their normal ability to trigger the orgasmic response in the opposite hemisphere. This implies intact interhemispheric connections. Pathological neural organization in the dominant hemisphere provides the neural substrate for the abnormal ideational representations of sexual deviations and leads to (or is associated with) perturbed interhemispheric interactions so that only these abnormal ideas are capable of eliciting, or have a high probability of inducing, the orgasmic response. The characteristic obsessional ruminations on sexual themes typical of sexual deviation are a natural consequence of impaired dominant hemispheric functions (Flor-Henry *et al.*, 1979).

In normal subjects sexual and erotic behavior can be inhibited by left hemisphere inhibitory modulations; in psychopathy and sexual deviation this inhibition is impaired or lost, a consequence of the left hemisphere hypofunction and right hemisphere hyperfunction characteristic of these conditions. Thus, we return to the aggression, emotionality, and sexuality of the left neocortical ablations and intact right hemisphere rodents of Denenberg (1981).

VI. Conclusion

The neuroanatomical organization of the brain, which is profoundly asymmetric and quite different in its structural characteristics in the left and right hemispheres is the infrastructure on which the complex interacting systems of lateralized cognitive, affective, and motor specialization are superimposed. Yakovlev and Rakic (1966) described the massive bias toward dextral motor activity in *Homo sapiens* as a consequence of (*a*) the left hemisphere–right pyramidal corticospinal projections being much more abundant than the converse right cortical–left pyramidal tracts and (*b*) the ipsilateral right cortical–right pyramidal projections being more abundant than the ipsilateral left hemispheric–spinal tracts. Thus, at the statistical level both hemispheres conspire, so to speak, in favor of right motor laterality. Studying upper limb motility impairment accompanying unilateral right and left hemispheric lesions, Wyke (1967) showed that with left hemisphere lesions there is bilateral impairment, whereas right hemisphere insults are associated only with contralateral defect. It is remarkable that the same situation is true for somatosensory impairment and cutaneous sensibility, as was demonstrated by Semmes (1968). Furthermore, at the level of sensory cortical organization the left hemisphere field (bilateral projections) is more restricted and punctuate than the right hemisphere field, which, purely contralateral, is diffuse. The diffuse organization of the right hemisphere, then, is related to the visuospatial, affective, erotic–orgasmic, and musical functions, for which that hemisphere is relatively specialized. The punctuate, discrete organization of the left hemisphere subtends the verbal–linguistic, bilateral, and, in a general sense, controlling functions characteristic of the dominant hemisphere. In *Homo sapiens* the male is a specialized female, and as a consequence of that specialization has acquired more lateralized and more efficient right hemisphere functions, visuospatial, musicogenic, and those related to emotional stability, than the female. The complete absence of great composers, the relative scarcity of great painters, but the very large number of outstanding writers among women cannot be attributed to social pressures alone. It reflects the differential cerebral organization of men and women, which hinges on different solutions to problems of cerebral laterality. The paradox is that in women the more bilateral cognitive system, for both verbal and spatial processes, is translated into verbal–linguistic superiority (compared with males) but more precarious visuospatial and affective modes.

This differential cognitive elaboration in men and women was first described by Lansdell and Urbach (1965). In cases of unilateral temporal lobe epilepsy, only the men showed a decrement in verbal IQ after left temporal lobectomy and of performance IQ following right temporal lobectomy, on the Wechsler scales. McGlone (1980) found the same laterality-by-sex interaction in patients with unilateral cerebrovascular lesions and in patients with lateralized cerebral tumors. Inglis and Lawson (1981) reanalyzed the left- and right-sided temporal lobectomy data reported by Meyer and Jones (1957) confirming these effects. They concluded that "the presence of sexual dimorphism in the functional asymmetry of the [damaged] human brain reflected as a test-specific laterality effect [is] present in male but not female patients [p. 693]." Thus, as far as cognitive, laterality, and gender interactions are concerned, the evidence derived from epilepsy and from nonepileptic lesional material is convergent. As we have seen the same is true for psychopathological parameters. In both epileptics and nonepileptics the psychopathy–left hemisphere–male interaction is found; in both epileptics and nonepileptics sadness (a right-hemisphere-dependent emotion) and depression, as syndrome complex, interact with the female gender, and again in both epileptics and nonepileptics pathological euphoria (a left-hemisphere-dependent emotion) is more frequent in men than in women. As far as schizophrenia is concerned the left hemisphere association is well documented in both epileptic and endogenous schizophrenias. The gender interaction that is so pronounced for the early-onset chronic dementia praecox-type deterioriating forms (male association) is much less evident in symptomatic schizophrenias, that is, in those occurring with epilepsy or in relation to monozygotic twinning. In epilepsy, as we have seen, Taylor (1975) found a significant female–left hemisphere interaction, whereas Lindsay *et al.* (1979) observed a strong male–left hemisphere association.

In monozygotic twins Boklage (1977) noted that concordance for schizophrenia was crucially related to concordance or discordance for handedness but was independent of gender effects. Perhaps what these complex relationships imply is that under certain circumstances the underlying pathogenesis and its repercussions on left hemisphere systems in schizophrenia may override the gender-determined lateralized predisposition. On balance, nevertheless, the evidence reviewed shows clearly that both in epileptic and in nonepileptic populations asymmetric lateralized disturbance of cerebral organization is reflected in similar psychopathological expressions and in similar patterns of cognitive impairment. Indeed, given the consistency of these trends, it seems probable that the cognitive and the psychopathological dimensions are themselves deeply interrelated and not as distinct from each other as is generally supposed.

References

Abrams, R., and Taylor, M. A. (1980). Psychopathology and the electroencephalogram. *Biol. Psychiatry* **15,** 871–878.

Alford, L. B. (1933). Localization of consciousness and emotion. *Am. J. Psychiatry* **89,** 789–799.

Bakan, P. (1975). Dreaming, REM sleep and the right hemisphere: A theoretical integration. *Lect., Int. Cong. Sleep Res., 2nd,* 1975.

Bear, D. M., and Fedio, P. (1977). Quantitative analysis of interictal behavior in temporal lobe epilepsy. *Arch. Neurol. (Chicago)* **34;** 454–467.

Bingley, T. (1958). Mental symptoms in temporal lobe epilepsy and temporal lobe gliomas. *Acta Psychiatr. Neurol. Suppl.* **33,** 136–151.

Boklage, C. E. (1977). Schizophrenia, brain asymmetry development, and twinning: Cellular relationship with etiological and possibly prognostic implications. *Biol. Psychiatry* **12,** 19–35.

Brumback, R. A., and Staton, R. D. (1980). Neuropsychological study of children during and after remission of endogenous depressive episodes. *Percept. Mot. Skills* **50,** 1163–1167.

Cohen, H. D., Rosen, R. C., and Goldstein, L. (1976). Electroencephalographic laterality changes during human sexual orgasm. *Arch. Sex. Behav.* **5**(3), 189–195.

Cohen, M. R., and Niska, R. W. (1980). Localized right cerebral hemisphere dysfunction and recurrent mania. *Am. J. Psychiatry* **137,** 847–848.

Davidson, R. J., Schwartz, G. E., Saron, C., Bennett, J., and Goleman, D. J. (1979). Frontal vs. parietal EEG asymmetry during positive and negative affect. *Psychophysiology* **16,** 202–203.

Deglin, V. L., and Nikolaenko, N. N. (1975). Role of the dominant hemisphere in the regulation of emotional states. *Hum. Physiol.* **1,** 394–402.

d'Elia, G., and Perris, C. (1973). Cerebral functional dominance and depression. *Acta Psychiatr. Scand.* **49,** 191–197.

DeMyer, M. K., Barton, S., Albern, G. D., Allen, J., Yang, E., and Steele, R. (1974). The measured intelligence of autistic children. *J. Autism Child. Schizophr.* **4,** 42–60.

Denenberg, V. H. (1980). General systems theory, brain organization and early experiences. *Am. J. Physiol.* **238,** R3–R13.

Denenberg, V. H. (1981). Hemispheric laterality in animals and the effects of early experience. *Behav. Brain Sci.* **4,** 1–49.

Dobrokhotova, T. A., and Braghina, N. N. (1975). Functional asymmetry of the cerebral hemispheres in psychopathological cases due to brain lesions. *Psychol. Abstr.* **53,** 9932–9939.

Falconer, M. A., and Taylor, D. C. (1970). Temporal lobe epilepsy: Clinical features, pathology, diagnosis and treatment. *In* "Modern Trends in Psychological Medicine" (J. H. Price, ed.), pp. 346–373. Butterworth, London.

Flor-Henry, P. (1966). Psychosis and temporal lobe epilepsy. Unpublished. Doctoral Thesis, University of Edinburgh.

Flor-Henry, P. (1969a). Psychosis and temporal lobe epilepsy—a controlled investigation. *Epilepsia* **10,** 363–395.

Flor-Henry, P. (1969b). Schizophrenic-like reactions and affective psychoses associated with temporal lobe epilepsy: Etiological factors. *Am. J. Psychiatry* **126,** 400–403.

Flor-Henry, P. (1974). Psychosis, neurosis and epilepsy. *Br. J. Psychiatry* **124,** 144–150.

Flor-Henry, P. (1976a). Epilepsy and psychopathology. *In* "Recent Advances in Clinical Psychiatry" (K. Granville-Grossman, ed.), pp. 262–295. Churchill-Livingstone, Edinburgh.

Flor-Henry, P. (1976b). Lateralized temporal–limbic dysfunction and psychopathology. *Ann. N.Y. Acad. Sci.* **280,** 777–795.

Flor-Henry, P. (1978). The endogenous psychoses: A reflection of lateralized dysfunction of the anterior limbic system. *In* "Limbic Mechanisms" (K. E. Livingston and O. Hornykiewicz, eds.). Plenum, New York.

Flor-Henry, P. (1979a). Laterality, shifts of cerebral dominance, sinistrality and psychosis. *In* "Hemisphere Asymmetries of Function in Psychopathology" (J. Gruzelier and P. Flor-Henry, eds.), pp. 3–19. Elsevier/North-Holland Biomedical Press, Amsterdam.

Flor-Henry, P. (1979b). On certain aspects of the localization of the cerebral systems regulating and determining emotion. *Biol. Psychiatry* **14,** 677–698.

Flor-Henry, P. (1980). Cerebral aspects of the orgasmic response: Normal and deviational. *In* "Medical Sexology" (R. Forleo and W. Pasini, eds.), pp. 256–262. Elsevier/North-Holland Biomedical Press, Amsterdam.

Flor-Henry, P., and Koles, Z. J. (1980). EEG studies in depression, mania and normals: Evidence for partial shifts of laterality in the affective psychoses. *Adv. Biol. Psychiatry* **4,** 21–43.

Flor-Henry, P., and Koles, Z. J. (1981). The effect of lithium on the EEG in mania and in normals. *World Congr. Biol. Psychiatry, 3rd, 1981* Abstract.

Flor-Henry, P., Yeudall, L. T., Koles, Z. J., and Howarth, B. G. (1979). Neuropsychological and power spectral EEG investigations of the obsessive–compulsive syndrome. *Biol. Psychiatry* **14,** 119–130.

Folstein, M. F., Maiberger, R., and McHugh, P. R. (1977). Mood disorder as a specific complication of stroke. *J. Neurol., Neurosurg. Psychiatry* **40,** 1018–1020.

Fromm-Auch, D. (1982). Selective memory impairment with ECT. *Br. J. Psychiatry* **141,** 608–613.

Gainotti, G. (1972). Emotional behavior and hemispheric side of the lesion. *Cortex* **8,** 41–55.

Gasparrini, W. G., Satz, P., Heilman, K. M., and Coolidge, F. L. (1978). Hemispheric asymmetries of affective processing as determined by the Minnesota Multiphasic Personality Inventory. *J. Neurol., Neurosurg. Psychiatry* **41,** 470–473.

Giannitrapani, D., Sorkin, A. I., and Enenstein, J. (1966). Laterality preference of children and adults as related to interhemispheric EEG phase activity. *J. Neurol. Sci.* **3,** 139.

Golden, C. J., Graber, B., Coffman, J., Berg, R. A., Newlin, D. B., and Bloch, S. (1981). Structural brain deficits in schizophrenia. *Arch. Gen. Psychiatry* **38,** 1014–1017.

Goldstein, L. (1979). Some relationships between quantified hemispheric EEG and behavioral states in man. *In* "Hemisphere Asymmetries of Function in Psychopathology" (J. Gruzelier and P. Flor-Henry, eds.), pp. 237–254. Elsevier/North-Holland Biomedical Press, Amsterdam.

Goldstein, L., Stolzfus, N. W., and Gardocki, J. F. (1972). Changes in interhemispheric amplitude relationships in the EEG during sleep. *Physiol. Behav.* **8,** 811.

Goode, D. J., Manning, A. A., and Middleton, J. F. (1981). Cortical Laterality and Asymmetry of the Hoffmann reflex in psychiatric patients. *Biol. Psychiatry* **16,** 1137–1152.

Gregoriadis A., Fragos, E., Kapslakis, Z., and Mandouvalos, B. (1971). A correlation between mental disorders and EEG and AEG findings in temporal lobe epilepsy. *World Congr. Psychiatry, 5th, 19* Prensa Medica Mexicana, p. 325.

Gruzelier, J. (1981a). Hemispheric imbalances masquerading as paranoid and nonparanoid syndromes? *Schizophr. Bull.* **7,** 663–673.

Gruzelier, J. (1981b). Cerebral laterality and psychopathology: Fact and fiction. *Psychol. Med.* **11,** 219–227.

Gruzelier, J., and Hammond, N. (1976). Schizophrenia: A dominant hemisphere temporal–limbic disorder? *Res. Commun. Psychol., Psychiatry Behav.* **1,** 33–72.

Gruzelier, J., and Venables, P. (1974). Bimodality and lateral asymmetry of skin conductance orienting activity in schizophrenics: Replication and evidence of lateral asymmetry in patients with depression and disorders of personality. *Biol. Psychiatry* **8,** 53–73.

Hara, T., Hoshi, A., Takase, M., and Saito, S. (1980). Factors related to psychiatric episodes in epileptics. *Folia Psychiatr. Neurol. Jpn.* **34** (3), 329–330.

Hoffman, E., and Goldstein, L. (1981). Hemispheric quantitative EEG changes following emotional reactions in neurotic patients. *Acta Psychiatr. Scand.* **63,** 153–164.

Humphrey, M. E., and Zangwill, O. L. (1951). Cessation of dreaming after brain injury. *J. Neurol., Neurosurg. Psychiatry* **14,** 322.

Inglis, J., and Lawson, J. S. (1981). Sex differences in the effects of unilateral brain damage on intelligence. *Science* **212,** 693–695.

Ischlondsky, N. D. (1955). The inhibitory process in the cerebro-physiological laboratory and in the clinic. *J. Nerv. Ment. Dis.* **12,** 5–18.

Ishiguro, T. (1981). EEG and polygraphic findings in periodic psychosis of puberty. *Electroencephalogr. Clin. Neurophysiol.* **52,** 107.

Jensen, I., and Larsen, J. K. (1979). Psychoses in drug-resistant temporal lobe epilepsy. *J. Neurol., Neurosurg. Psychiatry* **42,** 948–954.

Kemali, D., Vacca, L., Marciano, F., Nolfe, G., and Iorio, G. (1981). EEG findings in schizophrenic, depressives, obsessives, heroin addicts and normals. *In* "Electroneurophysiology and Psychopathology" (C. Perris, D. Kemali and L. Vacca, eds.), Vol. 6, 17–28. Karger, Basel.

Koukkou, M., Angst, J., and Zimmer, D. (1979). Paroxysmal EEG activity and psychopathology during the treatment with clozapine. *Pharmakopsychiatr./Neuro-Psychopharmakol.* **12,** 173–183.

Kriss, A., Blumhardt, L. D., Halliday, A. M., and Pratt, R. T. C. (1978). Neurological asymmetries immediately after unilateral ECT. *J. Neurol., Neurosurg. Psychiatry* **41,** 1135–1144.

Kristensen, O., and Sindrup, E. H. (1978a). Psychomotor epilepsy and psychosis. I. Physical aspects. *Acta Neurol. Scand.* **57,** 361–377.

Kristensen, O., and Sindrup, E. H. (1978b). Psychomotor epilepsy and psychosis. II. Electroencephalographic findings (sphenoidal electrode recordings). *Acta Neurol. Scand.* **57,** 370–379.

Landsell, H., and Urbach, N. (1965). Sex differences in personality measures related to size and side of temporal lobe ablations. *Proc. Am. Psychol. Assoc.* **73,** 113–114.

Lindsay, J., Ounsted, C., and Richards, P. (1979). Long-term outcome in children with temporal lobe seizures. III. Psychiatric aspects in childhood and adult life. *Dev. Med. Child Neurol.* **21,** 630–636.

Lishman, W. A. (1966). Psychiatric disability after head injury: The significance of brain damage. *Proc. R. Soc. Med.* **59,** 261–266.

Lishman, W. A. (1968). Brain damage in relation to psychiatric disability after head injury. *Br. J. Psychiatry* **114,** 373–410.

McGlone, J. (1980). Sex differences in human brain asymmetry: A critical survey. *Behav. Brain Sci.* **3,** 215–263.

McIntyre, M., Pritchard, P. B., and Lombroso, C. T. (1976). Left and right temporal lobe epileptics: A controlled investigation of some psychological differences. *Epilepsia* **17,** 377–386.

Marin, R. S., and Tucker, G. J. (1981). Psychopathology and hemispheric dysfunction: A review. *J. Nerv. Ment. Dis.* **169,** 546–557.

Matousek, M., Capone, C., and Okawa, M. (1981). Measurement of the interhemispheral differences as a diagnostic tool in psychiatry. *In* "Electroneurophysiology and Psychopathology" (C. Perris, D. Kemali, and L. Vacca, eds.), Vol. 6, 76–80. Karger, Basel.

Meyer, V., and Jones, H. G. (1957). Patterns of cognitive test performance as functions of the lateral localization of cerebral abnormalities in temporal lobe. *J. Ment. Sci.* **103,** 758–772.

Mignone, R. J., Donelly, E. F., and Sadowsky, D. (1970). Psychological and neurological comparisons of psychomotor and nonpsychomotor epileptic patients. *Epilepsia* **11,** 345–359.

Mnoukhine, S. S., and Dinabourg, E. Y. (1965). Epileptiform manifestations in early right sided and left sided lesions of the brain in children. *Zh. Nevropatol. Psikhiatrim. S. S. Korsakova* **65,** 1073–1077.

Myslobodsky, M. S., and Horesh, N. (1978). Bilateral electrodermal activity in depressive patients. *Biol. Psychol.* **6,** 111–120.

Myslobodsky, M. S., Mintz, M., Yedid-Levi, B., and Ben-Mayor, V. (1977). Electrophysiological evidence of hemispheric asymmetry in non-REM sleep. *Electroencephalogr. Clin. Neurophysiol.* **43,** 460.

Newlin, D. B., Carpenter, B., and Golden, C. J. (1981). Hemispheric asymmetries in schizophrenia. *Biol. Psychiatry* **16,** 561–582.

Nielsen, H., and Kristensen, O. (1981). Personality correlates of sphenoidal EEG-foci in temporal lobe epilepsy. *Acta Neurol. Scand.* **64,** 289–300.

Nielsen, J. M. (1955). Occipital lobes dreams and psychosis. *J. Nerv. Ment. Dis.* **121,** 50.

Onuma, T., Sekine, Y., Komai, S., and Akimoto, H. (1980). Epileptic Psychosis: Its electroencephalographic manifestation and follow-up study. *Folia Psychiatr. Neurol. Jpn.* **34,** 338–339.

Paul, R. (1973). The changes induced by phenelzine in the human encephalogram: a longitudinal study correlating these with the outcome of therapy and certain psychological tests. *Acta Psychiatr. Scand.* **49,** 611–646.

Perez, M. M., and Trimble, M. R. (1980). Epileptic psychosis—Diagnostic comparison with process schizophrenia. *Br. J. Psychiatry* **137,** 245–249.

Robinson, B. W. (1976). Limbic influences on human speech. *Ann. N.Y. Acad. Sci.* **280,** 761–771.

Rochford, J. M., Weinapple, M., and Goldstein, L. (1981). The quantitative hemispheric EEG in adolescent psychiatric patients with depressive or paranoid symptomatology. *Biol. Psychiatry* **16,** 47–54.

Ross, E., and Rush, A. J. (1981). Diagnosis and neuroanatonomical correlates of depression in brain damaged patients. *Arch. Gen. Psychiatry* **38,** 1344–1354.

Rossi, G. F., and Rosadini, G. (1967). Experimental analysis of cerebral dominance in man. *In* "Brain Mechanisms Underlying Speech and Language" C. H. Millikan and F. L. Darley, eds.), pp. 167–184. Grune & Stratton, New York.

Rutter, M. (1981). Psychological sequelae of brain damage in children. *Am. J. Psychiatry* **138**(12), 1533–1544.

Sackeim, H. A., Greenberg, M. S., Weiman, A. L., Gur, R. C., Hungerbuhler, J. P., and Geschwind, N. (1982). Hemispheric asymmetry in the expression of positive and negative emotions: Neurological evidence. *Arch. Neurol.* (*Chicago*) **39**, 210–218.

Sai-Halasz, A., Brunecker, G., Szara, S. (1958). Dimethyltryptamine: Ein neues psychoticum. *Psychiatr. Neurol.* **135**, 285–301.

Schenk, L., and Bear, D. (1981). Multiple personality and related dissociative phenomena in patients with temporal lobe epilepsy. *Am. J. Psychiatry* **138**(10), 1311–1316.

Schwartz, G. E., Davidson, R. J., and Maer, F. (1975). Right hemisphere lateralization for emotion in the human brain: Interactions with cognition. *Science* **190**, 286–288.

Semmes, J. (1968). Hemispheric specialization: A possible clue to mechanism. *Neuropsychologia* **6**, 11–26.

Shaffer, D., Bijur, P., Chadwick, O. F. D., and Rutter, M. L. (1981). Localized cortical injury and psychiatric symptoms in childhood. Cited in Rutter (1981).

Sheldrick, C., Jablensky, A., Sartorius, N., and Shepherd, M. (1977). Schizophrenia succeeded by affective illness: Catamnestic study and statistical enquiry. *Psychol. Med.* **7**, 619–624.

Sherwin, I. (1977). Clinical and EEG aspects of temporal lobe epilepsy with behavior disorder, the role of cerebral dominance. *McLean Hosp. J. Spec. Issue* June, pp. 40–50.

Sherwin, I. (1981). Psychosis associated with epilepsy: Significance of the laterality of the epileptogenic lesion. *J. Neurol., Neurosurg. Psychiatry* **44**, 83–85.

Sherwin, I., Peron-Magnan, P., Bancaud, J., Bonis, A., and Talairach, J. (1982). Prevalence of psychosis in epilepsy as a function of the laterality of the epileptogenic lesion. *Arch. Neurol.* **39**, 621–625.

Shukla, G. D., and Katiyar, B. C. (1980). Psychiatric disorders in temporal lobe epilepsy: The laterality effect. *Br. J. Psychiatry* **137**, 181–182.

Shukla, G. D., Srivastava, O. N., Katiyar, B. C., Joshi, V., and Mohan, P. K. (1979). Psychiatric manifestations in temporal lobe epilepsy: A controlled study. *Br. J. Psychiatry* **135**, 411–417.

Sironi, V. A., Franzini, R. A., Ravagnati, L., and Marossero, F. (1979). Interictal acute psychoses in temporal lobe epilepsy during withdrawal of anticonvulsant therapy. *J. Neurol., Neurosurg. Psychiatry* **42**, 724–730.

Staton, R. D., Wilson, H., and Brumback, A. (1981). Cognitive improvement associated with tricyclic antidepressant treatment of childhood major depressive illness. *Percept. Mot. Skills* **53**, 219–234.

Takahashi, R., Inaba, Y., Inanaga, K., Kato, N., Kumashiro, H., Nishimura, T., Okuma, T., Otsuki, S., Saki, T., Sato, T., and Shimazono, Y. (1981). CT scanning and the investigation of schizophrenia. *Proc. World Congr. Biol. Psychiatry, 3rd, 1981* (in press).

Taylor, D. C. (1969). Aggression and epilepsy. *J. Psychosom. Res.* **13**, 229–236.

Taylor, D. C. (1975). Factors influencing the occurrence of schizophrenia-like psychosis in patients with temporal lobe epilepsy. *Psychol. Med.* **5**, 249–254.

Taylor, D. C., and Marsh, S. (1979). The influence of sex and side of operation on personality responses after temporal lobectomy. *In* "Hemispheric Asymmetries of Function in Psychopathology" (J. Gruzelier and P. Flor-Henry, eds.), pp. 391–400. Elsevier/North-Holland Biomedical Press, Amsterdam.

Terzian, H. (1964). Behavioral and EEG effects of intracarotid sodium amytal injection. *Acta Neurochir.* **12**, 230–239.

Terzian, H., and Cecotto, C. (1957). Su un nuovo metodo per la determinazione e lo studio della dominanza emisferica. *G. Psichiatr. Neuropatol.* **87**, 889–924.

Toone, B. D., and Driver, M. V. (1980). Psychosis and epilepsy. *Res. Clin. Forums* **2**, 121–127.

Toone, B. D., Dawson, J., and Driver, M. V. (1982). Psychoses of epilepsy: A radiological evaluation. *Br. J. Psychiatry* **140**, 244–248.

Trimble, M. R., and Perez, M. D. (1982). The phenomenology of the chronic psychoses of epilepsy. *In* "Seizures, Psychosis, Mania and the Hippo-campal Link." (W. Koella and M. R. Trimble, eds.), Vol. 8, pp. 98–105. Karger, Basel.

Tucker, D. M. (1981). Lateral brain function, emotion and conceptualization. *Psychol. Bull.* **89**(1), 19–46.

Tucker, D. M. (1982). Asymmetrical coherence topography and relationship to various cognitive and emotional affects. *Int. Conf. Laterality Psychopathol. 2nd,* 1982. *In* "Laterality and Psychopathology." (P. Flor-Henry and J. H. Gruzelier, eds.) Elsevier/North Holland, Amsterdam (1983; in press).

Tucker, D. M., Stenslie, C. E., Roth, R. S., and Shearer, S. L. (1981). Right frontal lobe activation and right hemisphere performance. *Arch. Gen. Psychiatry* **38,** 169–174.

von Knorring, L. (1982). Interhemispheric EEG differences in affective disorders. *Int. Conf. Laterality Psychopathol., 2nd,* 1982. *In* "Laterality and Psychopathology" (P. Flor-Henry and J. H.Gruzelier, eds.) Elsevier/North Holland, Amsterdam (1983; in press).

von Knorring, L., and Goldstein, L. (1982). Quantitative hemispheric EEG differences between healthy volunteers and depressed patients. *Res. Commun. Psychol., Psychiatry Behav.* **7,** 57–67.

Wexler, B. E. (1980). Cerebral laterality and psychiatry: A review of the literature. *Am. J. Psychiatry* **137**(3), 279–291.

Wyke, M. (1967). Effect of brain lesions on the rapidity of arm movement. *Neurology* **17,** 113–120.

Yakovlev, P., and Rakic, P. (1966). Patterns of decussation of bulbar pyramids and distribution of pyramidal tracts on two sides of the spinal cord. *Trans. Am. Neurol. Assoc.* **91,** 336–367.

8: Laterality of Affect: The Emotional Behavior of Right- and Left-Brain-Damaged Patients

GUIDO GAINOTTI

Institute of Neurology
Catholic University
Rome, Italy

I. Introduction 175
II. Clinical Aspects of Emotional Reactions Associated with Unilateral Brain Lesions 177
III. Experimental Studies of Emotional Comprehension, Emotional Appropriateness, and Emotional Expression in Right- and Left-Brain-Damaged Patients 181
IV. Meaning of the Emotional Behavior of Right- and Left-Brain-Damaged Patients 184
References 189

I. Introduction

The hypothesis that the division of labor between the right and left hemispheres, rather than being limited to language, motor planning, and perceptual analysis, may also involve emotions and affects is a recent one. For more than a century studies of behavioral defects produced by unilateral cerebral lesions had focused on aphasic, apraxic, and agnosic disorders, ignoring the possibility that the human brain is also laterally specialized for emotions. In reality, the emotional behavior of some patients affected by extensive lesions of the right hemisphere is so striking that it had attracted the attention of such important neurologists and psychiatrists as Babinski (1914), Schilder (1935), and Critchley (1955, 1957). However, the intriguing observations of these authors were generally included in the confusing and perhaps misleading category of the so-called disorders of the body schema, in which, being mixed with dis-

HEMISYNDROMES:
Psychobiology, Neurology,
Psychiatry

ISBN 0-12-512460-0

turbances of a very different nature, they lost their specificity. Consequently, until the beginning of the 1960s the implicit assumption of an equivalence between right and left hemispheres in the modulation of emotions and affects was accepted by almost all students of brain–behavior relationships.

In the past two decades and above all in the past 10 years the situation has changed radically because a large number of clinical and experimental studies conducted with brain-damaged patients, normal subjects, and psychiatric patients have provided increasing support for the hypothesis that the right hemisphere may be critically involved in emotional functions. Reviews of the problem have been published by Galin (1974), Flor-Henry (1976), Gainotti (1979), Seron and Vanderlinden (1979), Bruyer (1980), Dimond (1980), Wexler (1980), Ladavas (1982), Ley and Bryden (1981), Tucker (1981), and Borod *et al.* (1982), and there has been a steadily growing number of studies directed at clarifying the implications of these results for psychopathology and clinical psychiatry.

The relationship between emotions and cerebral dominance remains controversial, however. In fact, even if we do not take into account the controversial problem of the relationship between hemispheric asymmetries of function and psychopathology (Gruzelier and Flor-Henry, 1979; Merrin, 1981) and we limit ourselves to the more restricted problem of the relationship between emotions and cerebral dominance, we still find two contrasting points of view. Some authors (e.g., Seron and Vanderlinden, 1979; Bruyer, 1980; Dimond, 1980; Tucker, 1981) assume the existence at the level of the right and left hemispheres of two neural mechanisms subsuming opposite aspects of mood, with a dominance of the right hemisphere for negative emotions and a prevalence of the left hemisphere for positive affects. Other authors (e.g., Galin, 1974; Gainotti, 1979; Ley and Bryden, 1981) maintain the view of an overall dominance of the right hemisphere for various kinds of emotions and affects. Since the body of data relevant to the problem of laterality of affects is large, we do not take into account in this chapter a number of aspects of this intricate problem. Rather, we focus our attention on a more circumscribed part of this topic, namely, the emotional behavior of right- and left-brain-damaged patients, because we hope that an accurate analysis of this line of research will provide deeper insight into the entire problem of laterality of affects.

We have adopted this type of approach for two reasons. The first is that the clinical studies that have been interpreted as showing that a different emotional reaction is often associated with right and left hemispheric lesions are generally reported in the literature in an overschematic manner, which distorts their meaning. We intend to review in some detail the results of these investigations, since an accurate description of the emotional behavior of right- and left-brain-damaged patients is a useful starting point from which to evaluate the results of subsequent, more focused experimental investigations.

The second reason for focusing on results obtained in right- and left-brain-damaged patients is that a large number of experimental investigations dealing with the recognition, expression, and memory of affects have been conducted in patients with unilateral cerebral lesions. A careful review of these data could help to clarify the link between emotions and cerebral dominance.

This discussion of the meaning of emotional reactions associated with unilateral brain lesions is divided into three parts: In the first we report the clinical aspects of emotional reactions shown by right- and left-brain-damaged patients. In the second we summarize the results of experimental investigations that have studied more focal aspects of the emotional behavior associated with unilateral cerebral lesions. In the third part we discuss the meaning of emotional reactions associated with lesions of the right or left hemisphere with reference both to data reported in the first two sections and to experimental results obtained in normal subjects.

II. Clinical Aspects of Emotional Reactions Associated with Unilateral Brain Lesions

Although careful descriptions of the emotional behavior of patients affected by right or left brain lesions can incidentally be found in many old neuropsychological reports, no systematic study of this problem was undertaken until the end of the 1960s. Thus, about 15 years ago, when I was repeatedly impressed by the contrasting emotional behavior of right- and left-brain-damaged patients, I could find no systematic study of this problem in the neuropsychological literature. The only results available at that time were experimental data derived from pharmacological inactivation of the right and left hemispheres by intracarotid amytal injection. Terzian and Ceccotto (1959) had noticed that a depressive–catastrophic reaction follows the pharmacological inactivation of the left hemisphere, whereas a "euphoric–maniacal" reaction can be observed after barbiturization of the right side. These observations had been confirmed by other authors (Perria *et al.*, 1961; Alemà and Rosadini, 1964) and seemed consistent with the clinical findings that had attracted my attention during the neuropsychological examination of brain-damaged patients. Therefore, I began a systematic study of this phenomenon by taking into account, in large groups of unselected brain-damaged patients, (*a*) the patterns of emotional behavior shown by patients with lesions restricted to the right or left cerebral hemisphere, (*b*) the clinical context and the neuropsychological correlates of these different patterns of behavior, and (*c*) the longitudinal evolution of the most striking emotional reactions observed in patients with extensive lesions of the right hemisphere. The first step of this research (Gainotti, 1969) consisted in studying the incidence of two opposite types of emotional reaction that seemed characteristic of the lesions of the dominant and of the minor hemispheres, namely, depressive–catastrophic reactions and indifference reactions, respectively. Patients were considered to be presenting a *catastrophic reaction* when, in the face of repeated failures, either in verbal communication or in neuropsychological test situations, they showed increasing signs of anxiety or sudden bursts of tears. In contrast, patients were considered to be presenting an *indifference reaction* when they showed an apparent indifference toward failures and seemed to ignore the obvious consequences of their disabilities or treated them with cheerful acceptance, sometimes even jokingly.

A double dissociation was found between right- and left-brain-damaged patients; catastrophic reactions were significantly more frequent in left- than in right-hemisphere-damaged patients, whereas indifference reactions prevailed in patients with lesions restricted to the right hemisphere. Furthermore, the clinical context of catastrophic reactions, showing that this kind of emotional reaction is closely related to important defects in verbal communication and to severe sensori-motor disorders at the level of the right hand, seemed to suggest that catastrophic reactions can be considered a dramatic but psychologically appropriate emotional reaction. In contrast, it seemed difficult, on the basis of the clinical context, to consider the indifference reaction of right-brain-damaged patients to be an attenuated emotional reaction to a less biologically relevant cerebral injury, since the severity of sensorimotor impairment was even greater in this group of right-brain-damaged patients than in left-hemisphere-damaged patients with catastrophic reactions. Furthermore, it was not possible to consider indifference reactions to be due to a demential lack of awareness, since the association between indifference reactions and mental impairment did not reach the level of statistical significance.

Because the meaning of indifference reactions shown by right-brain-damaged patients was not clear, we thought it useful to undertake a more detailed analysis of the patterns of emotional behavior shown by right- and left-brain-damaged patients during neuropsychological examination. In this new study (Gainotti, 1972) the patterns of behavior previously described under the heading of "catastrophic reactions" were divided into two groups, trying to distinguish the patterns directly linked to the emotional storm of the catastrophic reaction, from the patterns due to a more elaborate expression of anxiety and suggestive of a depressed mood. The first group included anxiety reactions, bursts of tears, swearing and sharp or depressed refusals to go on with the examination, whereas the second group included expressions of discouragement, anticipations and declarations of incapacity, rationalizations, and glorification of past abilities.

Furthermore, in addition to the patterns characteristic of the indifference reaction (which included anosognosia, minimization of the disability, indifference to failures, and a tendency to joke in a fatuous, ironic, or euphoric manner), we also took into account a certain number of attitudes toward the disability that seemed to be due to a strong need for denial of illness. These attitudes included delusions about parts of the body, confabulations of denial, and expressions of hatred toward the paralyzed limbs.

With this more detailed study of the patterns of emotional behavior shown by right- and left-brain-damaged patients we intended to test a hypothesis advanced by Terzian (1964) and Rossi and Rosadini (1967) to explain the contrasting emotional behavior observed after pharmacological inactivation of the right and left cerebral hemispheres. These authors had attributed depressive–catastrophic and euphoric–maniacal reactions to the inactivation of two distinct neurophysiological mechanisms subsuming the positive and negative aspects of mood and had located the first in the left and the second in the right hemisphere. This interpretation, however, was not in accordance with the clinical impression we had obtained in our previous work, since the catastrophic reaction of left-brain-damaged patients seemed to us a psychologically appropriate emotional reaction and since the analogy between indifference reaction and euphoric orientation of mood seemed rather superficial. Our expectation was that, if we were to draw a distinction between depressive and catastrophic reactions, that is, between patterns of behavior suggestive of a depressive orientation of the mood and patterns directly linked to the emotional storm of the catastrophic reaction (in the sense originally put forward by Goldstein, 1939), this could help to clarify the meaning of the emotional behavior of left-brain-damaged patients. At the same time we expected that an analytical study of the attitudes toward illness and disability of right-brain-damaged patients could cast some light on the meaning of the "indifference reactions" shown by patients with lesions restricted to the right hemisphere. The results supported, in part at least, these expectations, since it was found that only patterns directly linked to the emotional storm of the catastrophic reaction were significantly more frequent within the left-brain-damaged patients, whereas patterns pointing to a depressive mood were not significantly more highly represented in this group. In contrast, when patients' attitudes toward failures and disability were taken into account, it was found that not only attitudes pointing to an indifference reaction (namely, anosognosia, minimization of the disability, indifference toward failures, and tendency to joke), but also expressions of hatred toward the paralyzed limbs were significantly more frequent among the right-brain-damaged patients.

Because in our previous study we had found that catastrophic reactions are almost always associated with aphasia and that indifference reactions are highly associated with neglect phenomena for the left half of the body and of extrapersonal space, the relationships between patterns of emotional reaction, aphasia, and neglect phenomena were also considered. Among the left-brain-damaged patients some patterns linked to the emotional storm of the catastrophic reaction (namely, anxiety reactions, bursts of tears, swears, and sharp refusals to go on with the examination) were significantly more frequent in aphasic than in nonaphasic patients. Furthermore, depressive–catastrophic reactions assumed distinctive qualitative features according to the different clinical forms of aphasia. They were particularly sharp and violent in Broca's aphasic patients, in whom bursts of tears were frequent (68%) and showed a dramatic but transient phenomenology. Anxiety reactions were most prevalent among amnesic aphasic patients (50%), in whom fits of tears appeared only when compensative boasting or attempts to rationalize or glorify past abilities had failed to discharge the emotional strain. Still different was the emotional behavior of patients with Wernicke's aphasia, since swears, refusals, and expressions of discouragement were frequent among these patients, but no subject of this group showed a tendency to weep. The results for right-brain-damaged patients generally confirmed our earlier results. Verbal denial, minimization of the disability, indifference to failures, a tendency to joke, and expressions of hatred toward the paralyzed limbs were all significantly related to the presence of hemiasomatognosia or of unilateral spatial neglect.

Because indifference toward failures and denial of the disability are generally observed in patients with extensive lesions of the right hemisphere and are particularly frequent in the early postictal stages, we followed the temporal evolution of emotional behavior in 10 patients affected by acute and extensive lesions of the right hemisphere (Gainotti, 1968). The results of this study showed that the emotional behavior of right-brain-damaged patients often follows a predictable evolutionary pattern. Anosognosia and delusions about parts of the body were observed only in the acute postictal periods and were generally associated with a low level of vigilance and, sometimes, with sarcasm and hostility. In the subacute stage anosognosic patients began to admit the presence of hemiplegia but showed a tendency to minimize its importance or became fatuous, indifferent, and sometimes frankly euphoric. Finally, in the chronic stage some patients became much more conscious of their disability and showed a depressed mood, with anxiety, tears, and expressions of discouragement, whereas the behavior of other patients alternated between indifference or apathy and expressions of hatred toward the paralyzed limbs.

Even though the exact meaning of the paradoxical emotional behavior of right-brain-damaged patients was not clear, this form of emotional reaction to the disability was considered to be psychologically inappropriate and was attributed to the disruption of a structure critically involved in emotions and affects.

III. Experimental Studies of Emotional Comprehension, Emotional Appropriateness, and Emotional Expression in Right- and Left-Brain-Damaged Patients

Wechsler (1973) was the first author to study experimentally the problem of emotional behavior associated with unilateral brain lesions. In this study right- and left-brain-damaged patients were asked to recall neutral and emotionally charged stories. A significant interaction was found between hemispheric side of lesion and type of memory disturbance, since recall of emotionally charged material was more impaired in right- than in left-brain-damaged patients, but there was no difference between patient groups in recall of neutral narrative texts. Finlayson and Rourke (1975) and Gardner *et al.* (1975) obtained, with very different experimental procedures, results consistent with the hypothesis that an abnormal or inappropriate emotional (and social) reaction may result from lesions of the right hemisphere. Finlayson and Rourke (1975) found that right-brain-damaged patients achieve particularly poor scores on a test of social judgment, and Gardner *et al.* (1975) noticed that these patients, although perfectly able to explain verbally the meaning of humorous cartoons, often react to them with an inappropriate emotional reaction. Results in line with the hypothesis of an inappropriate reaction to the disability of right-brain-damaged patients were also obtained by Denes *et al.* (1977) in a rehabilitation study. These authors showed that, when right- and left-brain-damaged patients of comparable sensorimotor impairment were enrolled in a program of physical rehabilitation, the worst results were achieved by right-brain-damaged patients with indifference reaction, anosognosia, and unilateral spatial neglect. This could suggest that a motivational defect is responsible for the poor improvement shown after attempts at physical rehabilitation by right-brain-damaged patients.

Other studies have focused on the issue of whether damage to the right hemisphere impairs the ability to comprehend emotional information and to express emotions. In this group of investigations we distinguish between two lines of research: The first attempted to study the capacity of brain-damaged patients to perceive and to produce the affective components of speech; the second aimed to assess the patients' ability to recognize and produce facial (and gestural) emotional expressions.

Heilman *et al.* (1975) reported that right-brain-damaged patients with unilateral spatial neglect, although perfectly able to understand the meaning of a sentence, are unable to perceive the mood of the person reading the sentence on the tape recorder. These results were not confirmed by Schlanger *et al.* (1976), who found that right-brain-damaged patients do not achieve lower scores than aphasic subjects on a task requiring subjects to match emotional voices with emotional faces.

However, the findings of Heilman *et al.* (1975) were replicated and extended by Tucker *et al.* (1977), who showed that patients with temporoparietal lesions of the right hemisphere are unable both to perceive the emotional components of speech and to express emotions through propositional speech, and by Ross and Mesulam (1979), who reported the anatomoclinical observation of two patients who had suddenly lost the capacity to express emotions through speech and gestures after vascular lesion of the right hemisphere.

The entire problem of the relationships between right hemisphere lesions and disruption of the affective components of language has been systematized by Ross (1981), who has claimed that these components of speech are subsumed above all by the right hemisphere and that their functional–anatomical organization mirrors in the right hemisphere the anatomical organization of propositional language in the left hemisphere. Even if the clinical data reported by Ross (1981) seem too weak to support fully his contention that a clear anatomoclinical correspondence exists between disorders of affective language ("aprosodias") and of propositional language, his contribution certainly supports the claim that the right hemisphere plays a dominant role in the recognition and production of the affective components of speech.

Results parallel to those obtained in studies of the affective component of speech have been obtained in studies of the nonverbal communication of affects through facial expression. It has been shown that right-brain-damaged patients are often unable to recognize facial expressions (or emotional scenes) and to express emotions through facial and gestural expressions. Dekosky *et al.* (1980), Cicone *et al.* (1980), and Goldblum (1980) showed that patients with right hemisphere lesions (and especially those with unilateral spatial neglect) show significantly more impairment than left-brain-damaged patients when they are asked to recognize an emotional facial expression or to comprehend the emotion represented in a picture. To be sure, results obtained by Dekosky *et al.* (1980) and by Cicone *et al.* (1980) do not necessarily prove that right-brain-damaged patients are specifically impaired in recognizing emotions, since a more general defect in processing faces or other complex visual material could also account for the poor scores obtained by their right-brain-damaged patients. In the study reported by Dekosky *et al.* (1980), in fact, the intergroup differences disappeared when "prosopagnosia" scores were covariated against the "emotional" test scores.

Similarly, in a study reported by Cicone *et al.* (1980) the difference between right- and left-brain-damaged patients disappeared when subjects were asked to evaluate the emotional content of a given situation on the basis of its verbal description and not its pictorial representation. This criticism, however, does not apply to the study of Goldblum (1980) since this author presented two types of faces to right- and left-brain-damaged patients: (*a*) faces expressing an emotion; and (*b*) faces with a conventional characteristic (i.e., with an intentional communicative aspect). With this experimental procedure Goldblum (1980) demonstrated that the emotional and not the visuoperceptual characteristic of the stimuli is the critical factor in determining the poor scores of right-brain-damaged patients. These patients were selectively impaired in the recognition of emotional faces, whereas left-brain-damaged patients were significantly more impaired in the comprehension of conventional faces.

If we proceed now from the recognition of emotional faces to the facial expression of emotions, we find some interesting results in a study by Buck and Duffy (1980). These authors studied the spontaneous nonverbal expressiveness of right- and left-brain-damaged patients, Parkinson's disease patients, and control subjects by means of a slide-viewing paradigm in which affective-loaded color slides were presented to the patients, while a hidden camera videotaped their facial and gestural responses. Different types of affective slides were shown to the patients, and judges, who were watching the videotapes without sound, were asked to guess the type of affective slide shown to the patients. The accuracy with which the judges identified the slides presented to the patients was taken as an index of the spontaneous nonverbal expressiveness of the various groups. The results showed that aphasic patients are even more expressive than controls, whereas right-brain-damaged and Parkinson's disease patients are significantly less expressive than the other patients. The interest of this study consists, in our opinion, of the fact that, in addition to showing that right hemispheric lesions often impair the ability to express emotions through facial and gestural expressions, it also suggests that left hemispheric lesions, far from disrupting emotional expressiveness, may even enhance it.

The last line of research to be reviewed briefly in this survey of experimental investigations of the emotional behavior of right- and left-brain-damaged patients deals with the autonomic arousal of patients with unilateral cerebral lesions. Heilman *et al.* (1978) demonstrated that right- and left-brain-damaged patients show a very different galvanic skin response to painful stimuli applied to the limbs ipsilateral to the damaged hemisphere. Right-brain-damaged patients with unilateral spatial neglect showed significantly less response than control subjects, whereas aphasic patients with lesions involving the left hemisphere showed a significantly greater response to stimuli than did either the controls or the right-brain-damaged patients.

This last finding is consistent with the observation of Buck and Duffy

(1980) that aphasic patients with left hemispheric lesions show an even greater emotional expressiveness than normal controls do. Results obtained by Heilman *et al.* (1978) were replicated by Morrow *et al.* (1981) and by Zoccolotti *et al.* (1982) by means of a slide-viewing procedure in which galvanic skin responses were monitored in right- and left-brain-damaged patients during the random presentation of neutral and emotionally loaded visual stimuli. In the control group and in patients with left hemispheric damage, galvanic skin responses were significantly greater for the emotional than for the neutral stimuli, whereas in right-brain-damaged patients only a small galvanic skin change was obtained in response to either stimuli. These results suggest that the reduced emotional reactiveness of right-brain-damaged patients could be due either to an overall defect in arousal or to a disorder in the emotional arousal.

IV. Meaning of the Emotional Behavior of Right- and Left-Brain-Damaged Patients

Since the attention of researchers appears to have been attracted mainly by the strange emotional behavior that accompanies lesions of the right hemisphere, most of the interpretations advanced to explain the meaning of emotional reactions shown by right- and left-brain-damaged patients have focused on the indifference reaction of right-brain-damaged patients. This emotional behavior has been interpreted in at least three different ways.

The first interpretation assumes the existence at the level of the right and left hemispheres of two specific neural mechanisms subsuming opposite aspects of mood. This interpretation was first advanced by authors who had observed a depressive–catastrophic reaction after pharmacological inactivation of the left hemisphere and a euphoric–maniacal reaction after injection of sodium amytal into the right carotid artery (Terzian, 1964, Rossi and Rosadini, 1967).

More recently, data supporting this interpretation were obtained in normal subjects by Dimond and Farrington (1977), who observed, using a contact-lens method devised to direct visual stimuli to either the right or left half of the brain, that the right hemisphere shows an enhanced response to unpleasant emotional stimuli, whereas the left hemisphere shows the highest level of response to humorous material. Dimond and Farrington (1977) interpreted these data as suggesting a different emotional specialization of the two halves of the brain, with a dominance of the right hemisphere for negative, unpleasant emotions and a prevalence of the left hemisphere for positive affects. Some indirect support for this interpretation was given by Ahern and Schwartz (1979) and Natale and Gur (1980), who interpreted the direction of lateral eye movements in response to positive and negative emotional questions as an index of relative hemispheric activation. Positive-emotion questions evoked a greater number of right looks (suggestive of a relative left hemisphere involvement), whereas negative-emotion questions tended to elicit a greater number of left looks (suggestive of a relative right hemisphere involvement). Similar results were obtained by Schwartz *et al.* (1979) using asymmetries in facial electromyographic activity as a further index of hemispheric activation. Also in this case, there was a greater electromyographic activity in right-side facial muscles following questions about positive emotions and a greater activity in left-side facial muscles following questions about negative emotions.

Even if the validity of these data remains to be demonstrated [Ehrlichman and Weinberger (1978) have shown, for example, that the direction of lateral eye movements is not a reliable index of relative hemispheric activation], the assumption of a different emotional specialization of the right and left hemispheres seems, at first glance, capable of explaining in a simple manner the different emotional reaction of patients with unilateral brain lesion. According to this interpretation, catastrophic reactions of left-brain-damaged patients could be provoked by the lesion of a center subsuming positive affects (with shift of mood toward the depression), whereas the emotional reaction of right-brain-damaged patients could be considered a euphoric–maniacal reaction resulting from inactivation of the center subsuming negative affects. In reality, the analogy between catastrophic reaction and depressive orientation of mood is rather superficial, and even less convincing is the equivalence between indifference reaction and the excited, euphoric behavior of manic patients. In fact, in our study only patterns of behavior directly linked to the emotional storm of the catastrophic reaction were found to be significantly associated with left hemisphere lesions, but we did not find a similar relationship for patterns suggesting a depressive orientation of the mood. Similarly, the analysis of patterns of behavior significantly associated with right hemispheric lesions confirmed Critchley's claim that patients with indifference reactions are "not euphoric in the ordinary way" (Critchley, 1955), since their tendency to joke coexisted with apathy and with exaggerated feelings of hatred toward the paralyzed limbs.

Furthermore, the hypothesis that the two halves of the brain may subsume opposite aspects of mood is also at variance with the results of some recent investigations in normal subjects of either the processing of positive and negative emotional information in the right and left half-fields or the expression of positive and negative emotions on the right and left sides of the face. On the one hand, Butchel *et al.* (1978), Campbell (1978), Ladavas *et al.* (1980), Strauss and Kaplan (1980), and Strauss and Moscovitch (1981) have shown that the left visual field (right hemisphere) is consistently superior to the right one (left hemisphere) in processing both positive and negative emotions. On the other hand, Chaurasia and Goswami (1975), Campbell (1978), Borod and Caron (1980), and Heller and Levy (1981) have shown that the left side of the face is more expressive than the right not only in expressing negative emotions (such as sadness or fear) but also in expressing positive emotions (such as happiness).

These results clearly argue against the hypothesis of a right hemisphere dominance for negative emotions and a left hemisphere dominance for positive affects.

The second interpretation assumes that the indifference reaction of right-brain-damaged patients may be due to an attention–arousal defect leading to a sort of "flattened affect." This interpretation was proposed by Heilman *et al.* (1978), who, struck by the correlation between indifference reaction and neglect phenomena, advanced the hypothesis that an attention–arousal defect may be responsible for both these symptoms. According to Heilman *et al.* (1978) this attention–arousal defect could be provoked by the disruption of a corticolimbic–reticular loop similar to that proposed by Sokolov (1963). This hypothesis is supported by studies of the galvanic skin response to painful stimuli (Heilman *et al.*, 1978) or to emotional visual scenes (Morrow *et al.*, 1981; Zoccolotti *et al.*, 1982) in patients with unilateral brain lesions. In both cases, right-brain-damaged patients showed the smallest response to stimuli.

The hypothesis that an attention–arousal defect may be responsible both for the indifference reaction and for the neglect syndrome shown by right-brain-damaged patients is of great interest, since it would explain some of the most important symptoms resulting from right hemispheric lesions. However, this hypothesis cannot account for some important features of the emotional behavior shown by right-brain-damaged patients. It is difficult, indeed, to explain the tendency to joke in a fatuous, ironic, or euphoric manner or the occasional strong aversion toward the paralyzed limbs by considering the emotional disturbance of right-brain-damaged patients only in terms of hypoarousal or "flattened affect." Furthermore, this theory can hardly explain the results of other studies, conducted in patients with unilateral brain lesions, which have shown an elective impairment of right-brain-damaged patients in the perception, appreciation, and memory of emotionally loaded material. Finally, this theory cannot explain the results of investigations conducted in normal subjects that have consistently shown that the intact right hemisphere is superior to the left both in the recognition and in the expression of emotional information.

The last interpretation, and the one this author favors, assumes that the right hemisphere may be dominant for emotions and affects. From this viewpoint the emotional behavior of right-brain-damaged patients could be considered an abnormal or inappropriate emotional reaction determined by damage to a system critically involved in emotions and affects. The advantage of this interpretation is that it can explain in a simple way the results of the clinical and experimental investigations that have consistently shown a major involvement of the right hemisphere in various emotional situations.

Speculative attempts have been made to explain the relative dominance of the right hemisphere for affects. Bogen (1969) and Galin (1974) proposed, for example, two distinct modes of thought characteristic of the right and of the left hemisphere, assuming that the former may be based on a "holistic" or "*gestalt*" processing capacity, whereas the latter might be based on a verbal–analytical–logical mode of thought. The "appositional mind" of the right hemisphere could be viewed as being similar to Freud's primary process, whereas the "propositional mind" of the left hemisphere could be considered analogous to Freud's secondary process.

From a slightly different perspective the author has advanced the hypothesis that the presence or absence of a complex linguistic mediation could be the factor that is critical for a different organization of the highest cortical functions at the level of the right and left cerebral hemispheres (Gainotti, 1972). In the left hemisphere, sensory data could undergo a complex conceptual elaboration, because of the presence of language mediation, whereas at the level of the right hemisphere, where language is not represented, they should be processed in a more primitive way, preserving characteristics of immediateness and of rich affective value. Some support for this view comes from data (Giannitrapani, 1967) that suggest a more rapid development of the right hemisphere until the age of 18 to 24 months, when language appears and the specialization for language of the left hemisphere begins. Because of these maturational differences, the right hemisphere might be involved mainly in the treatment of important prelinguistic experiences (such as visuospatial relations, emotional situations, and so on). The left hemisphere could therefore be considered to be more important from the verbal–conceptual viewpoint, whereas the right hemisphere could be viewed as being more involved in nonlinguistic visuospatial and emotional functions.

A more composite interpretation has been advanced by Ley and Bryden (1981), who have proposed that at least three characteristics of the right hemisphere functioning (i.e., a diffuse organization of sensorimotor functions, a holistic or *gestalt* processing style, and a greater capacity for producing imagic material) might bias this hemisphere for processing affective information. We do not think it possible, given the present state of affairs, to decide which of the previously mentioned interpretations gives a better explanation of the emotional behavior of right-brain-damaged patients and of the results obtained in other clinical and experimental investigations. Two points, however, seem to be worth stressing.

The first is that, even if we concur with the hypothesis of a right hemisphere dominance for emotions, we do not consider this interpretation to be exclusive and antithetical to other theories discussed in this section. Heilman's hypothesis of an attention–arousal defect in right-brain-damaged patients could be complementary, for example, to that of an abnormal emotional reaction of these patients. In the same manner the hypothesis of an emotional disorder resulting from a lesion of the right hemisphere does not rule out the possibility that the intact left hemisphere may make an important contribution to the elaboration of the verbal defenses necessary to cope with the disability.

The second and conclusive point is that, in addition to the possibility of using powerful verbal defenses to control the anxiety provoked by the disability, the left hemisphere might also have other important mechanisms of control over emotional expression. In fact, it has been observed (Gainotti, 1972) that the sharp bursts of tears of Broca's aphasic patients resemble in some aspects, such as the low level of elicitation and the dramatic but transient phenomenology, the spasmodic bursts of tears of pseudobulbar palsy. This suggests, by analogy, that an important mechanism for the control of emotional discharge may exist in the anterior regions of the left hemisphere and that inactivation of this mechanism may be responsible for the sharp and violent aspects of the catastrophic reaction shown by this group of aphasic patients. We have reported in previous sections other data that might support this interpretation. On the one hand, Heilman *et al.* (1978) observed that aphasic patients showed significantly greater galvanic skin responses to painful stimuli than did either right-brain-damaged patients or normal controls and interpreted this finding as being due to a disinhibited sympathetic activity resulting from the left hemisphere lesion. On the other hand, Buck and Duffy (1980) observed that, while viewing emotional slides, aphasic patients were even more expressive than normal controls and that emotional expressiveness was positively correlated with the severity of aphasia. The authors explained this finding by assuming that the left hemisphere may normally exert an inhibitory influence over emotional expression and that damage to the left hemisphere, decreasing this inhibition, may allow a greater nonverbal expression.

Taken together, these clinical and experimental data might therefore suggest that the division of labor between the two halves of the brain consists of a separation between structures subserving recognition and elaboration of affects (located mainly in the right hemisphere) and mechanisms responsible for emotional control (located mainly in the left hemisphere). Further investigations are, in any case, required to confirm the validity of this more speculative than proved interpretation of the emotional behavior of right- and left-brain-damaged patients.

Note Added in Proof

After the present chapter had been sent to the typesetter Sackeim Greenberg, Weiman, Gur, Hungerbuhler, and Geschwind (1982) published an article that seems to support substantially the hypothesis that the right side of the brain subserves negative emotions and the left side subserves positive emotions. These authors conducted a retrospective study of all the published cases of uncontrollable outbursts of laughing and crying resulting from destructive brain lesions or observed as ictal manifestations in epilepsy. They found that in cases of destructive lesions pathological laughing was associated with predominantly right brain damage and pathological crying with predominantly left brain damage, whereas in epileptic patients with ictal outbursts of laughing (gelastic epilepsy) foci were predominantly left sided. According to the authors, these data show that "the experience of positive mood and outbursts of uncontrollable laughing are most often due to excitation or disinhibition of regions in the left side of the brain . . . whereas the reverse holds for negative emotions [p. 216]." In our opinion, the data reported by Sackeim *et al.* (1982) clearly suggest that a hemispheric asymmetry exists in the production of positive and negative emotional outbursts, but do not prove the existence of a lateral specialization in the experience of positive and negative emotions. As a matter of fact, pathological laughing and crying (either of lesional or epileptic nature) may well be dissociated from the corresponding subjective mood, since patients who present these symptoms often claim that their concurrent moods are unrelated to the displayed emotions. Thus data reported by Sackeim *et al.* (1982) about patients with uncontrollable emotional outbursts suggest a different hemispheric localization of the mechanisms involved in the expression of positive and negative emotions, but are not conclusive in the lateralization of structures subserving positive and negative emotional experiences. Data obtained by Williams (1956) seem much more relevant. Williams observed the laterality of foci causing fear, depression, pleasure, or displeasure as ictal manifestations, but could find no relationship between laterality of focus and type of positive or negative ictal experience.

References

Ahern, G. L., and Schwartz, G. E. (1979). Differential lateralization for positive versus negative emotion. *Neuropsychologia* **17,** 693–698.

Alemà, G., and Rosadini, G. (1964). Données cliniques et EEG de l'introduction d'amytal sodium dans la circulation encéphalique, concernant l'état de conscience. *Acta Neurochir.* **12,** 240–257.

Babinski, J. (1914). Contribution à l'étude des troubles mentaux dans l'hémiplégie cérébrale (Anosognosie). *Rev. Neurol.* **27,** 845–847.

Bogen, J. E. (1969). The other side of the brain: An appositional mind. *Bull. Los Angeles Neurol. Soc.* **34,** 135–162.

Borod, J., and Caron, H. (1980). Facedness and emotion related to lateral dominance, sex and expression type. *Neuropsychologia* **18,** 237–242.

Borod, J., Koff, E., and Caron, H. (1982). Right hemisphere specialization for the expression and appreciation of emotion. A focus on the face. *In* "Cognitive Processing in the Right Hemisphere" (E. Perecman, ed.), pp. 83–110. Academic Press, New York.

Bruyer, R. (1980). Implication différentielle des hémisphères cérébraux dans les conduites émotionnelles. *Acta Psychiatr. Belg.* **80,** 266–284.

Buchtel, H. A., Campari, F., De Risio, C., and Rota, R. (1978). Hemispheric differences in discriminative reaction time to facial expressions. *Ital. J. Psychol.* **5,** 159–169.

Buck, R., and Duffy, R. J. (1980). Nonverbal communication of affect in brain-damaged patients. *Cortex* **16,** 351–362.

Campbell, R. (1978). Asymmetries in interpreting and expressing a posed facial expression. *Cortex* **14,** 327–342.

Chaurasia, B. D., and Goswami, H. K. (1975). Functional asymmetry in the face. *Acta Anat.* **91,** 154–160.

Cicone, M., Wapner, W., and Gardner, H. (1980). Sensitivity to emotional expressions and situations in organic patients. *Cortex* **16,** 145–158.

Critchley, M. (1955). Personification of paralysed limbs in hemiplegics. *Br. Med. J.* **30,** 284–286.

Critchley, M. (1957). Observations on anosodiaphoria. *Encephale* **46,** 540–546.

Dekosky, S. T., Heilman, K. M., Bowers, D., and Valenstein, E. (1980). Recognition and discrimination of emotional faces and pictures. *Brain Lang.* **9,** 206–214.

Denes, G. F., Semenza, C., Stoppa, E., Galli, G., and Turco, R. (1977). Influence of neuropsychological deficit on recovery of sensorimotor functions following brain damage. *Int. Congr. Ser.—Excerpta Med.* **147,** 73.

Dimond, S. J. (1980). "Neuropsychology." Butterworth, London.

Dimond, S. J., and Farrington, L. (1977). Emotional response to films shown to the right or left hemisphere of the brain measured by heart rate. *Acta Psychol.* **41,** 255–260.

Ehrlichman, H., and Weinberger, A. (1978). Lateral eye movements and hemispheric asymmetry: A critical review. *Psychol. Bull.* **85,** 1080–1101.

Finlayson, M. A. J., and Rourke, B. P. (1975). Personality correlates of lateralized cerebral vascular disease. *Pap., Am. Psychol. Assoc. Conv.* 1975.

Flor-Henry, P. (1976). Lateralized temporal limbic dysfunction and psychopathology. *Ann. N. Y. Acad. Sci.* **280,** 777–795.

Gainotti, G. (1968). Aspetti qualitativi ed evolutivi della sintomatologia conseguente a lesioni dell'emisfero destro. *Ann. Neurol. Psichiatr.* **62,** 1–29.

Gainotti, G. (1969). Réactions "catastrophiques" et manifestations d'indifférence au cours des atteintes cérébrales. *Neuropsychologia* **7,** 195–204.

Gainotti, G. (1972). Emotional behavior and hemispheric side of the lesion. *Cortex* **8,** 41–55.

Gainotti, G. (1979). The relationship between emotions and cerebral dominance: A review of clinical and experimental evidence. *In* "Hemisphere Asymmetry of Function in Psychopathology" (J. Gruzelier and P. Flor-Henry, eds.), pp. 21–34. Elsevier, Amsterdam.

Galin, D. (1974). Implications for psychiatry of left and right cerebral specialization. *Arch. Gen. Psychiatry* **31,** 572–583.

Gardner, H., King, P. D., Flamm, L., and Silverman, J. (1975). Comprehension and appreciation of humorous material following brain damage. *Brain* **98,** 399–412.

Giannitrapani, D. (1967). Developing concepts of lateralization of cerebral functions. *Cortex* **3,** 353–370.

Goldblum, M. C. (1980). La reconnaissance des expressions faciales émotionnelles et conventionnelles au cours de lésions corticales. *Rev. Neurol.* **136,** 711–719.

Goldstein, K. (1939). "The Organism: A Holistic Approach to Biology, Derived from Pathological Data in Man." American Books, New York.
Gruzelier, J., and Flor-Henry, P., eds. (1979). "Hemisphere Asymmetry of Function in Psychopathology." Elsevier, Amsterdam.
Heilman, K. M., Scholes, R., and Watson, R. T. (1975). Auditory affective agnosia. *J. Neurol., Neurosurg. Psychiatry* **38,** 69–72.
Heilman, K. M., Schwartz, H. D., and Watson, R. T. (1978). Hypoarousal in patients with the neglect syndrome and emotional indifference. *Neurology* **28,** 229–232.
Heller, W., and Levy, J. (1981). Perception and expression of emotion in right-handers and left-handers. *Neuropsychologia* **19,** 263–272.
Ladavas, E. (1982). Specializzazione emisferica ed emozioni. *Ric. Psicol.* **18,** 255–273.
Ladavas, E., Umiltà, C., and Ricci-Bitti, P. E. (1980). Evidence for sex differences in right-hemisphere dominance for emotions. *Neuropsychologia* **18,** 361–366.
Ley, R. G., and Bryden, M. P. (1981). Consciousness, emotion, and the right hemisphere. *In* "Aspects of Consciousness" (G. Underwood and R. Stevens, eds.), Vol. 2, pp. 216–239. Academic Press, New York.
Merrin, E. L. (1981). Schizophrenia and brain asymmetry—an evaluation of evidence for dominant lobe dysfunction. *J. Nerv. Ment. Dis.* **169**(7), 405–416.
Morrow, L., Vrtunski, B. P., Kim, Y., and Boller F. (1981). Arousal responses to emotional stimuli and laterality of lesion. *Neuropsychologia* **19,** 65–71.
Natale, H., and Gur, R. (1980). Differential hemispheric lateralization of positive and negative emotions in normals. *INS Bull.*, 24–25.
Perria, L., Rosadini, G., and Rossi, G. F. (1961). Determination of side of cerebral dominance with amobarbital. *Arch. Neurol.* (*Chicago*) **4,** 173–181.
Ross, E. D. (1981). The aprosodias: Functional-anatomic organization of the affective components of language in the right hemisphere. *Arch. Neurol.* (*Chicago*) **38,** 561–569.
Ross, E. D., and Mesulam, M. M. (1979). Dominant language functions of the right hemisphere: Prosody and emotional gesturing. *Arch. Neurol.* (*Chicago*) **36,** 144–148.
Rossi, G. F., and Rosadini, G. (1967). Experimental analysis of cerebral dominance in man. *In* "Brain Mechanisms Underlying Speech and Language" (C. H. Millikan and F. L. Darley, eds.), pp. 167–184. Grune & Stratton, New York.
Sackeim, H. A., Greenberg, M. S., Weiman, A. L., Gur, R. C., Hungerbuhler, J. P., and Geschwind, N. (1982). Hemispheric asymmetry in the expression of positive and negative emotions: Neurologic evidence. *Arch. Neurol.* **39,** 210–218.
Schilder, P. (1935). "The Image and Appearance of the Human Body." K. Paul, London.
Schlanger, B. B., Schlanger, P., and Gerstman, L. J. (1976). The perception of emotionally toned sentences by right-hemisphere damaged and aphasic subjects. *Brain Lang.* **3,** 396–403.
Schwartz, G. E., Ahern, G. L., and Brown, S. L. (1979). Lateralized facial muscle response to positive and negative emotional stimuli. *Psychophysiology* **16,** 561–571.
Seron, X., and Vanderlinden, M. (1979). Vers une neuropsychologie humaine des conduites émotionnelles? *Ann. Psychol.* **79,** 229–252.
Sokolov, Y. N. (1963). "Perception and the Conditioned Reflex." Pergamon, Oxford.
Strauss, E., and Kaplan, E. (1980). Lateralized asymmetries in self-perception. *Cortex* **6,** 283–293.
Strauss, E., and Moscovitch, M. (1981). Perception of Facial Expressions. *Brain Lang.* **13,** 308–332.
Terzian, H. (1964). Behavioural and EEG effects of intracarotid sodium amytal injection. *Acta Neurochir.* **12,** 230–239.
Terzian, H., and Ceccotto, C. (1959). Su un nuovo metodo per la determinazione e lo studio della dominanza emisferica. *G. Psichiatr. Neuropatol.* **87,** 889–924.
Tucker, D. M. (1981). Lateral brain function, emotion and conceptualization. *Psychol. Bull.* **89,** 19–46.

Tucker, D. M., Watson, R. T., and Heilman, K. M. (1977). Discrimination and evocation of affectively intoned speech in patients with right parietal disease. *Neurology* **27,** 947–950.

Wechsler, A. (1973). The effect of organic brain disease on recall of emotionally charged versus neutral narrative texts. *Neurology* **23,** 130–135.

Wexler, B. E. (1980). Cerebral laterality and psychiatry: A review of the literature. *Am. J. Psychiatry* **137,** 279–291.

Williams, D. (1956). The structure of emotions reflected in epileptic experience., *Brain* **79,** 29–67.

Zoccolotti, P., Scabini, D., and Violani, C. (1982). Electrodermal responses in patients with unilateral brain damage. *J. Clin. Neuropsychol.* **4,** 143–150.

9: Is There Hemi-aging?

MARGO B. LAPIDOT

School of Communication Disorders
Chaim Sheba Medical Center
Tel-Hashomer, Israel

I. Introduction ... 193
II. Aging Cognitive Abilities: Evidence for Asymmetric Decline ... 194
A. Intelligence ... 194
B. Visuospatial Abilities ... 195
C. Dichotic Listening ... 199
III. Central Measures of the Aging Brain: Known and Unexplored Territory ... 201
A. Electrophysiology ... 201
B. Neurotransmitters ... 202
C. Exploration of Time Sharing with an Older Population ... 203
IV. Concluding Remarks ... 206
References ... 208

I. Introduction

Chapter titles that pose questions obligate authors to furnish answers, and it seems fitting to do just that, here, at the outset, before any of the relevant material is presented. Not surprisingly, the answer at this stage of development of the field of hemi-aging must be an equivocal yes and no.

Hemi-aging, or the selective decline of activity of one cerebral hemisphere, is a relatively new concept, discussed rarely in the literature, whereas hemispheric development in children (e.g., Kinsbourne, 1981) and functioning in young adults (e.g., McGlone, 1980; Bradshaw and Nettleton, 1981) have and continue to receive a good deal of attention. Apart from several sparks of information concerning the presence or absence of signs of hemidecline of certain cognitive functions and components of

HEMISYNDROMES:
Psychobiology, Neurology,
Psychiatry

ISBN 0-12-512460-0

the electroencephalogram (EEG), the idea of hemi-aging is not referred to directly in most of the serious work being done in gerontology.

The purpose of this chapter is twofold: to present a case for hemidecline of the right hemisphere, insofar as it is involved with visuospatial processing, and to review the research with human beings pertinent to hemi-aging, with the hope that it will spur further investigations of the subject and with the belief that such endeavors are, indeed, worthwhile.

II. Aging Cognitive Abilities: Evidence for Asymmetric Decline

In this section the verbal–performance dichotomy, crystallized–fluid intelligence differences, visuospatial abilities, and dichotic memory are reviewed. Aspects of memory, the major cognitive components that decline with age, have been reviewed extensively elsewhere (Craik, 1977; Kubanis and Zornetzer, 1981) and are not directly discussed here except where pertinent to spatial, tactual, and dichotic tasks that may imply certain hemisphere decline.

A. Intelligence

Verbal intelligence, as tested by such measures as the Wechsler Adult Intelligence Scale (WAIS), increases until the seventh decade and then gradually declines. Performance scores increase until the fifth decade, gradually decline until the seventh, and thereafter decline more sharply (Siegler, 1980). Verbal and performance subtests are considered by most neuropsychologists to reflect predominantly left hemisphere and predominantly right hemisphere functioning, respectively (see Chapter 15). When the element of speed is neutralized (Doppelt and Wallace, 1955), performance scores of older adults on the WAIS remain lower than verbal scores.

This verbal–performance difference is regarded as the "classic aging pattern" (Albert and Kaplan, 1980) and, to the extent that it can be superimposed on the now also classic model of hemisphericity, it is in itself an indicator of hemi-aging and has probably been the prime motivator of investigations of right hemisphere decline.

The WAIS scores of normal older subjects were found by Schaie and Schaie (1977) to be indistinguishable from those of chronic and acute right-brain-damaged patients. They refrained from implying that the right hemisphere selectively declines with age and asserted that tests developed with young populations should not be employed with older people.

Albert and Kaplan (1980) raised the possibility of a scoring artifact leading to the aging pattern in light of evidence that using qualitative in addition to quantitative criteria for the scoring of verbal subtests, such as giving synonyms graded value rather than simply counting them, produces results that do indicate verbal decline with age. Nevertheless, the WAIS, or parts of it, continues to be widely used as an assessment tool with older populations.

Another categorization of intelligence, that of crystallized and fluid abilities, is frequently discussed in the aging literature (e.g., Horn and Cattell, 1966, 1967; Hayslip and Sterns, 1979). Crystallized intelligence includes abilities that depend on knowledge accumulated over a long time (i.e., experience), whereas fluid intelligence is exhibited in abilities that are not modified by learning and that involve reliance on spontaneously applied strategy (Botwinick, 1981). Of the two, fluid intelligence is the more vulnerable to aging (Botwinick, 1981), although Hayslip and Sterns (1979) found higher correlations between crystallized and fluid abilities in elderly subjects (59–76 years) than in middle-aged subjects (39–51 years).

It is tempting to draw a parallel between the verbal–performance differences already mentioned and crystallized and fluid intelligence and to claim that they, in turn, respectively reflect left and right hemisphere performance. However, the space subtest of Thurstone's Primary Abilities Test (PMA) is considered to be an example of crystallized ability, and the PMA word fluency subtest appears to be a fluid measure (Siegler, 1980, p. 181), so the verbal visuospatial division cannot be strictly adhered to and it is not possible to fully equate verbal with crystallized and nonverbal with fluid.

B. Visuospatial Abilities

Spatial memory is considered to be a predominantly right hemisphere ability (see Hécaen, 1978). Using data from the Baltimore Longitudinal Study, Arenberg (1978) reported that male subjects' WAIS vocabulary scores were maintained over a 6-year period, whereas memory for geometric designs declined. Error increases were moderate for 50- to 70-year-olds but were substantially greater beyond 70 years. Siegler (1980, p. 182) noted that these findings are "consistent with increased age deficits in intellectual functions that involve spatial relationships and increased memory loads" and can be considered fluid intelligence.

Additional studies reporting an age-related decrement in spatial memory are those of Park *et al.* (1982), in which individuals had to remember the location of target items, of Andersen (1976), in which subjects reproduced complex designs based on geometric figures, and of Riege and Inman (1981), who used the WAIS block design subtest and a recurrent recognition task based on geometric designs.

Memory for faces, another predominantly right hemisphere ability (Yin, 1970; Hilliard, 1973), was found to decline with normal aging by Ferris *et al.* (1980). Encoding, storage, and retrieval, that is, presumably all the strategies underlying recognition memory, were implicated in the deficit. Smith and Winograd (1978) reported a similar decrement in recognition memory for unfamiliar faces.

Imagery, or the ability to generate internally a pictorial representation of a verbal or otherwise nonvisual signal or to create a modification of a visual stimulus, is also considered to be a right hemisphere task (Bogen, 1969) and has shown a decrement with age. Hulicka and Grossman (1967) and more recently Treat *et al.* (1981) reported that elderly subjects used fewer spontaneous mediators than younger subjects in paired-associate learning, and when instructed to use mediators they employed more verbal than visual ones. Whitbourne and Slevin (1978) found that older people used significantly fewer visual mediators on a sentence retention task when items were graded as either abstract or concrete. The latter are usually encoded visually by young adults (Paivio *et al.*, 1968).

Mental manipulation of visual information, such as by scanning, superimposition, mental rotation, or successive additions of segments to create a whole, is attributed to the right hemisphere's repertoire as well (Bogen, 1969). Gaylord and Marsh (1975) had male subjects rotate spatial images in order to arrive at a same–different judgment. They reported a reduction in reaction time and a marked slowing with age of rate of mental rotation. It is pertinent here to cite evidence, based on patients with unilateral cerebral lesions, that the right hemisphere plays a major role in the control of reaction time (Howes and Boller, 1975; Isagoda *et al.*, 1981). Results such as those of Gaylord and Marsh (1975) may reflect right hemisphere involvement in reaction time, which may decline in normal aging. However, see the discussion later of Elias and Kinsbourne's (1974) work, which does not support this conjecture.

Krauss *et al.* (1980) suggested that the slower processing observed by Gaylord and Marsh (1975) may confound results by reducing the total number of stimuli that a subject will attempt to process. They examined older subjects' spatial rotation abilities but with no younger comparison group because their purpose was to observe individual differences and to ascertain which factors contribute to reduced rotation skill. They found that sequential presentation (memory load) caused more difficulty than simultaneous presentation, that practice improved performance, and that stimulus characteristics (mirror image or angle of rotation) affected responses and concluded that elderly subjects "possess the requisite skills but do not know how to use them [p. 205]." That conclusion does not seem to be acceptable in order to fully account for aging deficits with rotation tasks. We are still obliged to ask why older people do not take advantage of the rotation skills they possess and to wonder how a younger group would be affected by practice, angle of rotation, etc. Then the nonexistence of residual age differences would be enlightening.

A study by Herman and Coyne (1980) provides further evidence of decline with age on a mental manipulation task that they termed "perspective-taking." Subjects were taken to one of four objects placed in a room and instructed to imagine that they were at each of the others, each time pointing to the imagined position of the remaining three objects. Older subjects had significantly more difficulty with the task.

Jacewicz and Hartley (1979) examined the effects of familiarity on rotation of images by using English (familiar) and Greek (unfamiliar) letters as stimuli. In this study stimlui were presented simultaneously, a factor that Krauss *et al.* (1980) claim should improve older people's performance (see earlier). Plane rather than depth rotation was used, the former being the easier of the two; yet there remained a significant age difference. Regardless of the factors that might improve performance, rotation of mental images may be more difficult for older people because of reliance on the supposedly more deteriorated right hemisphere.

In a frequently cited study, Elias and Kinsbourne (1974) recorded reaction time and accuracy of performance for a verbal and visual same–different task. They found that older individuals, particularly women, made significantly more errors on the nonverbal (visual) stimuli than on the verbal. However, measures of reaction time did not reflect the age-by-sex-by-stimulus material interaction.

Nonverbal memory in the tactual modality was investigated in a study by Riege *et al.* (1980), in which 120 right-handed people with an age range of 20 to 84 years were asked to recognize nonmeaningful wire shapes. There was a significant age decrement, expressed by poor left hand performance, implicating diminished superiority of the right hemisphere in processing tactual memory. Support for these results can be found in Riege and Inman (1981).

Studies comparing normal aged with brain-damaged groups are perhaps the most convincing for establishing a model of hemi-aging. Ben Yishai *et al.* (1971) reported similarity in the inability of older normal and right-brain-damaged patients to reproduce WAIS block designs.

Albert and Kaplan (1980) also compared degraded drawings of normal elderly and brain-damaged individuals with focal right frontal lesions and found similarities sufficient to implicate the right frontal lobe in normal aging. They, in turn, claimed that results of similar work by Farver demonstrate right frontal aging rather than right parietal aging as Farver originally suggested. The point to be stressed, of course, is that the right hemisphere is the common side of decline.

Smith and Milner (1980) found that patients with right temporal lobectomy including excision of the hippocampal region were impaired in the recall of location of objects in comparison with left temporal lobectomy patients and normal controls.

The work of Klisz has been reviewed by Albert and Kaplan (1980) and Botwinick (1981). Using the Halstead–Reitan Neuropsychology Test Battery, Klisz found that adults in their early forties could best be differentiated from adults in their fifties by subtests sensitive to right hemisphere impairment. Those subtests sensitive to left hemisphere impairment least differentiated between the two age groups. Klisz proposed that these results "may indeed reflect a faster decline in right hemisphere functions [cited in Botwinick, 1981, p. 142]." The work of Schaie and Schaie (1977) mentioned earlier is also pertinent here.

Until now, the case for right hemisphere decline has been argued. At this point those studies which present evidence that is either contradictory or simply not in agreement will be cited.

The one study that suggests possible vulnerability of verbal processes with superior performance of right hemisphere visuospatial processing in older people is that of Charman (1981). Subjects were required to recall tachistoscopically presented matrices of letters, and for older subjects the right hemisphere demonstrated superiority whereas for younger ones left hemisphere scores were better. This hemispheric difference, termed a "turn-about" by the author, supposedly reflecting hemispheric processing of the decaying iconic trace, invites further investigation.

Schear and Nebes (1980) found differences between young (mean age 18.8 years) and older (mean age 69.5 years) subjects for both verbal (letter identification) and spatial (letter location) tasks; that is, the performance of older subjects was uniformly poorer on both verbal and visual tasks.

Testing imagery effects with abstract and concrete nouns that were presented for short- and long-term retention, Bruning *et al.* (1975) concluded that "imagery effects appear to be relatively consistent across age [p. 316]." This result is particularly convincing in light of their extreme age groups; young persons were 18–27 years of age, and two older groups were 65–79 and 80–94 years of age. McCormack (1982) also reported uniformity of results with young and older participants in a spatial location memory task.

In comparing recall of words with recall of pictures in young and older individuals, Winograd *et al.* (1982) concluded that their results do not support the hypothesis that imagery (picture recall) declines at a steeper rate with age than verbal recall. They suggested that evidence to the contrary may be based on research designs with inherent methodological problems. The authors, citing the work of Poon *et al.* (Winograd *et al.*, 1982, p. 70), stressed the importance of further clarification of the issue due to the potential value of mnemonic training based on imagery for remediating the memory problems associated with aging. The majority of adult aphasics, with intact right hemispheres, may also benefit from the application of mnemonic cues to language stimulation techniques.

Using the technique of assigning a Cognitive Laterality Profile (reflecting relative performance of the hemispheres) to patient and control groups, Bentin *et al.* (1981) found that profiles for both young and older normal controls showed no hemispheric preference. This study is classified here with those demonstrating uniformity of hemispheric activity with normal aging. However, the reader is referred to the last section of this chapter, where results from patient groups from this study are described and applied in a completely different context.

Elias *et al.* (1977) noted asymmetric performance decrements of older subjects, particularly older men, during a same–different decision task involving competition for time and space using the auditory channel. Both hemispheres were implicated in the aging process, in general the right being the more vulnerable for women and the left for men. In a similar study using the visual modality, Elias *et al.* (1979) again found asymmetric decline and an interaction with gender. However, there was a reversal of pattern: older men showed poorer right hemispheric processing, and the left hemisphere of older women reflected the effects of the time and space competition. An unequivocal, consistent result obtained by Elias and co-workers in both studies was the poor performance of the right hemisphere on the "different" task, a task that is presumed to entail serial or sequential processing, a cognitive style not primarily attributed to the more holistic right hemisphere. This interesting result did not interact with age.

If we were to tally those studies suggesting differential right hemisphere decline against those providing evidence of uniformity or equivocal results, it is clear that the case for hemidecline would rest on the weightier side of the scales.

C. Dichotic Listening

We now briefly discuss the question of aging effects with the dichotic listening paradigm, and it will be seen that in these studies there is more convincing evidence refuting hemidecline—the perfect fuel for an already flaming controversy.

Dichotic listening techniques have been applied appropriately to aging research under the assumption that, if changes in the proportion of right over left ear advantage observed in young adults were discovered, the hemisphere reflecting the reduced ear advantage would be responsible for the aging effect. Dichotic studies have been reviewed by Craik (1977) with emphasis on explaining how aspects of memory can influence results. The reader is referred to Craik's review for a description of the dichotic listening design and detailed treatment of the studies to that date. Here, it is important to note, in general, two methodological procedures that can influence ear effects in dichotic studies and that explain why, with few exceptions, the dichotic paradigm has not been adequately applied to aging populations.

The first is order of report from ears. If competitive verbal material is simultaneously presented to ears, individuals tend to report first what the right ear heard, since that ear has stronger contralateral connections to the verbal left hemisphere than the ipsilateral left ear. In order to neutralize the natural superiority of the right ear in reporting verbal material, order of report from ears must be controlled. The early studies of dichotic listening, which did not counterbalance for order of report, give the impression that left ear performance declines with age. However, when order of ear report is controlled, it is seen that all subjects tend to report with greater accuracy the material from the first ear reported, regardless of left or right, with the second ear being particularly vulnerable due to the rapidity with which echoic memory decays.

The second procedure that can influence results of dichotic listening studies with older groups in particular is auditory screening of subjects. The hearing loss so commonly accompanying aging was reported by Borod and Goodglass (1980) to effect the left ear more than the right. In the absence of additional studies confirming this finding, it can be assumed, tentatively, that if people self-report on hearing acuity, results of dichotic tests might enhance the normal right ear advantage due to greater hearing loss (with or without subject awareness) on the left side. This confounding of results would occur even if order of report from ears were controlled.

Taking into account both of these crucial points so frequently overlooked in studies of aging dichotic listening, Borod and Goodglass (1980) controlled order of report from ears and used rigorous audiometric screening for participants and found no interaction with age of degree of right ear advantage on a dichotic digits task or of degree of left ear advantage for dichotic melodies.

Another study controlling order of ear report and screening subjects audiometrically is that of Parkinson *et al.* (1980), who found that digit span and dichotic memory declined with age, but no ear effects were observed. In addition, the authors reported that, when young and older individuals were matched for digit span, the performance of the older people greatly improved, so that the aging effect was eliminated.

McCoy *et al.* (1977), using the Staggered Spondaic Word test, demonstrated how correction for peripheral ear sensitivity altered results to such an extent that age-by-ear interactions were greatly reduced. They did report that older men exhibited poorer right ear performance.

Johnson *et al.* (1979) observed a decline with age of verbal material reported from the left ear with no right ear decline. However, subjects self-reported on hearing acuity, so these results must be held in abeyance pending duplication of the paradigm with adequate audiometric screening included.

If dichotic listening is to be considered a suitable investigative approach to aging central auditory function and hence to possible hemispheric decline (and it should be), the methodological "misdemeanors" disqualifying some of the work from serious consideration will have to be amended.

III. Central Measures of the Aging Brain: Known and Unexplored Territory

A. Electrophysiology

The one asymmetric finding that consistently appears in normal, healthy, aging subjects is a slowing of EEG of θ or δ type in the left temporal lobe, usually the anterior portion (Marsh and Thompson, 1977; Obrist, 1979; Soininen *et al.*, 1982a).

In their extensive review, Marsh and Thompson (1977) cited numerous references that report on "focal" slowing, collectively in 30–50% of elderly subjects. This slowing "appears 75 percent of the time in the left hemisphere and predominantly in the anterior temporal region [p. 222]."

Obrist (1979, p. 105) cited the work of Silverman *et al.* as the "first to report a high incidence of focal slow activity" in 30 to 40% of individuals over 60 years of age. Eighty percent of focal slowing in the left hemisphere (which comprised three-fourths of the slowing observed) "appeared maximally over the anterior portion of the temporal lobe [p. 105]."

Soininen *et al.* (1982a) reported that 33% of their normal subjects (mean age 74.7 years) showed slowing of the θ type in the left temporal region, without specifying which portion of that lobe is involved. Computed tomography of normal elderly individuals showing cortical atrophy of the left temporal region may be related to the EEG findings (Soininen *et al.*, 1982b).

This asymmetric focal slowing so commonly seen in older neurologically normal people has no behavioral correlates, whereas the diffuse slowing occurring in both hemispheres frontally and posteriorally is related to senile intellectual deterioration (Obrist, 1979, 1980) and occurs only in about 20% of normal individuals over 80 years of age. Therefore, symmetric and diffuse EEG slowing has prognostic value for gerontopsychiatry, whereas the asymmetric findings, with no overt behavioral counterparts, remain a puzzlement.

Motivated by the verbal–nonverbal dichotomy discussed in the previous section, Marsh and Thompson (in Woodruff, 1978, pp. 162–163) raised and investigated the possibility of nonuniformity in aging of the hemispheres. Asymmetries in the contingent negative variation (CNV) were demonstrated as a result of a psychological set for verbal or nonverbal perception in young and old adults. However, age differences did not contribute to the effect. "After extensive attempts to find age differences in EEG asymmetry as a function of age differences in spatial and verbal information processing, Thompson suggested that the hypothesis that the right and left brain aged at different rates could not be supported [Woodruff, 1978, p. 163]." Similarly, no asymmetry of hemispheres with age was found by Marsh in recordings from temporal and parietal areas (in Marsh and Thompson, 1977).

Dustman *et al.* (1981) investigated visual evoked potentials (VEPs) elicited by patterned and unpatterned flash stimuli in male subjects from 4 to 90 years of age. From central scalp recordings, VEPs reflected better differentiation of patterned and unpatterned flashes by the right hemisphere, but this finding did not interact with age.

Only those electrophysiological studies directly addressing the question of laterality and aging have been presented here. Obviously, there is a wealth of material on the symmetric changes with age of waking and sleep EEG, CNV, and auditory, visual, and somatosensory evoked potentials; however, it is not relevant to this chapter.

B. Neurotransmitters

The study of the asymmetric organization of different neurotransmitter systems in the human brain is in its infancy (see Chapters 2, 5, and 17). It is not surprising, then, that the extensive literature on age-related neurochemical changes does not include specific reference to asymmetric modifications of neurotransmitters. Whether animal or human brains are studied, the distinctive intrahemispheric regional patterns of change are discussed with no mention of which hemisphere was observed. One must conclude that hemispheres were arbitrarily chosen and therefore not specified. There is one exception. Corkin (1981) reported on alterations in central cholinergic functions with Alzheimer's disease, presumably resulting from morphological changes of brain tissue. "These changes usually occur on both sides of the brain but are not necessarily symmetrical, though there is no evidence of a systematic difference [p. 287]."

Possibly given impetus by the pioneering work of Glick with animals (see Chapter 2 for review) Oke *et al.* (1978) reported on asymmetric distribution of norepinephrine (NE) in the human thalamus. Findings were based on five brains with an average age of 62 years. The question that immediately and quite naturally arises is, Could Oke and co-workers have been unintentionally reporting an aging effect? Subsequently, Oke *et al.* (1980) reported similar thalamic asymmetry of NE in rats. Their animals were "24 male or female albino rats (approximately 250 g) [p. 270]." With no details as to strain or breakdown of gender number, the fact that female rats weighing 250 g may be considered old leaves us with the same possibility of age confounding results.

It is interesting to glance at the continuum of aging and senility due to cerebral blood flow changes offered by Obrist (1980) and to consider it an analog of the depletion with normal aging of dopamine (DA) in the basal ganglia. Here, too, a specific amount of depletion must be reached before the symptoms of Parkinsonism appear clinically (Bernheimer *et al.*, 1973). Hemi-Parkinsonism, of course, is the ideal model for hemi-decline with age (Chapter 10). Another suggested analog is that "Alzheimer's disease represents an accelerated form of the deterioration of memory and the cholinergic system which accompany normal aging [Kubanis and Zornetzer, 1981, p. 151; see also Gottfries, 1981]." However, with the exception of hemi-Parkinsonism, there is no evidence of asymmetric neurotransmitter depletion with age.

Notice should be made of an article in which Bridge *et al.* (1978) report an alteration of schizophrenic symptoms with age (55–64 years). Symptoms are reduced or diminished in what the authors term a "burn-out" phenomenon. The need for further work on this subject is stressed by Bridge and co-workers. The cumulative effects of neuroleptic drugs on DA and other neurotransmitter systems and the chronicity of schizophrenia are factors that we have to consider when viewing the longitudinal aspect of the disease. However, for those who regard schizophrenia as a hemisyndrome (see Chapters 12 and 14 for discussion), the implications for hemi-aging of this "burn-out" of symptoms are inviting.

Other investigations of neurochemical asymmetries are based on young animals or human beings (see Table 17.1). Whether these asymmetries continue or alter with age awaits investigation.

C. Exploration of Time Sharing with an Older Population

In an attempt to elucidate the question of heterochrony of hemisphere aging a study incorporating a time-sharing design was undertaken by this writer. Time-sharing paradigms are based on the assumption that competition for the same cerebral space will result when two tasks targeted for the same hemisphere are performed by subjects simultaneously (Hiscock and Kinsbourne, 1978; Dalby, 1980). Mutual interference of the tasks (or lack of it) as indicated by performance enables one to draw conclusions implicating the hemisphere involved.

Young and older right-handed individuals (Table 9.1) screened for hearing, central nervous system disease, drug use, psychopathology, and ability to perform smooth pursuit eye movements tracked a horizontal moving light, alternately in both directions, while concurrently furnishing either verbal (left hemisphere) or imagery-mediated (right hemisphere) associations to single word stimuli presented through earphones. Eye tracking was monitored by electrooculogram.

Although the complex central mechanisms controlling eye movements are not completely understood, there is increasing clinical evidence, based on unilateral cerebral lesions, suggesting ipsilateral occipital

TABLE 9.1
Distribution of Subjects (N = 98) by Age and Gender

	Young		Old	
	Males ($N = 24$)	Females ($N = 24$)	Males ($N = 25$)	Females ($N = 25$)
Mean age (years)	23.4	22	66	65.8
Range	21–27	20–26	60–73	60–73

regulation of horizontal pursuit movements (Hoyt and Daroff, 1971; Troost *et al.*, 1972; Estañol *et al.*, 1980; Larmande *et al.*, 1980; Kimura *et al.*, 1981; Sharpe and Lo, 1981). It was therefore assumed that degraded tracking, characterized by saccadic interference or arrest of pursuit movement (PA), would indicate when the word association tasks proved to be competitive maneuvers. Analysis of variance and covariance with repeated measures showed that older subjects performed more poorly than younger ones in that they produced significantly more saccades and instances of PA (Table 9.2).

The effects of aging on pursuit eye movements have been investigated (Kuechenmeister *et al.*, 1977; Spooner *et al.*, 1980), and such movements are considered to be an age-dependent motor system (Sharpe and Sylvester, 1978). The age effect in these results, however, cannot be attributed to that because all participants were able to do saccade- and arrest-free pursuit during preliminary practice sessions. Only when tracking was coupled with a task did the older subjects show significant deficit in comparison with the young.

As can be seen in Table 9.2 the imagery-mediated association task ("visual") proved to be more difficult for all subjects, but a most interesting task-by-age interaction was also found. Older subjects made significantly more arrests of tracking while conjuring up images to word stimuli than while furnishing simple single word associations.

Tasks that divide attention in laboratory settings are difficult for old people, particularly when stimuli are presented through two sensory modalities or when two distinctly different activities are required (Craik, 1977; Wright, 1981). In the present study stimuli arrived through two modalities, and the tasks were entirely different activities. If conditions of divided attention per se were the sole cause of the difficulty experienced by the older subjects, we would expect the verbal and visual tasks to be similarly affected. This was not the case. Image-mediated associations were more difficult for older subjects.

Task complexity, another important factor in age-related performance deficits, is usually measured in terms of memory load or increasing number of items to be processed. Neither of the tasks in the present experiment required a memory load or produced increments of difficulty. Subjects had maximally to retain a single word in order to produce a ver-

TABLE 9.2
Mean Number of Saccades and Instances of Pursuit Arrest for Age and Task Main Effects and Task-by-Age Interaction

	Saccades	Pursuit arrest
Age effect		
Young	24.4^{a}	0.187^{b}
	($N = 32$)	($N = 48$)
Old	28.0^{a}	6.28^{b}
	($N = 36$)	($N = 50$)
Task effect		
Verbal	7.78^{c}	1.26^{d}
	($N = 68$)	($N = 98$)
Visual	13.05^{c}	1.97^{d}
	($N = 68$)	($N = 98$)
Task-by-age interaction ($N = 98$)		
Young verbal	—	0.08^{e}
Young visual	—	0.10^{e}
Old verbal	—	2.44^{e}
Old visual	—	3.84^{e}

[a] $F(1,64) = 15.03, p < 0.0003$.
[b] $F(1,94) = 42.06, p < 0.0000$.
[c] $F(1,64) = 38.32, p < 0.0000$.
[d] $F(1,94) = 8.49, p < 0.0045$.
[e] $F(1,94) = 8.0, p < 0.0057$.

bal or visual associate, and the tracking task is stable over time. Although the effect of fatigue on eye tracking is known (Troost *et al.*, 1972), a count of saccades and PA over time revealed no correlation. The visual association task, although devoid of memory load, did require reorganization of the single word input, and such reorganization of input, before responding, is known to cause difficulty for older people (Craik, 1977). Our task required conversion of the strictly verbal stimulus to an internal visualization and, subsequently, to an oral encoding for response. To use Kinsbourne's (1977) terminology, the brains of our older subjects apparently could not "insulate" the two competitive visual activities from each other.

The results presented here, then, can be added to the evidence presented earlier in the chapter which implicates the right hemisphere in aging.

If degree of attention (arousal) as opposed to division of attention is considered, then an explanation for right hemisphere vulnerability can be presented, because that seems to be the common denominator among various age-related behavioral manifestations. For instance, cases of pseudodementia, which are well documented in the aging literature (e.g., Comfort, 1980), present clinically with such symptoms as confusion and disorientation. However, the problem can be reversed with antidepressive drugs and is actually an endogenous depression. Depression is the most common psychiatric disorder associated with age (Comfort, 1980), probably due to the basic neuroendocrine shifts involving DA, NE, serotonin, and acetylcholine, which are most vulnerable to the aging process (Gottfries, 1980; Enna *et al.*, 1981). In other words, the pseudodementias and depression of aging essentially represent a deficit of arousal created by the depletion of certain neurotransmitters (Adolfsson *et al.*, 1979).

The mechanisms of arousal and in turn depression have been related predominantly to right hemisphere control (Flor-Henry *et al.*, 1979; see also Chapter 7; Myslobodsky *et al.*, 1979; Heilman and Van Den Abell, 1980; Ross and Rush, 1981; Tucker, 1981a). The prevalence of depression in Parkinsonism has been clarified (Mayeux *et al.*, 1981). Mintz and Myslobodsky (Chapter 10) found that their right hemi-Parkinson patients were nonresponders during an attention task for which measurements of electrodermal activity were recorded. Bentin *et al.* (1981) reported that patients with right hemi-Parkinsonism, bilateral Parkinsonism, and dementia were assigned better left hemisphere cognitive profiles than right after neuropsychological testing. They claimed that subcortical (basal ganglion) damage can produce alterations in spatial orientation, which led to the lower right cognitive scores.

Tucker (1981b), working with induced depressive state in young college students, found impaired imagery, as he and co-workers did in students who self-reported depression.

Thus, by linking deficits of arousal with DA depletion and subsequently with depression and other disorders of aging (Parkinsonism, dementia) and, in turn, by relating these with lowered right hemisphere performance, we come back full circle to the original contention that the right hemisphere expresses the effects of aging more than the left. Our subjects' poorer eye tracking during visual task can be considered a right hemisphere arousal-related disruption [see Kubanis and Zornetzer (1981) for a discussion of an "overarousal" (sic) hypothesis of age-related deficits in performance].

In the absence of EEG correlates with the behavior of normal aging (Obrist, 1980), hemi-Parkinson pathology (Chapter 10), or depression (Perris and Monakhov, 1979), covert age changes that preface pathology can be observed only through the poorer performance of older subjects on most activities that tap right hemisphere processing.

IV. Concluding Remarks

It was stated initially that the question of whether aging differentially affects hemispheres requires a noncommittal answer. In retrospect, the obvious precondition to a discussion of hemi-aging is that we specify which behaviors or central mechanisms are under scrutiny. Certainly, there is more evidence based on behavior than on central mechanisms, which are so much more difficult to observe and record.

For instance, if EEG is considered, there is a definite asymmetric change with age. Change and decline cannot necessarily be considered synonymous in this case in light of the fact that the focal left anterior temporal slowing observed in normal elderly individuals is not indicative of pathology in any way.

Behaviorally, we have the evidence based on the performance of older people on visuospatial tasks and based on the eruption of hemi-Parkinsonism, depression, or pseudodementia which has been presented here, albeit in abbreviated form, as being intimately connected to the right hemisphere.

Several methodological issues are unique to studies of aging, and mention is made of them here in what is essentially a call for uniformity of approach to studies of nonuniformity of the aging hemispheres.

Foremost among the points to be considered is subject selection. Botwinick (1973) wrote, "It comes as a surprise to many that only five percent of old people live in institutions [p. 2]." Older, independent people living in their own homes are more representative of the aging population than are those living in retirement communities or homes for the aged. Although it is easier to obtain volunteers *en masse* from residential communities for older people, investigators should opt for those living at home. Gathering places for the elderly such as pensioner clubs are more advantageous sources of volunteers for aging research.

Strict screening for health status is another basic issue in subject selection. If individuals suffering from various chronic disorders (cardiac, metabolic, etc.) or those who consume drugs indiscriminately are grouped with those free of such ailments or medication, a concept of normal aging cannot emerge.

Grouping individuals for age is another sensitive issue because of the wide variability found when the elderly are tested in laboratory situations. Ideally, subjects should be grouped by half-decade spans that include the middle adult years (35–55) since declines in performance have been observed for people in the fifth decade of life (e.g., Talland, 1968). This also diminishes the range of cohorts characterizing each group.

The augmented cautiousness and preference for self-paced tasks that may characterize older people (see Siegler, 1980) should be considered when research paradigms are designed. Reaction time tasks should be avoided in light of the evidence presented regarding right hemisphere involvement with basic reaction time.

Finally, the hand preference of subjects, including handedness of blood relations, determined by a laterality questionnaire, must be controlled in any study of hemi-aging.

When such requirements are met, providing for the accumulation of more extensive data, it will be easier to form a conclusion regarding hemi-aging. However, even though there was a commitment at the beginning of the chapter to present a case for selective right hemisphere decline, it does not have to be exclusive of the presentation of evidence of left hemisphere decline. In fact, it seems unreasonable to assume that aging could be so one-sided. The more conservative view allows the question to remain open until future contributions to the field provide more evidence implicating one hemisphere and/or the other. Such a coupling of aging with a look to the future is by no means incongruous.

Acknowledgments

Assistance with statistical analysis was provided by the Department for Statistical Consultation of Tel-Aviv University. The author is grateful for the helpful comments of Michael S. Myslobodsky and Rachel Tomer and for the technical assistance of Matti Mintz.

The preparation of this manuscript was partially supported by a grant from the American Jewish Joint Distribution Committee No. 812–02.

References

Adolfsson, R., Gottfries, C. G., Roos, B. E., and Winblad, B. (1979). Post-mortem distribution of dopamine and homovanillic acid in human brain, variations related to age, and a review of the literature. *Neural Transm.* **45**, 81–105.

Albert, M. S., and Kaplan, E. (1980). Organic implications of neuropsychological deficits in the elderly. *In* "New Directions in Memory and Aging: Proceedings of the George Talland Memorial Conference" (L. W. Poon, J. L. Fozard, L. S. Cermak, D. Arenberg, and L. W. Thompson, eds.), pp. 403–432. Lawrence Erlbaum Assoc., Hillsdale, New Jersey.

Andersen, R. (1976). Verbal and visuo-spatial memory. *Scand. J. Psychol.* **17**, 198–204.

Arenberg, D. (1978). Differences and changes with age in the Benton Visual Retention test. *J. Gerontol.* **33**, 534–540.

Bentin, S., Silverberg, R., and Gordon, H. (1981). Asymmetrical cognitive deterioration in demented and Parkinson patients. *Cortex* **17**, 533–544.

Ben Yishai, Y., Diller, L., Mandelberg, J., Gordon, W., and Gerstman, L. J. (1971). Similarities and differences in Block Design performance between older normal and brain-injured persons: A task analysis. *J. Abnorm. Soc. Psychol.* **78**, 17–25.

Bernheimer, H., Birkmayer, W., Hornykiewicz, O., Jellinger, K., and Seitelberger, F. (1973). Brain dopamine and the syndromes of Parkinson and Huntington, Clinical, morphological and neurochemical correlations. *J. Neurol. Sci.* **20**, 415–455.

Bogen, J. E. (1969). The other side of the brain. II. An appositional mind. *Bull. Los Angeles Neurol. Soc.* **34**, 135–162.

Borod, J., and Goodglass, H. (1980). Lateralization of linguistic and melodic processing with age. *Neuropsychologia* **18**, 79–83.

Botwinick, J. (1973). "Aging and Behavior." Springer-Verlag, New York.

Botwinick, J. (1981). Neuropsychology of aging. *In* "Handbook of Clinical Neuropsychology" (S. B. Filskov and T. J. Boll, eds.), pp. 135–171. Wiley, New York.

Bradshaw, J. L., and Nettleton, N. C. (1981). The nature of hemispheric specialization in man. *Behav. Brain Sci.* **4**, 51–92.

Bridge, T. P., Cannon, H. E., and Wyatt, R. J. (1978). Burned-out schizophrenia: Evidence for age effects on schizophrenic symptomatology. *J. Gerontol.* **33**, 835–839.

Bruning, R. H., Holzbauer, I., and Kimberlin, C. (1975). Age, word imagery and delay interval: Effects on short-term and long-term retention. *J. Gerontol.* **30**, 312–318.

Charman, D. K. (1981). A note on the aging of hemispheric asymmetries. *B. J. Clin. Psychol.* **20**, 67–68.

Comfort, A. (1980). "Practice of Geriatric Psychiatry." Am. Elsevier, New York.

Corkin, S. (1981). Acetylcholine, aging and Alzheimer's disease. Implications for treatment. *Trends Neurosci.* **4**, 287–290.

Craik, F. I. M. (1977). Age differences in human memory. *In* "Handbook of the Psychology of Aging" (J. E. Birren and L. W. Schaie, eds.), pp. 384–420. Van Nostrand-Reinhold, New York.

Dalby, J. J. (1980). Hemispheric time-sharing: Verbal and spatial loading with concurrent unimanual activity. *Cortex* **16**, 567–573.

Doppelt, J. E., and Wallace, W. L. (1955). Standardization of the Wechsler Adult Intelligence Scale for older persons. *J. Abnorm. Soc. Psychol.* **51**, 312–330.

Dustman, R. E., Snyder, E. W., and Schlehuber, C. J. (1981). Life-span alterations in visually evoked potentials and inhibitory function. *Neurobio. Aging* **2**, 187–192.

Elias, J. W., Wright, L. L., and Winn, F. J. (1977). Age and sex differences in cerebral asymmetry as a function of competition for "time" and "space" in a successive auditory matching task. *Exp. Aging Res.* **3**, 33–48.

Elias, J. W., Winn, F. J., and Wright, L. L. (1979). Age, sex and hemisphere asymmetry difference induced by a concurrent memory processing task. *Exp. Aging Res.* **5**, 217–237.

Elias, M., and Kinsbourne, M. (1974). Age and sex differences in the processing of verbal and non-verbal stimuli. *J. Gerontol.* **29**, 162–171.

Enna, S. J., Samorajski, T., and Beer, B. (1981). "Brain Neurotransmitters and Receptors in Aging and Age-Related Disorders." Raven Press, New York.

Estañol, B., Romero, R., Sáenz de Viteri, M., Mateos, J. H., and Corvera, J. (1980). Oculomotor and oculovestibular functions in a hemispherectomy patient. *Arch. Neurol. (Chicago)* **37**, 365–368.

Ferris, S. H., Crook, T., Clark, E., McCarthy, M., and Rae, D. (1980). Facial recognition memory deficits in normal aging and senile dementia. *J. Gerontol.* **35**, 707–714.

Flor-Henry, P., Kiles, Z. J., Howarth, B. G., and Burton, L. (1979). Neurophysiology studies of schizophrenia, mania and depression. *In* "Hemisphere Asymmetries of Function in Psychopathology" (J. Gruzelier and P. Flor-Henry, eds.), pp. 189–222. North-Holland, Amsterdam.

Gaylord, S. A., and Marsh, G. R. (1975). Age differences in the speed of a spatial cognitive process. *J. Gerontol.* **30**, 674–678.

Gottfries, C. G. (1980). Biochemistry of dementia and normal aging. *Trends Neurosci.* **3**, 55–57.

Gottfries, C. G. (1981). Levels of monoamines, monoamine metabolites, and activity in related enzyme systems correlated to normal aging and in patients with dementia of Alzheimer type. *In* "Apomorphine and Other Dopaminomimetics" (G. U. Corsini, and G. L. Gessa eds.), Vol. 2, pp. 243–249. Raven Press, New York.

Hayslip, B., Jr., and Sterns, H. L. (1979). Age differences in relationships between crystallized and fluid intelligences and problem solving. *J. Gerontol.* **34**, 404–414.

Hécaen, H. (1978). "La dominance cérébrale: Une anthologie." Mouton, Paris.

Heilman, K. M., and Van Den Abell, T. (1980). Right hemisphere dominance for attention: The mechanism underlying hemispheric asymmetries of inattention (neglect). *Neurology* **30**, 327–330.

Herman, J. F., and Coyne, A. C. (1980). Mental manipulation of spatial information in young and elderly adults. *Dev. Psychol.* **16**, 537–538.

Hilliard, R. D. (1973). Hemispheric laterality effects on a facial recognition task in normal subjects. *Cortex* **9**, 246–258.

Hiscock, M., and Kinsbourne, M. (1978). Ontogeny of cerebral dominance: Evidence from time-sharing asymmetry in children. *Dev. Psychol.* **14**, 321–329.

Horn, J. L., and Cattell, R. B. (1966). Age differences in primary mental abilities factors. *J. Gerontol.* **21**, 210–229.

Horn, J. L., and Cattell, R. B. (1967). Age differences in fluid and crystallized intelligence. *Acta Psychol.* **26**, 107–129.

Howes, D., and Boller, F. (1975). Simple reaction time: Evidence for focal impairment from lesions of the right hemisphere. *Brain* **98**, 317–332.

Hoyt, W. F., and Daroff, R. B. (1971). Supranuclear disorders of ocular control systems in man: Clinical, anatomical and physiological correlations. *In* "The Control of Eye Movements" (P. Bach-y-Rita, C. C. Collins, and J. E. Hyde, eds.), pp. 175–235. Academic Press, New York.

Hulicka, I. M., and Grossman, J. L. (1967). Age-group comparisons for the use of mediators in paired-associate learning. *J. Gerontol.* **22**, 46–51.

Isagoda, A., Nakamura, R., and Sajiki, N. (1981). Dependence of reaction time on visual fields in patients with unilateral hemispheric lesions. *Tohoku J. Exp. Med.* **134**, 295–299.

Jacewicz, M. M., and Hartley, A. A. (1979). Rotation of mental images by young and old college students: The effects of familiarity. *J. Gerontol.* **34**, 396–403.

Johnson, R. C., Cole, R. E., Bowers, J. K., Foiles, S. V., Nikaido, A. M., Patrick, J. W., and Woliver, R. E. (1979). Hemispheric efficiency in middle and later adulthood. *Cortex* **15**, 109–119.

Kimura, Y., Kato, I., Watanabe, Y., and Mizukoshi, K. (1981). Modification of saccade by various central nervous system dysfunctions. *Ann. N.Y. Acad. Sci.* **374**, 755–763.

Kinsbourne, M. (1977). Cognitive decline with advancing age: An interpretation. *In* "Aging, and Dementia" (W. L. Smith and M. Kinsbourne, eds.), pp. 217–235. Spectrum Publ., New York.

Kinsbourne, M. (1981). The development of cerebral dominance. *In* "Handbook of Clinical Neuropsychology" (S. B. Filskov and T. J. Boll, eds.), pp. 399–417. Wiley, New York.

Krauss, I. K., Quayhagen, M., and Schaie, K. W. (1980). Spatial rotation in the elderly: Performance factors. *J. Gerontol.* **35**, 199–206.

Kubanis, P., and Zornetzer, S. F. (1981). Age-related behavioral and neurobiological changes: A review with an emphasis on memory. *Behav. Neural Biol.* **31**, 115–172.

Kuechenmeister, C. A., Linton, P. H., Mueller, T. V., and White, H. B. (1977). Eye tracking in relation to age, sex, and illness. *Arch. Gen. Psychiatry* **34**, 578–579.

Larmande, P., Prier, S., Masson, M., and Cambier, J. (1980). Perturbations de la poursuite oculaire et lésions pariéto-occipitales unilatérales. *Rev. Neurol.* **5**, 345–353.

McCormack, P. D. (1982). Coding of spatial information by young and elderly adults. *J. Gerontol.* **37**, 80–86.

McCoy, C., Butler, M., and Broekhoff, J. (1977). Effects of age and sex on dichotic listening: The SSW test. *J. Audit. Res.* **17**, 263–268.

McGlone, J. (1980). Sex differences in human brain asymmetry: A critical survey. *Behav. Brain Sci.* **3**, 215–263.

Marsh, G. R., and Thompson, L. W. (1977). Psychophysiology of aging. *In* "Handbook of the Psychology of Aging" (J. E. Birren and K. W. Schaie, eds.), pp. 219–248. Van Nostrand-Reinhold, New York.

Mayeux, R., Stern, Y., Rosen, J., and Leventhal, J. (1981). Depression, intellectual impairment, and Parkinson disease. *Neurology* **31**, 645–650.

Myslobodsky, M., Mintz, M., and Tomer, R. (1979). Asymmetric reactivity of the brain and components of hemispheric imbalance. *In* "Hemisphere Asymmetries of Function in

Psychopathology" (J. Gruzelier and P. Flor-Henry, eds.), pp. 125–148. Elsevier/North-Holland, Amsterdam.

Obrist, W. D. (1979). EEG changes in normal aging and dementia. *In* "Brain Function in Old Age" (F. Hoffmeister and C. Müller, eds.), pp. 102–111. Springer-Verlag, Berlin.

Obrist, W. D. (1980). Cerebral blood flow and EEG changes associated with aging and dementia. *In* "Handbook of Geriatric Psychiatry" (E. W. Busse and D. G. Blazer, eds.), pp. 83–101. Van Nostrand-Reinhold, New York.

Oke, A., Keller, R., Mefford, I., and Adams, R. N. (1978). Lateralization of norepinephrine in human thalamus. *Science* **200**, 1411–1413.

Oke, A., Lewis, R., and Adams, R. N. (1980). Hemispheric asymmetry of norepinephrine distribution in rat thalamus. *Brain Res.* **188**, 269–272.

Paivio, A., Rogers, T. B., and Smythe, P. C. (1968). Why are pictures easier to recall than words? *Psychon. Sci.* **11**, 137–138.

Park, D. C., Puglisi, J. T., and Lutz, R. (1982). Spatial memory in older adults: effects of intentionality. *J. Gerontol.* **37**, 330–335.

Parkinson, S. R., Lindholm, J. M., and Urell, T. (1980). Aging, dichotic memory, and digit span. *J. Gerontol.* **35**, 87–95.

Perris, C., and Monakhov, K. (1979). Depressive symptomatology and systemic structural analysis of the EEG. *In* "Hemisphere Asymmetries of Function in Psychopathology" (J. Gruzelier and P. Flor-Henry, eds.), pp. 223–236. Elsevier North-Holland, Amsterdam.

Riege, W., Metler, E. J., and Williams, M. V. (1980). Age and hemispheric asymmetry in nonverbal tactual memory. *Neuropsychologia* **18**, 707–710.

Riege, W., and Inman, V. (1981). Age differences in nonverbal memory tasks. *J. Gerontol.* **36**, 51–58.

Ross, E. D., and Rush, A. J. (1981). Diagnosis and neuroanatomical correlates of depression in brain-damaged patients. *Arch. Gen. Psychiatry* **38**, 1344–1354.

Schaie, K. W., and Schaie, J. P. (1977). Clinical assessment and aging. *In* "Handbook of the Psychology of Aging" (J. E. Birren and K. W. Schaie, eds.), 692–723. Van Nostrand-Reinhold, New York.

Schear, J. M., and Nebes, R. D. (1980). Memory for verbal and spatial information as a function of age. *Exp. Aging Res.* **6**, 271–281.

Sharpe, J. A., and Lo, A. W. (1981). Voluntary and visual control of the vestibulo-ocular reflex after cerebral hemidecortication. *Ann. Neurol.* **10**, 164–172.

Sharpe, J. A., and Sylvester, T. O. (1978). Effects of aging on horizontal smooth pursuit. *Invest. Ophthalmol. Visual Sci.* **17**, 465–468.

Siegler, I. C. (1980). The psychology of adult development and aging. *In* "Handbook of Geriatric Psychiatry" (E. W. Busse and D. G. Blazer, eds.), pp. 169–221. Van Nostrand-Reinhold, New York.

Smith, A. D., and Winograd, E. (1978). Adult age differences in remembering faces. *Dev. Psychol.* **14**, 443–444.

Smith, M. L., and Milner, B. (1981). The role of the right hippocampus in the recall of spatial location. *Neuropsychologia* **19**, 781–793.

Soininen, H., Partanen, V. J., Helkala, E. L., and Riekkinen, P. J. (1982a). EEG findings in senile dementia and normal aging. *Acta Neurol. Scand.* **65**, 59–70.

Soininen, H., Puranen, M., and Riekkinen, P. J. (1982b). Computed tomography findings in senile dementia and normal aging. *J. Neurol., Neurosurg. Psychiatry* **45**, 50–54.

Spooner, J. W., Sakala, S. M., and Baloh, R. W. (1980). Effect of aging on eye tracking. *Arch. Neurol. (Chicago)* **37**, 575–576.

Talland, G. (1968). Age and the span of immediate recall. *In* "Human Aging and Behavior: Recent Advances in Research and Theory" (G. Talland, ed.), pp. 92–129. Academic Press, New York.

Treat, N. J., Poon, L. W., and Fozard, J. L. (1981). Age, imagery, and practice in paired-associate learning. *Exp. Aging Res.* **7**, 337–342.

Troost, B. T., Daroff, R. B., Weber, R. B., and Dell'Osso, L. F. (1972). Hemispheric control of eye movements. *Arch. Neurol. (Chicago)* **27**, 449–452.

Tucker, D. M. (1981a). Lateral brain function, emotion, and conceptualization. *Psychol. Bull.* **89**, 19–46.

Tucker, D. M. (1981b). Asymmetrical frontal lobe function during a transient depressive state. *Adv. Biol. Psychiatry* **6**, 68–71.

Whitbourne, S. K., and Slevin, A. E. (1978). Imagery and sentence retention in elderly and young adults. *J. Genet. Psychol.* **133**, 287–298.

Winograd, E., Smith, A. D., and Simon, E. W. (1982). Aging and the picture superiority effect in recall. *J. Gerontol.* **37**, 70–75.

Woodruff, D. S. (1978). Brain electrical activity and behavior relationships over the life span. *In* "Life Span Development and Behavior" (P. B. Baltes, ed.), pp. 111–179. Academic Press, New York.

Wright, R. E. (1981). Aging, divided attention, and processing capacity. *J. Gerontol.* **36**, 605–614.

Yin, R. (1970). Face recognition by brain-damaged patients: A dissociable ability? *Neuropsychologia* **8**, 395–402.

10: Two Types of Hemisphere Imbalance in Hemi-Parkinsonism Coded by Brain Electrical Activity and Electrodermal Activity

MATTI MINTZ and MICHAEL S. MYSLOBODSKY

Psychobiology Research Unit
Department of Psychology
Tel-Aviv University, Israel

I. Introduction 213
II. Hemi-Parkinsonism 214
III. Debut of the Syndrome 215
IV. Symmetry of Sleep Electroencephalogram Abnormalities in Hemi-Parkinsonism 216
V. Visual Evoked Potentials in Hemi-Parkinsonism 219
VI. Attention-Related Visual Evoked Potentials Asymmetry Reduction 222
VII. Components of Hemisphere Interdependence 223
VIII. Asymmetries of Electrodermal Activity 229
IX. Summary 234
References 235

I. Introduction

Whenever a new approach becomes available for exploration, there emerges the possibility that something worth knowing will be discovered. This happened with the model of postlesion gyratory locomotion introduced by Arbuthnott and Ungerstedt (1975) when Glick's group started exploring pharmacologically induced rotation in normal rodents (Glick *et al.*, 1976). Ungerstedt's rats rotated because of an imbalance in the dopamine-carrying nigrostriatal system inflicted by unilateral electrolytic lesion or administration of the neurotoxin 6-hydroxydopamine. Normal rats rotated because of a small but rather stable intrinsic lateral asymmetry of the nigrostriatal system (see Chapter 2).

Initially, circling rodents were looked upon largely as instruments for

HEMISYNDROMES:
Psychobiology, Neurology,
Psychiatry

ISBN 0-12-512460-0

unveiling various aspects of Parkinsonism. However, Glick's discovery of dopamine (DA) asymmetry, very soon supplemented by findings of an asymmetric distribution of other neurotransmitters (Chapters 2 and 17; Oke *et al.*, 1978, 1980; Knapp and Mandell, 1980; Starr and Kilpatrick, 1981), along with a recognition of the role of DA in the control of sleep and wakefulness, attention and spatial orientation, brain laterality, emotions, cognitive functions, and aberrant behaviors, has made the rotating rodent a welcome and virtually omnipresent model.

The model's connection with Parkinsonism, although never lost (Chapter 4), has become far less obvious. Due to an overwhelming interest on the part of researchers, multiplied by an unexpected complexity of gyration control systems, circling today has acquired all the attributes of a prosperous and independent research area (see Pycock, 1980). Also, it has been recognized that circling does not answer the questions concerning the very extrapyramidal pathology that originally spurred its study. A parallel, clinically based endeavor is necessary to meet the requirements of neurologists. Ideally, it should be a pathology that emulates the best features of the model, that is, lateralized deficit of a known transmitter system with an easily assessed motor imbalance. This chapter is an attempt to initiate exploration of such a syndrome caused by brain dopaminergic hemideficit, namely, hemi-Parkinsonism.

II. Hemi-Parkinsonism

Hemi-Parkinsonism seems to be an ideal model for laterality research in schizophrenia and depression for the following reasons:

1. Parkinsonism is often accompanied by depression (Mayeux *et al.*, 1981), and hemi-Parkinsonism may shed some light on brain imbalance developing during affective psychosis.
2. Rewarded behavior is intimately related to the dopaminergic system. Given that Parkinsonism is associated with DA deficit, an anhedonic state, which is believed to be associated with schizophrenia (Meehl, 1975), may be more typical of Parkinsonism.
3. We often see Parkinsonian symptoms in the course of neuroleptic medication, whereas subclinical alterations of brain reactivity associated with the DA receptor blockade may long remain undetected. Given that the extrapyramidal symptoms are either unilateral or distinctly lateralized, the advantage of investigating hemi-Parkinsonism lies in the possibility of comparing the supposedly normal brain reactivity, largely reflecting age-related changes, with reactivity of the hemisphere displaying the first signs of the failing DA system. In full agreement with the recommendations of the Classification of Extrapyramidal Disorders

(1981), hemi-Parkinsonism provides a chance to "compare the patient with himself" rather than with other patients or control subjects.

4. The extrapyramidal symptoms and cognitive abnormality of Parkinsonism respond to L-dopa medication. This allows *in vivo* analysis of the asymmetry of the DA system in the human brain by the exploration of postmedication brain reactivity changes.

5. Animal experiments show that lesions in the nigrostriatal system and the administration of DA agonists and antagonists produce a profound and lasting alteration of locomotion accompanied by changes in electroencephalogram (EEG), evoked potentials, and cellular activity. It is hoped, therefore, that by means of electrophysiological methods the lateralized abnormality of DA transmission and its posttreatment improvement will be detected. Specifically, we believe that visual evoked potentials (VEPs) and EEG may be adequate instruments for testing brain reactivity in Parkinsonism inasmuch as DA projections from the mesencephalic tegmentum are known to reach the posterior neocortex (Törk and Turner, 1981).

6. Finally, nowhere in neurology or psychiatry has the anatomy, physiology, or biochemistry of a single disease been so handsomely delineated as in Parkinsonism. Its major pathophysiological mechanism is related to the failure of DA neurotransmission in the nigrostriatal tract (Hornykiewicz, 1966; Bernheimer *et al.*, 1973). The hemideficit of DA in the hemi-Parkinsonian patient has been verified by Barolin *et al.* (1964).

III. Debut of the Syndrome

The only disadvantage of using this syndrome as a model is that it is believed to be relatively rare. However, a study conducted by V. Ben-Mayor, H. Radwan, and M. Mintz (1980, unpublished) showed that, within the span of approximately one decade in two hospitals in the Tel-Aviv area, 191 patients were treated for unilateral or lateralized extrapyramidal syndrome. It should be remembered that, even in Parkinson's (1817) original sample of 6 patients, 2 had a strongly lateralized abnormality.

Table 10.1 shows that the incidence of left-sided hemi-Parkinsonism in Ben-Mayor *et al.*'s sample was significantly higher ($p<0.01$). This result is attributed largely to the female group, in which the left-sided debut of the disease occurred in 71.0% of the cases, whereas among males the left-sided debut of the disease occurred in 58.2% of the cases.

Rothman and Glick (1976) demonstrated that lesions in the striata caused a different intensity of effects depending on whether the lesion was inflicted on the side of a higher or lower DA content. Also, systemic administration of metrazol caused bilaterally asymmetric spike–wave

TABLE 10.1
Distribution of Patients by Sex and Side of Hemi-Parkinsonian Symptoms[a]

		Side of Parkinsonian symptoms			
		Left		Right	
Sex	Age range	*N*	%	*N*	%
Male	34–80	71	58.2	51	41.8
Female	34–74	49	71.0	20	29.0
Total	—	120[b]	62.8	71	37.2

[a]The incidence and laterality of hemi-Parkinsonism were reviewed among patients admitted consecutively to the Departments of Neurology at Beilinson Hospital (from 1968 to 1981) and Meir Hospital (from 1974 to 1981), Tel-Aviv. Care was taken to exclude conditions that resembled classical Parkinson's disease: essential tremor, "Parkinson's disease" with atypical features—without rigidity and with pyramidal signs—cranial trauma, cerebral infarcts, etc. None of the patients was on drug treatment at the time of admission. All of the patients were eventually diagnosed as having idiopathic Parkinsonism.

[b]$z = 3.54$, $p < 0.01$ (test for significance of proportions).

discharges; greater discharges were noticed on the side homolateral to dominant rotation directionality in the preconvulsive screening tests (Myslobodsky and Rosen, 1979).

The preceding findings are therefore interpreted as favoring the hypothesis of intrinsic asymmetry of nigrostriatal DA in the human brain. The higher incidence of women presenting a right hemisphere (left-sided) Parkinsonism implicates gonadal steroids in alterations of dopaminergic activity.

The injection of large doses of estrogen has been noted to increase the duration of stereotypy (Lal and Sourkes, 1972), suggesting an estrogen-related increase in DA receptor sensitivity. Indeed, like neuroleptics, estrogen leads to the development of a withdrawal supersensitivity (Bedard *et al.*, 1978; Naik *et al.*, 1978; Chiodo *et al.*, 1979; Hruska and Silbergeld, 1980; Gordon and Diamond, 1981). Robinson *et al.* (Chapter 5) analyzed a growing body of evidence indicating a close interaction between gonadal steroids and the nigrostriatal DA system. Further exploration of the sexual variation of hemi-Parkinsonian symptoms is clearly indicated. If these findings were replicated, they would help in understanding the intriguing interaction between psychopathology and hemisphere asymmetries.

IV. Symmetry of Sleep Electroencephalogram Abnormalities in Hemi-Parkinsonism

Our first study of hemi-Parkinsonism was conducted with a small sample of patients who displayed sleep abnormalities. It was inspired by a small but reliable asymmetry of secondary VEP components and σ spindles occurring in non-REM sleep in normal individuals (Myslobodsky,

1976; Myslobodsky *et al.*, 1977). Given that σ spindles are modulated by the dopaminergic system (Neal and Keane, 1980) and that DA is known to participate in EEG synchronization, one may predict that electrical activity in sleeping and waking patients should be asymmetric. Moreover, this asymmetry should be corrected by L-dopa treatment. With this prediction in mind, waking and sleep EEG patterns were recorded during two nights in 4 male and 3 female patients drawn from a larger sample (described in Table 10.3).

Considering that the hemisphere contralateral to Parkinsonian symptomatology is largely involved, it will be designated as the Parkinsonian (P) hemisphere in order to differentiate between the EEG patterns generated over it and the control, non-Parkinsonian (NP) hemisphere. The first night EEG was monitored before the initiation of L-dopa medication; the second night EEG was monitored not less than 2 months after. The techniques employed were described by Myslobodsky *et al.* (1977, 1982).

Visual analysis showed considerable abnormalities of EEG in presleep wakefulness and night sleep. Waking EEG was of low amplitude. Sleep EEG showed reduced stage 2 σ spindles and underrepresentation of stages 3 to 4. Because during sleep most of the EEG intensity falls within the δ band (Johnson *et al.*, 1969) the sleep pattern also looked strikingly flat. The administration of L-dopa caused an improvement in the quality of sleep, consisting of decreased latency to sleep onset, enhanced amount of slow-wave sleep, and increased number of REM periods. This notwithstanding, EEG patterns were rather symmetric. To verify this observation the duration of different sleep patterns was assessed and expressed as an asymmetry index (AI). Positive index values indicate that values of the P hemisphere exceed those of the NP side. Table 10.2 indicates that the AI was positive for α (α rhythm was a consequence of frequent EEG arousals by intermittent awakenings) and negative for sleep

TABLE 10.2
Asymmetry Index[a] of Duration of Selected EEG Patterns over the Parkinsonian and Non-Parkinsonian Hemispheres during Pretreatment and Post-L-dopa Medication Nights

EEG pattern	Pretreatment night	Posttreatment night
α	0.16	−0.28
α during REM	−0.29	0.07
Spindles (σ)	−0.32	0.35
θ	−0.06	0.12
δ	−0.03	0.03

Source: Myslobodsky *et al.*, 1982.

[a] Computed as the net difference between the values of the two hemispheres over their sum, (P − NP)/(P + NP).

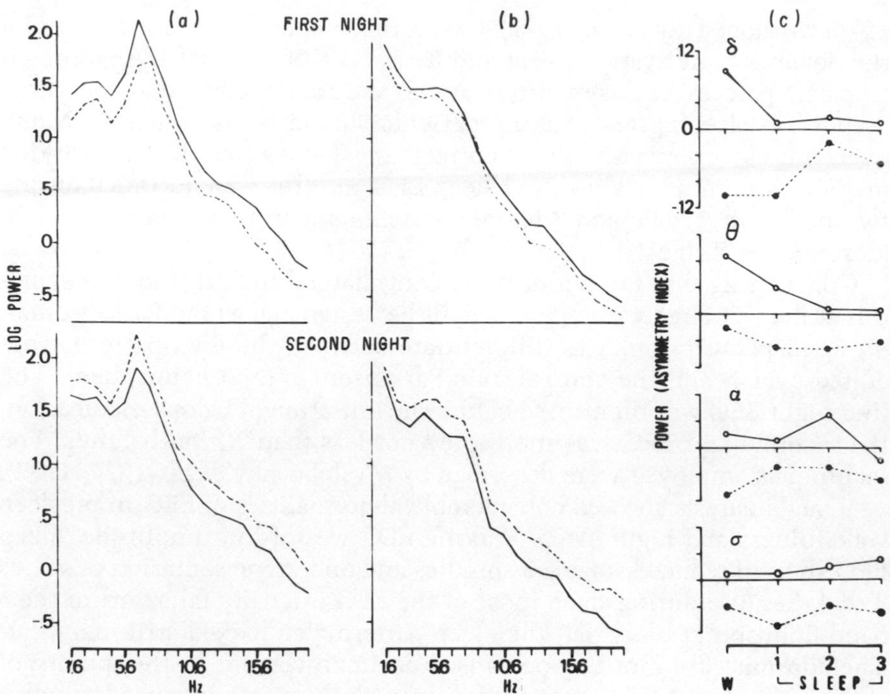

FIG. 10.1. Power spectrum of EEG (in arbitrary units), recorded from P3 and P4 sites and referred to joint mastoids, of a typical hemi-Parkinsonian patient in the first and second nights, during presleep wakefulness (a) and during the first period of night sleep (b). In graphs (a) and (b) the abscissa represents the frequencies analyzed in 1-Hz steps, and the ordinate represents the log values of power plotted for Parkinsonian (- - -) and non-Parkinsonian (—) hemispheres separately. Note the relative change in power across the hemispheres during the second night as compared with the first night. In graph (c) this change is represented as a group AI, computed separately for δ (1.1–4.0 Hz), θ (4.1–7.0 Hz), α (7.1–12.0 Hz), and σ (12.1–16.0 Hz) spectra for presleep wakefulness (W) and three consecutive arbitrary sleep periods (1, 2, 3) of about 2 hr each (•---•, first night; ○—○, second night). The AI is the net difference between the values of the two hemispheres over the maximal value [(P-NP)/maximum]. Each point is the mean of seven patients. Note that, although in individual and group graphs lateral asymmetry is visible in nonmedicated patients and reversed after L-dopa treatment in wakefulness and sleep, the treatment-by-hemispheres interaction proved significant only for the δ spectrum during sleep ($F(1,6) = 11.65$, $p < 0.014$). Adapted from Myslobodsky, M., Mintz, M., Ben-Mayor, V. and Radwan, H. (1982). Unilateral dopamine deficit and lateral EEG asymmetry: Sleep abnormalities in hemi-Parkinson's patients. *EEG Clin. Neurophysiol.* **54**, 227–231.

EEG patterns. A reversal of the index sign was seen after L-dopa medication, indicating increased duration of σ spindles, θ and δ patterns, and reduced duration of waking α pattern, especially over the P hemisphere, albeit not to a statistically significant extent.

The mean σ, α, θ, and δ power values from both hemispheres before and after L-dopa treatment, during wakefulness and three arbitrary periods of NREM sleep, were then compared. The most noteworthy change was a consistent reduction of EEG power in all frequencies over the P hemisphere and its recovery after L-dopa medication (Fig. 10.1 A and B). Statistical analysis showed marginally significant hemisphere-by-treatment interaction only for the δ range in wakefulness ($p<0.058$), which reached significance in NREM sleep ($p<0.014$). These findings became more visible when the AI was computed and plotted as a function of sleep periods. Figure 10.2C demonstrates that pre- and posttreatment values of the index have different signs, especially for δ and θ bands, indicating a relative increase of EEG power after L-dopa medication over the P hemisphere.

V. Visual Evoked Potentials in Hemi-Parkinsonism

Studies on VEPs were conducted in the two groups of hemi-Parkinson patients described in Table 10.3. One group was seen twice for VEP examination, before and after chronic L-dopa medication (hereafter referred to as group A). Another group of patients (referred to as group B) was seen only once, either before or after chronic L-dopa medication.

The techniques employed were described by Mintz *et al.* (1981). The VEP components (P_{100}, N_{130}, P_{300}, and N_{400}) were identified on the basis of

TABLE 10.3
Description of the Two Subgroups of Hemi-Parkinsonian Patients[a]

Group	Drug-free session	Treatment duration: L-dopa (250–500 mg/day), carbidopa (25–50 mg/day)	L-dopa session
Group A (N = 11)			
Sex (F/M)	4/7	2–8 months	Same patients
Handedness (L/R)	1/10		Same patients
Parkinsonian side (L/R)	5/6		Same patients
Group B (N = 18)			
N	6	5 months to 6 years	12
Sex (F/M)	1/5		4/8
Handedness (L/R)	1/5		1/11
Parkinsonian side (L/R)	2/4		7/5

[a]Patients, ranging from 40 to 75 years of age (mean age 62 ± 8 years), were screened for stage 1 Parkinson's disease at the Department of Neurology, Meir Hospital, Tel-Aviv. The diagnosis was based on patient's complaints that clearly indicated the laterality of their abnormality and on the presence of the following lateralized symptoms: rigidity of the limbs (N = 16), tremor at rest (N = 20), and slowing (N = 19). In 20 patients strictly unilateral symptoms were diagnosed, whereas in 9 only initial signs of involvement of the other side were noted. None of the patients had, at the time of examination, significant symptoms of pulmonary or heart disease. Their EEG patterns were normal, except for that of one patient, in which occasional bursts of θ waves were observed.

TABLE 10.4

Peak Latency of Selected VEP Components Recorded from Parkinsonian (P) and Non-Parkinsonian (NP) Hemispheres during Pre- and Post-L-dopa Medication[a]

Treatment condition	N	P_{100}		N_{130}		P_{300}		N_{400}	
		P	NP	P	NP	P	NP	P	NP
Pre-L-dopa	11	$100.9^{b} \pm 22.8$	94.1 ± 23.7	135.4 ± 21.4	133.2 ± 22.8	253.0 ± 43.0	250.2 ± 51.9	349.4 ± 91.8	346.1 ± 96.4
	(6)	(92.5 ± 16.0)	(90.8 ± 13.6)	(129.2 ± 25.0)	(125.0 ± 17.6)	(308.3 ± 49.3)	(319.2 ± 40.9)	(443.3 ± 66.3)	(438.3 ± 63.2)
Post-L-dopa	11	91.4 ± 24.5	94.5 ± 20.5	135.5 ± 23.8	139.5 ± 33.6	266.4 ± 66.1	261.8 ± 64.3	355.0 ± 87.1	356.4 ± 93.0
	(12)	(81.2 ± 16.5)	(81.5 ± 14.4)	(115.0 ± 24.9)	(115.8 ± 23.8)	$(315.8 \pm 44.3$	(312.9 ± 56.1)	(430.8 ± 77.2)	(422.9 ± 76.4)

[a]The findings were based on VEP values of group A, seen before and after chronic L-dopa treatment, and of group B, seen once, either before or after L-dopa medication (values in parentheses). Peak latencies are expressed as milliseconds ± SD.

[b]Treatment-by-hemisphere interaction, $F(1,10) = 11.00$, $p < 0.008$ (group A).

TABLE 10.5

Amplitude of Selected VEP Components Recorded from Parkinsonian (P) and Non-Parkinsonian (NP) Hemispheres during Pre- and Post-L-dopa Medication[a]

Treatment condition	N	P_{100}		P_{300}		VEP_{max}	
		P	NP	P	NP	P	NP
Pre-L-dopa	11	12.9 ± 9.6	13.7 ± 7.4	$14.2^{b} \pm 8.2$	16.0 ± 7.3	$15.2^{c} \pm 8.2$	17.3 ± 8.2
	(6)	(7.3 ± 4.7)	(7.7 ± 5.2)	(16.8 ± 9.9)	(17.8 ± 9.1)	(16.8 ± 9.9)	(18.0 ± 9.3)
Post-L-dopa	11	16.2 ± 9.2	15.7 ± 8.5	16.6 ± 4.3	15.1 ± 5.8	17.2 ± 5.3	15.1 ± 5.8
	(12)	(20.4 ± 16.3)	(19.1 ± 15.2)	(20.7 ± 10.4)	(18.4 ± 10.2)	(21.5 ± 11.7)	(20.2 ± 11.9)

[a]The findings are based on VEP values of group A, seen before and after chronic L-dopa treatment, and of group B, seen once, either before or after L-dopa medication (values in parentheses). Amplitudes of VEP components (expressed as microvolts ± SD) were determined by measuring the vertical distance (in microvolts) between adjacent positive (P_{100} and P_{300}) and negative (N_{130} and N_{400}) peaks and troughs; VEP_{max} is the maximal amplitude of the secondary VEP components (see text).

[b]Treatment-by-hemisphere interaction, $F(1,10) = 8.16$, $p < 0.017$ (group A).

[c]Treatment-by-hemisphere interaction, $F(1,10) = 19.31$, $p < .001$ (group A).

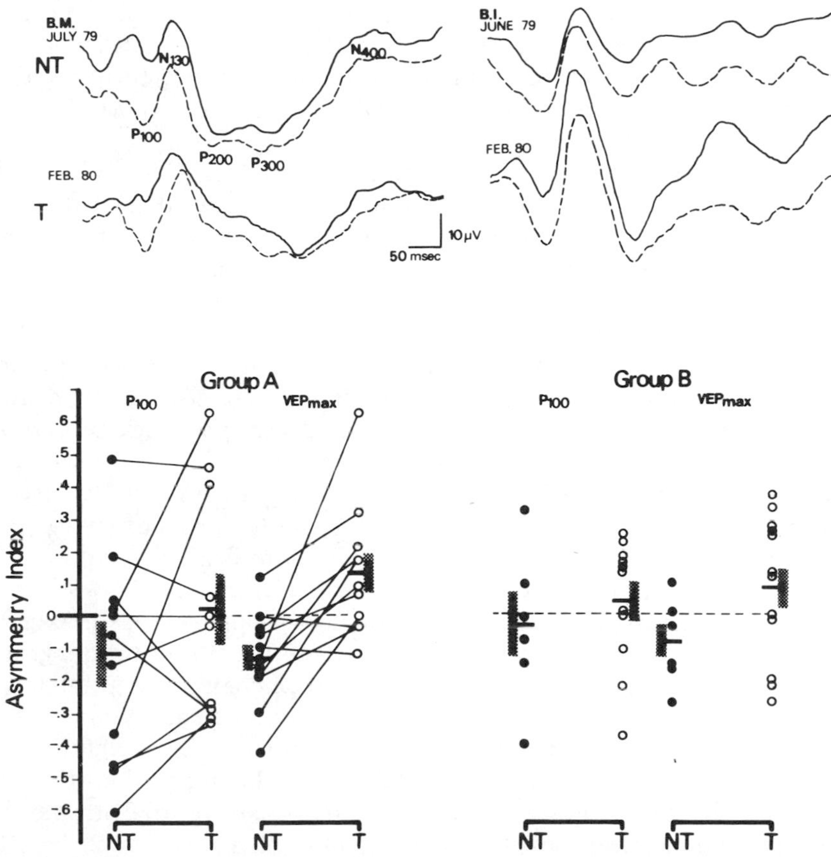

FIG. 10.2. Examples of VEPs recorded from P3 and P4 sites in the open-eyes state, from two hemi-Parkinsonian patients (B.M. and B.I.), in a nontreated (NT) condition and after L-dopa treatment (T), at dates specified. Stroboscopic flashes were presented binocularly, with a 3–15-sec interval between the stimuli. The lamp was positioned 150 cm in front of the subjects' eyes at 13° above the fixation point. Solid and dashed traces represent the VEPs over the Parkinsonian and non-Parkinsonian hemispheres, respectively. Each tracing was derived from an average of 20 trials. Stimuli presentation coincides with the beginning of the averages. Scalp positivity is down. Nontreatment (NT) and posttreatment (T) conditions were analyzed separately for group A (repeated measures in the same patients) and group B (two different samples). Each circle represents individual values of AI before (•) and after (o)L-dopa medication. The AI is the net difference between the values of the two hemispheres over the maximal value [(P–NP)/maximum]. Horizontal lines and the stippled vertical bars represent the mean ± SEM for each condition. (Adapted from Mintz *et al.*, 1981.)

sequence, polarity, and latency range (see Fig. 10.2). Latency findings, summarized in Table 10.4, show that the VEP components were somewhat delayed over the P hemisphere before medication. The L-dopa had a tendency to shorten the P_{100} latency more over the P hemisphere. This observation was supported by a significant ($p<0.008$) treatment-by-hemisphere interaction for group A. Increased VEP latencies are in agreement with findings reported by Bodis-Wollner and Yahr (1978) in response to patterned stimulus. These authors are inclined to relate this phenomenon to the abnormal DA-related modulation of sensory transmission.

Table 10.5 represents amplitude values for early and later VEP components. It shows that in group A the later positive wave (P_{300}) is reduced over the P hemisphere in nonmedicated patients and is relatively enhanced after L-dopa treatment. This finding was supported by a significant ($p<0.017$) treatment-by-hemisphere interaction.

It is important to mention that the reversal of asymmetry of the P_{300} cautions against the interpretation of the preceding findings as being related to motor imbalance (as, in fact, might happen; see Gevins *et al.*, 1979). Tremor is a rather stubborn symptom and in most patients can be easily detected despite L-dopa therapy.

Since P_{300} and the preceding positive peak (P_{200}) are often very close to each other and sometimes merge into a single broader positivity (Fig. 10.2), the amplitude of the entire "secondary complex" [the "most positive point" of Seales (1973), designated hereafter as VEP_{max}] was measured as the vertical distance from P_{300} or P_{200} (whichever was maximal) to the N_{400} wave. Analysis proved that, by the use of this criterion, group A shows similar and highly significant amplitude changes. In group B the asymmetry of later components before and after medication changed in the same direction, although not to the extent of statistical significance (Table 10.5). This finding was supported by the AI computed for the amplitude of early and secondary VEP components. As Fig. 10.2 shows, the AI of VEP_{max} underwent post-L-dopa reversal of polarity.

It is known that striatal stores show a considerable loss of DA with age, so that Parkinsonism builds up on age-related alterations of dopaminergic transmission in both hemispheres. That notwithstanding, owing to data obtained in group A, Parkinsonism-related VEP alterations proved to be detectable in both groups. It is important to acknowledge at this point that, had only group B patients been examined, interhemispheric asymmetry of VEPs would not have been noticed.

VI. Attention-Related Visual Evoked Potentials Asymmetry Reduction

However meager are the VEP asymmetries described earlier, they are a real manifestation of the degree of imbalance of the two sensory systems. Unfortunately, one can only further decrease the magnitude of this asymmetry to prove the point.

Some severely disabled Parkinson patients show temporary motor improvement ("paradoxical kinesia") under conditions of stress. The nature of this phenomenon is obscure, and it would be interesting to investigate whether effects similar to paradoxical kinesia could be detected in the sensory system during a simple cognitive task. Therefore, after the medication-related VEP enhancement in hemi-Parkinson patients was documented, we reasoned that if moderate stress caused by task demands were capable of overcoming insufficient DA transmission by mobilizing DA from remaining presynaptic terminals, then the effect of an attentive state should resemble that of L-dopa treatment.

Table 10.6 (in which the technical details are described) shows that attentional factors did not affect early VEP components [which are believed to reflect processes occurring during signal identification (Buchsbaum *et al.*, 1974)], either before or after treatment. Whereas in some patients (25%) the early components were clearly facilitated, in most of the patients the later VEP components changed in the anticipated direction. This change, however, proved to be marginally significant before L-dopa treatment.

In the L-dopa-medicated sample, the task caused a bilateral VEP enhancement that was significant for P_{300} ($p<0.037$). When treated patients with right and left hemi-Parkinsonism were separated, it was noted that individuals with left-sided symptoms made fewer counting errors than those with right-sided symptoms (5.6 versus 13.5%). In view of this finding the treated sample was regrouped into patients with left ($N=9$) and right ($N=8$) Parkinsonian symptoms. Table 10.7 shows that the task-related enhancement of the later components was contributed to mainly by the NP hemisphere of patients with left-sided symptoms. Indeed, in this group all 9 patients showed attention-related enhancement of P_{300} over the NP hemisphere. In patients with right-sided symptoms the enhancement of P_{300} (albeit not significant) was noted over the P hemisphere. It was seen in 4 of 8 patients in this subgroup.

VII. Components of Hemisphere Interdependence

Given that patients had an advanced unilateral or distinctly lateralized extrapyramidal syndrome, the practically symmetric EEG and the rather special efforts required to detect its small asymmetries were surprising. Visual evoked potential asymmetry was often barely visible and was far from the asymmetry required to substantiate the lateralized neurological abnormality. Why were the electrophysiological asymmetries so meager compared with a very profound and stable unilateral or strongly lateralized motor imbalance? One possibility is that, although dopaminergic abnormality is not below the limits of resolution of the electrophysiological methods employed in the present study, the visibility of asym-

TABLE 10.6
Effect of Attention Task on Amplitude of Selected VEP Components Recorded from the Parkinsonian (P) and Non-Parkinsonian (NP) Hemispheres during Pre- and Post-L-dopa Medication[a]

Treatment condition	N	P_{100}		P_{300}		VEP_{max}	
		P	NP	P	NP	P	NP
Pre-L-dopa							
Relaxation	8	8.6 ± 6.6	11.0 ± 7.7	18.4[b] ± 8.8	18.9 ± 7.3	18.4 ± 8.8	19.3 ± 7.8
Attention task	8	9.0 ± 7.7	10.1 ± 8.0	18.8 ± 6.6	16.5 ± 5.0	18.8 ± 6.6	16.8 ± 5.2
Post-L-dopa							
Relaxation	17	19.6 ± 13.8	19.8 ± 13.1	20.3[c] ± 8.7	18.1 ± 8.7	20.8 ± 9.8	19.4 ± 10.2
Attention task	17	19.8 ± 17.2	19.4 ± 17.2	24.5 ± 12.1	23.8 ± 11.8	24.8 ± 12.1	24.2 ± 12.1

[a] Patients (from either group A or B) were asked to perform in an attention task. They were first given several training trials in which they learned to discriminate between "regular" (intensity 8 of the photostimulator) and "weak" (intensity 1) flashes. Thereafter, 30–35 "regular" and 20–25 "weak" flashes were delivered in random order, and the patients were asked to count the number of flashes of either intensity. Three patients not receiving L-dopa and eight who were receiving L-dopa had difficulty in discriminating between the two intensities and were therefore asked to count all flashes, of either intensity. Active involvement of the patients in the task was indicated by the accuracy of counting. The techniques employed were described by Mintz *et al.* (1982). Amplitude expressed as microvolts ± SD.

[b] Task-by-hemisphere interaction, $F(1,7) = 3.94$, $p < 0.087$.

[c] Task effect, $F(1,16) = 5.19$, $p < 0.037$.

TABLE 10.7

Effect of Attention Task on Amplitude of Selected VEP Components Recorded from Patients with Left- and Right-sided Parkinsonian Symptoms after L-dopa Medication

Patients	N	P_{100}		P_{300}[a,b]		VEP_{max}	
		P	NP	P	NP	P	NP
Left-sided symptoms							
Relaxation	9	21.5 ± 17.7	23.0 ± 15.9	18.3 ± 9.1	15.3 ± 7.7	18.7 ± 9.9	17.3 ± 11.1
Attention task	9	22.4 ± 18.9	24.5 ± 20.2	23.0 ± 13.0	24.2 ± 11.9	23.3 ± 13.0	25.0 ± 12.4
Right-sided symptoms							
Relaxation	8	17.7 ± 9.4	16.6 ± 9.7	22.5 ± 8.3	21.2 ± 9.2	23.2 ± 9.8	21.7 ± 9.2
Attention task	8	17.2 ± 16.3	14.2 ± 12.8	26.2 ± 11.5	23.4 ± 12.3	26.5 ± 11.5	23.4 ± 12.3

Source: Mintz *et al.*, 1982.

[a] Task effect, $F(1,15) = 4.87$, $p < 0.043$.

[b] Task-by-hemisphere-by-group interaction, $F(1,15) = 3.64$, $p < 0.075$.

metries may be lessened by the reduced amplitudes of the signals that we process. Reduced slow-wave amplitude in sleep is a striking example of the evolution of brain reactivity caused by DA deficit.

The generators of diffuse δ waves are located in the lower layers of the cortex (Nakamura *et al.*, 1968; Ball *et al.*, 1977). Ball *et al.* (1977) found a strong relationship between δ waves and unit discharges in the neocortex. Typically, surface positivity was associated with unit firing, whereas surface negativity was associated with a decrease in the probability of cellular discharges. Also, δ waves showed laminar profiles indicating that they are generated by radially oriented neurons. Positivity of the waves represents a passive source related to an active sink produced by summated deep EPSPs. The surface negative waves represent a passive sink caused by an active source of summated deep IPSPs generated most likely by axosomatic synapses located on pyramidal cells in layer V. Most cells of layers IV–VI are DA sensitive (see Bunney, 1979, for review), and DA failure would be expected to reduce the electrical activity generated by these cells. Conceivably, age-related reduction of slow-wave sleep (Agnew *et al.*, 1967; Kahn and Fisher, 1969; Feinberg, 1974; Smith *et al.*, 1977) and the decline of δ waves in Parkinsonism are associated with selective abnormalities of the DA-mediated activity of the cortex. In fact, a decrease in endogenous DA in elderly rhesus monkeys has been reported to occur in the prefrontal area (Goldman-Rakic and Brown, 1981), which normally generates the largest number of δ waves. However, negative correlations (although not significant) were obtained between asymmetry and amplitude scores. Thus, because we failed to obtain a reduction of EEG and VEP asymmetry as a function of reduced amplitude of these measures, the preceding conjecture can be rejected.

Another hypothesis should consider the argument that nigrostriatal abnormality, even if strictly unilateral, may not be sufficiently represented by the activity of neocortical neurons. Neocortex is the major (if not the only) layer of active tissue the responsiveness of which is accessible for examination by our EEG–VEP technique. This conjecture further implies that the mesocortical DA system either is not involved (at least initially) in Parkinsonism or, on the contrary, may suffer to a similar extent on both sides, creating a deceptively balanced pattern of neocortical activity.

It should be remembered that the extrapyramidal symptoms, although the major feature of the disease, are not the only abnormality. There are other troublesome symptoms, the most common of which are depression, recognized originally by James Parkinson (1817), and intellectual impairment (Lieberman *et al.*, 1979; Boller *et al.*, 1980; Mayeux *et al.*, 1981). These are hardly caused by nigrostriatal abnormality alone, especially since signs of dementia may be associated with only mild extrapyramidal symptoms (Purdy *et al.*, 1978). It is possible that considerable deficits in the mesofrontal and mesolimbic DA systems accompany the degeneration of nigrostriatal pathways. Experimental depletion of DA in the prefrontal cortex of rhesus monkeys produced by the injection of microquantities of the catecholaminergic toxin 6-OHDA into the cortex leads to a selective cognitive deficit similar to that produced by surgical ablation of the region (Brozoski *et al.*, 1979). Javoy-Agid and Agid (1980) have shown that brain tyrosine hydroxylase activity, examined postmortem in Parkinson's patients in order to identify catecholaminergic neurons, was decreased in the ventral tegmental area. This finding has been interpreted as suggesting a dysfunction of the mesocortical (mesofrontal) DA system. Although the present data give no indication that the mesocortical system suffers bilateral DA deficit, the generalized involvement of this system cannot be ruled out. The deficit of the "noninvolved" mesocortical system may not reveal itself clinically until the DA deficit reaches a certain threshold level. In fact, the DA-mediated control of locomotion has a peculiar "all-or-none" mode of action. Age-related loss of the dopaminergic neurons may be profound and reach 70% (Carlsson and Winblad, 1976; Riederer and Wuketich, 1976; McGeer *et al.*, 1977) without clinical abnormalities of locomotion or cognitive impairment. Major extrapyramidal signs of Parkinsonism may not show up until the nigrostriatal deficit exceeds 70–80% (Bernheimer *et al.*, 1973). Seen in this perspective the lack of EEG asymmetry may be a symptom of the tacit (preclinical) involvement of the "control" side. However, Barolin *et al.* (1964) demonstrated that hemi-Parkinsonism is accompanied by a considerable DA (but not 5-hydroxytryptamine) imbalance, uncomparable to "physiological" DA asymmetry. The level of DA in the caudate nucleus of the P hemisphere was about half of that on the noninvolved side; the amount of DA in the putamen was one-seventh of that in the same structure on the supposedly healthy side. Unfortunately, Barolin *et al.* had a single case of senile hemi-Parkinsonism. More data would be required to reject the loss of DA in either system of the noninvolved hemisphere of patients with unilateral extrapyramidal syndrome. Robinson *et al.* (Chapter 5) made an interesting step toward showing that pathological dopaminergic asymmetry may not override the intrinsic locomotion imbalance of nonlesioned animals. They found that more than 90% of the DA input to the "dominant" hemisphere (the hemisphere contralateral to the dominant side of amphetamine-induced circling of the naive rat) should be destroyed by 6-OHDA in order to disrupt the tendency of the rat to turn away from that side.

Still another conjecture rests on the evidence that the dopaminergic nerve terminals to the cerebral cortex originate not only from A_{10} group neurons but from cells of the rostral mesencephalic A_9 system (Lidbrink *et al.*, 1974; Lindvall *et al.*, 1974; Hökfelt *et al.*, 1976) and that nigrostriatal projections are partially crossed (Fass and Butcher, 1981). These data imply that with DA hemideficit the neighboring hemisphere should always display signs of involvement. Hahn *et al.* (1981) noted that unilateral chemical (6-OHDA) and electrolytic lesioning in the substantia nigra in rats was followed within a week by a considerable bilateral decrease in the striatal DA content. In addition, the DA content was reduced bilaterally in the substantia nigra. Although these changes were transient, they were interpreted as supporting the concept of an interdependence of the DA systems of the two sides. Correspondingly, the lesioned and the nonlesioned sides might be expected to undergo similar processes of compensatory readjustment, triggered by DA deficiency. According to Lloyd (1977) the most prominent of these are (*a*) a reduction in synthesis and release of acetylcholine (ACh) by striatal neurons in order to maintain a normal DA–ACh balance and (*b*) decreased synthesis and release of γ-aminobutyric acid allowing maximal firing of the remaining DA neurons (see also Finch, 1980). A weakening of the corticostriatal pathway of the P hemisphere might also cause a release of DA-mediated activity. One of the earliest attempts to alleviate Parkinsonism involved the removal of the prefrontal cortex. In addition, a loss of striatal neurons accompanying a loss of substantia nigra cells may reduce the risk of Parkinsonism (Bugiani *et al.*, 1978). To a certain extent a compensatory hypersensitivity to the DA of cells in the basal ganglia (Lee *et al.*, 1978) may preserve relatively equal responsiveness of the two sensory areas. Another possibility is that the intact hemisphere provides the deficient one with a variety of stimuli, via dopaminergic and nondopaminergic pathways directed to reduce the disparity between their excitability.

There are several crossed pathways shown electrophysiologically and neurochemically (Fig. 10.3; see also Chapter 3): caudate–caudate (Mensah and Deadwyler, 1974), pallidopallidal (Nauta and Mehler, 1966), nigrostriatal projections (Fass and Butcher, 1981), nigrothalamic (Rinvik *et al.*, 1976; Deniau *et al.*, 1978; Pritzel and Huston, 1981), and nigrotectal fibers (Rinvik *et al.*, 1976; Deniau *et al.*, 1977). Until recently the role of these crossed pathways was not recognized, probably because normally they remain functionally dormant and are activated only by unilateral dopaminergic deficiency (Pritzel and Huston, 1981). In addition, neocortical callosal fibers should be considered (Cavada and Reinoso-Suarez, 1981). Most callosal fibers represent axons of neurons located largely in deep cortical layers (Pines and Maiman, 1939; Jacobson and Trojanowski, 1974), which, as mentioned earlier, respond predominantly to dopaminergic activation (Bunney, 1979). Finally, messages originating from the motor areas project to both caudate nuclei (Carman *et al.*, 1965; Kunzle, 1975). Unilateral electrical stimulation of the motor cortex (area 4) in cats induced a long-lasting activation of [^{3}H]DA release in both caudates (Nieoullon *et al.*, 1978). Given this evidence the lack of pronounced EEG asymmetry may suggest that a variety of within- and between-hemisphere circuits and mechanisms operate as a single *interdependence system* in response to a lesion inflicted on one hemisphere. It is tempting

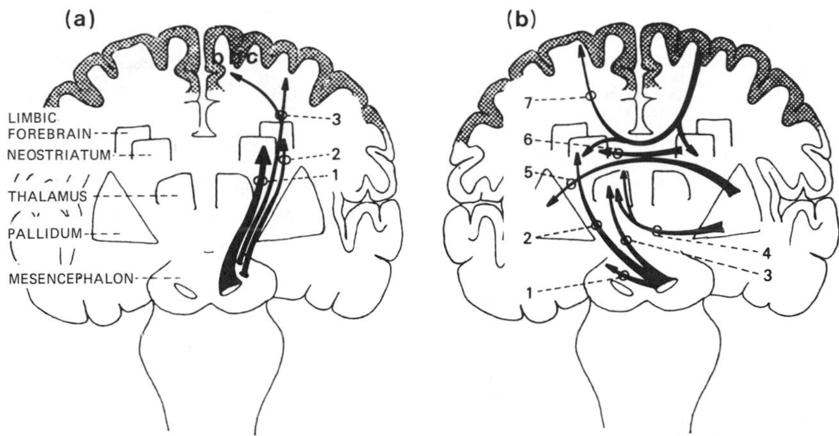

FIG. 10.3. Diagrammatic representation of major DA systems. (a) Our initial hypothesis was based on the assumption that the nigrostriatal pathway projects almost exclusively homolaterally (Andén *et al.*, 1964), and the sparsely crossed nigrostriatal pathway (Royce, 1978) would not significantly alter interhemispheric imbalance due to brain DA hemideficit. 1: Nigrostriatal tract, the largest and most thoroughly investigated DA system. The cell bodies are located in the pars compacta of the substantia nigra. Their axons terminate on the neurons in the neostriatum. 2: Mesolimbic system begins in the ventral tegmental area and projects to the limbic system (the nucleus accumbens, nucleus of the stria terminalis, amygdala, and olfactory tubercle). 3: Mesocortical system projects to the gyrus cinguli, entorhinal cortex, frontal cortex (mostly basal layers). It originates partially in the ventral tegmental area and partially in the substantia nigra. (b) Crossed pathways suggested to balance the reactivity of the hemispheres in cases of DA hemideficit. 1: Crossed nigrotectal pathways (Deniau *et al.*, 1977; Wright and Arbuthnott, 1981). 2: Nigrostriatal projections (Fass and Butcher, 1981). 3: Nigrothalamic connections (Rinvik *et al.*, 1976; Deniau *et al.*, 1978; Pritzel and Huston, 1981; Wright and Arbuthnott, 1981). 4: Connections of the pallidum (entopeduncular nucleus) with the thalamus and lateral habenular nucleus (Jackson and Crossman, 1981). 5: Pallidopallidal (Nauta and Mehler, 1966). 6: Caudate–caudate connections (Cahndu-Lall *et al.*, 1970; Mensah and Deadwyler, 1974). 7: Corticocortical (Cavada and Reinoso-Suarez, 1981) and bilateral corticostriatal connections (Carman *et al.*, 1965; Kunzle, 1975; Nieoullon *et al.*, 1978).

to hypothesize that part of this system in the form of a complicated web interconnects the hemispheres (Fig. 10.3), thus compensating for a reduced efficiency of the DA-sensitive callosal neurons. In other words, Parkinson's disease may be postulated to have features of both the hemisphere hyperconnection and disconnection syndromes.

VIII. Asymmetries of Electrodermal Activity

We soon came to realize that the "interdependence conjecture" may have limited relevance. It was inspired by changes in such codes of intrinsic hemisphere activity and reactivity as EEG and VEP; functions (and their codes) controlled predominantly by one or the other hemisphere may be considerably altered by damage to the respective hemisphere. Alterations of electrodermal activity (EDA) in hemi-Parkinsonism may illustrate this point.

The assessment of EDA was not initially an independent goal of this project. However, difficulties encountered by some patients during the attention task suggested that VEP (P_{300}) abnormalities may be related to an orienting–arousal deficit created by the dysfunction of the dopaminergic system, that is, to the patients' inability to generate and sustain sufficient levels of attention in order to differentiate between the stimuli and memorize their number. It was desirable, therefore, to obtain an independent measure of orienting response, and this was done by recording EDA.

Reactive EDA was investigated in response to nonsignal stroboscopic flashes (relaxation) and to photic stimuli employed to evoke visual potentials in the simple attention task described in the previous section. Technical details have been reported elsewhere (Myslobodsky and Rattok, 1977; see also Chapter 14) and are described briefly in Table 10.8.

Among the medicated sample two categories of patients were isolated: those who failed to produce any EDA-orienting response or were unresponsive in the initial three trials of a single experimental session are referred to as *nonresponders*, whereas patients who produced consistent EDA-orienting response or habituated after three or more trials are referred to as *responders*.* Table 10.8 shows that nonresponders are typically patients with a left-sided extrapyramidal syndrome. The two responders of this group generated a relatively small amount of EDA. Conversely, right-sided Parkinsonians were largely responders, with a significantly higher amount of EDA generated on both hands during the task ($p<0.02$ for P hand and $p<0.01$ for NP hand) as compared with the relaxation session. These findings are hardly an artifact of motor abnormality since a comparable intensity of tremor and rigidity was noted among nonresponders and responders.

Two major aspects of this finding merit discussion: (*a*) the association of bilateral nonresponding with nondominant hemisphere dysfunction; and (*b*) the DA deficit underlying this abnormality.

The right hemisphere is believed to be intimately involved in the mediation of bilateral control of arousal and EDA-orienting activity (Myslobodsky and Rattok, 1977; Heilman and Valenstein, 1978; Heilman and Van Den Abell, 1979; Myslobodsky *et al.*, 1979). In Chapter 8 Gainotti reviews the evidence that right hemisphere damage leads to a general-

*Some of these patients were actually "underresponsive," and a low level of responding was sometimes noted in the attention task. This was similar to observations of Gruzelier (Chapter 12) in schizophrenic patients who exhibited EDA when attention to stimuli was required.

TABLE 10.8

Mean EDA (±SEM) during Relaxation and Task Conditions in Patients Receiving L-dopa and Showing Right and Left-sided Parkinsonian Symptoms[a]

Patients	Relaxation				Task			
	N	P hand	NP hand	AI	*N*	P hand	NP hand	AI
Right-sided Parkinsonism[b]								
Responders	8	482 ± 159	429 ± 161	0.20 ± 0.11	9	833[c] ± 164	797[d] ± 179	0.06 ± 0.07
Nonresponders	2	—	—	—	0	—	—	—
Left-sided Parkinsonism[e]								
Responders	2	168 ± 128	111 ± 104	0.53 ± 0.26	2	96 ± 69	60 ± 37	0.28 ± 0.12
Nonresponders	5	—	—	—	3	—	—	—
Total responders	10	419 ± 131	365 ± 132	0.27 ± 0.10	11	690 ± 164	663 ± 171	0.10 ± 0.06

[a] Asymmetry index (AI) was calculated as EDA values recorded from the Parkinsonian (P) hand minus EDA values recorded from the non-Parkonsonian (NP) hand, divided by the maximal EDA value. With a constant current of 10 μA applied to the index and ring fingers, reactive changes of resistance were measured. The EDA values were monitored by electronic counters. A response was defined as the resistance decrement starting up to 5 sec after stimulus presentation and the amplitude of which resulted with at least 20 counts of the EDA counter (20 counts were equal to 330 Ω per 5 sec of resistance decrement).

[b] Data for task session were not available for one patient.

[c] For seven patients, task effect, $t(6) = 3.4$, $p < 0.02$.

[d] For seven patients, task effect, $t(6) = 3.9$, $p < 0.01$.

[e] Data for task session were not available for two patients.

ized, systemic abnormality of emotional input processing and responding. The present findings extend this concept, suggesting that it is the dopaminergic circuitry of the right hemisphere that may be critically responsible for bilateral control of EDA-orienting activity.

The results of this study contradict the predictions of Gruzelier *et al.* (1981), based on Lacroix and Comper's (1979) model. In this model the EDA control system consists of two identical circuits that share responsibility for bilateral EDA control. The model presented in Fig. 10.4 conceptualizes our findings as suggesting that the integrity of right hemisphere machinery is indispensible for EDA manifestation. Left hemisphere circuits are seen as providing integratory or modulatory influences on the right hemisphere "pathways" to the hypothetical mechanisms arbitrarily designated as EDA command neurons.

Moreover, Fig. 10.4 shows that right hemisphere dopaminergic regulation reaches EDA command neurons via an "intermediate system." The presence of this system is assumed because L-dopa failed to promote EDA responding. It is proposed that the "intermediate system" was irreparably damaged by the progressive loss of DA-related neural transmission.

A word of caution is in order. The weight of this diagram is borne almost entirely by the present experimental observations. It was not intended to represent an anatomical reality. For instance, left hemisphere mechanisms are depicted as acting via right hemisphere pathways and as having no hold of their own over EDA control. It is possible that the two hemispheres have about equal share of control over the bilateral EDA. However, mutual connections between the hemispheres along with a special role for the right hemisphere in directing attention to both sides of space may create a situation in which EDA deteriorates bilaterally due to a deficit of some form of facilitatory influences provided by the right hemisphere. A study of EDA elicited under conditions of stimulation ac-

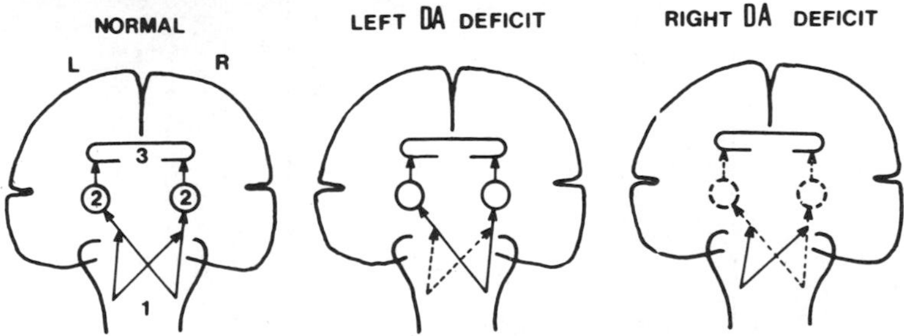

FIG. 10.4. Diagram showing that right hemisphere DA deficit leads to EDA nonresponding in L-dopa-medicated patients. It is suggested that only dopaminergic pathways (1) originating on the right side control "EDA command neurons" (3) via an interneuronal system (2). Pathways originating on the left side largely modulate the activity of the neighboring control system. Key: a solid line refers to normal DA pathways; a broken line refers to deficient DA pathways.

tivating predominantly one hemisphere at a time (field stimulation) is required to examine this conjecture.

It is yet to be specified which portion of the DA system is critically involved in EDA regulation. Despite the venerable history of psychogalvanic reflex, the role of DA in EDA modulation remains practically unknown. Even circumstantial evidence suggesting that various portions of the dopaminergic system produce dissimilar effects is meager. The neostriatum seems to exert largely inhibitory effects on EDA (Wang and Brown, 1956); the tuberoinfundibular region is reportedly a facilitatory center (Langworthy and Richter, 1930; Celesia and Wang, 1964), whereas the areas that are recognized today as related to the mesocortical system (the premotor cortex and the anterior cingulate cortex) may produce a bimodal (facilitatory and inhibitory) action in relation to EDA (Schwartz, 1937; Isamat, 1961; Wilcott, 1969).

Because of this multilevel control of EDA, the present findings cannot be employed to specify the locus of DA-mediated EDA control. In addition, it is known that Parkinsonism does not guarantee that the deficit of DA is restricted only to the nigrostriatal system (Javoy-Agid and Agid, 1980).

The other theoretical prediction of Gruzelier *et al.* (1981), that a prepotency of right hemisphere activity would lead to a higher EDA on the right than on the left side, is more complicated. Right-sided Parkinsonism (left hemisphere DA deficit) is an ideal model with which to test this prediction, because it gives "right hemisphere superiority," which is less contaminated by modulatory left hemisphere influences. As Table 10.8 shows, in these patients slight, albeit nonsignificant, EDA enhancement was noted over the P hand, which is consistent with Gruzelier *et al.*'s prediction. This phenomenon becomes more pronounced toward the end of the relaxation session ($p<0.05$) due to a faster habituation of left-hand (*NP*) responses ($p<0.01$) (data not shown).

One might anticipate that task-induced involvement of the spared right hemisphere would sharpen EDA asymmetry due to activation-related contralateral EDA suppression (Lacroix and Comper, 1979). However, contrary to this prediction EDA increased bilaterally, whereas its asymmetry actually decreased slightly throughout the task session (Table 10.8).

We turned to findings represented in Table 10.7, in order to determine whether in left hemisphere Parkinsonism the attention task would engage the right hemisphere, as evidenced by the P_{300} enhancement. Such facilitation (albeit not reaching a significant level) was obtained. The correlation between individual EDA and VEP asymmetries was also examined. It proved to be weak and unreliable.

In summary, we showed that the right and left hemispheres control EDA in distinctly dissimilar ways. However, they seem to provide this control over the two sides. We failed to obtain any conclusive evidence of EDA asymmetry suggesting the predominance of either a contralateral or homolateral EDA regulation in responders.

IX. Summary

The analysis of hemi-Parkinsonism began with the realistic assumption that the hemideficit of the dopaminergic system may be an ideal condition for causing a detectable imbalance of brain reactivity. It ends with the terse conclusion that clinical manifestations of the lateralized extrapyramidal syndrome are *not* matched by robust unilateral brain reactivity changes and that EDA and VEP measures do not show a similar profile of abnormalities with right versus left hemisphere dysfunction.

Several explanations were proposed to account for these results. The one based on EEG and VEP findings suggested that a chronic unilateral pathology triggers a complex response activating a web of compensatory pathways that reduce the disparity of hemisphere reactivity. This hypothetical web may be conceived as a structural basis of the "functional system," a constellation of bilaterally represented circuits (Luria, 1966; Kok, 1967) leading to hemisphere interdependence.

It should be understood that we use such terms as *functional system* and *interdependence* as stipulative definitions to suggest the link between compensatory machinery emerging after the infliction of a unilateral brain lesion and the existing pattern of hemispheric relations. Admittedly, our definition may not conform to what Kok and Luria intended, but our usage of these terms is not wrong as long as in most cases the *emerging* machinery is not newly formed but merely becoming detectable. Finally, the interdependence hypothesis was selected by Occam's razor as that which best describes the difficulties encountered at this stage of research. However, this is by no means the only possible realistic explanation. Also, EDA nonresponding in patients with predominant right hemisphere DA deficit seemed to suggest that the interdependence principle hardly operates when the premorbid sharing of control by the two hemispheres over certain functions is unequal.

Acknowledgments

A shorter preliminary version of this chapter is being published in the "Proceedings of the Second International Conference on Laterality and Psychopathology, Banff, Canada, April 1982" (P. Flor-Henry and J. Gruzelier, Eds.).

This study was supported in part by a gift from the H. Pardee Foundation (M. Myslobodsky) and by the Israel Foundations Trustees (M. Mintz). E. Kot, H. Sroka, H. Radwan, H. Braun, V. Ben-Mayor, and R. Tomer collaborated in different stages of this study.

References

Agnew, H. W., Webb, W. B., and Williams, R. L. (1967). Sleep patterns in late middle-age males: An EEG study. *Electroencephalogr. Clin. Neurophysiol.* **23,** 168–171.

Andén, N.-E., Carlsson, A., Dahlström, A., Fuxe, K., Hillarp, N.-A., and Larsson, K. (1964). Demonstration and mapping out of nigro-neostriatal dopamine neurons. *Life Sci.* **3,** 523–530.

Arbuthnott, G. W., and Ungerstedt, U. (1975). Turning behavior induced by electrical stimulation of the nigro-striatal system of the rat. *Exp. Neurol.* **47,** 162–172.

Ball, G. J., Gloor, P., and Schaul, N. (1977). The cortical electromicrophysiology of pathological delta waves in the electroencephalogram of cats. *Electroencephalogr. Clin. Neurophysiol.* **43,** 346–361.

Barolin, G. S., Bernheimer, H., and Hornykiewicz, O. (1964). Seitenverschiedenes Verhalten des Dopamine (3-Hydroxytyramin) im Gehirn eines Falles von Hemiparkinsonismus. *Schweiz. Arch. Neurol., Neurochir. Psychiatr.* **94,** 241–248.

Bedard, P., Dankova, R., Boucher, R., and Langelier, P. (1978). Effects of estrogens on amphetamine-induced circling behavior in rats. *Can. J. Physiol. Pharmacol.* **56,** 538–541.

Bernheimer, H., Birkmayer, W., Hornykiewicz, O., Jellinger, K., and Seitelberger, F. (1973). Brain dopamine and the syndromes of Parkinson and Huntington: Clinical, morphological and neurochemical correlations. *J. Neurol. Sci.* **20,** 415–455.

Bodis-Wollner, I., and Yahr, M. D. (1978). Measurement of visual evoked potentials in Parkinson's disease. *Brain* **101,** 661–671.

Boller, F., Mizutani, T., Roessmann, U., and Gambetti, P. (1980). Parkinson disease, dementia and Alzheimer disease: Clinicopathological correlations. *Ann. Neurol.* **7,** 329–335.

Brozoski, T. J., Brown, R. M., Rosvold, H. E., and Goldman, P. S. (1979). Cognitive deficit caused by regional depletion of dopamine in prefrontal cortex of rhesus monkey. *Science* **205,** 929–932.

Buchsbaum, M., Coppola, R., and Bittker, T. (1974). Differential effects of "congruence" stimulus meaning and information on early and late components of the averaged evoked response. *Neuropsychologia* **12,** 533–544.

Bugiani, O., Salvarani, S., Perdelli, F., Mancardi, G. L., and Leonardi, A. (1978). Nerve cell loss with aging in the putamen. *Eur. Neurol.* **17,** 286–291.

Bunney, B. S. (1979). The electrophysiological pharmacology of midbrain dopaminergic systems. *In* "The Neurobiology of Dopamine" (A. S. Horn, J. Korf, and B. H. C. Westerink, eds.), pp. 417–452. Academic Press, New York.

Carlsson, A., and Winblad, B. (1976). Influence of age and time interval between death and autopsy on dopamine and 3-methoxytyramine levels in human basal ganglia. *J. Neural. Transm.* **38,** 271–276.

Carman, J. B., Cowan, W. M., Powell, T. P. S., and Webster, K. E. (1965). A bilateral cortico-striate projection. *J. Neurol. Neurosurg. Psychiatry* **28,** 71–77.

Cavada, C., and Reinoso-Suarez, F. (1981). Interhemispheric cortico-cortical connections to the prefrontal cortex in the cat. *Neurosci. Lett.* **24,** 211–214.

Celesia, G. G., and Wang, G. H. (1964) Sudomotor activity induced by single shock stimulation of the hypothalamus in anesthesized cats. *Arch. Ital. Biol.* **102,** 587–598.

Chandu-Lall, J. A., Haase, G. R., Zivanovic, D., and Szekely, E. G. (1970). Dopamine interdependence between the caudate nuclei. *Exp. Neurol.* **29,** 101–110.

Chiodo, L. A., Caggiula, A. R., and Saller, C. F. (1979). Estrogen increases both spiperone-induced catalepsy and brain levels of [^{3}H]spiperone in the rat. *Brain Res.* **172,** 360–366.

Classification of Extrapyramidal Disorders (1981). *J. Neurol. Sci.* **51,** 311–327.

Deniau, J. M., Hammond-Le Guyader, C., Feger, J., and McKenzie, J. S. (1977). Bilateral projection of nigro-collicular neurons: An electrophysiological study in the rat. *Neurosci. Lett.* **5,** 45–50.

Deniau, J. M., Hammond, C., Riszk, A., and Feger, J. (1978). Electrophysiological properties of identified output neurons of the rat substantia nigra (pars compacta and pars reticulata): Evidence for the existence of branched neurons. *Exp. Brain Res.* **32,** 409–422.

Fass, B., and Butcher, L. L. (1981). Evidence for a crossed nigrostriatal pathway in rats. *Neurosci. Lett.* **22,** 109–113.

Feinberg, I. (1974). Changes in sleep cycle patterns with age. *J. Psychiatr. Res.* **10,** 283–306.

Finch, C. E. (1980). The relationship of aging changes in the basal ganglia to manifestations of Huntington's chorea. *Ann. Neurol.* **7,** 406–411.

Gevins, A. S., Zeitlin, G. M., Doyle, J. C., Schaffer, R. E., and Callaway, E. (1979). EEG patterns during "cognitive" tasks. II. Analysis of controlled tasks. *Electroencephalogr. Clin. Neurophysiol.* **47,** 704–710.

Glick, S. D., Jerussi, T. P., and Fleisher, L. N. (1976). Turning in circles: The neuropharmacology of rotation. *Life Sci.* **18,** 889–896.

Goldman-Rakic, P. A., and Brown, R. M. (1981). Regional changes of monoamines in cerebral cortex and subcortical structures of aging rhesus monkeys. *Neuroscience* **6,** 177–187.

Gordon, J. H., and Diamond, B. I. (1981). Antagonism of dopamine supersensitivity by estrogen: Neurochemical studies in an animal model of tardive dyskinesia. *Biol. Psychiatry* **16,** 365–371.

Gruzelier, J., Eves, F., and Connolly, J. (1981). Reciprocal hemispheric influences on response habituation in the electrodermal system. *Physiol. Psychol.* **9,** 313–317.

Hahn, Z., Karádi, Z., and Lénárd, L. (1981). Striatal dopamine levels after unilateral lesions of the substantia nigra. Evidence for a contralateral decrease. *Acta Physiol. Acad. Sci. Hung.* **57,** 249–253.

Heilman, K. M., and Valenstein, E. (1978). Mechanisms underlying hemispatial neglect. *Ann. Neurol.* **5,** 166–170.

Heilman, K. M., and Van Den Abell, T. (1979). Right hemisphere dominance for mediating cerebral activation *Neuropsychologia* **17,** 315–321.

Hökfelt, T., Johansson, O., Fuxe, K., Goldstein, M., and Park, D. (1976). Immunohistochemical studies on the localization and distribution of monoamine neurone systems in the rat brain. I. Tyrosine hydroxylase in the mes- and diencephalon. *Med. Biol.* **54,** 427–453.

Hornykiewicz, O. (1966). Dopamine (3-hydroxytyramine) and brain function. *Pharmacol. Rev.* **18,** 925–964.

Hruska, R. E., and Silbergeld, E. K. (1980). Estrogen treatment enhances dopamine receptor sensitivity in the rat striatum. *Eur. J. Pharmacol.* **61,** 397–400.

Isamat, F. (1961). Galvanic skin responses from stimulation of limbic cortex. *J. Neurophysiol.* **24,** 176–181.

Jackson, A., and Crossman, A. R. (1981). The efferent projections of the entopeduncular nucleus in the rat: A study using anterograde and retrograde transport of HRP. *Neurosci. Lett., Suppl.* **7,** S127.

Jacobson, S., and Trojanowski, J. Q. (1974). The cells of origin of the corpus callosum in rat, cat, and rhesus monkey. *Brain Res.* **74,** 149–155.

Javoy-Agid, F., and Agid, Y. (1980). Is the mesocortical dopaminergic system involved in Parkinson disease? *Neurology* **30,** 1326–1330.

Johnson, L., Lubin, A., Naitoh, P., Nute, C., and Austin, M. (1969). Spectral analysis of the EEG of dominant and non-dominant alpha subjects during waking and sleeping. *Electroencephalogr. Clin. Neurophysiol.* **26,** 361–370.

Kahn, A., and Fisher, C. (1969). The sleep characteristics of the normal aged male. *J. Nerv. Ment. Dis.* **148,** 477–494.

Knapp, S., and Mandell, A. J. (1980). Lithium and chlorimipramine differentially alter bilateral asymmetry in mesostriatal serotonin metabolites and kinetic conformations of midbrain tryptophan hydroxylase with respect to tetrahydrobiopterin cofactor. *Neuropharmacology* **19,** 1–7.

Kok, E. (1967). ["Visual agnosias."] Medizine, Leningrad (in Russian).

Kunzle, H. (1975). Bilateral projections from precentral motor cortex to the putamen and other parts of the basal ganglia: An autoradiographic study in macaca fasicularis. *Brain Res.* **88,** 195–209.

Lacroix, J. M., and Comper, P. (1979). Lateralization in the electrodermal system as a function of cognitive/hemispheric manipulations. *Psychophysiology* **16,** 116–129.

Lal, S., and Sourkes, T. L. (1972). Potentiation and inhibition of the amphetamine stereotypy in rats by neuroleptics and other agents. *Arch. Int. Pharmacodyn. Ther.* **199,** 289–301.

Langworthy, O. R., and Richter, C. P. (1930). The influence of efferent cerebral pathways upon the sympathetic neurons system. *Brain* **53,** 178–193.

Lee, T., Seeman, P., Rajput, A., Farley, I., and Hornykiewicz, O. (1978). Receptor basis for dopaminergic supersensitivity in Parkinson's disease. *Nature (London)* **273,** 59–61.

Lidbrink, P., Jonsson, G., and Fuxe, K. (1974). Selective reserpine resistant accumulation of catecholamines in the central dopamine neurons after DOPA administration. *Brain Res.* **67,** 439–456.

Lieberman, A., Dziatolowski, M., Kupersmith, M., Serby, M., Goodgold, A., Korein, J., and Goldstein, M. (1979). Dementia in Parkinson disease. *Ann. Neurol.* **6,** 355–359.

Lindvall, O., Björklund, A., Moore, R. Y., and Stenevi, U. (1974). Mesencephalic dopamine neurons projecting to neocortex. *Brain Res.* **81,** 325–331.

Lloyd, K. G. (1977). Neurochemical compensation in Parkinson's disease. *Excerpta Med. Int. Congr. Ser.* **429.**

Luria, A. R. (1966). "Higher Cortical Function in Man." Basic Books, New York.

McGeer, P. L., McGeer, E. G., and Suzuki, J. S. (1977). Aging and extrapyramidal function. *Arch. Neurol. (Chicago)* **34,** 23–35.

Mayeux, R., Stern, Y., Rosen, J., and Leventhal, J. (1981). Depression, intellectual impairment and Parkinson disease. *Neurology* **31,** 645–650.

Meehl, P. E. (1975). Hedonic capacity: Some conjectures. *Bull. Menninger Clin.* **39,** 295–307.

Mensah, P., and Deadwyler, S. (1974). The caudate nucleus of the rat: Cell types and the demonstration of a commisural system. *J. Anat.* **117,** 281–293.

Mintz, M., Tomer, R., Radwan, H., and Myslobodsky, M. S. (1981). Visual evoked potentials in hemiparkinsonism. *Electroencephalogr. Clin. Neurophysiol.* **52,** 611–616.

Mintz, M., Tomer, R., Radwan, H., and Myslobodsky, M. S. (1982). A comparison of levodopa treatment and task demands on visual evoked potentials in hemi-Parkinsonism. *Psychiatry Res.* **6,** 245–251.

Myslobodsky, M. S. (1976). "Petit Mal Epilepsy: A Search for the Precursors of Wave-Spike Discharges." Academic Press, New York.

Myslobodsky, M. S., and Rattok, J. (1977). Bilateral electrodermal activity in waking man. *Acta Psychol.* **41,** 273–282.

Myslobodsky, M. S., and Rosen, J. (1979). Hemispheric asymmetry of pentamethylenetetrazol-induced wave-spike discharges and motor imbalance in rats. *Epilepsia* **20,** 377–386.

Myslobodsky, M. S., Ben-Mayor, V., Yedid-Levy, B., and Mintz, M. (1977). Hemispheric asymmetry of EEG and averaged visual evoked potentials during non-REM sleep. *In* "Sleep" (W. P. Koella and P. Levin, eds.), pp. 295–297. Karger, Basel.

Myslobodsky, M. S., Mintz, M., and Tomer, R. (1979). Asymmetric reactivity of the brain and components of hemispheric imbalance. *In* "Hemisphere Asymmetries of Function and Psychopathology" (J. Gruzelier and P. Flor- Henry, eds.), pp. 125–148. Elsevier North-Holland, Amsterdam.

Myslobodsky, M. S., Mintz, M., Ben-Mayor, V. and Radwan, H. (1982). Unilateral dopamine deficit and lateral EEG asymmetry: Sleep abnormalities in hemi-Parkinson's patients. *Electroencephalogr. Clin. Neurophysiol.* **54,** 227–231.

Naik, S. R., Kelkan, M. R., and Sheth, U. K. (1978). Attenuation of stereotyped behavior by sex steroids. *Psychopharmacology* **57,** 211–214.

Nakamura, Y., Ohye, C., and Mano, N. (1968). Cortical polarization and experimentally-produced delta waves in the cat. *Electroencephalogr. Clin. Neurophysiol.* **24,** 42–52.

Nauta, W. J. M., and Mehler, W. R. (1966). Projections of the lentiform nucleus in the monkey. *Brain Res.* **1,** 3–42.

Neal, H., and Keane, P. E. (1980). Electrically and chemically induced spindling and slow waves in the encéphale isolé rat: A possible role for dopamine in the regulation of electrocortical activity. *Electroencephalogr. Clin. Neurophysiol.* **48,** 318–326.

Nieoullon, A., Cheramy, A., and Glowinski, J. (1978). Release of dopamine evoked by electrical stimulation of the motor and visual areas of the cerebral cortex in both caudate nuclei and in the substantia nigra in the cat. *Brain Res.* **145,** 69–83.

Oke, A., Keller, R., Mefford, I., and Adams, R. N. (1978). Lateralization of norepinephrine in human thalamus. *Science* **200,** 1411–1413.

Oke, A., Lewis, R., and Adams, R. N. (1980). Hemispheric asymmetry of norepinephrine distribution in rat thalamus. *Brain Res.* **188,** 269–272.

Parkinson, J. (1817). "An Essay on the Shaking Palsy." Sherwood, Neely & Jones, London.

Pines, L. J., and Maiman, R. M. (1939). Cells of origin of fibers of corpus callosum. *Arch. Neurol. Psychiatry* **42,** 1076–1082.

Pritzel, M., and Huston, J. P. (1981). Neural and behavioral plasticity: Crossed nigro-thalamic projections following unilateral substantia nigra lesions. *Behav. Brain Res.* **3,** 393–399.

Purdy, A., Hahn, A., Barnett, H. J. M., Bratty, P., Ahmed, D., Lloyd, K. G., McGeer, E. G., and Perry, T. L. (1978). Familial fatal parkinsonism with alveolar hypoventilation and mental depression. *Ann. Neurol.* **6,** 523–531.

Pycock, C. J. (1980). Turning behaviour in animals. *Neuroscience* **5,** 461–514.

Riederer, P., and Wuketich, S. (1976). Time course of nigrostriatal degeneration in Parkinson's disease. *J. Neural Transm.* **38,** 277–301.

Rinvik, E., Grofova, I., and Ottersen, O. P. (1976). Demonstration of nigro-tectal and nigro-reticular projections of the cat by axonal transport of protein. *Brain Res.* **112,** 388–394.

Rothman, A. H., and Glick, S. D. (1976). Differential effects of unilateral and bilateral caudate lesions on side preference and passive avoidance behavior in rats. *Brain Res.* **118,** 361–369.

Royce, G. J. (1978). Cells of origin of subcortical afferents to the caudate nucleus: A horseradish peroxidase study in the cat. *Brain Res.* **153,** 465–475.

Schwartz, H. G. (1937). Effect of experimental lesions of the cortex on the "psychogalvanic reflex" in the cat. *Arch. Neurol. Psychiatry* **38,** 308–320.

Seales, D. M. (1973). Cited by L. W. Poon, L. W. Thompson, and G. R. Marsh. Averaged evoked potential changes as a function of processing complexity. *Psychophysiology* **13,** 43–49.

Smith, J., Karacan, I., and Yang, M. (1977). Ontogeny of delta activity during human sleep. *Electroencephalogr. Clin. Neurophysiol.* **43,** 229–237.

Starr, M., and Kilpatrick, I. C. (1981). Bilateral asymmetry in GABA brain function? *Neurosci. Lett.* **25,** 167–172.

Törk, I., and Turner, S. (1981). Histochemical evidence for a catecholaminergic (presumably dopaminergic) projections from the ventral mesencephalic tegmentum to the visual cortex in the cat. *Neurosci. Lett.* **24,** 215–219.

Wang, G. H., and Brown, V. W. (1956). Suprasegmental inhibitions of an autonomic reflex. *J. Neurophysiol.* **19,** 564–572.

Wilcott, R. C. (1969). Electrical stimulation of the anterior cortex and skin potential responses in the cat. *J. Comp. Physiol. Psychol.* **69,** 465–472.

Wright, A. K., and Arbuthnott, G. W. (1981). Crossed efferent connections of the substantia nigra. *Neurosci. Lett., Suppl.* **7,** S126.

11: Epileptic Laughter

MICHAEL S. MYSLOBODSKY

Psychobiology Research Unit
Department of Psychology
Tel-Aviv University
Ramat-Aviv, Israel

I. Introduction 239
II. Symptoms of Gelastic Epilepsy 240
A. Role of Pleasure 240
B. Psychopathology 242
C. Electroencephalographic and Laterality Findings 244
D. Laughter and Adversive Epilepsy 246
E. Role of Antiepileptic Medication 249
III. Brain Pathology and Pathophysiology of Epileptic Laughter 251
IV. Postscript 256
References 258

I. Introduction

There is a great deal of evidence suggesting the involvement of the right hemisphere in the interpretation and expression of normal and abnormal affect (Chapters 7 and 8; Gardner *et al.*, 1975; Moscovitch and Olds, 1982). Cohen and Niska (1980) reported a case of recurrent mania accompanying right temporal lobe hematoma, and four similar cases have been found in the literature.

Episodes of paroxysmal "forced" laughter, christened *gelastic epilepsy* by Daly and Mulder (1957) (*gelos* being Greek for *mirth*), are often interpreted as fragments of emotional response accompanying epilepsy. Under the entry *laughing attack,* the "Dictionary of Epilepsy," edited by Gastaut (1973), states, "A brief and unmotivated attack of laughter constituting the essential manifestation of some affective epileptic seizures, usually of temporal lobe origin [p. 49]."

HEMISYNDROMES:
Psychobiology, Neurology,
Psychiatry

ISBN 0-12-512460-0

It can be argued that laughter alone is insufficient to diagnose an affective disorder to any appreciable extent. The latter diagnosis requires a spectrum of changes involving alterations in autonomic and neuroendocrine systems, somatic symptoms, specific cognitive schemata, and so on. Without these components, laughter may be related to parathymia, hysteroepilepsy, or epileptic psychosis. Within the framework of the aberrant laterality hypothesis of psychopathology (Chapter 7) this might implicate left rather than right hemisphere lesion. However, regardless of the core syndrome with which epileptic laughter is associated, it is undoubtedly an interesting pathology with which the concept of aberrant brain laterality might be probed.

II. Symptoms of Gelastic Epilepsy

A. Role of Pleasure

The incidence of gelastic episodes, ranging from a facile smile to violent laughter, is relatively low. In a series of 5000 consecutive cases of epilepsy examined at the University of Wisconsin Epilepsy Center, there were only 10 cases of gelastic epilepsy (Chen and Forster, 1973). However, a videotape recording of behavior revealed gelastic symptoms in about 42% of patients with psychomotor attacks (Dreyer and Wehmeyer, 1978). Since gelastic epilepsy most typically develops as an equivalent or a symptom of psychomotor fits (Chen and Forster, 1973), its incidence may indeed be much higher than is currently believed. Smiling and giggling may be occasionally noted in automatisms with absences of petit mal epilepsy (Roger *et al.*, 1967; Gascon and Lombroso, 1971). Penry and Dreifuss (1969) described a child (case 2) with seizure episodes of blank staring followed by fumbling movements with the hands and grinning, which lasted 10–15 sec.

The mechanisms responsible for the precipitation of epileptic laughter remain unknown. In one of the three cases of Battisti *et al.* (1965) (case 1) paroxysmal laughter was elicited by gustatory stimuli. This is reminiscent of a case reported by Scollo-Lavizzari and Hess (1967) concerning a boy (case 2) whose seizures were precipitated by mastication, swallowing, or the mere sight of food. Sinisi (1961) described two cases in which positive emotional arousal was a precipitating factor of laughing fits, whereas Loiseau *et al.* (1971) and Williams *et al.* (1978) reported fatigue or emotional disbalance as a trigger. Beneicke (1967) noted a patient who developed states resembling narcoleptic attacks in response to spontaneous or induced laughter. Laughter may be self-induced by posturing (Jacome *et al.*, 1980) and gaze deviation (Leopold, 1977). The latter patient also responded with gelastic episodes to a strong light. However, these episodes may have been associated with the lateral eye movement to the flash.

Most investigators believe, however, that laughter is an automatic reflectoral phenomenon without exogenous triggers and emotional content (Druckman and Chao, 1957). Indeed, paroxysmal laughter seems to be an isolated, encapsulated, so to speak, fragment of emotion that invites a guess about the emotional experience of the patient but provides no additional clues in bodily or autonomic indices of affect. Martin (1950) even designated paroxysms of laughter as "sham mirth," that is, a state symmetric to "sham rage," and a number of descriptions emphasize that the laughter has neither emotional charge nor the contagious quality of hilarity.

Considering the weight that this label has acquired in the area, it should be recalled here that the concept of "sham rage" (suggesting that hypothalamic activity induces objective signs of affect without corresponding subjective feeling) is no longer widely shared. Akert (1961) prepared a map of active "rage sites" of the hypothalamus in the cat which, he assures, leaves no doubt of the subjective feeling of the animal when it is stimulated in these sites: "Skeptics may convince themselves of this unambiguous behavior by being exposed to the ferocious and well-directed attack with his teeth and claws [p. 295]."

No doubt paroxysms of laughter may be related to a sense of well-being and merriment to the same extent that jerks are related to a purposeful muscular effort or gyratory fits to dancing, or the syndrome of crocodile tears to weeping. However, there are good reasons to trust reports that laughter and smiling may indeed reflect certain emotional experience, even though very often they are *both* enjoyable and unpleasant (Daly and Mulder, 1957; Stutte, 1963; Zecchini and Cecotto, 1967; Gascon and Lombroso, 1971; Loiseau *et al.*, 1971; Bancaud and Bacia, 1980). The reports of gelastic self-induced seizures (Jacome *et al.*, 1980) and of a feeling of mirth preceding epileptic laughter induced by pursuit eye movements (Leopold, 1977) demonstrate that, whereas emotional changes underlying gelastic fits cannot be taken indiscriminately to support the concept of ecstatic (Dostoevsky) epilepsy or "orgasmolepsy" (Martin, 1950), certain changes of emotions behind a grimace of inappropriate laughter would be impossible to dismiss. Yet it is puzzling why the latter cases are so unique. Among nine patients reported by Yamada and Yoshida (1977), only one experienced a "feeling of amusement or some sense of fun during the seizure [p. 131]." Of course, most patients may be completely or partially amnestic of the episode. Some patients who were initially amnestic of their experience eventually report orgastic feelings (Jacome *et al.*, 1980). Therefore, even though the "meaning" of laughter may not be obvious or be disconnected from the patients' recollection, it may still be triggered by a pleasurable experience. There is an excellent anecdote to illustrate this point.

William James, a great believer in nitrous oxide, or "laughing gas," was unable to document the moments of illumination and bliss he experienced while experimenting with this anesthetic and euphoriant gas. One night he managed to record his revelations before losing consciousness. Upon arising he rushed to read the protocol and found that he had produced the following:

Hogamus, Higamous
Man is polygamous,
Higamous, Hogamus
Woman is monogamous.

It is not unlikely that the attack of laughter is simply unretrievable in the conscious state but remembered in a state of confusion. The possibility that gelastic laughter is related to the category of dissociative experience is suggested by an interesting description of a patient (case 1) presented by Chen and Forster (1973). This 9-year-old girl with both gelastic and cursive epilepsy was able to repeat numerals, counting after the technician, but did so with a southern accent. Later, she could not recall that she had counted and was unable to speak with a southern accent. This phenomenon is strikingly similar to the cases of multiple personalities described by Mesulam (1981) and Schenk and Bear (1981) in patients with temporal lobe epilepsy.

Of course, from some other observations one might draw other conclusions. One might argue that laughter is erroneously interpreted as an indication that the patient is "feeling good." I find it difficult to dismiss the possibility that paroxysmal laughter is induced by "normal triggers" such as surprise, disapproval, or embarrassment. Sem-Jacobsen's (1976) patient manifested laughter during about 10 consecutive sessions of electrical brain stimulation until it became apparent that stimulation produced rhythmic contraction of certain pelvic muscles that "forced her to laugh," although she did not enjoy the sensation and in fact became increasingly annoyed with the study. The "inner life" remains obstinately inaccessible in individuals, even those with normal consciousness, let alone confused epileptic patients.

B. Psychopathology

Laughter is often seen as a conclusive stage of the cognitive act, with a strong context-related message, or "meaning." In psychotics, in which the *validity of meaning* (*Sinngesetzlichkeit*) of Schneiderians is lost, whereas the cognitive performance is *knocked out* (*ausgestanzt*) from the contextual frame, laughter is perceived as bizarre, misplaced, and irrelevant.

Given the ambiguity of laughter, the reader may be rightfully curious as to whether these patients have accompanying swings of mood, or rather schizophreniform symptoms. According to Stevens and Shorey (1965) the answer is unequivocal: Gelastic epilepsy belongs to the category of *masked epilepsies,* for example, a disease that can be and often is erroneously diagnosed as psychosis. The patient described by Erastus in 1581 (cited in Temkim, 1971) and referred to by Chen and Forster (1973) as suffering the first published episode of gelastic epilepsy can well be cited as the first case of epileptic psychosis. Giggling and laughter were frequently encountered in patients with epileptic psychosis resembling hebephrenic syndrome. The patient F. S. of Penfield and Erickson (1941) serves as an example of laughter and weeping against a background of schizophreniform symptoms. Among the patients of Slater and Beard (1963), one "was agitated, hilarious, excited" (case 6); others manifested "inappropriate giggling" (case 36), a "facile laugh and smile" (case 47), or foolish giggling (case 50). Similar to schizophreniform symptoms of temporal lobe epilepsy often developing insidiously, gelastic fits require some time before they appear. Chen and Forster (1973) wrote that gelastic components occurred rather early in the course of the patients' epilepsy. However, in one of the patients the delay of gelastic epilepsy was as long as 27 years (case 15). In others laughing occurred about 7 years (case 9), 3 years (case 12), and 5 years (case 13) after the onset of seizures. The patient of Woon and Vignaendra (1978) developed laughing fits about 4 years after his seizures began. Gelastic fits may debut at a time when some major epileptic conditions are controlled by medication (Yamada and Yoshida, 1977). Similarly, the debut of schizoid symptoms in temporal lobe epilepsy may develop when the frequency of seizures is reduced by antiepileptic treatment (Slater and Beard, 1963).

Chen and Forster (1973) have seen an above-average incidence of personality and psychiatric problems among gelastic patients. One of their patients (case 1) had dissociative experience; another (case 12) was diagnosed as schizophrenic. A patient of Gumpert *et al.* (1970) developed a negativistic attitude toward her family, became withdrawn, and refused to eat. At periods she was talkative, spoke of a nonexisting fiancé, and confused past and present events. Laughing fits and psychopathology in this patient were prominent during a twilight state (status psychomotoricus).

Yamada and Yoshida (1977) reported that in three of their patients (cases 1, 2, and 3) fits began with forced ideas, different from the ideas they usually held, and only then did an attack of laughter and confusion follow. One patient described by Weil *et al.* (1958) and three patients of Chen and Forster (1973) were diagnosed as having hyperkinetic behavior disorder. The child described by Woon and Vignaendra (1978) was initially seen at the psychiatry service of a hospital; this 8-year-old boy was hyperactive, antisocial, aggressive, and "attention-seeking." The patient of Jacome *et al.* (1980) gradually showed a personality change and became belligerent.

Parenthetically, it should be mentioned that in some patients, especially children, laughing attacks pose another problem. They may be interpreted as defiant behavior and lead to what has been known since the mid-1930s as "classroom psychopathology," which could act as an emotional trigger aggravating the original epileptic condition. Ames and Enderstein (1975) emphasized that the laughter in their patient was initially perceived by his teacher as "an attempt to gain attention," especially as his high school performance deteriorated.

C. Electroencephalographic and Laterality Findings

Although detailed electroencephalographic (EEG) studies of gelastic epilepsy are lacking, it would be unrealistic to expect a profile different from that of temporal lobe epilepsy. In fact, Druckman and Chao (1957) noted that interictal EEG abnormalities disappear during laughter and electrical activity becomes desynchronized. This pattern was probably identical to that designated later as "forced normalization" (Landolt, 1958), developing often in psychotic episodes of temporal lobe epilepsy.

Feindel (1961) wrote that an invariable feature of automatism set up by stimulation in the mesial portion of the temporal lobe in epileptic patients is "the remarkable obliteration of active spiking on the corticogram, with low-voltage rapid activity replacing the normal background activity [p. 529]."

Suzuki (1963) seems to have replicated EEG suppression in gelastic patients, whereas Gumpert *et al.* (1970) have reported that periodic suppression of hypersynchronous generalized paroxysmal discharges correlates with laughter during gelastic status epilepticus. Four patients of Gascon and Lombroso (1971) (N. M., D. R., G. C., and A. H.) had low-voltage fast EEGs during gelastic episodes.

Roger *et al.* (1967) described both desynchronized and synchronized electrical activity in gelastic attack. Ames and Enderstein (1975) and Jandolo *et al.* (1977) are inclined to interpret desynchronization as an initial response followed by a buildup of paroxysmal slowing. Although in both cases slowing was recorded during a period of vigorous locomotion, which might have distorted its actual pattern, hypersynchronized bursts of bilateral slow waves (Jacome *et al.*, 1980) or wave–spikes may be the only correlates of paroxysmal laughter (case 1 of Chen and Forster, 1973). In the case of Jacome *et al.* (1980) slow waves seem to have been preceded by and succeeded by a short-lasting period of EEG suppression. In petit mal patients, giggling was correlated with a regular pattern of spike–wave discharges (Penry and Dreifuss, 1969).

The role of laterality of epileptic discharges in the pathophysiology of gelastic epilepsy remains unknown. Stein and Dietze (1965) expressed their conviction that gelastic epilepsy is associated with abnormalities of the nondominant hemisphere. However, Dietze (1965) himself (in the neighboring paper) described at least one patient (of two) with paroxysms of laughter and left hemisphere atrophy. Table 11.1 summarizes cases extracted from the literature in which *asymmetric* discharges or grossly

TABLE 11.1
Laterality Findings in Patients with Gelastic Epilepsy

Case	Seizure type	EEG or neurological findings	Reference
—	Psychomotor	Left frontal lobe focus (?)	Hympan and Bozik (1948)
3	Psychomotor	Right temporal focus	Ironside (1956)
1	Psychomotor	Oligodendroglioma, left temporal–occipital region	Daly and Mulder (1957)
2	Psychomotor	Left temporal focus	
3	Psychomotor	Left temporal focus	Weil *et al.* (1958)
Ti, E.	Psychomotor	Left hemisphere paroxysmal activity	Lennox (1960)
Ce, H.	Psychomotor	Left anterior temporal spikes	
Cr, E.	Psychomotor	Left anterior temporal spikes	
—	Psychomotor	Left hemisphere atrophy	Dietze (1965)
2	Psychomotor	Right anterior temporal spikes, slow waves	Lehtinen and Kivalo (1965)
Five cases	Temporal lobe epilepsy (four left, one right)	—	Roger *et al.* (1967)
—	Psychomotor	Right temporal lobe focus	Zecchini and Cecotto (1967)
5	Psychomotor	Right anterior temporal spikes, sharp waves	Gascon and Lombroso (1971)
B.D.	Psychomotor	Right temporal focus, slow and sharp waves	Gascon and Lombroso (1971)
A.H.	Psychomotor	Right temporal spikes	
C.L.	Psychomotor	Right midtemporal spikes	
F.D.	Psychomotor	Right anterior temporal focal δ and spikes	
G.O.	Psychomotor	Right anterior temporal spike focus	
1	Psychomotor, epilepsia cursiva	Right hemisphere spikes, slow waves	Chen and Forster (1973)
2	Psychomotor, grand mal, epilepsia cursiva	Left temporal spikes	
9	Petit mal, grand mal	Left anterior temporal spikes	
11	Psychomotor	Left temporal spike–waves	
12	Psychomotor, adversive	Left temporal spikes	
13	Febrile convulsion, grand mal, petit mal, psychomotor	Left anterior temporal spikes	
14 and 15	Grand mal, psychomotor	Left temporal, sharp and slow waves	
16	Psychomotor, tonic drop attacks	Right anterior temporal, δ waves (pyramidal signs bilateral)	

(Continued)

TABLE 11.1 (*Continued*)

Case	Seizure type	EEG or neurological findings	Reference
1	Psychomotor	Paroxismal trains of slow activity, more in frontotemporal areas	Louiseau *et al.* (1971)
2	Jacksonian seizures	Spikes in the left rolandic area	
4	Psychomotor, grand mal	Diffuse slowing predominantly in the left temporal region	
5	Grand mal	Continuous polymorphic δ in the midregion of left hemisphere	
—	Psychomotor	Left anterior temporal, sharp and slow waves	Ames and Enderstein (1975)
4 (left-handed)	Grand mal	Right frontal and midtemporal foci	Ludwig *et al.* (1975)
—	Epilepsia cursiva	"Dynamic focus" right hemisphere atrophic changes	Jandolo *et al.* (1977)
3	?	Right frontal focus	Geier *et al.* (1977)
1, 2, 4, 6, and 7	Grand mal, psychomotor	Left anterior and midtemporal, spikes	Yamada and Yoshida (1977)
5	Grand mal, psychomotor	Right midtemporal, spikes	
8	Grand mal, psychomotor	Left temporal spikes	
9	Grand mal, psychomotor	Right temporal sharp waves	
—	Six episodes of loss of consciousness between 10 and 21 days	Right osteochrondroma	Leopold (1977)
—	Psychomotor, grand mal, akinetic falls	Left frontal region (?)	Lewis (1977)
—	Epilepsia cursiva	Left temporal spike–waves and sharp waves	Woon and Vignaendra (1978)
—	"Clouding of consciousness," EEG status	Left temporal focus	Bollea *et al.* (1980)
—	Psychomotor, grand mal	Right temporal spikes	Jacome *et al.* (1980)

asymmetric neurological findings were obtained. It does not include generalized and bilaterally synchronous abnormalities. The table demonstrates that epileptiform abnormalities were noted more frequently on the left side.

D. Laughter and Adversive Epilepsy

Gyratory (adversive) symptoms seem to be a rather frequent companion of laughing fits. Several phenomena are classified under the title of gyratory epilepsy (see Chapter 6 for review):

1. Eye deviation and head turning. These are typically in the same direction, although crossed deviation of the head and eyes has been noticed (Geier *et al.*, 1977).
2. Turning of an arm, or both arms and a shoulder, homolaterally to eye movements, followed by a general body turn of up to 180°.
3. Turning movement continuing into a frank rotation (Riser *et al.*, 1951; Geier *et al.*, 1977) or a more complicated (scenic) pseudo-spontaneous behavioral pattern reminding one of a dance (Geier *et al.*, 1976; Hallen, 1962).

Case 2 of gelastic and cursive epilepsy of Chen and Forster (1973) debuted with a frank gyratory attack directed toward the right side, and only thereafter did the patient begin running. The patient with gelastic status epilepticus described by Gumpert *et al.* (1970) initially exhibited conjugate eye deviation and head turning to the right, followed by a "high pitched, monotonous, cackling laugh."

Ludwig *et al.* (1975) described a patient (case 4) who had a "silly laugh" followed by head turning to the left and "purposeless" waving of the left arm. Geier *et al.* (1977) noted in one of their patients (a case illustrated in Fig. 2 of that article) grinning with gyratory symptoms toward the right. The other patient (case 3) had a history of gyratory fits. Hanson and Chodos (1978) described a child (4 months) who manifested conjugate eye deviation to the right while smiling during right-sided focal seizures. Yamada and Yoshida (1977) described a patient who had grand mal seizures since the age of 24; these were complicated by psychomotor attacks at age 27. Although behavioral automatisms were alleviated by medication, the seizure pattern changed to an attack that began with a period of confusion followed by "looking around" (directionality not specified) and terminated with about 20 sec of laughter.

The most common findings in adversive epilepsy are contralateral foci in the frontal area (Guidetti *et al.*, 1959; Yoshida, 1962; Ludwig and Ajmone-Marsan, 1975; Geier *et al.*, 1976, 1977). Findings of a focus in the occipital lobe are also fairly numerous (Ajmone-Marsan and Goldhammer, 1973; Huott *et al.*, 1974). Ludwig and Ajmone-Marsan (1975) reported head and eye adversion in 16 of 55 patients (29%) with occipital focus. The least common are temporal lobe lesions. In a sample of 666 patients with temporal lobe epilepsy only 5 (0.7%) had adversive phenomena. However, the majority of patients with both gelastic epilepsy and adversive symptoms had temporal lobe foci.

Adversive movements are most commonly directed away from the epileptic focus. Cohen *et al.* (1960) noticed contraversive movements in 11 of 13 patients; in 2 patients turning was homolateral to the lesion. Lacchin and Taury (1950) observed contraversive symptoms in 46 of 70 patients (66%); in 34% (24 cases) they were homolateral to the EEG focus. Homolaterally directed turning has been noted in patients with epileptic laughter (patient F.D. of Gascon and Lombroso, 1971; Hanson and Chodos, 1978). It should be noted that homolaterally directed gyratory symptoms have been detected in patients with rich organic pathology. Thompson and Raney (1949) described such a patient with protoplasmic astrocytoma of the left frontal lobe. Schader (1966) reported left-directed head turning in a patient with brain injury in the left parietooccipital area and right-sided spastic hemiplegia. In contrast, Gauthier and Belanger (1953) described a case of right frontoparietal tumor with turning movements away from the lesion.

Apparently, there is a complex interaction between the location of the focus and the directionality of gyratory symptoms. An interesting feature of the occipital focus is that head and eye deviation were faithfully contralateral to the involved region in most of the cases reported. Tonic posturing was a falsely localizing sign on only one occasion (Ludwig and Ajmone-Marsan, 1975). In contrast, in a group with frontocentroparietal foci, tonic phenomena and head and eye contraversion were shown to be of substantially less lateralizing value (Ajmone-Marsan and Goldhammer, 1973; Ludwig and Ajmone-Marsan, 1975). Geier *et al.* (1977) reported that homolateral turning was more commonly associated with anterior discharges, whereas contralateral deviations were noted with posterior discharges.

Epileptiform foci in the two hemispheres may shift in excitability from time to time, causing an effect designated as a "dynamic focus" (Gibbs and Gibbs, 1952; Strobos and Kavallinis, 1968; Myslobodsky, 1976). This quasi-periodical alteration of hemisphere excitability might alter the directionality of adversive symptoms. In fact, there are cases in which gyratory symptoms are made clockwise and then counterclockwise (Kotowicz and Scherpereel, 1968).

The last case report returns us to psychotic symptoms in epilepsy. Adversive symptoms seem to channel the formation of delusions, especially in children. The patient of Kotowicz and Scherpereel (1968), a 9-year-old child, had a visual hallucination with a visitant, a large black monster, which might have provoked eye deviations. Critchley (1979) hypothesized that some cases of adversive epilepsy may be "not so much an involuntary rotation as a willed and purposeful act of inspection [p. 4]" of something horrific happening behind one's back.

To summarize, in view of the limitations of available EEG documentation of gelastic fits, adversive symptoms were expected to provide important additional evidence of focus location. This might have been the case had a full description of epileptic seizures been provided. Although the impression is that adversive symptoms support the EEG findings of left hemisphere involvement in epileptic laughter, this conclusion is based on an admittedly small number of cases. Also, a careful examination of descriptions of gelastic fits suggests that the contralateral mouth pulling frequently encountered with eye and head deviation may be

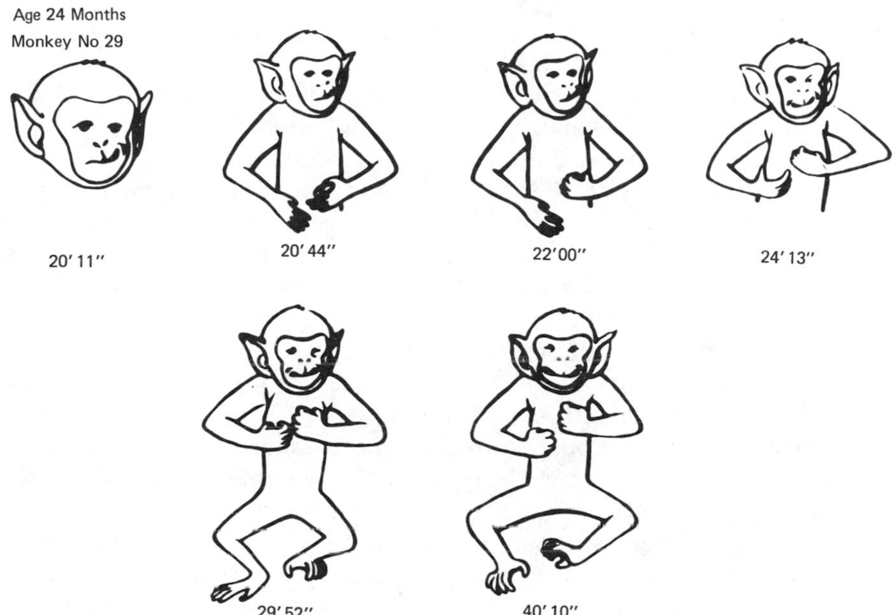

FIG. 11.1. Development of clinical expression at puberty. Note early rotatory movements of head, facial grimaces, and early fine movements of digits of left hand. With bilateral activity, greatest involvement remains on contralateral side. Loss of responsiveness was transient. [Adapted from W. F. Caveness (1969), Ontogeny of focal seizures. In "Basic Mechanisms of the Epilepsies" (H. H. Jasper, A. A. Ward and A. Pope, eds.), pp. 517–534. Little, Brown & Co., Boston, with kind permission of the publishers].

misinterpreted as an inadequate smile (see case 2 of Gascon and Lombroso, 1971). Figure 11.1 demonstrates an experimental adversive seizure with a facial grimace resembling a smile induced by penicillin administration into the motor (head–face) area of the monkey (Caveness, 1969).

E. Role of Antiepileptic Medication

Observations mentioned in Section II,B indicate that paroxysms of epileptic laughter may not accompany the underlying seizure condition until after a considerable delay. This may have to do with the action of antiepileptic drugs, at least in some patients. Most patients with gelastic epilepsy have various signs of organicity, and some are therapy resistant. It may be hypothesized that, due to a particular susceptibility of patients with brain damage, they develop idiosyncratic responses to antiepileptic medication.

Antiepileptic drugs are known to cause dyskinesias. Phenobarbitone, carbamazepine, phenytoin, and diphenylhydantoin medication has long been recognized to produce occasional facial grimacing, mouth movements, choreoathetoid movements of the limbs and trunk, etc. (Logan and Freeman, 1969; Kooiker and Sumi, 1974; McLellan and Swash, 1974; Ahmad *et al.*, 1975; Chadwick *et al.*, 1976).

Orofacial dyskinesia produced by antiepileptic treatment is indistinguishable from that developing in psychotic patients chronically medicated with neuroleptics. Similar symptoms are frequently noted in Parkinson patients treated with L-dopa or in individuals who chronically abuse amphetamine or amphetamine-like agents, which suggests that dyskinesias of various origins may result from excessive dopamine (DA) stimulation. It may be inferred from the phenomena occurring in epilepsy that they reflect a reactive supersensitivity of DA receptors, triggered by a lasting suppression of their function by anticonvulsants. Alternatively, there is a possibility of endogenous or acquired abnormalities within the dopaminergic nigrostriatal system in epilepsy.

There have been no reports of dyskinesias in gelastic epilepsy patients, although oral symptoms and choreoathetoid movements may have been overlooked, classified as psychomotor symptoms, or remained a subclinical locomotor difficulty. Phenytoin-induced choreoathetoid movements were once mistaken for status epilepticus, and the dose of phenytoin was even increased (Ahmad *et al.*, 1975). It is of interest that one patient of Chen and Forster (1973) (case 1) was characterized as a "moderately hyperactive child with a suspicious [sic] drifting of left leg when both legs were maintained in the air [p. 1022]."

It is not unlikely that laughter itself and some accompanying pseudogelastic symptoms such as grunting and hiccups may be equivalent to dyskinesia. Subclinical respiratory difficulties in patients with tardive dyskinesia are known (Jackson *et al.*, 1980). The patient of Faheem *et al.* (1982) who was treated with neuroleptics showed no evidence of orobuccal, limb, or trunk dyskinesia but had trouble with breathing, especially before speaking. He grunted, gulped air, regurgitated air, coughed, choked, and gasped. The connection of this abnormality with tardive dyskinesia was not immediately apparent, and only after several years was it discovered that these symptoms improved dramatically on the physostigmine test (and, later, after lithium medication) and substantially worsened after the patient received benztropine.

One may entertain the hypothesis that psychotic changes and gelastic symptoms result from a combination of antiepileptic treatment and some background neurological deficit, facilitating the development of supersensitivity of DA receptors. Indeed, iatrogenic complications are especially likely when there is an underlying organicity (Logan and Freeman, 1969; Ahmad *et al.*, 1975). It is tempting to speculate that the hyperactivity of the dopaminergic system can be aggravated by the capacity of seizures to promote the DA autoreceptor subsensitivity, as in Chiodo and Antelman's (1980) demonstration with electroconvulsive shock in rats. In addition, some anticonvulsants (e.g., diphenylhydantoin, Hadfield, 1972) may have, like phenothiazines, the paradoxical effect of blocking

DA uptake into the presynaptic terminal, thereby enhancing the already pronounced "hyperdopaminergia." This state may suppress generalized motor seizures at the price of the development of psychomotor attack with EEG suppression and frank psychotic symptoms (Stevens, 1973; Sato *et al.*, 1979).

III. Brain Pathology and Pathophysiology of Epileptic Laughter

Paroxysmal laughter may be associated with various neurological abnormalities. A number of writers emphasize "midline anomalies" (Lehtinen and Kivalo, 1965) due to inborn pathology or to tumors in the third ventricle, hypothalamus, and pituitary. Table 11.2 summarizes major abnormalitics detected in patients with gelastic epilepsy. It demonstrates that there is no common denominator for all the findings of brain pathology associated with fits of laughter.

The diversity of pathological findings suggests the multiplicity, and apparently a certain degree of equipotentiality, of neurochemical and neurophysiological triggers of epileptic laughter. The substrate underlying epileptic laughter may also be a part of a complicated system that can be activated through a number of structures and react as a whole. The high incidence of hypothalamic pathology (Martin, 1950; Money and Hosta, 1967; Gascon and Lombroso, 1971; Matustik *et al.*, 1981), along with abnormalities of the hypothalamic regulation of the pituitary gland (Lennox, 1960; Pines, 1963), may indicate that the hypothalamus is an important part of the "laughter system" (Fig. 11.2). In contrast, laughter associated with tumors localized in the temporooccipital cortex (Daly and Mulder, 1957), frontal lobe (Loiseau *et al.*, 1971), and interpeduncular region (Ironside, 1956) as well as diffuse brain abnormalities suggests that the system governing epileptic laughter overlaps with the limbic system and seems to interact with striopallidal, thalamic, and epithalamic activities. Clinical experience has long been interpreted as implicating at least two forms of laughter, one associated with affective syndromes, and the other one a rather automatic, reflectoral reaction. The gap between the two may not necessarily be wide. Nonemotional, "mechanical" laughter may be akin to a stereotypic display of the erect phallus to any environmental trigger in the squirrel monkey (Ploog and MacLean, 1963) or resemble an overlearned emotional cliché ("dammit") uttered by some aphasic patients rather inappropriately or the coprolalia of Gilles de la Tourette's patients. Some writers (Gascon and Lombroso, 1971; Yamada and Yoshida, 1977) hypothesize that there are two major mechanisms for the two clinical subtypes of laughter: hypothalamolimbic machinery governing emotional aspects of attacks and diencephalic (thalamocortical) circuitry responsible for pseudoaffective facial expression.

TABLE 11.2
Partial List of Brain Pathological Findings Associated with Gelastic Epilepsy

Pathological finding	Reference
Birth trauma	Chen and Forster (1973) Weil *et al.* (1958), Yamada and Yoshida (1977)
Metabolic disease	
Niemann–Pick	Chen and Forster (1973), Schneck (1965)
Tay–Sachs	
Diffuse cerebral lesion	Druckman and Chao (1951), Fukuyama *et al.* (1959), Suzuki (1963)
Encephalitis and meningitis	Chen and Forster (1973), Weil *et al.* (1958)
Head injury	Ames and Enderstein (1975), Chen and Forster (1973), Lehtinen and Kivalo (1965), Yamada and Yoshida (1977)
Brain tumor	
Third ventricle and hypothalamus	Dott (1938, reported in Williams *et al.*, 1978), Gascon and Lombroso (1971)
Mammilary bodies	Money and Hosta (1967), Matustik *et al.* (1981), Pines (1963), Weil *et al.* (1958), Williams *et al.*, (1978)
Hypohyseal	Martin (1950), Lennox (1960)
Cortical, callosal	Chen and Forster (1973), Daly and Mulder (1957), Loiseau *et al.* (1971)
Hemisphere atrophy (left)	Chen and Forster (1973), Dietze (1965)

Figure 11.2 describes the interconnection between the various sites the abnormality of which may occasionally be associated with epileptic laughter (see also Table 11.2). This diagram adds some weight to the notion that gelastic epilepsy is generated by a multiplicity of intimately interconnected centers. Considering the contemporary explanation of the concept of the limbic system (Nauta, 1979) one might reach the conclusion that the border between the "diencephalic" and "limbic" varieties of gelastic epilepsy has become anatomically blurred. In fact, they are so tied together that epileptic discharges originating in or propagated to the major station of the limbic system, the amygdala or periamygdaloid region, can produce behavioral and autonomic features of seizures obtained from various locations of this system (Gloor, 1955; Pribram, 1961).

However, laughter has been seldom obtained in response to electrical brain stimulation. Ludwig *et al.* (1975) reported typical clinical seizures along with "retraction of the left side of the mouth and smile" produced by electrical stimulation of the right orbital area (the classical cortical "laughter center") in a patient with gelastic epilepsy (case 4). Electrical stimulation in the amygdala and periamygdaloid areas conducted by Feindel (1961) in epileptic patients during brain surgery produced masticatory

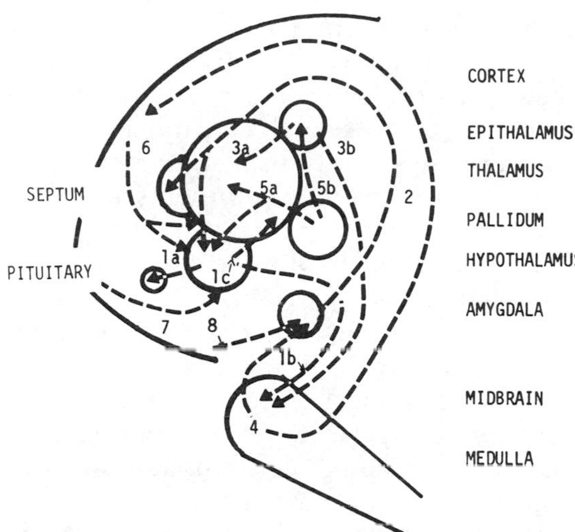

FIG. 11.2. Diagram of interconnections between some structures the pathology of which may be accompanied by epileptic laughter. 1, Hypothalamohypophyseal pathway (1a), mamillotegmental tract (1b), and mamillothalamic tract of Vicq d'Azyr (1c); 2, major amygdaloid projections via the stria terminalis to the hypothalamus and septum; 3, habenulothalamic (3a) and habenulopeduncular (3b) tracts; 4, mesolimbic and mesocortical dopaminergic system; 5, pallidal projections to the thalamus, hypothalamus (5a), and epithalamus (5b); 6, frontohypothalamic and frontodorsomedial (thalamic) projections; 7, orbitohypothalamic projections; 8, projections to amygdala from temporal cortex and parahippocampal gyrus. The disseminated character of lesions in some cases, the substantial extent of damage in others, mass effects, the involvement of surrounding or remote areas via the spread of epileptic afterdischarges, etc., render the interpretation of the anatomoclinical correlations problematic.

movements with contralateral pulling of the mouth (which might be reminiscent of a grin; compare with Fig. 11.1). Confusion, unresponsiveness, nonsensical speech, and amnesia of the entire episode were additional symptoms of the attack. Similar behavioral profiles associated with amygdaloid afterdischarge were seen by other writers (Roberts, 1961; Walker and Marshall, 1961). Electrocortical activity during induced psychomotor attack often resembles that of arousal (Feindel, 1961), although psychologically patients may be in a dreamlike state and experience fear, feelings of sorrow, and disgust. Roberts (1961) was puzzled to find a single instance of a pleasant sensation in response to electrical stimulation of the amygdala. However, stimulation of some points of the amygdala in the cat produces spasmodic expirations and inspirations (Kaada, 1951), which are the basic respiratory vehicle of laughter.

It is yet to be examined whether the infrequent occurrence of pleasurable sensations during brain stimulation are related to brain laterality and/or to variations in the background electrical activity of the stimulated sites, as seems to follow from the study by Walter *et al.* (1964).

Delgado (1969) observed that stimulation of the surface of the left temporal lobe made a patient increasingly friendly and talkative. This 11-year-old boy (case A. F.) became flirtatious with the male interviewer, expressed confusion about his sexual identity, and repeatedly requested that this enjoyable brain test continue. Another patient of Delgado (case V. P.) would giggle and make funny comments when stimulated in the right temporal lobe. A typically withdrawn patient (J. M.) would increase her verbal output when stimulated in the right temporal lobe.

The 26-year-old right-handed patient of Jacome *et al.* (1980) with self-induced epileptic laughter also had right temporal lobe focus. He was able to activate the orgastic seizure by hyperextending his back, a posture that seems to be a stereotyped and bizarre modification of the voluptuous stretch of one of Delgado's patients (A. F.). He then experienced sexual pleasure reminiscent of orgasm, although unaccompanied by penile erection, ejaculation, or copulatory movements.

Leopold's patient (1977) who had right-sided osteochrondroma experienced joy before uncontrolled giggling when he directed his gaze to the right. Bechtereva *et al.* (1975) reported a sexually flavored sensation during stimulation of the right centrum medianum. Given these findings, one might be tempted to suggest that emotionally charged laughter is associated with right hemisphere mechanisms, whereas laughter frequently occurring in epileptic patients is often related to accompanying psychopathology associated with left hemisphere abnormality. However, when Sem-Jacobsen (1976) compared the effect of left and right locations of the electrodes on emotions, no significant differences emerged between the sides.

Experimental analysis of this problem, in which so much depends on verbal communication and an interpretation of postural cues, remains cumbersome. Attempts to compare self-stimulation of the left and right hemispheres in monkeys (Hopkins and Kuypers, 1976) and catecholamine asymmetry during self-stimulation in rats (St.-Laurent *et al.*, 1976) also revealed no differences between the sides (see, however, Chapter 2).

The paucity of "positive points" in the temporal lobe is not important in itself. Under certain conditions the "points" associated with adversive effects may prove to mediate positive effects as well. Miller (1961) stated, "The fact that both the reward and aversion effects can be obtained from the same points in so many different parts of the brain shows that one must be cautious about saying that one system is primarily rewarding and another primarily aversive unless one has made extensive tests for both effects [p. 580]." Experimentally proved positive emotional reactions in animals during self-stimulation are so frequently accompanied by a spectrum of autonomic and behavioral signs of fearful and aggressive behaviors that Doty (1961) asked in surprise, "Is it pleasurable or a reward?" Valenstein (1976) reviewed evidence that primate aggression may be associated with both positive and negative emotions.

Still another possibility is that laughter may be a reaction to the cessation of pain or intense aversive experience produced by amygdaloid afterdischarge. This may happen, at least in some cases, toward the end of the epileptic attack, when paroxysmal discharges in the amygdala may have been terminated due to postictal depression. The temporary electrical inactivation of the amygdala may cause its removal. The latter has long been known to reduce the intensity of affective behavior and decreases responsiveness to noxious stimuli (Schreiner and Kling, 1953).

Heath *et al.* (1968) interpreted the sensation of well-being and happiness in response to electrical brain stimulation as being the result of pain alleviation. The most intensely pleasurable effects were obtained in patients who had been suffering intense pain or had been particularly distressed.

This experience cautions that there may be nothing enigmatically delightful behind the attack of laughter; rather, it might camouflage the cessation of a sensation of devastating loneliness and bewilderment. It is of interest that in some gelastic patients episodes of crying are observed (Stutte, 1963; Gumpert *et al.*, 1970; Gascon and Lombroso, 1971), even though sometimes this is a joyful weeping (Zecchini and Ceccotto, 1967).

The major problem with any attempt to reconstruct the "anatomy of laughter" is that the locations of the lesions are not unique. Madsen and Bray (1966) reviewed a number of cases of brain tumors leading to spike–wave paroxysms. Most of the locations were in the thalamus, hypothalamus, and hypophysis, third ventricle, basal ganglia, and both right and left temporal and frontal lobes. None of these patients seemed to manifest epileptic laughter.

The other locus of confluence between the striatal and limbic systems is the lateral habenular nuclei. These receive projections from the lateral preoptic–hypothalamic region and the entopeduncular nucleus, the homolog of the internal segment of the globus pallidus in primates (Nauta, 1979). The pallidum is the major recipient of striatal afferents and seems to be one of the major stations of γ-aminobutyric acid-carrying fibers operating in the feedback regulation of the dopaminergic nigrostriatal system (Hattori *et al.*, 1973). A spread of the epileptic discharge to the pallidum might produce adversive phenomena, as are so often seen in gelastic patients. Moreover, Hassler (1979) reproduced both a contraversive turning of eyes and smiling or even loud laughing, which began on the contralateral side of the face, by stimulating the globus pallidus.

Electrical stimulation of the globus pallidus or the entopeduncular nucleus in cats (Hassler, 1979) and rats (Crossman *et al.*, 1977) results in contraversive turning of the head. Hassler showed that in a restrained cat (*encephalé isolé*) stimulation of the pallidum produced a contraversive conjugate deviation of the eyes. Symmetric stimulation of both pallida activated a straightforward running (evoked cursive episode).

Lee and Slater (1981) examined some underlying pathophysiological mechanisms of contraversive head turning. They found that a discrete electrolytic lesion of the substantia nigra slowed down but did not eliminate the turning. Also, thalamic lesions (in ventromedial and centromedial nuclei), motor cortex decortication, electrolesion of the nucleus pedunculopontis, and the administration of micro amounts of 6-hydroxydopamine into the lateral hypothalamus were all without significant effect. The only lesion that abolished the head turning proved to be in the periaqueductal gray. The role of this area in adversive movements has also been suggested by Hassler (1979).

The neurochemical mechanisms of head turning remain obscure. A γ-aminobutyric acid (GABA) antagonist, picrotoxin, injected into the globus pallidus, failed to prevent head turning; rather, it facilitated the response (Crossman *et al.*, 1977). Apparently, adversive head movement is mediated by a system not necessarily using GABA as a neurotransmitter. Slater and Longman (1980) reported that ethylketocyclazocine, a selective agonist of κ-type opiate receptors, injected either intraperitoneally or into the pallidum, caused a pronounced naloxone-sensitive slowing of the contraversive head deviation. Although this result is in line with a conjecture that opiate κ receptors may play a role in the experimental adversive response, it is hardly the only mechanism involved.

Fariello and Mehendale (see Chapter 6) prefer to explain the gyratory symptoms of epilepsy using the model of the circling rodent (see Chapters 2, 4, and 5). The mechanisms of head turning and circling are not identical even though they seem to serve the same behavioral response. Head turning in response to stimulation of the pallidum may ultimately channel locomotion into a gyratory pattern (Hassler, 1979). Postural asymmetry (largely trunk flexion) is known to channel chaotic locomotion into circling (Pycock, 1980). However, microinjections of the GABA agonist muscimol into the substantia nigra or entopeduncular nucleus induced contraversive postural asymmetry with trunk flexion but no deviation of the head (Scheel-Krüger *et al.*, 1981).

IV. Postscript

Paroxysmal laughter is a symptom associated with a variety of conditions caused by temporal lobe epilepsy. It may be (*a*) combined with akinetic seizures: (*b*) develop during automatisms associated with petit mal; (*c*) precede grand mal seizures; (*d*) be encountered in psychomotor status, the postictal twilight state, or a twilight state not time-related to a seizure; or (*e*) be the chief feature of a short-lived psychomotor attack or a component of grossly inadequate behavior of patients with schizophrenia-like psychoses. The precise nature of certain attacks of laughter remains obscure and of doubtful validity in some cases. Laughter may occur with or without an external trigger; the route and the type of epileptic discharges leading to it have yet to be discovered. In certain patients laughter may occur through the mechanisms of conditioning, as were the hallucinatory episodes in patients J. C. and M. G. of Penfield and Erickson (1941), or as *de novo* automatisms, as in Penry and Dreifuss's patients (1969). One of the most detailed descriptions of gelastic epilepsy, presented by Ames and Enderstein (1975), cites a patient's recollection that his attack occurred about the time when he was listening to a radio program in which one of the actors had a peculiar laughter, which he tried to imitate. He suggested, "This laugh must have just 'come out' when I had an attack [p. 11]."

Although the involvement of the amygdala provides the causal link between temporal lobe psychosis and "gelastic micropsychosis," an explanation as to why the paroxysms of laughter so often (but not always) develop some time after the onset of seizures (and why they occur at all) is lacking. At this point one can only speculate that in some patients gelastic episodes may be a side effect of medication. It is virtually impossible to extract treatment data from case reports because of insufficient information about doses or blood levels. However, it has been reported that epileptic patients with psychomotor slowing, intellectual deterioration, personality changes, and psychotic symptoms have generally higher blood concentrations of phenytoin and phenobarbital than patients without these characteristics (Reynolds and Travers, 1974).

The link between antiepileptic treatment and paroxysmal laughter is tantalizing. Suggesting a reasonably discrete abnormality within a well-delineated dopaminergic system, it provides a bridge between a singular, rather unique symptom and the spectrum of psychotic symptoms of temporal lobe epilepsy. Moreover, it suggests that in nonmedicated patients with paroxysmal laughter there may be a more advanced abnormality within the same neurochemical locus and hints at the possibility of left hemisphere involvement in gelastic epilepsy. Indeed, among cases of asymmetric brain pathology, left hemisphere abnormalities were predominant, the ratio being about 2:1. Given that this group manifests a high incidence of psychopathology and personality changes, this finding is consistent with the hypothesis of Flor-Henry (see Chapter 7) relating psychopathology to left temporal lobe lesion. Unfortunately, the value of this finding is reduced because a number of patients (not included in Table 11.1) seem to have "symmetric" abnormalities. Also, a particular drawback of reports on gelastic epilepsy is the rather casual way in which psychiatric and neurological data are described; there is a lack of references to the handedness of patients, and the electrophysiological findings are inadequate and incomplete. It is small wonder that gelastic epilepsy remains a wholly mysterious syndrome.

Finally, the majority of writers believe that the name *gelastic* is inadequate because the patients are seldom cheerful, hilarious, or mirthful. Rather, their laughter is designated as *inappropriate*. Alas, Plato maintained that laughter was not at all appropriate in dignified men. Naturally, this criterion of pathology, especially used against a background of psychomotor attack, adds nothing. Admittedly, it is often pointed out that laughter is not always natural, sometimes it resembles a hiccup; the face remains frozen and unemotional; and the patient may have episodes of weeping or deny any positive experience even when recollecting the episode. These characteristics probably indicate that laughter in an attack of epilepsy, as in normal situations, may be related to pleasure, surprise, boredom, or pain. In other words, gelastic epilepsy may be gelastic indeed in some and devoid of overt or covert mirthful characteristics in others. As Lord Taylor (1978) noted, almost all honestly descriptive diagnoses are multiple. In this sense the diagnosis of gelastic epilepsy limited to two words may simply be a classificational error. This is why I join ranks with those who, like Roger *et al.* (1967), noncommittally designate this syndrome as epileptic laughter.

Note Added in Proof

The study by Sackeim *et al.* (1982), published after this chapter had been written, reached the identical conclusion regarding the preponderance of left hemisphere foci in patients with epileptic laughter. They interpret this phenomenon as an emotional outburst and propose that it "most often result[s] . . . from excitation of the left side of the brain [p. 215]." The present chapter demonstrates that the evidence marshaled to draw this conclusion is hardly sufficient.

References

Ahmad, S., Laidlaw, J., Houghton, G. W., and Richens, A. (1975). Involuntary movements caused by phenytoin intoxication in epileptic patients. *J. Neurol. Neurosurg. Psychiatry* **38,** 225–231.

Ajmone-Marsan, C., and Goldhammer, L. (1963). Clinical ictal patterns and electrographic data in cases of partial seizures in fronto-central-parietal origin. *In* "Epilepsy: Its Phenomena in Man" (M. A. B. Brazier, ed.), pp. 236–260. Academic Press, New York.

Akert, K. (1961). Diencephalon. *In* "Electrical Stimulation of the Brain" (D. E. Sheer, ed.), pp. 288–310. Univ. of Texas Press, Austin.

Ames, F. R., and Enderstein, O. (1975). Ictal laughter: A case report with clinical, cinefilm, and EEG observations. *J. Neurol. Neurosurg. Psychiatry* **38,** 11–17.

Bancaud, J., and Bacia, T. (1980). Does laughter epilepsy (gelastic epilepsy) exist? *Electroencephalogr. Clin. Neurophysiol.* **49,** P44.

Battisti, A., Monaci, G., and Leece, C. (1965). Sui rapporti tra le crisidi riso e le manifestazioni epilettiche (in particolare descrizione di un caso con crisi gelastiche spontanee e riflesse da stimoli sensoriali gustativi. *Riv. Neuro.* **11,** 708–722.

Bechtereva, N., Kambarova, D. K., Smirnov, V. M., and Sandurine, A. N. (1975). The principles and tactics of using the brain's latent abilities for therapy. Chronic intracerebral electrical stimulation. *Proc. World Congr. Psychiatr. Surg., 4th, 1975* p. 000.

Beneicke, U. (1967). Lachen als ausloser eines kleinen epileptischen anfalls. *Psychiat., Neurol. Med. Psychol.* **19,** 380–381.

Bollea, A., Manfredi, M., Sideri, G., and Vigevano, F. (1980). Gelastic epilepsy with EEG status. *Electroencephalogr. Clin. Neurophysiol.* **50,** P8.

Caveness, W. F. (1969). Ontogeny of focal seizures. *In* "Basic Mechanisms of the Epilepsies" (H. H. Jasper, A. A. Ward, and A. Pope, eds.), pp. 517–534. Little, Brown, Boston, Massachusetts.

Chadwick, D., Reynolds, E. H., and Marsden, C. D. (1976). Anticonvulsant-induced dyskinesias: A comparison with dyskinesias induced by neuroleptics. *J. Neurol., Neurosurg. Psychiatry* **39,** 1210–1218.

Chen, R. C., and Forster, F. M. (1973). Cursive epilepsy and gelastic epilepsy. *Neurology* **23,** 1019–1029.

Chiodo, L. A., and Antelman, S. M. (1980). Electroconvulsive shock: Progressive dopamine autoreceptor subsensitivity independent of repeated treatment. *Science* **210,** 799–801.

Cohen, B., Rey-Bellet, J., and Bergmand, P. S. (1960). Electroencephalographic and convulsive responses of patients with brain disease to methetharimide *Neurology* **10,** 1024–1030.

Cohen, M. R., and Niska, R. W. (1980). Localized right cerebral hemisphere dysfunction and recurrent mania. *Am. J. Psychiatry* **137,** 837–848.

Critchley, M. (1979). "The Divine Banquet of the Brain and Other Essays." Raven Press, New York.

Crossman, A. R., Lee, L. A., and Slater, P. (1977). Effects of manipulating pallidal and nigral GABA on striatally-mediated head-turning in the rat. *Br. J. Pharmacol.* **61,** 483P.

Daly, D. D., and Mulder, D. W. (1957). Gelastic epilepsy. *Neurology* **7,** 189–192.

Delgado, J. M. R. (1969). "Physical Control of the Mind." Harper & Row, New York.

Dietze, R. (1965). Accese de ris patologice in cadrul unei epilepsic simptomatice. *Neurologia* **10,** 535–540.

Doty, R. W. (1961). Conditioned reflexes formed and evoked by brain stimulation. *In* "Electrical Stimulation of the Brain" (D. E. Sheer, ed.), pp. 397–412. Univ. of Texas Press, Austin.

Dreyer, R., and Wehmeyer, W. (1978). Laughing in complex partial seizure epilepsy. A video tape analysis of 32 patients with laughing as symptom of an attack. *Fortschr. Neurol., Psychiatr. Ihrer Grenzgeb.* **46,** 61–75.

Druckmann, R., and Chao, D. (1957). Laughter in epilepsy. *Neurology* **7,** 26–36.

Erastus, T. (1581). Cited in Temkin, O. (1971).

Faheem, A. D., Brightwell, D. R., Burton, G. C., and Struss, A. (1982). Respiratory dyskinesia and dysarthria from prolonged neuroleptic use: Tardive dyskinesia? *Am. J. Psychiatry* **139,** 517–518.

Feindel, W. (1961). Response patterns elicited from the amygdala and deep temporo-insular cortex. *In* "Electrical Stimulation of the Brain" (D. Sheer, ed.), pp. 519–533. Univ. of Texas Press, Austin.

Fukuyama, Y., Arima, M., and Okada, Y. (1959). Pathologic laughter as an epileptic manifestation. *Recent Adv. Res. Nerv. Syst.* **3,** 675–695.

Gardner, H., Ling, P. K., Flamm, L., and Silverman, J. (1975). Comprehension and appreciation of numerous material following brain damage. *Brain* **98,** 399–412.

Gascon, G. G., and Lombroso, C. T. (1971). Epileptic (gelastic) laughter. *Epilepsia* **12,** 63–76.

Gastaut, H. (1973). "Dictionary of Epilepsy," p. 49. World Health Organ., Geneva.

Gauthier, C. A., and Belanger, C. (1953). Contribution à l'étude de l'épilepsie giratoire. *Laval Med.* **18,** 12–21.

Geier, S., Bancaud, J., Talairach, J., Bonis, A., Enjelvin, M., and Mossard-Bouchard, M. (1976). Automatisms during frontal lobe epileptic seizures. *Brain* **99,** 447–458.

Geier, S., Bancaud, J., Talairach, J., Bonis, A., Szikla, G., and Enjelvin, M. (1977). The seizures of frontal lobe epilepsy. A study of clinical manifestations. *Neurology* **27,** 951–958.

Gibbs, F. A., and Gibbs, E. L. (1952). "Atlas of Electroencephalography," Vol. 2. Addison-Wesley, Reading, Massachusetts.

Gloor, P. (1955). Electrophysiological studies on the connections of the amygdaloid nucleus of the cat. Part I. The neural organization of the amygdaloid projection system. *Electroencephalogr. Clin. Neurophysiol.* **7,** 223–242.

Guidetti, B., Fortuna, A., and Moscatelli, G. (1959). Sul valore localizzatorio della crisi avversative e giratorie. *Riv. Patol. Nerv. Ment.* **80,** 1113–1185.

Gumpert, J., Hansotia, P., and Upton, A. (1970). Gelastic epilepsy. *J. Neurol., Neurosurg. Psychiatry* **33,** 479–483.

Hadfield, M. G. (1972). Uptake and binding of catecholamines. Effects of diphenylhydantoin and a new mechanism of action. *Arch. Neurol.* (*Chicago*) **26,** 78–84.

Hallen, O. (1962). Zur differenzierung der psychomotorischen anfaelle in klinische formen. *Dtsch. Z. Nervenheilkd.* **183,** 199–217.

Hanson, P. A., and Chodos, R. (1978). Hemiparetic seizures. *Neurology* **28,** 920–923.

Hassler, R. (1979). Striatal regulation of adverting and attention directing induced by pallidal stimulation. *Appl. Neurophysiol.* **42,** 98–102.

Hattori, T., McGeer, P. L., Fibiger, H. C., and McGeer, E. G. (1973). On the source of GABA-containing terminals in the substantia nigra. Electron microscopic autoradiographic and biochemical studies. *Brain Res.* **54,** 103–114.

Heath, R. G., John, S. B., and Fontana, C. J. (1968). The pleasure response; studies by stereotaxic techniques in patients. *In* "Computers and Electronic Devices in Psychiatry" (N. S. Kline and E. Laska, eds.), pp. 178–189. Grune & Stratton, New York.

Hopkins, D. A., and Kuypers, H. G. J. M. (1976). Response lateralization and self-stimulation in normal and split-brain monkeys. *In* "Brain Stimulation Reward" (A. Wauquier and E. T. Rolls, eds.), pp. 577–579. Elsevier, Amsterdam.

Huott, A. D., Madison, D. S., and Niedermeyer, E. (1974). Occipital lobe epilepsy. A clinical and electroencephalographic study. *Eur. Neurol.* **11,** 325–339.

Hympan, J., and Bozik, L. (1948). Smiech ako epilepticky ekvivalent. *Bratisl. Lek. Listy* **28,** 958–964.

Ironside, R. (1956). Disorders of laughter due to brain lesions. *Brain* **79,** 589–609.

Jackson, I. V., Volavka, J., James, B., and Reker, D. (1980). The respiratory component of tardive dyskinesia. *Biol. Psychiatry* **15,** 485–487.

Jacome, D. E., McLain, L. W., and Fitzgerald, R. (1980). Postural reflex gelastic seizures. *Arch. Neurol.* (*Chicago*) **37,** 249–251.

Jandolo, B., Gessini, L., Occhipinti, E., and Pompili, A. (1977). Laughing and running fits as manifestation of early traumative epilepsy. *Euro. Neurol.* **15,** 177–182.

Kaada, B. R. (1951). Somato-motor, autonomic and electrographic responses to electrical stimulation of "rhinencephalic" and other structures in primates, cat and dog. *Acta Physiol. Scand.* **24,** Suppl. 83, 1–285.

Kooiker, J., and Sumi, S. M. (1974). Movement disorders as a manifestation of diphenylhydantoin intoxication. *Neurology* **24,** 68–71.

Kotowicz, A., and Scherpereel. P. (1968). L'épilepsie gyratoire à propos d'un nouveau cas. *Maroc Med.* **48,** 141–143.

Lacchin, R., and Taury, M. (1950). Etude de la localisation des anomalies électriques au cours des épilepsies presentant une deviation conjuguée de la tête et des yeux. *Rev. Neurol.* **82,** 517–519.
Landolt, H. (1958). Serial electroencephalographic investigation during psychotic episodes in epileptic patients and during schizophrenic attacks. *In* "Lectures on Epilepsy" (A. M. Lorentz de Haas, ed.), pp. 91–133. Elsevier, Amsterdam.
Lee, L. A., and Slater, P. (1981). Role of globus pallidus and substantia nigra efferent pathways in striatally evoked head turning in the rat. *Exp. Brain. Res.* **44,** 170–176.
Lehtinen, L., and Kivalo, A. (1965). Laughter epilepsy. *Acta Neurol. Scand.* **41,** 255–261.
Lennox, W. G. (1960). "Epilepsy and Related Disorders," Vol. 1, p. 280. Little, Brown, Boston, Massachusetts.
Leopold, N. A. (1977). Gaze-induced laughter. *J. Neurol., Neurosurg. Psychiatry* **40,** 815–817.
Lewis, J. A. (1977). Seizures characterized by laughter. *Electroencephalogr. Clin. Neurophysiol.* **43,** 904.
Logan, W. J., and Freeman, J. M. (1969). Pseudodegenerative disease due to diphenylhydantoin intoxication. *Arch. Neurology (Chicago)* **21,** 631–637.
Loiseau, P., Cohadon, F., and Cohadon, S. (1971). Gelastic epilepsy, a review and report of five cases. *Epilepsia* **12,** 313–325.
Ludwig, B. I., and Ajmone-Marsan, C. (1975). Clinical ictal patterns in epileptic patients with occipital electroencephalographic foci. *Neurology* **25,** 463–471.
Ludwig, B. I., Ajmone-Marsan, C., and Van Buren, J. (1975). Cerebral seizures of probable orbitofrontal origin. *Epilepsia* **16,** 141–158.
McLellan, D. L., and Swash, M. (1974). Choreo-athetosis and encephalopathy induced by phenytoin. *Br. Med. J.* **2,** 204–205.
Madsen, J. A., and Bray, P. F. (1966). The coincidence of diffuse electroencephalographic spike-wave paroxysms and brain tumors. *Neurology* **16,** 546–555.
Martin, J. P. (1950). Fits of laughter (sham mirth) in organic cerebral disease. *Brain* **73,** 453–464.
Matustik, M. C., Eisenberg, H. M., and Meyer, W. G. (1981). Gelastic (laughing) seizures and precocious pubergy. *Am. J. Dis. Child.* **135,** 837–838.
Mesulam, M. M. (1981). Dissociative states with abnormal temporal lobe EEG. *Arch. Neurol. (Chicago)* **38,** 176–181.
Miller, N. E. (1961). Implications for theories of reinforcement. *In* "Electrical Stimulation of the Brain" (D. E. Sheer, ed.), pp. 575–581. Univ. of Texas Press, Austin.
Money, J., and Hosta, G. (1967). Laughing seizures with sexual precocity: Report of two cases. *Johns Hopkins Med. J.* **120,** 326–336.
Moscovitch, M., and Olds, J. (1982). Asymmetries in spontaneous facial expressions and their possible relation to hemispheric specialization. *Neuropsychologia* **20,** 71–81.
Myslobodsky, M. S. (1976). "Petit Mal Epilepsy: A Search for the Precursors of Wave-Spike Activity." Academic Press, New York.
Nauta, W. J. H. (1979). Expanding borders of the limbic system concept. *In* "Functional Neurosurgery" (T. Rasmussen and R. Marino, eds.), pp. 7–23. Raven Press, New York.
Penfield, W., and Erickson, T. (1941). "Epilepsy and Cerebral Localization." Thomas, Springfield, Illinois.
Penry, J. K., and Dreifuss, F. E. (1969). Automatisms associated with the absence of petit mal epilepsy. *Arch. Neurol. (Chicago)* **21,** 142–149.
Pines, L. N. (1963). Laughter as an epileptic equivalent. *Zh. Nevropatol. Psikhiat. im. S. S. Korsakova* **63,** 1341–1348.
Ploog, D. W., and MacLean, P. D. (1963). Display of penile erection in the squirrel monkey (*Saimiri seiureus*). *Anim. Behav.* **11,** 32–39.
Pribram, K. H. (1961). Limbic system. *In* "Electrical Stimulation of the Brain" (D. E. Sheer, ed.), pp. 311–320. Univ. of Texas Press, Austin.

Pycock, C. (1980). Turning behaviour in animals. *Neuroscience* **5,** 461–514.

Reynolds, E. H., and Travers, R. D. (1974). Serum anticonvulsant concentrations in epileptic patients with mental symptoms. A preliminary report. *Br. J. Psychiatry* **124,** 440–445.

Riser, M., Geraud, J., Grezes-Rueff, C., Lavitary, S., and Rascol, A. (1951). A propos de 14 cas d'épilepsie giratoire. *Rev. Neurol.* **85,** 245–253.

Roberts, L. (1961). Activation and interference of cortical functions. *In* "Electrical Stimulation of the Brain" (D. E. Sheer, ed.), pp. 133–173. Univ. of Texas Press, Austin.

Roger, J., Lob, H., Waltregrny, A., and Gastaut, H. (1967). Attacks of epileptic laughter. Report of five cases. *Electroencephalogr. Clin. Neurophysiol.* **22,** 297.

Sackeim, H. A., Greenberg, M. S., Weiman, A. L., Gur, R. C., Hungerbuhler, J. P., and Geschwind, N. (1982). Hemispheric asymmetry in the expression of positive and negative emotions: Neurologic evidence. *Arch. Neurol.* **39,** 210–218.

St.-Laurent, J., Roizen, M. F., Beckman, H., Miliaressis, E., Goodwin, F. K., and Jacobowitz, D. M. (1976). Neurochemical changes in discrete areas of the brain after self-stimulation from the area ventralis tegmenti. *In* "Brain-Stimulation Reward" (A. Wauquier and E. T. Rolls, eds.), pp. 283–289. Elsevier, Amsterdam.

Sato, M., Hikasa, N., and Otsuki, S. (1979). Experimental epilepsy, psychosis, and dopamine receptor sensitivity. *Biol. Psychiatry* **14,** 537–540.

Schader, H. E. (1966). Zum subklinischen fokalem anfallsgeschehen. Ein kasuistischer Beitrag zur hemmung der anfallsaktivitat. *Nervenarzt* **37,** 319–321.

Scheel-Krüger, J., Magelund, G., and Olianas, M. C. (1981). Role of GABA in the striatal output system: Globus pallidus, nucleus entopeduncularis, substantia nigra and nucleus subthalamicus *Adv. Biochem. Psychopharmacol.* **30,** 165–186.

Schenck, L. (1965). The early electroencephalographic and seizure characteristics of Tay-Sachs' disease. *Acta Neurol. Scand.* **41,** 163–171.

Schenck, L., and Bear, D. (1981). Multiple personality and related dissociative phenomena in patients with temporal lobe epilepsy *Am. J. Psychiatry* **138,** 1311–1316.

Schreiner, L., and Kling, A. (1953). Behavioral changes following rhinencephalic injury in the cat. *J. Neurophysiol.* **16,** 643–659.

Scollo-Lavizzari, G., and Hess, R. (1967). Sensory precipitation of epileptic seizures. *Epilepsia* **8,** 157–161.

Sem-Jacobsen, C. W. (1976). Electrical stimulation and self-stimulation in man with chronic implanted electrodes. Interpretation and pitfalls of results. *In* "Brain-Stimulation Reward" (A. Wauquier and E. T. Rolls, eds.), pp. 505–520. Elsevier, Amsterdam.

Sinisi, C. (1961). Sulle crisi gelastiche parossistiche nell'epilepssia. *Osp. Psichiati.* **29,** 403–416.

Slater, E., and Beard, A. W. (1963). The schizophrenia-like psychoses of epilepsy. I. Psychiatric aspects. *Br. J. Psychiatry* **109,** 95–112.

Slater, P., and Longman, D. A. (1980). Effects of intrapallidal opiate receptor agonists on striatally evoked head turning. *Neuropharmacology* **19,** 1153–1156.

Stein, J., and Dietze, R. (1965). Data electroencefalografica in geloplegie. *Neurologia (Bucharest)* **10,** 541–547.

Stevens, H., and Shorey, M. (1965). Masked epilepsy. *Clin. Proc. Child. Hosp., Washington* **21,** 297–314.

Stevens, J. R. (1973). An anatomy of schizophrenia? *Arch. Gen. Psychiatry* **29,** 177–189.

Strobos, R. J., and Kavallinis, G. P. (1968). Changes in repeat electroencephalograms in epileptics. *Neurology* **18,** 622–633.

Stutte, H. (1963). Zwangsaffekte und paroxysmale Lach- und Weinausbruecke als Epilepsie-Symptom. *Nervenarzt* **34,** 290–295.

Suzuki, M. (1963). Fits of laughter as a symptom of epilepsy. *Psychiatr. Neurol. Paediatr. Jpn.* **3,** 20–27.

Taylor, S. (1978). Psychiatry and natural history. *Br. Med. J.* **2,** 1754–1758.

Temkin, O. (1971). "Falling Sickness," pp. 190–191. Johns Hopkins Press, Baltimore, Maryland.

Thompson, G. N., and Raney, R. (1949). Epileptic incident to protoplasmic astrocytome. Report of a case. *Bull. Los Angeles Neurol. Soc.* **14,** 46–49.

Valenstein, E. S. (1976). The interpretation of behavior evoked by brain stimulation. *In* "Brain-Stimulation Reward" (A. Wauquier and E. T. Rolls, eds.), pp. 557–575. Elsevier, Amsterdam.

Walker, A. E., and Marshall, C. (1961). Stimulation and depth recording in man. *In* "Electrical Stimulation of the Brain" (D. E. Sheer, ed.), pp. 498–518. University of Texas Press, Austin.

Walter, R. D., Chapman, L., Porter, R., Crandale, P., and Rand, R. (1964). Behavioral responses to stimulation of human hippocampus, hippocampal gyrus and amygdala. *Electroencephalogr. Clin. Neurophysiol.* **17,** 461.

Weil, A. A., Nosik, W. A., and Demmy, N. (1958). Electroencephalographic correlation of laughing fits. *Am. J. Med. Sci.* **235,** 301–308.

Williams, M., Schutt, W., and Savage, D. (1978). Epileptic laughter with precocious puberty. *Arch. Dis. Child.* **53,** 967–969.

Woon, T. H., and Vignaendra, V. (1978). Cursive and gelastic epilepsy—probable sequelae of physical abuse. *Postgrad. Med. J.* **5,** 821–824.

Yamada, H., and Yoshida, H. (1977). Laughing attack: A review and report of nine cases. *Folia Psychiatr. Neurol.* **31,** 129–137.

Yoshida, T. (1962). A clinical survey of epilepsy with special reference to electroencephalographic findings. *Psychiatr. Neurol. Jpn.* **64,** 1173–1191.

Zecchini, A., and Cecotto, C. (1967). Crisi parossistiche di riso e di natura epilettica. Presentazione di un caso. *Minerva Med.* **58,** 3405–3410.

12: A Critical Assessment and Integration of Lateral Asymmetries in Schizophrenia

JOHN H. GRUZELIER

Department of Psychiatry
Charing Cross Hospital Medical School
London, England

I. Introduction 265
A. Fixed Structure versus Dynamic Process 265
B. Clinical Syndromes Delineated by Lateral Asymmetries 267
C. Hemispheric Reversals and Computed Tomography 269
II. British Origins 270
A. Neuropsychiatry 270
B. Psychophysiology 272
C. Bipartite Laterality Model of Psychosis 273
D. Callosal Transmission 274
III. Experimental Approaches 275
A. Neuropsychiatry 275
B. Experimental Psychology 280
C. Psychophysiology 298
IV. Conclusions 311
A. Dynamic-Process Asymmetries 311
B. Fixed-Process Asymmetries 315
C. Locus of Dysfunction 315
References 318

I. Introduction

A. Fixed Structure versus Dynamic Process

This chapter presents a critical assessment of the many reports on hemispheric asymmetries of function in schizophrenia. To some extent the approach is chronological and addresses each of several general research techniques in the area. One departure from this plan is the

HEMISYNDROMES:
Psychobiology, Neurology,
Psychiatry

ISBN 0-12-512460-0

prefatory presentation of a model based on distinctions between different classes of lateralized processes. This is offered in an attempt to unravel some of the complexity in what follows and in the belief that advance knowledge of the theoretical model will enable the reader to judge its tenability more effectively.

The model is a simple one and arose when accumulated results from the author's laboratory were considered in the light of recent theoretical developments in cognitive psychology (Hellige *et al.*, 1979; Moscovitch, 1979; Bradshaw and Nettleson, 1981; Cohen, 1982). A clear exposition is offered by Cohen (1982), who draws a distinction between fixed-structure and dynamic-process models of hemisphere functions. The former hinge on the lateralization of structures that mediate the cognition, be it verbal or visuospatial, analytical or gestalt, serial or parallel process, or a lower or higher stage of processing. This class of model draws its main support from evidence of a coincidence between neuroanatomical and functional asymmetries, such as the larger planum temporale in the left hemisphere which converges on Wernicke's area for language comprehension (Geschwind and Levitsky, 1968). The fact that hemispheric specializations are seldom all or none is catered to by positing a relative degree of specialization, which permits graded individual differences. Nevertheless, this class of model falls down when faced with the frequently experienced trial-by-trial fluctuations in asymmetries.

Recourse is then conventionally made to the other class of model, which concerns dynamic-process asymmetries such as shifts in attention or activation. Kinsbourne (e.g., 1974) has been the most notable proponent here. In his view directing attention to a particular lateral input channel promotes the already existing structural asymmetry to the extent that it may be enhanced, reduced, or even reversed if attention is switched the other way. This dynamic prepotency can be achieved by the lateral focusing of attention, by stimulus set, by a concurrent task, or by practice. Such priming may be canceled by fatigue. Thus, the asymmetries of dynamic process are not independent of those of fixed structure and, in fact, may exert a controlling influence over the structural mechanism. Both models must be considered in combination. The problem then becomes one of making testable predictions. Concurrent bilateral monitoring of psychophysiological variables, using techniques that may be more familiar to experimental psychopathologists than to cognitive psychologists, may go some way toward resolving this dilemma.

The reason for urging consideration of this theoretical approach to schizophrenia is not an academic one but was compelled by the author's attempt to resolve a paradox when comparing old data with new. When we examined lateral asymmetries in electrodermal orienting responses to tones (for reasons given in Section II,B), schizophrenic patients who were selected on the basis of conservative case history diagnoses were found to be mostly homogeneous in lateral asymmetry (see Gruzelier, 1979a, for a review and group distributions). However, when we tested a new sample, which was selected because of florid symptoms that might respond to medication and differentiate two forms of drug treatment, patients showed electrodermal response asymmetries in either direction (Gruzelier, 1981a). A further paradox emerged when many of this group were examined for hemifield detection of verbal and visuospatial stimuli. Patients were found to be homogeneous for the hemisphere advantage in processing verbal stimuli, which, as it happened, was in the opposite direction to the one found in control subjects, and homogeneous for the visuospatial advantage, which corresponded to that of controls (Connolly *et al.*, 1979). This homogeneity contrasted with the heterogeneity observed on the electrodermal measure.

The detection of verbal and visuospatial stimuli presented to the nasal retina has produced results in keeping with fixed-structure theories of hemispheric specialization (Beaumont, 1982). What of electrodermal asymmetries? The psychophysiological measure involved the orienting response to indifferent stimuli, a process that may well reflect a state of hemispheric balance in dynamic processes. From this it may follow that asymmetries in a dynamic process may be in either direction, whereas asymmetries in a fixed-structure process are uniform. Hence, the nature of lateral asymmetries becomes a pressing issue.

The interpretation that the electrodermal asymmetry belongs to the dynamic-process class of functions is strengthened by considering the clinical syndromes of the two groups differentiated by opposite electrodermal asymmetries. Undeniable evidence emerges for an activation dimension that distinguishes the groups. Subtypes of schizophrenia, therefore, are as compelling an issue as the nature of the asymmetry itself. Accordingly, the character of the clinical syndromes is examined in some detail before the literature review is presented.

B. Clinical Syndromes Delineated by Lateral Asymmetries

Twenty-three schizophrenic patients, diagnosed with the help of the Present State Examination [PSE (Wing *et al.*, 1974)] and showing florid symptoms on the Brief Psychiatric Rating Scale [BPRS (Overall and Gorham, 1962)], were examined shortly after admission to hospital and before medication. Electrodermal responses to 90-dB tones were examined. Eleven patients had larger right hand responses (the asymmetry previously found in the majority of schizophrenic patients) and 12 had larger left hand responses. The two groups were compared on the syndromes of the CATEGO diagnostic system (based on PSE) and ratings on the BPRS. Striking differences emerged and were put to the test of replication in the next 25 consecutive admissions. Of these, 18 patients had larger right hand responses and 7 had larger left hand responses (Gruzelier and Manchanda, 1982; Gruzelier, 1981a). The main clinical distinctions between the groups are summarized in Table 12.1.

The groups differed on a bipolar dimension, which involved self-concepts, interpersonal behavior, affect, cognition, and motoric behavior. The group with larger right hand responses had more of the classical features of Bleulerian schizophrenia and, despite the small numbers in the asymmetry groups when the two samples were considered separately, it is noteworthy that the notoriously subjective features of blunted affect and emotional withdrawal significantly characterized the retarded syndrome in both samples. Emotional withdrawal coincided with interpersonal difficulties, retarded behavior, and reduced cognition and self-confidence. In contrast, patients with larger left hand responses had florid, hypomanic features including exaggerated self-concepts, heightened affect, and increased cognitive arousal. In terms of hemispheric specialization these patients showed left hemisphere overactivation, which contrasted with the abnormal reduction in left hemisphere activity shown by patients in the other group. The nature of the electrodermal lateral asymmetries suggests reciprocal hemispheric influences operating in seesaw fashion (see also Gruzelier *et al.*, 1981a), implying that with respect to right hemisphere function the retarded group would show right hemi-

TABLE 12.1
Syndromes Differentiated by Electrodermal Asymmetries

Syndrome of patients with larger right hand responses
Lack of self-confidence
Social withdrawal
Emotional withdrawal
Reduced emotional tone (blunted affect)
Depressed mood
Inefficient thinking (muddled, slow, not goal-directed)
Motor underactivity
Slow speech
Muteness
Restricted quantity of speech
Lack of cooperation (resistance, resentment, unfriendliness)
Irritability to hostility
Syndrome of patients with larger left hand responses
Heightened self-consciousness (simple ideas of reference)
Exaggerated self-opinion and conviction of unusual ability (grandiosity)
Exaggerated concern about bodily welfare (hypochondriasis)
Euphoria (hypomania)
Pressure of speech (hypomania)
Flight of ideas (hypomania)
Situational anxiety; avoidance of situations; phobias

sphere overactivation and the florid group right hemisphere underactivation.

It should be noted that these syndrome pictures are not full descriptions of the patients' symptoms. The patients had many other features of schizophrenia, including auditory hallucinations, which Schneider considered to be primary (Mellor, 1970), but these did not distinguish the groups. The character of the syndromes has a bearing on contemporary controversies about diagnosis and, in particular, the distinction Kety (1980) has drawn between classical Bleulerian schizophrenia, which has poor prognosis, and acute functional psychosis, which, in his view, is commonly treated as schizophrenia and responds to neuroleptic treatment. The syndromes also resemble (but are not to be confused with) the diagnostic subcategories of chronic, nonparanoid schizophrenia and acute, reactive, paranoid schizophrenia (Gruzelier, 1981a), a distinction that has been most productive in differentiating the paranoid cognitive deficit (Magaro, 1980).

The syndromes clearly represent hemispheric differences in dynamic processes, and, as will be seen, a dichotomy on other measures of hemispheric arousal and selective attention recurs persistently in the review that follows whenever contrasts are made between diagnostic subcategories approximating the syndromes defined by the electrodermal asymmetry. At the same time, lateral dysfunctions on many other measures appear to be common to both groups of patients, and the reader might consider the extent to which such unitary asymmetries reflect fixed-structural rather than dynamic hemispheric functions.

C. Hemispheric Reversals and Computed Tomography

One final methodological issue must be kept in mind. The discovery of anatomical asymmetries, with a larger planum temporale in the left hemisphere, gave impetus to the search for other morphological asymmetries with functional implications. Computed tomography (CT) studies, particularly those of Le May (1976), have revealed a wider occipital lobe on the left and frontal lobe on the right. A relation has been drawn between asymmetries in the occipital region and the planum temporale. Evidence is accruing to show that reversals in normal asymmetry occur in about 10% of the population and may augur well for recovery from aphasia, implying functional significance for the localization of language both between and within hemispheres (see the work of Pieniadz and colleagues reviewed by Luchins, 1983). Nevertheless, the logical sequel of a higher incidence of reversals in sinistrals is controversial. If reversals of function follow the anatomical reversals, then, whatever the measure, a small subgroup of subjects should be characterized by an atypical asymmetry. To what extent are hemispheric reversals associated with schizophrenia?

Luchins (1983) reviewed the seven studies that have examined this question. In three studies affirming hemispheric reversals, there were methodological flaws; two used controls derived from the literature (Luchins *et al.*, 1979; Naeser *et al.*, 1981), and the third used neurological controls but was not done blindly (Luchins *et al.*, 1982). Four studies failed to find differences between schizophrenic patients and controls (Andreasen *et al.*, 1982; Jernigan *et al.*, 1982; Nyback *et al.*, 1982; Weinberger *et al.*, 1982). Atrophy was found to be associated with reversals in both studies of Luchins *et al.*, but others have failed to replicate this finding. An association with discrepancies in verbal and performance IQ was shown by Luchins *et al.* (1982), with verbal deficits in those with reversed asymmetries. Although the implications of frontal and occipital lobe asymmetries are relatively uncharted territory at this stage, they may well hold promise when more incisively related to psychological variables. Nevertheless, one must be on the alert for small subgroups of patients with asymmetries in the direction opposite to that of the majority.

II. British Origins

A. Neuropsychiatry

The genesis of interest in psychopathological asymmetries is found appropriately in neuropsychiatry. Davison and Bagley (1969) surveyed all the available literature relating localized organic lesions to schizophrenia and based their psychiatric diagnoses on symptoms of thought disorder, shallow or incongruous affect, hallucinations, and delusions, because these retain diagnostic specificity in the presence of organic brain disorder (World Health Organization Study Group on Schizophrenia, 1959). They selected 80 cases with evidence of circumscribed lesions (arising notably from postencephalitis, posttrauma, cerebral neoplasm, narcolepsy, and symptomatic epilepsy) and concluded, "The main features are the association of left cerebral hemisphere and particularly temporal lobe lesions with primary delusions and catatonic symptoms, basal ganglia lesions with catatonic symptoms, diencephalic lesions (including basal ganglia) with auditory hallucinations, and brain stem lesions with thought disorder and Schneider's symptoms of the first rank [p. 151]." Flat, incongruous affect was also associated with left hemisphere lesions, and it is noteworthy that none of the schizophrenic features occurred with right hemisphere lesions.

At about the same time, but independently, Lishman (1966, 1968) published a survey of psychiatric disturbance occurring between 1 and 5 years after soldiers had sustained penetrating head injuries in World War II. Of the 345 soldiers in whom evidence about location and extent of damage could be ascertained, 117 had right-sided lesions and 154 left-sided lesions. When the cases were classified as having "nil," "mild," or "severe" psychiatric disability, there was a nonsignificant trend for left-sided lesions to be associated with increasing psychopathology. When regional differences were examined, the relation between left-sided wounds and symptom severity was preserved in the temporal and parietal lobes but not in the frontal or occipital lobes. The right frontal area was also implicated in the severity of symptoms. Whereas the association of the left parietal lobe with sensorimotor defects was particularly marked, the temporal lobe was related to symptom severity over and above sensorimotor or visual field defects or dysphasia, leading to the conclusion that "temporal lobe wounds are more closely associated with psychiatric disability than frontal, parietal or occipital lobe wounds. This association is very largely due to injuries of the *left* temporal lobe [Lishman, 1968, p. 399]."

Individual symptoms and signs were related to the location of brain damage and its extent in the 144 patients categorized as manifesting severe psychiatric disability. A general relationship was found between the left hemisphere and intellectual disorders, with the exception of concentration difficulties, whereas other features were related to the right hemisphere. Although this general impression was not always confirmed when the lobes were considered individually (in which case the left frontal lobe was also implicated in behavior disorders involving crime, sexual abnormalities, and lack of judgment), left-sided disturbance was predominantly intellectual and temporoparietal in location with the one exception of a link between anxiety and the occipital lobe. Right-sided psychiatric disturbances included affective features and difficulty in concentration. Thus, although schizophrenic symptoms as such were not referred to specifically, the association of cognitive symptoms and the left hemisphere was in keeping with Davison and Bagley's survey of a relation between schizophrenia and the left hemisphere.

The essential distinction in lateralization between syndromes involving predominantly cognitive symptoms and those involving predominantly affective symptoms was further emphasized by Flor-Henry's (1969) survey of temporal lobe epileptics with concomitant psychotic features. Of the 100 patients surveyed, half were diagnosed as psychotic according to traditional Kraepelinian criteria. The diagnosis of schizophrenia hinged on the presence of thought disorder and disturbance of affect with or without secondary symptoms such as hallucinations ($N=21$). Manic–depressive states were characterized by euphoric or depressive alterations of mood that exhibited periodicity and left the personality intact between phases ($N=9$). States in which the psychotic episodes were of short duration, with schizophrenic, manic–depressive, or mixed features accompanying pervasive clouding of consciousness and disorientation, were called confusional ($N=9$). Patients were diagnosed as mixed or schizoaffective when there were atypical features of an affective type ($N=11$).

Results having a bearing on laterality were as follows. Bilateral involvement was more common in the psychotic group, occurring in 22 of 50 psychotics as opposed to 11 of 50 nonpsychotics. Of the unilateral cases, 19 of 28 psychotics had dominant hemisphere foci and only 9 of 28 nondominant foci, comparable figures for nonpsychotic patients being 13 of 38 and 25 of 38, respectively. The percentage of cases in the diagnostic groups were ordered along a continuum of right hemisphere involvement as follows: manic–depressive/mixed/confusional/schizophrenic. In cases of bilateral involvement, left hemisphere dysfunction was interpreted as being more closely related to the severity of psychopathology and psychosis. Accordingly, when bilateral and left-sided cases were combined, 82% of psychotics and 48% of nonpsychotics ($p<0.001$) were accounted for.

Although statistical analysis and the inferences drawn from the data have been criticized (Alpert and Martz, 1977; Marin and Tucker, 1981), the main trend aligning Kraepelinian schizophrenia and manic-depressive disorders with the left and right hemispheres, respectively, is both unmistakable and consistent with the surveys of Lishman and Davison and Bagley. If anything, what has been overlooked is the evidence of the nondiscriminating bilateral involvement that is common to both major psychoses.

B. Psychophysiology

In response to Flor-Henry's (1969) report Gruzelier and Venables adapted a study of schizophrenic patients to include bilateral monitoring of frontoamygdaloid and hippocampal influences as revealed by electrodermal responses to incidental stimuli. Lateral asymmetries in electrodermal activity had been reported in schizophrenia previously but were not referred to hemispheric involvement (Syz, 1926; Fisher and Cleveland, 1959; Dykman *et al.*, 1968). In neurological cases, bilateral recording by Luria and Homskaya (1963) showed an absence of responses to stimuli on the left hand in a patient with left frontal tumor; and Sourek (1965), with pre- and postoperative electrodermal recordings in patients undergoing partial lobectomies and coagulations of the thalamus for the control of focal epilepsy or tumors, found reliable postoperative changes only after the removal of medial or basal parts of the frontal lobe or rhinencephalon. These changes were expressed as a diminution of influences on the homolateral hand, which, in view of an increase in responsivity postoperatively, could reflect a loss of contralateral inhibition, a relative reduction of excitatory influences on the ipsilateral hand, or both. Despite the neurophysiological ambiguity, operationally the prediction is clear; a left-sided, frontotemporolimbic disturbance leads to fewer or smaller responses on the ipsilateral hand.

Two studies were conducted involving 107 patients (in the main, chronic or institutionalized) with unambiguous case note diagnoses of schizophrenia (Gruzelier, 1973; Gruzelier and Venables, 1974; reviewed by Venables, 1977, and by Gruzelier, 1978, 1979a). The patients were presented with short, indifferent auditory stimuli to which amygdalectomized monkeys had been under- or overresponsive and hippocampal monkeys overresponsive (Pribram and McGuinness, 1975). Fifty-seven patients exhibited no response and, in the 50 who did, bilateral asymmetries were predominantly in the direction of less responsivity on the left hand, an asymmetry that was more pronounced in institutionalized patients. A group of unipolar depressives, included in a replication study (Gruzelier and Venables, 1974), showed asymmetry opposite to that found in schizophrenia.

Drawing on further evidence from Luria and Homskaya (1970) that a comparison of responses to indifferent and signal stimuli distinguished neurological patients on an anterior–posterior axis, it was found that almost all of the underresponsive schizophrenic patients exhibited electrodermal responses when attention to stimuli was required (Gruzelier and Venables, 1973). Moreover, the lateral asymmetry in these cases was in the same direction as that found in patients overresponsive to indifferent stimuli. This pattern of response—underresponsive to indifferent stimuli yet responsive to signal stimuli—resembled that seen with temporoposterior involvement rather than frontal involvement and, together with the lateral asymmetry, provided psychophysiological support for left temporolimbic dysfunction in schizophrenia.

C. Bipartite Laterality Model of Psychosis

The first theoretical review was provided by Flor-Henry (1974). To summarize, he associated schizophrenic and paranoid psychoses with temporolimbic dysfunction of the dominant hemisphere and the affective disorders of mania and depression with a corresponding dysfunction of the nondominant hemisphere. Other forms of psychopathology were incorporated, with psychopathy and hysteria included as left hemisphere disorders and dysthymia and neurotic depressions as right hemisphere disorders. Gender differences in the incidence and development of psychoses were related to hemispheric organization. In view of neuropsychological evidence of weaker dominant hemisphere development in men and nondominant hemisphere development in women, it was thought significant that schizophrenia and related childhood psychopathologies occur predominantly in men under 30 years of age, whereas affective disorders occur predominantly in women. In martialing evidence to support these views, particular emphasis was placed on the temporolimbic locus of the disorders. However, it was the distinction between schizophrenic and manic–depressive psychoses in terms of lateral dysfunction that was to provide the spearhead for the experimental approaches that followed.

D. Callosal Transmission

Given the impetus to perform research on lateralized function from studies of commisurotomy patients (Sperry, 1968; Gazzaniga, 1970; Trevarthen, 1974; Gazzaniga and Le Doux, 1978), theories of hemispheric dysfunction in schizophrenia would be incomplete without a hypothesis of impairment within the interhemispheric pathways. Beaumont and Dimond (1973) drew an analogy between schizophrenia and the brain disconnection syndrome seen after commisurotomy. Twelve schizophrenic patients, 12 patients with mixed psychiatric diagnoses, and 12 normal controls were tested on a task requiring within- or between-hemisphere matching of stimuli (letters, digits, or abstract shapes) presented to visual half-fields. The results, published in abstract form, indicated that schizophrenic patients had no difficulty in identifying letters or digits but were deficient in matching letters and shapes between hemispheres and in matching letters within the left hemisphere. Otherwise, they did not differ from normal controls. Whereas they were inferior to the psychiatric controls in matching digits and shapes in the right hemisphere, the psychiatric controls actually exceeded the normal subjects in performance. These data indicate interhemispheric transfer problems in schizophrenia for two of the three classes of stimuli and problems in left hemisphere functions for the matching of letters. The study has also been widely misquoted as providing evidence for abnormal right hemisphere functions.

In support of an anomaly in callosal transmission, Rosenthal and Bigelow (1972) had earlier reported postmortem results showing that the mean thickness in the width of the corpus callosum was larger in the brains of 10 schizophrenic patients than in those of 10 control patients. In looking for other abnormalities, they concentrated only on the right hemisphere. This report has been replicated in part (Bigelow *et al.*, 1983) in an examination of 29 schizophrenic brains. Twenty-one of the patients in this study had an onset of illness before the age of 30 years and most of the remainder had good premorbid histories and paranoid illness of middle age. Comparison was made with 13 neurological controls with either a chronic organic brain syndrome or paresis and 14 psychiatric controls, all but one of whom had affective features. In cases of early-onset schizophrenia, the corpus callosum in the anterior and medial aspects (which interconnect the frontal and temporal lobes) was wider than normal. In fact, about one-third of the group had values outside the range of the control groups. It was also found that, the younger the age at death, the thicker the callosum, a relation that held only for the schizophrenic groups. When comparisons were made with the earlier study, the mean callosal thickness was less than before, a fact that was attributed to the lower age of the patients of the previous report. The authors speculated that the abnormality may reflect increased tissue volume that is due to a subclinical viral infection and that resolves later, after cell loss. The callosal transmission hypothesis will be returned to in the discussion of the behavioral approaches that follows.

III. Experimental Approaches

A. Neuropsychiatry

1. HANDEDNESS

An obvious sign of possible lateral reorganization in hemispheric specialization is sinistrality or ambidexterity. Whereas about 96% of dextrals are left hemisphere dominant for linguistic abilities, it is estimated that this dominance holds for only 60% of sinistrals, with speech lateralized to the right hemisphere in 20% and bilateral speech in the remaining 20% (Satz, 1980). Although there have been numerous reports on the handedness of schizophrenic patients, the simplicity of the approach is coming under increasing scrutiny (Taylor *et al.*, 1982), especially because findings have been far from conclusive. There are reports of a higher incidence of sinistrality in schizophrenia (Dvirskii, 1976; Gur, 1977; Flor- Henry, 1979), of stronger dextrality (Bolin, 1953; Fleminger *et al.*, 1977), and of no difference from controls (Chandler, 1934; Oddy and Lobstein, 1972; Wahl, 1976; Kameyama *et al.*, 1983). There is also anecdotal evidence of reversals in handedness with different phases of illness (Flor-Henry, 1979).

Similarly, reports on eye dominance and its degree of concordance with handedness in schizophrenia are inconclusive (Chandler, 1934; Oddy and Lobstein, 1972; Lishman and McMeekan, 1975; Gur, 1977; Kameyama *et al.*, 1983). Taylor *et al.* (1982) made adjustments for differences in methods and sampling in two apparently discrepant reports (Lishman and McMeekan, 1976; Fleminger *et al.*, 1977) and concluded that "there was no overall excess of left-handedness among schizophrenics, but trends towards excess sinistrality in men and full dextrality in women approached significance [p. 166]." This reinforces the view expressed elsewhere (Gruzelier, 1981b) that differences in handedness between patients and controls are marginal at best and that the measure is therefore rather insensitive to altered cerebral organization in psychopathology. Shifts in lateral organization may well occur, but handedness may be too crude a measure to reflect them.

These qualifications aside, handedness has been shown to have a bearing on schizophrenia in twins and may thus play a part in pathogenesis in some patients. There is agreement in studies by Boklage (1977) and Luchins *et al.* (1980) that less severe forms of psychosis occur in sinistral twin pairs, or when one of a pair is sinistral, than in dextral pairs. If twins are discordant for schizophrenia and handedness, the psychotic twin tends to be left-handed rather than right-handed. Not all the implications are genetic, however. Luchins *et al.* observed that the psychotic twin of right-handed pairs discordant for schizophrenia had the lower birth weight, suggesting the possible contribution of intrauterine factors. Whereas the association of sinistrality and psychosis supports the abnormal lateralization hypothesis, the authors noted that a failure to develop clear lateralization predisposes an individual to a wide range of psychopathologies (Zangwill, 1960). Thus where sinistrality occurs in the absence of a family history, persuasive evidence is provided by altered cerebral organization.

2. ORGANIC LESIONS

Etiological implications are taken a stage farther in Taylor's (1975) study of temporal lobe epileptics who had undergone temporal lobectomy. Cases of "alien tissue," such as small tumors, hematomas, and focal dysphasia, in the resected lobe were compared with those of sclerosis on demographic and clinical variables, and significant differences were found in handedness, gender, and incidence of schizophrenic-like psychosis. Psychosis was more common in the alien tissue group, and sinistrality occurred in just over half of the psychotic cases but only in about one-seventh of the nonpsychotic cases. Trends suggested that the likelihood of psychosis was increased in left-handed lesion cases and in women. Taylor suggested that, although it is unlikely that alien tissue per se produces psychosis, alien tissue tends to be more discrete than sclerotic tissue and a nonfunctional lobe may withstand psychosis better than a dysfunctional one. Given that many alien tissue lesions occur at early stages of brain development, the relatively late occurrence of psychosis may involve the breakdown of compensatory mechanisms. This breakdown may be due to a variety of factors such as aging and may be facilitated by the "unusual" organization of cerebral functions reflected in sinistrality.

3. NEUROPSYCHOLOGICAL TESTS

Neuropsychological test batteries have proved to be remarkably sensitive to dysfunction. Filskov and Goldstein (1974), for example, reported that the Halstead–Reitan battery was superior to angiography, electroencephalography, air-encephalography, and brain scan and X-ray techniques in diagnosing brain damage in 171 heterogeneous neurological cases. This approach, however, is not without pitfalls, although some common reservations may be unwarranted. One is the view that these tests are inapplicable to psychiatry because they have been validated on neurological patients. This objection is illogical. More to the point is whether the tests in current use are effective in detecting a subtle neurotransmitter imbalance that may well underly psychosis, as opposed to the comparatively gross lesions caused by sclerosis, hematomas, ventricular enlargement; and so on. It is apparent, for example, that a fair number of patients do not score over the cutoff points denoting "impairment," and exactly what "impairment" means in process terms is not clear.

Although the distinction between dynamic and fixed processes has little currency in clinical neuropsychology, it may well turn out to be a key issue in the applicability of such tests to schizophrenia. Different etiologies within a narrowly defined brain region may have different consequences for psychological function, a current concern in amnesia research (Butters and Cermak, 1980). Bingley (1958) and colleagues differentiated between tumors and epileptic foci of the temporal lobe and showed that generalized slowness in the former and perseveration in the latter produced identical scores on some tests. Etiological implications apart from this example also indicate that psychological tests are seldom pure in process terms. The complete results of a battery of tests are usually required if interpretations are to be valid. Even so, as Boll (1981) cautioned in relation to the lateralizing implications of many tests included in the Halstead–Reitan, "parts of neuropsychological test batteries . . . despite clinical hunches to the contrary, have been found equally sensitive to right, left and generalized brain impairment and not specifically indicative of lateralization or location of cerebral lesion [p. 602]."

Gruzelier and Hammond (1976) conducted a 12-week study of chronic hospitalized male schizophrenic patients stabilized by means of chlorpromazine, the sole medication. Patients were examined 4 weeks after stabilization, 4 weeks after chlorpromazine had been replaced by a matched placebo, and 4 weeks after chlorpromazine had been reinstated in the original dose. A battery of measures testing largely auditory functions was administered (Section III, B, 1) and performance on the Wechsler Adult Intelligence Scale (WAIS) was examined for evidence of lateralized pathology. The WAIS was administered at the end of the 12-week period, when the laboratory procedures had become a regular, and in most cases a looked forward to, event. Performance on the right hemisphere function tests of block design and object assembly was superior to that on the left hemisphere function tests of vocabulary, comprehension, and similarities. This discrepancy between visuospatial and verbal abilities was mirrored in the performance of the offspring of schizophrenic parents on the children's version of the test but not to the same extent in the offspring of parents with other forms of psychiatric disorder or without psychopathology (Gruzelier *et al.*, 1979).

The WAIS and an extensive neuropsychological battery including the Halstead–Reitan were employed in Flor-Henry and Yeudall's (1979) examination of 114 consecutive referrals with schizophrenia, mania, hypomania, or depression, about half of whom were medicated. Nondominant hemisphere dysfunction was implicated in schizophrenia, mania, and depression and did not distinguish the psychoses. Schizophrenia, however, was differentiated by virtue of dominant hemisphere disturbance. Although parietal involvement failed to distinguish schizophrenia from affective disorders, when patients were classified according to the relative degree of left- or right-sided impairment, 41 of 53 schizophrenics showed greater left-sided involvement in the frontotemporal region, and 41 of 49 affective disorders showed the opposite asymmetry. Severity of dysfunction proved to be critical for lateralized pathology, with consistent laterality effects emerging only in severe cases and involving the frontal region more than the temporal. The finding that "The strongest association relates schizophrenia to left frontal dysfunction [p. 347]." constitutes a departure from Flor-Henry's original model, placing the target area for schizophrenia in severe cases in the left frontal rather than temporal region.

Abrams and Taylor (1979), using the Halstead–Wepman Aphasia Screening Test and the Trail Making Test with 191 patients, of whom 31 were schizophrenic, 120 manic, and 40 depressed, confirmed some of Flor-Henry and Yeudall's schizophrenic–affective distinctions. Although unable to demonstrate a marked association between left frontal dysfunction and schizophrenia, they found that, whereas all groups showed bilateral impairment, the schizophrenics showed three times the dominant temporal and parietal dysfunction of the affective disorders.

Silverstein (1983) reported preliminary findings on 44 schizophrenic patients [Research Diagnostic Criteria (RDC), (Spitzer and Robins, 1975)], and 31 with schizoaffective or affective disorders. On administration of the Luria–Nebraska battery, patients were categorized as neuropsychologically intact or impaired (Golden *et al.*, 1982); 18 schizophrenic and 14 affective patients fell in the former category, and 26 schizophrenic and 17 affective patients in the latter. Patients in the two categories were comparable in age, sex, and drug status, but patients in the impaired group included more non-Caucasians and sinistrals and were more chronic and less well educated. A subgroup of these patients, too small to warrant discussion here, was also tested on the Halstead–Reitan battery.

Lateralized dysfunction was shown on the left in only six schizophrenic and five affective patients and on the right in eight schizophrenic and six affective patients. Evidence of elevated left frontal pathology in schizophrenia differentiated between diagnostic groups. There were nonsignificant tendencies for schizophrenic patients to score higher on left sensorimotor and parietal–occipital scales and affective patients on equivalent right hemisphere scales. The premorbid adjustment of impaired patients was poorer, a result in keeping with demographic differences. Clinical improvement on the BPRS was more marked in the impaired patients, a counterintuitive result that questions the extent to which factors such as education, practice, motivation, and intelligence may have confounded performance on the first test occasion. It is noteworthy that the battery was insensitive to dysfunction in 59% of schizophrenic patients; the left frontal region was implicated in some.

Scarone *et al.* (1981, 1983) employed the Short Aphasia Screening Test of Heinburger and Reitan (1961) and the Quality Extinction Test (Schwartz *et al.*, 1977, 1979), which involves simultaneous bilateral palmar stimulation with different textures. Schwartz and colleagues showed that a loss of right hand sensitivity (right extinction) almost always follows left hemisphere damage and involves the parietal region, whereas left extinction accompanies lesions of either hemisphere, showing particular prevalence with right parietal involvement but also accompanying left parietal and left frontal damage. Tactile extinction, therefore, is open to a number of interpretations, and the need for a patterning approach incorporating tests of aphasia is clear.

In a letter to the *British Journal of Psychiatry,* Scarone *et al.*(1981) summarized the results of a study of 30 schizophrenic patients and 30 handedness- and age-matched controls. Patients made 97 dominant hemisphere errors and no nondominant hemisphere errors on the tactile test and 63 dominant and 17 nondominant errors on the aphasia test. In combination, the results were interpreted as reflecting left frontal dysfunction. A larger study of 91 schizophrenic patients and 60 controls subdivided according to age (Scarone *et al.*, 1983) found a higher number of extinctions in patients than in controls and no deficit in just over 50% of controls (35 of 60) and under 25% of patients (20 of 91). Left extinction, more common than right in both groups, was shown by approximately 55% of patients and 25% of controls. This contrasted with right extinction, found in only 20 of 91 patients and 8 of 60 controls. Apart from the higher incidence of extinction in patients, there was also an age effect, with right extinction occurring more frequently in patients under the age of 29 years and left in patients over the age of 40 years.

These results, in light of the neurological evidence of Schwartz, may be variously interpreted. There is little doubt that the right extinction is almost certain to result from left hemisphere dysfunction; hence, left parietal involvement is clearly implicated in the younger patients. The more frequent left extinction, however, may result from right parietal, left parietal, left frontal, or, conceivably, right frontal disturbance. Some elucidation is offered by the aphasia test, which, by including left hemisphere writing abilities and right hemisphere geometric abilities, is sensitive to bilateral parietal damage. Geometric errors in the absence of writing errors were made by 24 patients, 17 of whom showed left extinction. Right hemisphere involvement is thus indicated on both counts. Seven patients made writing errors only, implying a left hemisphere locus for the extinction phenomenon, and 18 made both geometric and writing errors, implying bilateral involvement. The authors's interpretation of left hemisphere dysfunction in schizophrenia, therefore, appears to hold for the majority of younger patients but for only a minority of patients over the age of 40 years.

The age effect might indicate a transition from one state of hemispheric imbalance to the other or a spread of pathological influences beginning on the left and progressively involving the right. Alternatively, the test may reflect different dynamic-process asymmetries in focused attention which may coincide with different subtypes of schizophrenia. Prognosis is indicative here. One might infer that, by and large, younger patients have a good prognosis and present an acute, remitting syndrome, whereas older patients, whose chronicity is evidence of poor prognosis, present a classical schizophrenic syndrome. It is not clear how sensory inattention of the right hand might coincide with left hemisphere overactivation and inattention of the left hand with right hemisphere overactivation—premises of the model offered in Section I—unless it is postulated that overactivation leads to an occlusion of contralateral somatosensory pathways.

The studies reviewed in this section promote the impression that the more extensive the test battery, the greater the likelihood that bilateral impairment will feature in the results. Whether this is a reflection of schizophrenia generally or of schizophrenic subtypes is not clarified by the methodological approaches adopted to date. The majority of approaches support left temporoparietal involvement that extends to the frontal area in schizophrenia in which either neuropsychological dysfunction or symptoms are severe. Further delineation of the correspondence between regional involvement and syndromes is required and the failure of the conventional test batteries to detect dysfunction in many patients suggests the need for more flexible approaches with sensitive measures.

B. Experimental Psychology

1. AUDITORY STUDIES

Auditory functions in schizophrenia have received the most extensive and penetrating examination of all laterality issues, a reflection of the interest engendered by the predominantly auditory phenomenology of schizophrenia and the temporal lobe involvement implied by the early reports on organic lesions. The present treatment of auditory studies is subdivided according to some of the themes that are emerging.

a. Left Hemisphere Temporal Variation and a Limbic Locus. In an examination of bilateral auditory acuity, preliminary to tests of higher-level function, chronic schizophrenic patients being treated with chlorpromazine showed better right than left ear acuity (Gruzelier and Hammond, 1976). Curiously, when examined 8 and 12 weeks later the right ear showed progressive loss of acuity, whereas the left ear remained stable. The first retest was performed in the fourth week of drug withdrawal, and the second 4 weeks after drug reinstatement; neither withdrawal of the drug nor recrudescence of symptoms affected acuity. The ear difference was found to be reliable for 2 years and was shown to reflect sensory rather than cognitive factors. Acute patients showed the effect, and temporal variation in right ear sensitivity was found in the course of the day (Gruzelier and Hammond, 1979a).

In a replication study Kugler *et al.* (1982) examined the auditory thresholds of 20 chronic schizophrenic patients in a drug trial comparing pindolol and placebo as adjuvants to conventional neuroleptics. Patients were examined on four occasions spanning 30 weeks. Initially, right ear acuity was superior to left ear acuity, after which there was a linear decline in right ear acuity while left ear thresholds remained stable.

In Pavlovian personality theory (e.g., Gray,1964) some individuals are typified as more susceptible to stimulation, with low absolute thresholds, and as more susceptible to fatigue with continuing stimulation. These dynamics characterize the right ear thresholds of schizophrenic patients and, assuming the functional dominance of contralateral pathways, reflect left hemisphere functions. The locus of the dysfunction, along with some other psychophysiological phenomena in schizophrenia, was attributed to hippocampal–reticular influences (see Gruzelier, 1978, 1979b, for reviews). Since Pavlov, a susceptibility to inhibition has been ascribed to schizophrenia (Epstein and Coleman, 1970) and, more recently, to nonparanoid patients (Gruzelier *et al.*, 1972). Concurrent monitoring of electrodermal activity by Gruzelier and Hammond (1979b) revealed greater interaural threshold differences in less reactive patients. Thus, an asymmetry in dynamic processes is represented. This asymmetry, which denotes an inhibitory left hemisphere susceptible to fatigue, is enhanced in poor-prognosis, autonomically unresponsive, and nonparanoid patients. All three features are consistent with the retarded syndrome outlined in Section I, as is the depiction of an inhibitory left hemisphere.

Japanese investigators (Niwa *et al.*, 1983) also have reported data illustrating a lateralized auditory processing decrement over time. In the first experiment 11 RDC-diagnosed schizophrenic patients were required to detect a target sound presented in a random sequence with non-target sounds at interstimulus intervals of 2 sec. The stimuli were pitch contours and consisted of a 50-msec frequency-modulated sound followed by a tone burst of 100 msec. The counterbalancing of two target stimuli (500 or 100 Hz), one per condition, together with requirements to direct attention to either ear and manual responses of either hand gave eight conditions, which were presented in a fixed order. The most marked difference between patients and controls was in the detection of the 1000-Hz sequence; not only was patient performance poorer overall, but patients showed a laterality effect in the direction of poorer right ear detection. Reaction times to correct response showed no laterality differences.

Although the right ear loss was attributed to left hemisphere inability to sustain vigilance (Dimond and Beaumont, 1973) and interhemispheric pathway incompetency in modulating attention (Dimond, 1976; Ellenberg and Sperry, 1979), other interpretations are plausible. In fact, there was no evidence of poorer performance accompanying responses of the hand ipsilateral to the attended ear, an effect that would be expected in both patients and controls if interhemispheric control mechanisms were critical. Although performance was poorest under the condition in which attention was focused on the right ear, this condition unfortunately was the last tested in all subjects, and the lateral decrement may therefore reflect order.

The last issue was clarified in a follow-up experiment in which 14 medicated schizophrenic patients, diagnosed with Diagnostic and Statistical Manual III (DSM III), were compared with 17 normal controls. This time, 1000-Hz sounds were presented, and responses were made with the hand ipsilateral to the attended ear in a counterbalanced design. A detection index was computed combining errors of omission and commission. As before, poor right ear performance was found in the patient group. This was most marked in the last three of the five right ear conditions and was not paralleled by performance decrements in the corresponding left ear conditions. It is also of interest that right ear performance in the first condition was, on the average, superior to left ear performance. Thus, on two counts the temporal variation in right ear detection is consistent with the auditory threshold data.

Kugler (1983) adopted a configurational approach based on diagnostic audiometric techniques incorporating tests of pure tone sensitivity, impedance, auditory adaptation, and speech discrimination. Five patients from the preceding study (Kugler *et al.*, 1982) were examined with five additional patients who were male, chronic, and dextral. Nine had nuclear schizophrenia and one paranoid schizophrenia (Wing *et al.*, 1974). All were medicated, and comparisons were made with 10 normal controls.

As before, patients showed better right than left ear absolute thresholds. Impedance audiometry conducted on half the patients revealed no evidence of middle ear disorders. A tone decay test showed none of the auditory adaptation difficulties that characterize cochlear or seventh nerve damage. The Synthetic Sentence Identification Test (Jerger, 1973), whereby competing messages at various intensity levels are presented to the same or contralateral ear, produced evidence consistent with dysfunction of the temporal lobe rather than the brainstem: schizophrenic patients, like temporal lobe patients, produced bilateral speech perception deficits, which were more apparent with dichotic than monaural hearing, the reverse of that expected in brainstem disorders. The last result was substantiated with a dichotic phoneme identification test wherein phonemes with different initial stop consonants were judged to be the same or different, a task chosen because phonemic hearing and discrimination of stop consonants are both left hemisphere abilities (Luria, 1973; Brown and Deffenbacher, 1979). Of the 10 patients, 5 were unable to do the task because all phonemes sounded identical to them. Of the remainder, 4 of 5 failed to show the normal right ear advantage, and their performance was reduced bilaterally.

Thus, the pattern of results obtained in Kugler's small group of chronic patients was consistent with temporal lobe dysfunction as distinct from peripheral or brainstem disorders. It could also be tentatively distinguished from callosal damage and, in the light of Noffsinger and Kurdziel's (1979) survey of central nervous system auditory dysfunction, localized to either diffuse left hemisphere damage or left posterior temporoparietal damage rather than an anterior locus. This interpretation must be treated cautiously because a larger study with less chronic patients (Kugler and Caudrey, 1983) produced different results. Neither study showed an ear asymmetry but, whereas Kugler reported a bilateral decrement, Kugler and Caudrey found that right ear performance was reduced to the level of unimpaired left ear ability. The latter result would be compatible with left anterior temporal or temporofrontal damage.

In a study overlapping that of Kugler (1983), 15 schizophrenic patients were compared with 10 normal controls on Hebb's Recurring Digits Test, which examines left hemisphere short- and long-term memory processes. The groups were matched by digit span for short-term memory capacity. As expected, the normal subjects showed cumulative learning of recurring strings of digits that exceed by 1 each individual's immediate memory span. Such learning was absent in schizophrenic patients and was indicative of a long-term memory deficit. Examining patients with various degrees of hippocampal damage, Corsi (1967) showed performance on this test to be negatively correlated with the extent of left hippocampal lesions. Again, limbic dysfunction in the form of hippocampal involvement is implicated in schizophrenia.

Green and Kotenko (1980) required subjects to listen to monaurally and binaurally presented stories and to answer corresponding questions. Twenty patients on maintenance medication were selected on the basis of a hospital diagnosis of schizophrenia and case history evidence of Schneiderian auditory hallucinations. Comparisons were made with 10 normal and 10 neurotic controls, half of the latter being drug free. Four schizophrenic patients were excluded retrospectively, two because of poor overall performance and two because they obtained distinct left ear advantages on the test. Following these exclusions, schizophrenic patients showed poorer left than right ear performance, an asymmetry not shared by the control groups. Larger than normal left ear deficits in schizophrenia were confirmed with a laterality index, which also showed that the effect was particularly marked in female schizophrenic patients. Unexpectedly, whereas control subjects performed better when stories were presented to both ears, schizophrenic patients performed worst of all in the binaural condition, a result that implies a problem in integrating input from two auditory channels. Green and Kotenko interpreted their findings as evidence of defective callosal transmission in schizophrenia.

Kugler (1983) reviewed an unsuccessful attempt to replicate the preceding study, which reported a bilateral deficit in schizophrenia in the absence of the previously reported asymmetry (Abbott, 1982). Reasoning that simultaneous presentation of different, and hence competing, stories in a dichotic listening task should be especially sensitive to ear dominance and general performance deficit effects, Kugler and C. Green (see Kugler, 1983) tested subjects under two conditions. In one, subjects were asked to listen to both competing stories and, in the other, to shadow one story while ignoring the other. Checklists of words from both stories, occurring at approximately equal intervals within the stories but not time-aligned to overlap, were presented before comprehension testing. In both conditions, schizophrenic patients did not differ from controls in word recognition but were poorer at comprehension. In the shadowing condition, whereas 67% of patients and 58% of controls showed a right ear advantage for comprehension, the main group interaural difference was significant only for the controls, suggesting that the right ear advantage in patients was negligible. Groups differed in comprehension performance over time, controls scoring higher on questions relating to the second half of the story and patients scoring lower. Otherwise, the number of word intrusions from the unattended channel was similar for both groups, suggesting that patients had no more difficulty than controls in directing attention to one ear or the other. The temporal variation in patients' performance is consistent with a deficient left hemisphere dynamic process, although in the absence of a right hemisphere task the specificity of this deficit is not tested.

Green and Kotenko (1980) raised the possibility of atypical right hemisphere speech lateralization in a subgroup of schizophrenic patients. A similar implication about subgrouping can be drawn from the report of Colbourn and Lishman (1979), who tested normal controls and patients on a left hemisphere verbal task, namely, recognition of syllable pairs comprising a stop consonant and vowel, and a right hemisphere nonverbal task, namely, recognition of tone contours. Schizophrenic, manic–depressive, neurotic, and psychopathic patients (diagnoses according to PSE criteria) were medicated, and florid symptoms were controlled. On the nonverbal task the schizophrenic patients were no different from controls. On the verbal dichotic task the 16 schizophrenic patients exhibited no mean ear preference in contrast to all other groups, who showed the expected right ear advantage. Comparisons of the two ears separately indicated that the groups differed only for the right ear. However, when individual results were examined a more complex impression emerged. The reduction in right ear performance was especially true of male schizophrenic patients; females, in fact, showed a right ear advantage ($N=5$). When reliable ear differences were considered, a bimodal distribution in male patients was found, with five showing a reliable left ear advantage and two a right ear advantage, in keeping with the left hemisphere nature of the task. Thus, a larger proportion of male schizophrenic patients showed a right hemisphere advantage for an essentially verbal task.

Finally, Yozawitz *et al.* (1979) employed a clinical audiometry test to examine hospitalized patients who were medicated but apparently refractory to treatment as indicated by the continued presence of marked psychotic symptoms. Ten schizophrenic and 9 affective patients were compared with 10 normal controls and 2 patients with right temporal lesions. On the Staggered Spondaic Word Test, in which dichotically presented words are staggered so that the last syllable of the first word overlaps the second syllable of the second, reduced accuracy in the contralateral ear was expected in the presence of structural brain disorder. Accordingly, the normal group was virtually error free, whereas the right temporal patients showed reduced left ear performance. Reduced left ear performance also characterized affective, but not schizophrenic patients. In schizophrenia the performance of both ears was reduced, possibly reflecting a general, non-lateralized performance decrement or, alternatively, deficient left hemisphere word comprehension. Because no patients with left temporal lesions were tested, these interpretations are untested. On a dichotic click perception test no evidence of impairment was found in schizophrenic patients, whereas affective patients again showed the same results as right temporal patients.

In summary, evidence has accumulated supporting a temporal decrement in left hemisphere auditory functions in schizophrenia influencing low and high levels of processing (Gruzelier and Hammond, 1976, 1979a; Kugler *et al.*, 1982; Kugler, 1983; Niwa *et al.*, 1983). The locus of dysfunction appears to reside in temporolimbic systems, with the hippocampus repeatedly implicated with respect to asymmetries of fixed structure

(Kugler, 1983) and dynamic process (Gruzelier, 1978). Evidence recurs of subgroups of patients with verbal processing asymmetry opposite to that of the majority, suggesting a reliance on right hemipshere linguistic functions. In general, no deficit is found with right hemisphere functions of either a dynamic or a fixed nature, and problems of interhemispheric connections arose only in the study of Green and Kotenko (1980), in which greater deficits were apparent with binaural than with monaural hearing.

b. Left Hemisphere Overactivation in Paranoid Schizophrenia: A Trait Factor. A clear distinction has emerged between paranoid and nonparanoid patients in dichotic listening studies of cerebral asymmetries. Lerner *et al.* (1977) examined 30 paranoid and 30 nonparanoid schizophrenic patients, two-thirds of each group being acute, and compared them with 20 normal controls. The groups were equated for gender, and all patients were medicated. The dichotic test consisted of strings of three or four digits. Recall was inferior in patients generally, but there was no difference between paranoid and nonparanoid patients, although paranoid patients showed a larger right ear preference ($\bar{x} = 38.56$) than nonparanoid patients ($\bar{x} = 17.53$), who in turn showed a larger preference than controls ($\bar{x} = 10.25$). Calculating the number of shifts in attention by the number of alternations between left and right ear in order of recall, fewer shifts of attention away from the right ear ($\bar{x} = 2.50$) occurred in paranoid than occurred in nonparanoid patients ($\bar{x} = 8.42$), who did not differ from controls ($\bar{x} = 10.32$). This is consistent with a left hemisphere bias in paranoid patients. The acute–chronic distinction produced no significant differences. Exaggerated right ear preferences in patients were later interpreted (Nachson, 1980) as compatible with left hemisphere overactivation in schizophrenia, a proposition questioned by Walker *et al.* (1981), who preferred a callosal impairment hypothesis.

A similar technique was incorporated by Gruzelier and Hammond (1976, 1978) in their chlorpromazine withdrawal study. In addition to examining free recall, they manipulated attentional bias through instructions and varied stimulus intensity between the ears. The outcome of such strategies resolves the theoretical dispute between Nachson and Walker *et al.*

In comparing normal controls with the 18 patients, all of whom were well familiarized with the task beforehand, there was no group difference in ear advantages, and the withdrawal and reinstatement of the drug had no effect on ear differences in free recall. When patients were subgrouped according to evidence of delusions in their present state, evidence of a paranoid subdiagnosis in their case history, and electrodermal responsiveness, larger differences in favor of the right ear were found in some subgroups. There was a tendency for electrodermally responsive patients to show larger ear differences than nonresponsive patients, with reduced left ear recall in responsive patients lowering overall performance. Patients with a paranoid subdiagnosis similarly showed larger right ear preferences (24.7%) than nonparanoid patients (−0.41%), yet their level of performance in free recall was superior to that of nonparanoid patients: $\bar{x}$ =77% for paranoid and $\bar{x}$ =65% nonparanoid patients. The presence of delusions had no bearing on ear differences. Thus, paranoid patients showed an exaggerated right ear bias in line with Lerner *et al.*, as did autonomically reactive patients, who in most cases had paranoid subdiagnoses.

In agreement with other reports, patients in general were able to direct their attention to either ear as effectively as controls, and inequalities of intensity had no substantial impact on performance. However, when the order of recall was in competition with differences in intensity—in other words, when the recall of louder digits was to be withheld until quieter ones had been recalled—schizophrenic patients showed impairment in withholding louder right ear words in favor of left ear words, an effect true of 13 of 18 patients. Controls showed the reverse tendency, namely, greater difficulty in withholding louder left ear words in favor of right ear words, a result true of 10 of 16 subjects. Thus, patients showed a suppression deficit implicating left hemisphere inhibitory processes, the opposite tendency to controls.

Serial position curves were examined to shed light on processing strategies. The curves of controls were bow-shaped, exhibiting superior recall of the first digit heard (primacy) and of the last digit heard (recency). The curves of patients were asymmetric, depending on recency more than controls and revealing an absence of primacy from one ear at a time. This appeared to reflect a reliance on automatic storage processes in patients that might involve low-level phonemic encoding due to a deficiency in higher-level semantic (left hemisphere) encoding.

Turning to the effects of focused attention and intensity differences on the paranoid–nonparanoid classification, when there were no instructions to direct attention paranoid patients behaved as if instructions had been given to focus on the right ear. The same ear bias was just as pronounced with inequalities of intensity. Despite a 20-dB advantage to the left ear, the effect on recall was marginal. In contrast, nonparanoid patients were capable of larger left ear advantages than either normal controls or paranoid patients under the condition in which words were louder in the left ear. An analysis of shifts in attention between the ears supported the interpretation of a right ear bias in paranoid schizophrenia and the results of Lerner *et al.* Evidence of the reversible nature of the right ear bias rules out the view of Walker *et al.* (1981) that the ear advantage represents structural impairment in callosal transmission and instead places the phenomenon in the class of dynamic-process asymmetries. The inability to suppress the recall of louder right ear words in favor of quieter left ear words suggests an impairment in an inhibitory mechanism with origins either in the left hemisphere or in a transcallosal inhibitory mechanism that leads to an overactivation of left hemispheric processes.

Diagnostic issues are also relevant to the results of a dichotic test used by Lishman *et al.* (1978) examining recall of triplets of monosyllabic consonant–vowel–consonant common words. Fifteen staff members, 15 schizophrenic patients, of whom 7 were paranoid, and 13 affective patients, of whom 10 showed manic features, were tested. Florid symptoms had been contained by medication to the extent that 4 patients were in complete remission and the remainder had only residual symptoms. They were either outpatients or were awaiting discharge. On the whole, recall was poorer in patients but, after due allowance for this, a larger than normal right ear advantage was found to be a reliable characteristic of psychosis. When subgroups were examined, the ear advantage was reliably found only with males. Within the schizophrenic group suggestive trends indicated that complete remission, an absence of auditory hallucinations in the case history, and a family history of schizophrenia were factors associated with normal asymmetries.

Approximately half of the schizophrenic patients were paranoid, and the results are thus consistent with those of the previously described studies. The relation between the right ear advantage and symptoms reported in the medical histories accords with the report of Gruzelier and Hammond. Trait factors as well as current state (electrodermal responsiveness) are implicated in these findings, an erstwhile diagnosis of paranoid schizophrenia in the Gruzelier and Hammond study and evidence of auditory hallucinations in the study by Lishman *et al.* In fact, as expounded in the next section, there is evidence that acute symptoms on admission to hospital sometimes coincide with an absence of normal asymmetries.

c. Hemispheric Equivalence and Acute Symptoms. By examining acute patients twice weekly throughout their hospital stay, Wexler and Heninger (1979) traced the association between asymmetric function and symptom exacerbation and recovery. They examined RDC-diagnosed psychotic patients admitted to a research ward initially drug free and, subsequently, in all but a few cases, on medication. Patients were schizophrenic ($N=8$), were schizoaffective ($N=6$), or had a primary depressive disorder ($N=12$). Tests involved the recall of dichotically presented nonsense syllables consisting of stop consonants preceded and followed by the vowel *a*.

There was no overall difference between patients and 23 normal controls. The estimate of asymmetry (laterality index) proved to be reliable, as shown by high test–retest correlations within weeks in patients and throughout the study in controls. Five patients (diagnoses unspecified) consistently had left ear preferences. Nevertheless, on the whole, ear differences in patients were labile, with the emergence of the normal right ear advantage on recovery.

The relationship between symptoms and shifts in lateral organization was elucidated by regarding one as a dependent variable and the other as an independent variable, and vice versa, and comparing times of maximum and minimum laterality in one analysis and symptom severity in another. Ratings of global illness showed important relations to laterality. Ear advantages were lost when symptoms were most severe. Otherwise, some individual symptoms showed a relationship when in the role of dependent variable. These included both positive and negative symptoms (Crow, 1980) but were predominantly of the positive type: paranoid behavior, hallucinations, odd and unusual thoughts, thought disorder, verbal anxiety, and expressed anger (positive) and psychomotor retardation and depressive mood (negative). Again ratings were highest when lateral differences were minimal.

Features of this report were replicated by Johnson and Crockett (1982), who examined 16 control subjects and 32 DSM III-diagnosed patients, 16 with schizophrenia and 16 with a major depressive disorder. Patients were examined unmedicated on admission to hospital, up to 2 weeks on medication before discharge, and up to 4 weeks on medication, when symptoms on both DSM III and the Beck Depression Scale had fallen to within normal limits. Tests of verbal fluency and spatial perceptual ability were administered in addition to a dichotic test involving words and musical chords. Patients showed no deficits in verbal fluency and, somewhat curiously, depressive patients were more fluent than controls. No evidence was found of left frontal dysfunction, which would have been indicated by an impairment in verbal fluency (see Section III,A,3). In contrast to these results both patient groups showed impairment of spatial ability, an impairment that implies right hemisphere dysfunction. The authors' attempt to discount the latter implication is unconvincing in that their explanation of psychomotor retardation should apply equally to verbal fluency, unless the retardation was hemisphere specific, in which case the right hemisphere would again be implicated. Performance on these tests, which have been used to reflect fixed-structural anomalies, did not vary with medication, a finding that is consistent with the view that medication influences dynamic rather than fixed processes (see Section IV).

Performance on the dichotic tests did vary with symptomatic improvement. Depressed patients showed no consistent group asymmetry at first but did show appropriate ear advantages for words and chords on recovery. In contrast, schizophrenic patients on admission showed an appropriate left ear advantage for chords and no ear advantage for words and, on recovery, an appropriate left ear advantage for words but an inappropriate one for chords. Levels of ability in both dichotic tasks did not vary.

One interpretation would be that, in schizophrenia, allocation of attention to the right ear was altered by medication or recovery, resulting in an inflexible left hemisphere advantage for words and chords, whereas, in depression, expected hemisphere advantages and a corresponding flexibility in directing attention were restored. Given that the schizophrenic patients were of the remitting type, a left hemisphere bias for stimuli that are ordinarily processed by the right hemisphere is consistent with the model outlined in Section I.

d. Lateralized Drug Influences. In their chlorpromazine study Hammond and Gruzelier (1978) had utilized an auditory detection task with some features in common with the task of Niwa *et al.* (1983) (Section III,B,1,a). Patients detected target tones randomly presented within a sequence of standard tones. Standard tones were of 1000 Hz, 80 dB, and 100 msec, and target tones differed in duration, being of 150, 200, or 300 msec. The tones were presented monaurally. The level of difficulty was determined by an acceptable level of performance (about 75% correct) in practice trials. In separate conditions the rate at which the target switched from ear to ear was set at 0.3 or 0.7 and the rate of presentation at 1 or 2 tones per second. Subjects changed hands halfway through the session. Patients were compared with normal controls and nonpsychotic patients. Schizophrenic patients were tested on six occasions at fortnightly intervals, twice while being treated with chlorpromazine, twice while being treated with a placebo, and twice after the reinstatement of drug treatment.

Whereas performance remained constant across sessions, the relative performance of the two ears altered in that, if the sessions were ordered from maximum time on placebo to maximum time on continuous chlorpromazine administration, right ear performance, compared with left ear performance, improved with increasing drug dosage. The degree of lateral asymmetry, computed as a laterality index, correlated with drug dose both on drug and on placebo. The higher the dose, the larger the right ear advantage on drug and the right ear decrement on placebo. Thus the neuroleptic produced an advantage in left hemisphere processing.

There were no laterality effects in other groups and, unlike other subjects, schizophrenic patients were not affected by the rate at which the target switched from ear to ear, but were impaired by the increase in presentation rate, which improved performance in other groups. This prompted the conclusion that problems in the selection and organization of responses, rather than in shifting attention, influenced the performance of schizophrenic patients on this task.

A bias toward left hemispheric processes in patients on medication is also mentioned later (Section III,C,3) in relation to the behavioral tests Goode *et al.* (1979) ran in conjunction with the Hoffman reflex. Similarly, Wexler and Heninger (1979), although finding no lateralized effects of lithium carbonate or tricyclics, did find an increase in lateral asymmetry in the direction of a left hemisphere advantage that approached significance.

2. SOMESTHETIC STUDIES AND THE CALLOSAL HYPOTHESIS

With few exceptions, tests of somesthetic function have involved intermanual transfer and have been designed to test the hypothesis of impaired callosal transmission. Green (1978) compared 20 mainly outpatient medicated schizophrenic patients with 18 neurotic patients and 20 nurse controls. Subjects had to learn without looking to which box a series of objects belonged. Feedback in the form of a hand tap was given to the same or opposite hand. The number of trials to a criterion of 100% success was calculated for each of four possible conditions. The stability of learning was also examined by both reversing and repeating hands and noting errors and the number of retraining trials required if mistakes were made. Schizophrenic patients required more trials to criterion in the two-handed conditions and more relearning trials when reversing hands than when repeating hands. None of these difficulties were experienced by the comparison groups. Although the results were interpreted as evidence for deficiencies in interhemispheric transfer, other explanations in terms of drugs, task complexity, and intelligence were tenable.

Carr (1980) examined 10 chronic, medicated, schizophrenic patients and 10 controls matched for sex, handedness, age, socioeconomic status, and employment. Blindfolded subjects were required to remember which of an array of objects had been presented up to 3 min previously. Patients made more errors when the retention interval increased, when recognition involved intermanual transfer, and when objects were unfamiliar. With the exception of the one involving intermanual transfer, these difficulties were also experienced by controls.

Dimond *et al.* (1980) examined 24 institutionalized schizophrenic patients with a mean age of 52 years and made comparisons with 6 patients with severe anxiety or depressive illnesses requiring long-term care and 6 normal controls. Tests included touch localization on both the finger and lateral body surfaces, hand tapping with or without intermanual transfer, and touch localization of the hand and forearm for which transfer was required. In most instances the results are difficult to evaluate because the errors for all subjects were pooled, and thus a few unrepresentative subjects may have exerted an undue influence on the results. Schizophrenic patients made more errors in finger localization on trials that required intermanual transfer. This was true of about one-third of patients, and it was noted that "more errors were made when the experimenter touched the left hand and the subject indicated with the right hand than vice versa [p. 506]." Only a few errors were made on the body surface transfer task, although hand and forearm transfer produced a substantial and symmetric error rate, which, however, was virtually eliminated by the fourth trial. More errors were made in hand tapping when transfer was required, and again there were no lateral differences. The authors interpreted these results as reflecting a problem in interhemispheric transfer rather than one of conceptual difficulty. They noted that impairments varied from task to task and patient to patient, implying an inefficient channel of communication in some patients rather than a total disconnection.

In another study (Dimond *et al.*, 1979) the same patients were examined for their ability to name common objects placed in either hand. Again, about one-third of schizophrenic patients showed naming deficits, which were more frequent for objects placed in the left hand. The patients were tested four times at monthly intervals. It is noteworthy that no errors were made on the second occasion because this provides further evidence of the transient nature of the putative callosal problem. The authors also noted that some patients were unable to do the task at all.

Dixon and Henley (1974), in a pilot study with normal subjects, found that the matching of information involving shape discrimination was more efficient if spatial features of the problem were presented to the right hemisphere and verbal features to the left. When schizophrenic patients were examined on the same task no laterality effects were found (Kugler and Henley, 1979), and the authors hypothesized that a callosal impairment may have dissipated any advantage resulting from the presentation of stimulus material to the more "competent" hemisphere. To elucidate this hypothesis they went on to test 12 medicated schizophrenic patients and 12 normal controls on a spatial task. Patients showed slower sorting times for shapes, letters, and numbers with the right hand and a higher incidence of errors in sorting letters and numbers with the right hand. Because the task involved active touch, a contralaterally mediated process, the results indicate a predominantly left hemisphere processing deficit.

Weller and Kugler (1979) examined three tests in which split-brain patients are shown to be impaired: touch localization, reproduction of imposed posture, and identification of inscribed digits. Although the authors chose these to reflect increasing difficulty of interhemispheric integration, they could be differentiated on other grounds. The first involved passive touch, which is bilaterally represented; the second involved proprioception, often implicated in the schizophrenic deficit; and the third involved a verbal component requiring left hemisphere processing. The authors examined up to 24 acute and 16 chronic schizophrenic, 8 schizoaffective, and 11 depressed patients and normal controls. Some of the schizophrenic patients were free of neuroleptics. In touch localization there were no significant differences in accuracy among groups, and it was concluded that there was nothing suggestive of a callosal or lateralized impairment. However, a close inspection of the results shows that the chronic schizophrenic group did not show an advantage of ipsilateral over contralateral localization when this involved the right hand. Thus, in some patients at least, when somatosensory information was mediated by the direct sensory pathway to the left hemisphere, it was less accurate when the same hand executed the response than when the contralateral hand executed the response and information had to traverse the callosum. This is analogous to the difficulties found in the tachistoscopic studies. In the second task, involving the reproduction of imposed posture, patients performed more poorly than controls, although this was significant only with chronic schizophrenic patients. The authors suggested that this may reflect a callosal transmission deficit, but there was no ipsilateral control condition, and it may therefore reflect a bilateral proprioception deficit. In the third task blindfolded patients had to identify verbally digits inscribed on either hand. Here, the schizophrenic patients, whether chronic or acute, showed poorer performance than controls, which the authors attributed to a combined callosal and left-sided deficit. However, the relative difference between the hands, which is the test of a callosal deficit, was of the same order in patients and controls, suggesting that the difference between them was due to a lateralized deficit, a process such as proprioception common to both hemispheres, or some other factor such as medication.

Tress *et al.* (1979) examined the interocular transfer of movement aftereffects, the transfer of which is absent in patients with agenesis of the corpus callosum. Sixteen chronic male patients, all but one on drugs, were tested, and two-thirds reported reliable aftereffects. The difference between the ipsilateral and contralateral conditions was smaller in patients than in controls. This was unexpected and was interpreted as evidence of greater transfer in patients. If the results are reliable (see Gruzelier, 1979b) and the interpretation valid, the phenomenon suggests an inhibitory callosal deficit in many chronic schizophrenic patients, such that too much information rather than too little is transmitted across the callosum. Such a phenomenon could coexist with, or stem from, a lateralized inhibitory deficit.

Thus, in the somesthetic modality a left hemisphere problem, although often masked by authors' interpretations, persistently emerges (Beaumont and Dimond, 1973; Section II,D; Dimond *et al.*, 1979; Kugler and Henly, 1979; Weller and Kugler, 1979). Evidence of a problem in callosal transmission is more ephemeral, and together the studies suggest dysfunction of a labile nature pertaining to a subgroup of patients.

3. VISUAL STUDIES

There have been about a dozen studies investigating hemispheric function by means of visual processing, either by using half-field stimulation to capitalize on the unilateral projections from the nasal hemiretina, or by encouraging different modes of processing and hemispheric predilections for processing different types of stimuli, for example, verbal (left) versus spatial (right), or by combinations of these approaches. The purely cognitive approaches (Gur, 1979; Pic'l *et al.*, 1979) have been inconclusive for reasons discussed elsewhere (Gruzelier, 1981b), and therefore this section concentrates on the use of the divided-field technique.

Gur (1978) compared 24 medicated, dextral, schizophrenic patients with the same number of controls matched for education and socioeconomic background. There were an equal number of men and women, and half the patients were paranoid (diagnostic procedures unspecified). Subjects first reported a number that appeared in a central field to control for fixation and then the stimulus that occurred to either side. In one session this involved the position of a dot in a rectangle, and in another the identification of consonant–vowel–consonent nonsense syllables. Whereas both patients and controls showed a left visual field–right hemisphere advantage in accurately locating dots, only the controls showed the expected right visual field–left hemisphere advantage for identifying syllables. The patients showed greater accuracy in the left visual field. In addition, patients' performance was poorer overall on the spatial task but poorer only for the right visual field on the verbal task. Gur reasoned that, since phonetic analysis can be executed only by the left hemisphere, the left visual field advantage indicates superior left hemisphere analysis of material that proceeds via the indirect transcallosal route. Accordingly, the right visual field deficiency reflects an inadequacy in direct left hemisphere input before the stage at which callosal input is dealt with, and consequently this represented a problem at a lower stage of processing.

These results were in most respects confirmed by Connolly *et al.* (1979) with 15 schizophrenic patients diagnosed with the help of the PSE and compared with 6 patients with affective disorders, 14 patients with nonpsychotic disorders, and 20 normal controls. The spatial task was essentially the same as Gur's, whereas the verbal task involved identifying numbers in sequences of letters and numbers. The subjects responded vocally, and no strategy apart from instruction was adopted to control fixation. The dependent variable was reaction time rather than accuracy; there were no lateral advantages or group differences in accuracy.

Schizophrenic patients showed the expected left visual field–right hemisphere advantage for spatial stimuli at a level that approached significance but also showed the same, atypical advantage for verbal stimuli. These results were true of more than 75% of schizophrenic patients and also of affective patients. Normal controls and nonpsychotic patients showed the same right hemisphere advantage for spatial processing but no visual field advantage for verbal stimuli, results that may reflect a lack of specificity in the left hemisphere requirements of the task. The psychotic groups were slower overall on both tasks, and the normal controls were faster on the verbal task than the nonpsychotic controls.

There was no support for the callosal deficit model. Absolute differences between visual fields were no different for schizophrenic patients than for normal controls, despite the fact that spatial processing in the right visual field required two crossings of the corpus callosum, the first for spatial analysis and the second for access to the speech production mechanism for verbal report. It is noteworthy that no lateral differences in accuracy or group differences in performance level were reported (cf. Gur, 1978).

Subsequently, Connolly *et al.* (1983b) reexamined these issues using unmedicated patients and modified the verbal task so that it required distinguishing vowels from consonants, thus placing greater emphasis on left hemisphere processes. The reaction times of 16 controls were compared with those of 12 patients, 10 of whom were diagnosed as schizophrenic (Wing *et al.*, 1974). Whereas 75% of controls showed the expected left hemisphere advantage on the verbal task, virtually all the patients showed a right hemisphere advantage. As before, both patients and controls showed a right hemisphere advantage for the discrimination of dot patterns. An estimate of processing time was calculated by the subtraction of response time, which had been determined in a practice condition in which subjects simply responded to the stimuli as quickly as they could. Effects that in the previous experiment had been attributed to hemispheric specialization were confirmed as such in the analysis of processing times. Furthermore, verbal processing in the patients' right hemisphere was faster than that in the left hemisphere of controls, and this right hemisphere advantage was found to be true of all patients. Regarding the spatial task, faster right hemisphere processing was found in 13 of 16 controls and 8 of 12 patients.

After the approach of Beaumont and Dimond (1973) (Section II,D), Eaton (1979) required matching of stimulus pairs within and between fields while subjects fixated centrally. In an unpublished doctoral dissertation, Eaton (1977) examined 51 unmedicated schizophrenic patients and controls and found that patients were poorer at name matching, a left hemisphere task, than at matching forms, a right hemisphere task, or digits, a task involving either hemisphere. Nevertheless, the schizophrenic patients showed the expected hemisphere advantages for spatial as well as verbal stimuli (cf. Gur, 1978; Connolly *et al.*, 1979, 1983b). Bilateral presentation conferred an advantage on controls on all tasks, but not on schizophrenic patients on the spatial task, a result interpreted as evidence for an impairment in hemispheric integration of spatial stimuli.

In Eaton's second study (Eaton, 1979; Eaton *et al.*, 1979), 24 patients fulfilling Feighner's criteria for schizophrenia were initially examined drug free or after having been withdrawn from medication, and a second time after a mean of 2 weeks of treatment with neuroleptics. Reaction time was slowest for name matching, and no task showed a visual field advantage. Reactions and clinical symptoms were improved in patients on medication. Regarding the accuracy of detection, when patients were unmedicated, name matching showed a hemisphere advantage opposite to that of digit and form matching, with advantages in the expected direction. In patients being treated with drugs, there was a general improvement in accuracy which involved the left hemisphere more than the right, except for verbal stimuli, in which case, the original asymmetry was reversed following an improvement in left visual field–right hemisphere detection. An improvement in left hemisphere processing in medicated patients is a common theme of this chapter, and so the asymmetry reversal that occurred in digit and form matching is not inconceivable. However, the improvement in right hemisphere matching of letters in medicated patients is unexpected and is further evidence of the anomalous lateralization of verbal processing in schizophrenia. All in all, there is some support for left hemisphere dysfunction and little support for the results obtained with the same paradigm by Beaumont and Dimond.

Hillsberg (1979) employed a matching task that involved pairs of arrows pointing in the same or opposite directions. Ten controls showed no lateral asymmetry, whereas five male schizophrenic patients who were all on drugs and were tested repeatedly on five occasions over 3 days showed slower reaction times to stimuli presented to the left hemisphere. This was true of 4 of 5 patients and was stable over sessions. Hillsberg found slower processing to bilateral and unilateral stimuli and no disparity between groups. Thus, a left hemisphere impairment was revealed, which, regardless of the way in which the material is categorized on nonverbal dimensions, is unlikely to be drug-mediated because drugs appear to produce a relative right hemisphere advantage only for letters (Eaton, 1979).

Colbourn and Lishman (1979) combined the auditory study mentioned earlier (Section III,B,1,b) with a divided-field tachistoscope measure and tested 13 schizophrenic, 9 manic-depressive, and 11 nonpsychotic patients and 19 normal controls. Although none of the groups showed the expected right hemisphere advantage for the spatial task, they all showed a left hemisphere advantage for the accuracy of word recognition. When gender differences were examined it was the male schizophrenic and nonpsychiatric patients who failed to show this advantage.

An intriguing series of studies was carried out by Kostandov (1980) in eastern Europe. In the first experiment thresholds for the recognition of letters were estimated for both visual fields using a dichotic method of presentation; that is, letters were presented simultaneously while the subject fixated centrally. Stimulus durations were initially of 10 msec and increased incrementally with successive presentations until there was correct identification in either visual field. Fifteen controls showed thresholds within the range of 20 to 40 msec, with greater accuracy in the right visual field–left hemisphere. In contrast, 14 patients (described as having schizophrenia of the nonprogressive form and with symptoms in remission) showed higher thresholds of 50 to 80 msec with no advantage to either visual field; accurate bilateral recognition occurred on more than half the trials. It is conceivable that the results reflect a sensory-processing advantage to the left hemisphere in normal subjects but the patients' twice as high thresholds and their bilateral accuracy make the operation of attitudinal factors plausible. A more conservative attitude toward acknowledging detection may have masked hemispheric effects.

The second experiment employed a backward masking technique whereby a sensory trace left by a stimulus after its offset is terminated by a second stimulus. This makes it possible to control the perception time of the first stimulus. Having first determined the recognition threshold for each stimulus, the interval preceding a masking flash was varied in 10-msec steps from a minimum 20-sec interval until letters in either field were recognized. Earlier detection occurred more frequently in the left visual field–right hemisphere for normal subjects. Patients showed the same pattern of results as before. On the majority of trials there was no advantage, and on the remainder there was a roughly equal distribution between visual fields.

Although in this case threshold data were not provided, the results might conceivably be interpreted in the same way as those of the first experiment. Assuming the absence of nonsensory confounding factors in controls, the results implicate a right hemisphere visuospatial analysis preceding higher-level left hemisphere analysis in the perception of letters. Some collaboratory evidence is provided by the analysis of occipital evoked potentials, which were monitored concurrently in normal subjects but not patients. Latencies of the N_{200} and P_{300} components were shorter in the right hemisphere. If the same sensory interpretation is applied to the results with patients, the hemispheres appear to be equipotential in both their visuospatial and semantic analyses, a possibility that requires further exploration.

In sum, left hemisphere deficits in schizophrenia were a common feature of the half-field studies. Left visual field–right hemisphere advantages for verbal material were representative of the samples of Gur, 1978; Connolly *et al.*, 1979; 1983b; Eaton, 1979. This may reflect a problem at low levels of analysis for stimuli transmitted over direct pathways to the left hemisphere, with as a consequence superior left hemisphere analysis of stimuli proceeding via the right hemisphere and transcallosal route as Gur suggests. Alternatively, it could reflect an abnormal reliance on right hemisphere verbal processes (Searleman, 1977). The callosal dysfunction model drew little support from the visual studies, unless the elementary forms of analysis required by these studies involved posterior aspects that interconnect the occipital lobes, a region free of abnormalities in recent studies of schizophrenia (Bigelow *et al.*, 1983).

C. Psychophysiology

1. ELECTROENCEPHALOGRAM

While visual inspection of recordings by early workers disclosed no gross lateral asymmetries, a reexamination by Small *et al.* (1979) of the electroencephalograms (EEGs) of 1494 adult patients revealed right-sided disorders to be more common in schizophrenia and left-sided disorders in depression. Recordings taken during waking, sleeping, photic stimulation, and hyperventilation were more often abnormal in organic, neurotic personality and bipolar affective disorders than in schizophrenia. The schizophrenic patients ($N=759$) were diagnosed with DSM I or II, and 343 fulfilled Feighner's criteria. Whether the right-sided disorder in schizophrenia characterized a subgroup was not elucidated. Abnormalities discernible "by eye" were also revealed in 29% of recordings in Abrams and Taylor's (1979) analysis of 159 psychotic patients. Of 27 schizophrenic patients, 13 (45%) showed abnormalities, with disturbance in temporal areas occurring in 8 cases, 5 lateralized to the left and 3 to the right.

Rodin *et al.* (1968) performed a spectral analysis of posterior parietal and occipital activity in 25 drug-withdrawn, chronic, male schizophrenic patients under 40 years of age. In control subjects power throughout the spectral range (2–33 Hz) was higher on the right. In patients, however, an overall reduction in power was accompanied by relatively higher δ and β activity on the left than the right, reflecting either overactivity on the left or, alternatively, underactivity on the right. From a study of cortical evoked potentials (EPs) to flashes and correlations between clinical ratings and empirically salient features of EP components, the highest association was found between pathology and low negativity in right-sided EPs. Features associated only with the right hemisphere were poor nonverbal accessibility, no sexual interest in student nurses, and poor body image perception. Poor touch-mediated body image showed a relatively stronger association with the right side than the left, whereas decreased psychomotor activity and speech showed equally strong correlations with both sides. Considered in relation to the potential range of schizophrenic symptoms, features related to the right hemisphere are those with a retarded, anhedonic character.

The opposite directionality in mean power was shown in the spectral analyses of Giannitrapani and Kayton (1974), who found that asymmetries occurring in control subjects showed higher left-sided power, whereas the less frequently occurring asymmetries in schizophrenic patients showed higher right-sided power. The left-sided excess in controls extended from the lateral frontal region to the temporal, posttemporal, and parietal area, peaking in the temporal region. Discrepancies between this and the report of Rodin *et al.* (1968) may have arisen from a number of factors, including differences in gender, age, medication, clinical subtype, and recording conditions. Furthermore, both reports paid special heed to individual differences. Rodin *et al.* stated that "all the results mentioned hold true only for a group of patients and cannot be used for reliably differentiating individuals." Giannitrapani and Kayton (1974) emphasized that this "homologous symmetry is not characteristic of individual patients but is the result of averaging the diverse asymmetrical patterns [p. 382]."

In an evolving study to which data on new patients have been added cumulatively, Flor-Henry and Koles (1982) have compared 53 schizophrenic, 63 depressed psychotic, and 75 manic patients with 60 normal controls. The patients were unmedicated, and recordings were taken from bilateral temporal and parietal placements. Nine measures were recorded for the α band alone, providing 34 different characterizations of the EEG from each patient. The EEG was recorded with the patients' eyes open and closed and during the Wechsler vocabulary and block design subtests, giving a total of 136 variables per bandwidth. The paucity of differences between patients and normal subjects is perhaps the most striking result. Some differences were observed. Schizophrenic and manic patients showed less bilateral α power while resting than controls, and schizophrenic patients showed less intrahemispheric coherence on right hemisphere recordings than all the other groups. Interhemispheric coherence between temporal sites was lower than normal in both schizophrenic and mania. Although the latter effect carried over to the verbal task, the EEG was similar to that of controls for other forms of cognitive activation in all but phase relationships. In schizophrenic patients activity led from the parietal site, whereas in controls this was true only of resting records, the temporal site leading with cognitive engagement.

The laterality results that distinguished schizophrenic patients in the penultimate report in the series (Flor-Henry *et al.*, 1979) together with studies by Shaw *et al.* (1979) and Weller and Montague (1979) have been reviewed (Gruzelier, 1979b). The earlier report of Flor-Henry and colleagues involved their first 20 schizophrenic patients and controls. Weller and Montague examined 5 unmedicated patients soon after admission. Patients in the Shaw *et al.* study were on medication, and 6 of the 18 schizophrenic patients were outpatients. The latter study compared the resting EEG recorded with the patients' eyes closed with the EEG recorded during two forms of cognitive activation: a mental imagery task to engage primarily the right hemisphere and a mental arithmetic task to engage the left hemisphere. In general, there was little consistency between studies with atypical recordings in schizophrenia most common with slow and fast frequency activity. Only in the 1982 report of Flor-Henry and Koles was α found to distinguish schizophrenic patients from controls, implying that possibly because of between-subject variability a large number of subjects are required to achieve a reliable α effect.

Telemetry involving ambulatory recording of EEG has revealed some lateral differences in activity contemporaneous with psychotic events. Stevens *et al.* (1979) examined 38 schizophrenic patients who had been withdrawn from drugs for between 1 month and 5 years, were on medication that failed to control their symptoms, or had never been medicated. Recordings were taken from central parietal and anterior temporal derivations. Although no clear relation between abnormal EEGs and the time at which symptoms occurred was evident, left-sided changes coincided with psychotic manifestations in four of the five vignettes reported.

Left-sided involvement is also implicated in a detailed report (Stevens and Livermore, 1982) on 18 of these patients during free ward activity, a psychiatric interview, two verbal tests (serial subtraction and word fluency), and two spatial tasks (the Seguin form board with the patient's eyes closed and a jigsaw puzzle). Hallucinations coincided with increased left central parietal slow activity. When abnormal behaviors such as hallucinations, psychomotor blocking, lateral eye movements, and catatonia were pooled, a relation was found with the suppression of anterior temporal α activity on the left. Lateral shifts in α activity coincided with verbal tests and were similar in both patients and controls, but the six patients tested on the spatial tests did not show the reduction in right-sided α activity found in controls. Syndromes within schizophrenia were mentioned in passing, and it is noteworthy that all three catatonic patients showed pathological EEG signs from the right anterior temporal region, and half (4 of 8) of the chronic paranoid patients with active auditory hallucinations and lateralized signs in left cerebral parietal placements, which extended to the anterior temporal regions in two cases.

Lateral asymmetries in electrocortical activity in either direction in different syndromes are supported by two other reports. Coger and Serafetinides (1983) selected patients considered to have a pure dominant hemisphere profile ($N=8$) or a nondominant profile ($N=6$) from a large sample of 30 schizophrenic patients. Hemisphericity was inferred from ratings on the BPRS. The dominant hemisphere profile was characterized by conceptual disorganization, grandiosity, hostility, suspiciousness, lack of cooperation, and unusual thought content, and the nondominant profile by somatic concern, anxiety, tension, mannerisms and posturing, and depressive mood. All patients were dextral and male. Whereas controls showed a nonsignificant asymmetry in the direction of higher right hemisphere power, elevated β activity (20–32 Hz) was found on the left side only in patients with dominant hemisphere profiles and bilaterally in nondominant profile patients. Statistical analysis revealed that the left-sided elevation was significant with both patient groups in the frontotemporal area, but the right-sided increase in the nondominant group did not reach significance; hence, only the dominant group showed a clear lateral asymmetry, which was in the 24- to 30-Hz range. In the posterior central occipital leads a bilateral elevation was seen in low β 16- to 18-Hz activity in both groups, and the nondominant group showed a right-sided elevation in the range 26–30 Hz. Thus, the left and right hemisphere groups were distinguished by some features of fast frequency power, with elevations more pronounced on the left in the "dominant" group and on the right in the "nondominant" group.

Examining drug-withdrawn schizophrenic patients and normal controls, Etevenon *et al.* (1983) made comparisons between controls, who were classified according to evidence of high ($N=15$) and low ($N=16$) α activity in parietooccipital leads. Patient subgroups were compared if they fulfilled DSM III criteria for paranoid schizophrenia ($N=7$) and residual schizophrenia ($N=10$). Recordings were taken from central parietal and parietal–occipital leads. Comparisons of low- and high-α-activity groups showed elevations in low and high frequencies in the low-α-activity group. There were similarities between the low-α-activity and paranoid groups in the distribution of spectral power, but any lateral differences were always on the *left* side, with paranoid patients showing relatively more anterior than posterior activity and greater elevations in low and high frequencies centrally. The residual patients had more in common with the high-α-activity group, and any differences were mainly on the *right* side, occurring as elevations in low and high frequencies with a notable increase in high frequency activity centrally.

In summary, EEG evidence of dynamic-process asymmetries clearly implicates both hemispheres in schizophrenia. There is some suggestion that hemispheric involvement is related to different syndromes, with all subgroups classed as paranoid (Stevens and Livermore, 1982; Etevenon *et al.*, 1983) or as dominant hemisphere profile (Coger and Serafetinides, 1983) manifesting left-sided activation, and all those classed as residual (Etevenon *et al.* 1983), nondominant hemisphere profile (Coger and Serafetinides, 1983), or anhedonic (Rodin *et al.*, 1968) manifesting right-sided dysfunction. The failure to examine group distributions has been noted to cancel out evidence of individual differences in lateral asymmetries. Otherwise, the results are confusing, and delineation of the nature of the EEG abnormality is likely to remain elusive until standardized procedures are adopted and the vast potential range of measures and analyses reduced.

2. CORTICAL EVOKED POTENTIALS

In a methodologically interesting study Buchsbaum *et al.* (1979) examined EPs in response to dim and bright flashes presented hemiretinally while subjects followed their sequential pattern or attempted to ignore them during a serial subtraction task. Sixteen schizophrenic patients withdrawn from medication for 2 weeks were compared with 17 patients with a primary affective disorder, 15 epileptic patients with temporal lobectomy of the left ($N=6$) or right ($N=9$) hemisphere, and 30 normal subjects. Placements were temporoparietal and occipital. Only the temporoparietal region differentiated the tasks with differences in the N_{120} component, a result consistent with previous studies. The pattern of results seen in schizophrenic patients was similar to that seen in left temporal cases. Whereas amplitudes to stimuli transmitted over direct pathways were similar to those of controls, those transmitted over indirect pathways were smaller than normal. When responses to low-intensity flashes only were compared between patients and normal subjects, the patients' failure to show an attentional increase in the N_{120} in response to stimuli transmitted over indirect pathways occurred only with transmission to the left hemisphere. Together the results imply a schizophrenic dysfunction of the left temporal lobe and of the passage or reception of stimuli transmitted indirectly via the callosum to the left temporoparietal region.

Possible impairments in callosal transmission were the concern of Tress *et al.* (1979), who compared 12 chronic male schizophrenic patients receiving neuroleptic drugs with 7 normal volunteers. Evoked potentials were recorded from somatosensory cortex in response to a repetitive tactile stimulus delivered to the forearm. In fact, patients and controls were differentiated by the latencies of early components, particularly those recorded from the left hemisphere in response to right arm stimulation, thus suggesting a sensory processing problem when transmission is via direct pathways to the left hemisphere.

More recently Jones and Millar (1981) examined interhemispheric conduction time following Salamy's (1978) deduction that ipsilateral EPs in response to a vibratory stimulus applied to the forefinger required callosal transmission and that a comparison of contralateral and ipsilateral latencies of the early components of the EP would therefore reveal callosal conduction time. Salamy had shown reduced conduction time with maturation. Jones and Millar concluded that their 12 schizophrenic patients admitted to an acute ward, half of whom were drug free, showed neither a difference between ipsilateral and contralateral latencies nor the expected reduction in amplitudes of ipsilateral EPs. This was interpreted as a functional occlusion of the corpus callosum compensated for by ipsilateral pathways. However, reservations have been expressed about the reliability of the methods used (Connolly, 1982), and Shagass *et al.* (1983) have failed to replicate the results in a small group of mostly medicated schizophrenic patients.

Shagass and colleagues (Roemer *et al.*, 1978; Shagass *et al.*, 1979, 1983) have reported left-sided EP anomalies in schizophrenia. Their focus is on the variability of waveforms and concerns schizophrenic patients described as chronic ($N=25$), latent ($N=12$), or "other" ($N=12$). Greater than normal variability was found in the early components of left-sided visual evoked responses (51–150 msec), an affect less pronounced in those with latent symptoms. When later components (post-150 msec) were examined, the left-sided variability was found only in chronic cases and, whereas the asymmetry in the early epoch was generalized throughout the left hemisphere, the later epoch showed asymmetry only in the temporal and occipital regions. These results found a parallel in the auditory modality insofar as variability of the early components (15–100 msec) in left-sided responses occurred in patients with overt symptoms of schizophrenia. Regarding the later epoch (101–450 msec) increased variability was found in both hemispheres. Thus, the left-sided anomaly was most common in the early components, suggesting a problem in lower stages of analysis.

Connolly and colleagues examined both visual (Connolly *et al.*, 1983a,b) and auditory (Connolly *et al.*, 1983c) evoked responses in two separate groups of schizophrenic patients tested shortly after hospital admission. A similarity was noted between lateral asymmetries at temporal sites in both modalities. In the visual study 22 normal controls and 16 unmedicated PSE-diagnosed schizophrenic patients received six levels of flash intensity. The P_{100}–N_{120} peak-to-trough amplitude showed a hemispheric imbalance in schizophrenia, with smaller T_3 and larger T_4 amplitudes, whereas in normal subjects it was symmetric. Another lateralized feature that characterized some patients was the stimulus intensity–EP amplitude relationship. Whereas all controls showed a reduction in left hemisphere P_{100} amplitudes at higher intensities, 6 of 16 schizophrenics failed to show the reduction at the temporal placement (T_3). Clinically, these patients were characterized by higher scores on the nuclear schizophrenia syndrome. Another subgroup ($N=4$) showed the same phenomenon over the left occipital region (0_1) and was characterized by features of hypomania and situational anxiety, a result in keeping with the association that Lishman (Section II,A) found between anxiety and left occipital lesions.

In the auditory study (Connolly *et al.*, 1983c) 10 normal subjects tested at weekly intervals for 6 weeks were compared with 10 unmedicated PSE-diagnosed schizophrenic patients tested once after hospital admission. Tones were 1000 Hz, 90 dB, and 100 msec duration with interstimulus intervals of 2 to 4 sec. There were no response requirements. For a period of weeks controls reliably displayed larger N_{120} amplitudes and shorter N_{120} latencies over temporal placements contralateral to the ear stimulated, a result consistent with the functional dominance of contralateral auditory pathways. The patients showed the expected larger left hemisphere amplitudes in response to right ear stimuli but no difference between ipsilateral and contralateral response amplitudes in response to left ear stimuli because of a reduction in contralateral EPs. The latency patterns shown by patients were also abnormal, being shorter than normal on the left and longer on the right. A large latency asymmetry between temporal placements was evident in the patients with latencies markedly reduced on the left and increased on the right. When ears were considered separately, the same normal contralateral-to-ipsilateral advantages were found. The involvement of the middle N_{120} component indicates an anomaly in input processing, the functional implications of which warrant further elucidation.

In a study methodologically similar to that of Buchsbaum *et al.* (1979), with EPs recorded in a focused attention condition, Saito *et al.* (1983) produced striking but complex results using a dichotic listening paradigm (Niwa *et al.*, 1983; Section III,B,1,a). Ten schizophrenic patients and 10 controls listened for target stimuli randomly presented with nontarget stimuli while attention was directed to one ear at a time. Bilateral monitoring involved temporal sites (T_3 and T_4) with analysis of the N_{100} and P_{200} components as well as the mean of the late positive component encompassing the P_{300} component. Concern here is with bilateral differences.

The N_{100} component, thought to reflect processes of selective attention, was reported for target stimuli only. Essentially, the responses of controls were symmetric when attention was directed to either ear, whereas the responses of patients, although reduced overall, were asymmetric when attention was directed to the right ear, with a marked reduction at the left temporal site. This condition should reflect the functional dominance of the left hemisphere. After the correction of lateral differences for EP magnitude, the responses of controls remained more or less symmetric, whereas the patients showed a paradoxical effect, with larger left-sided responses when attention was directed to the left and the converse with rightward attention. A reliable interpretation requires behavioral data. The results could reflect a failure of selective attention, although reports of behavioral experiments requiring focused attention to either ear have generally found no problem that would be compatible with the EP configuration here. Alternatively, the results could reflect an abnormal activation of ipsilateral pathways.

For the P_{200} component only an analysis of nontarget responses was provided. The one response in the normal range was on the right side when attention was directed to the left ear. Otherwise, responses were reduced in size, with smaller responses on the left than the right and smaller responses when attention was directed to the right ear rather than the left; the controls showed the opposite asymmetry. An abnormal reduction in the late positive component was also more apparent when attention was directed to the right ear. Thus, the later components revealed more left hemisphere abnormalities when bilateral electrode placements were compared and when conditions differing in hemispheric functional involvement were compared. A full interpretation of the electrophysiological results awaits integration with behavioral data.

No coherent picture emerges from the EP results. This is not surprising given the variation in components, measures quantified, stimulus conditions, task demands, and variables chosen for analysis, to name but a few issues. Both left- and right-sided abnormalities were reported, which may involve direct contralateral pathways (Tress *et al.*, 1979; Niwa *et al.*, 1983) or ipsilateral and indirect pathways (Buchsbaum *et al.*, 1979; Jones and Millar, 1981; Niwa *et al.*, 1983). Connolly *et al.* (1983c) as well as Niwa *et al.* (1983) found a reduction in middle components (N_{100} or N_{120}) at the left temporal site. However, Connolly's task requirements were of a passive nature, whereas the anomalies that Niwa *et al.* reported were in response to a target stimulus in a discrimination task or involved late (≥ 200 – msec) components. Only Connolly and colleagues have considered syndrome differences and here, although the numbers were small, there is tentative support for an association between left-sided abnormalities in the form of augmented temporal and occipital responses associated with Schneiderian hallucinations and delusions or situational anxiety.

3. NEUROMUSCULAR REFLEXES (HOFFMAN)

The Hoffman (H) reflex is an electromyographic response that provides some indication of α motor excitability in response to afferent stimulation. It is monosynaptic, involving afferent fibers from muscle spindles that terminate directly through a single synapse on the α motor neuron. The reflex occurs in response to electrical stimulation of the posterior tibial nerve, which innervates the gastrocnemius and the soleus, producing, first, a direct response within 5 msec and, second, a reflexive response 35 msec after stimulation. The critical measure is the recovery curve when a second H response follows the first. This is expressed as the ratio of the second response to the first and is produced by a series of stimulus pairs at intervals varying between 30 and 1000 msec. Typically, there is a facilitatory peak at about 300 msec followed by a postfacilitatory trough. Abnormalities in the reflex have been found in Parkinson's disease, in which recovery curves are enhanced. This and other evidence indicates that dopamine exerts an inhibitory effect on α motor neuron excitability, a feature that contributes to its relevance to schizophrenia. Although peripheral factors are by no means unimportant, it is thought that a major influence stems from cortical efferents.

Goode *et al.* (1977) subdivided schizophrenic patients into acute and chronic (more than 1 year's hospitalization) and paranoid and nonparanoid (Feighner's criteria). The results were presented descriptively. Five unmedicated acute schizophrenic patients exhibited recovery curves indicative of reduced α motor neuron excitability, as shown by the facilitatory peak, its latency, and the latency and extent of postfacilitatory recovery. Eleven unmedicated chronic patients had exaggerated recovery curves. After 1 week of receiving chlorpromazine at 200 mg/day and another week at 400 mg/day both groups showed recovery curves closer to those found in normal controls. In one chronic patient who remained resistant to this treatment the addition of L-dopa normalized the curve. Thus, an excess of dopamine is implicated in acute cases, but an insufficiency is indicated in chronic cases. Paradoxically, perhaps, unmedicated manic–depressive patients ($N=5$) showed exaggerated curves, that is, curves with a close resemblance to those found in chronic schizophrenia. The correlation between prognosis ratings and the deviation from the norm of the peak facilitation value was significant, poor prognosis being associated with a large deviation. The authors noted that, because the chronic patients were largely of the nonparanoid type with negative symptoms, the distinction above may not be related to chronicity but to symptoms.

Lateral differences were first examined in normal subjects tested twice (Goode *et al.*, 1980). They were found in either direction in a sample of seven subjects and remained reliable on retesting. Individual differences were of a greater magnitude than test–retest differences. The direction of the asymmetry was unrelated to handedness; all subjects were dextral, and 4 of 7 had larger recovery curves on the right leg. In a second study 27 schizophrenic or schizoaffective patients, all refractory to treatment, were examined. Some were tested more than once, and the second test was chosen as the more reliable in at least 18, all of whom were then on drugs. In addition to the H reflex, three measures of cortical laterality were examined: visual half-field presentation of four-letter words exposed in pairs, one to each half-field; dichotic presentation of monosyllabic nouns; and behavioral tests of motor preference.

The various laterality measures were correlated. The most informative H-reflex variable was the mean value spanning the postfacilitatory trough between 400 and 800 msec. This showed a correlation of -0.38 with the dichotic listening ear preferences and a correlation of -0.43 with an index combining the various behavioral measures. Thus, the greater the left hemisphere preference, the lower the recovery curve on the contralateral leg. Although such a relation would be compatible with a hemispheric model of contralateral inhibition of the motor neuron system, whether it constituted an abnormality is a matter of speculation in the absence of control data.

Goode *et al.* (1981) subsequently reported on up to 36 patients, at least 30 of whom were specified as chronic and 3 as acute. Twenty of 36 were schizoaffective, and, of these, 5 were in a manic phase and 15 depressed. Five of the chronic patients were paranoid. In contrast to results described in the preceding paper, the interval between 400 and 800 msec did not relate to clinical and behavioral measures. Visual, auditory, and motor tests comprising the latter were supplemented in this study by finger-tapping speed. Patients were examined twice: after drug withdrawal and after 1 month of drug treatment. Not all patients were examined on all the tests, the numbers for individual tests ranging between 12 and 18. Given the predominance of chronic patients, the reports that the H reflex of patients and controls did not differ indicates a failure to replicate the exaggerated recovery curves found previously in chronic cases. Instead, greater variability in patients was reported, indicative of more extremes in both directions. The height of the recovery curve was positively correlated with the number of Feighner's schizophrenic criteria. In addition, the authors related the BPRS to the H reflex, not in terms of individual items but as a total score and subscales concerning withdrawal–retardation, paranoid–interpersonal, thinking–disturbance, and anxiety–depression. In unmedicated patients the larger the facilitation on the right leg the higher the withdrawal–retardation rating. This relationship was also found with the magnitude of the lateral difference. The opposite asymmetry was associated with the anxiety–depression scale. In medicated patients these relations did not hold. Instead, relations were found with the behavioral laterality measures. The lower the recovery curves on the right leg the greater the left hemisphere preference in the visual test and, to a lesser extent, the auditory test.

Thus, whereas initially opposite deviations from the norm were associated with the acute–chronic dimension, it was the nature of symptoms that later proved to be more relevant. Symptoms of poor prognosis, Feighner's criteria for schizophrenia, and the BPRS withdrawal–retardation scale were all associated with elevated recovery curves that were larger on the right. The opposite asymmetry was associated with the anxiety–depression scale, good prognosis, and left hemisphere advantages on the behavioral measures. To a large extent the results are congruent with the model outlined in Section I. The negative correlations between the H reflex and the behavioral cortical asymmetries indicate, first, that corticofugal inhibitory influences are mediated contralaterally and, second, that hemispheric influences are reciprocal. Juxtaposing the syndromes associated with the opposite H-reflex asymmetries, on the one hand, and the relation between cortical and H-reflex asymmetries, on the other, it follows that the poor-prognosis retarded syndrome coincides with right hemisphere advantages and corresponding left hemisphere disadvantages, whereas the opposite state of hemisphere balance underpins the good-prognosis anxiety–depression syndrome.

4. CONJUGATE LATERAL EYE MOVEMENTS

Lateral eye movements, or "searching," was a category that Stevens and Livermore (1982) included among abnormal behaviors that coincided with left-sided EEG abnormalities. Lateral eye movements in response to thoughts have been used as an index of hemispheric activation (Kinsbourne, 1974) and have been studied extensively in their own right.

Gur (1978) utilized this as one estimate of abnormal hemispheric function in schizophrenia by examining 24 normal controls and 48 medicated schizophrenic patients, half of whom were paranoid; the number of men and women were equal in both diagnostic groups. Lateral eye movements were contingent on questions that had either a verbal or spatial content, half of the words in each category having emotional connotations. The experimenter sat in front of the subject for half the time and behind for the other half. In line with predictions, verbal questions elicited more rightward eye movements, indicative of left hemisphere activation, and spatial questions more leftward movements. Positioning the experimenter in front of the subject had the effect of enhancing the emotional effect of the questions and produced more leftward movements. In addition to these effects, schizophrenic patients, irrespective of diagnosis, showed more rightward movements than controls. Schizophrenic patients also manifested more "stares" than controls, a phenomenon that in normal subjects is more frequent with emotional questions. Although the greater frequency of rightward movements was interpreted as indicative of more left hemisphere activation in schizophrenia, "stare" responses were more puzzling and were thought to reflect no activation or an equilibrium between the hemispheres.

Using Bleulerian criteria for diagnosis, Schweitzer *et al.* (1978) examined 29 right-handed schizophrenics and 31 controls. Question categories were as for Gur's experiment, and patients again showed more rightward movements than controls with most question categories. When the 9 medicated patients were compared with unmedicated patients, no drug effect was apparent. Schweitzer followed this (1979) by comparing 13 additional schizophrenic patients and 13 psychotic unipolar depressives (DSM III) with the preceding groups. All new patients were medicated. The schizophrenic groups, who in fact did not differ, were combined, and spatial emotional questions were found to be particularly effective in producing rightward movements, a result contrary to the normal leftward tendency. Depressives differed from schizophrenics for all categories and also from controls when all categories were combined. Nevertheless, because differences between question categories were generally slight and patient–control differences were also small, although statistically significant, this technique appears to uncover relative hemispheric imbalance, with left hemisphere overactivation suggested by the results of both Gur and Schweitzer.

On a number of counts the report of Tomer *et al.* (1979) represented a methodological advance over the previous ones. Eye movements were recorded with the electrooculogram, which not only allowed blind scoring but also permitted a more careful delineation of the response. In previous approaches direction of gaze was determined by watching which way the eyes moved and was accomplished with full knowledge of diagnosis. Psychophysiological monitoring revealed that eye movements fell into two categories according to their latency and that the direction of the longer-latency movements alone had some bearing on the type of question. Another methodological advance was the concern with individual differences among the controls, who were subdivided into left and right movers.

In comparing 20 female outpatient schizophrenics with 13 female students in response to questions categorized as verbal–analytical and spatial–emotional, a higher percentage of left movements in controls and right movements in patients was found. The subdivision of controls into right and left movers indicated parallels between control right movers and patients. Both had a low constant rate of short-latency responses, whereas left movers showed an increase in responses across trials. Furthermore, the direction of short- and long-latency responses coincided only in the case of right movers, whether patients or controls. These findings cast a different light on the significance of the phenomenon, indicating that there is nothing inherently pathological about left hemispheric overactivation as reflected in conjugate eye movements.

The functional significance of lateral eye movements was interpreted as follows. Because question category did not influence the results in this experiment, cognitive constraints were interpreted as secondary to the prevailing state of hemispheric activation (cf. Kinsbourne, 1974). In the case of orientational responses to novel stimuli, the right hemisphere was considered to produce a generalized response and the left a localized response focusing on details. Ideally, the right hemisphere response should precede the left because a focused reaction could be quite haphazard without the advantage of an overall appraisal and so could contribute to processing difficulties in schizophrenia. A high incidence of "stares" and blinking was also found in schizophrenia. Tomer *et al.* placed a different interpretation on "stares" than Gur, referring to the reports of Day (1964) and Hiscock (1977) of fewer eye movements as well as more blinking in states of fear and anxiety.

Tomer *et al.* (1981) also recorded smooth pursuit movements of the eyes during the solving of spatial and nonspatial syllogisms, a task employed with schizophrenic patients by Hartlage and Garber (1976), who reported that patients experienced greater difficulty with spatial problems. Twenty hospitalized schizophrenic patients of both sexes and 25 normal controls were examined. Patients had florid symptoms and were dextral, and 16 were receiving some form of medication. Normal controls were selected from a larger sample in order to subcategorize left and right movers, as before. Similarities were again apparent between control right movers and schizophrenic patients. Tracking was significantly more disrupted when subjects proceeded from right to left during the syllogism task and, of the two types of problems, patients experienced more difficulty with the spatial than the verbal. Only on this feature was there no parallel with the control right movers, although, of the two control groups, the right movers performed less successfully than the left.

From neurological evidence the authors concluded that whereas the localizing value of impairments in smooth pursuit, which incidentally are well documented in schizophrenia (e.g., Holtzman *et al.*, 1974), are unclear, lateralized lesions, as in hemidecortication, lead to homolateral disruption. Thus, the impairment in patients and control right movers during leftward tracking indicates a left hemisphere impairment and "also implies that the left hemisphere performs in an inhibited fashion [p. 141]. To reconcile inhibition with hyperalertness, recourse was made to models suggesting a limited processing capacity with consequent information overload, arising in this case from the dual task requirement of tracking at the same time as solving syllogisms.

The clear pattern of a predominance of rightward movements in schizophrenia that emerges in these studies is called into question by the report of Sandel and Alcorn (1980) on 100 male dextral subjects. In their study one group consisted of 13 nonparanoid schizophrenics and 12 depressives, a second group of 20 manic–depressives and 5 schizoaffectives, a third of 25 alcoholics, and a fourth of 25 patients with antisocial personality disorders. Patients "were not overtly symptomatic." Eye movements were observed in response to questions, and a scoring procedure ranging from 0 to 200 provided three categories: 0–60, left hemisphericity; 61–139, bilaterality; 140–200, right hemisphericity. From the total sample the incidence of the three categories was 14, 41, and 45%, respectively. Nonparanoid and depressive patients had a mean score of 160.38, placing them in the right hemisphere category, whereas manic–depressives and schizoaffectives had a mean score of 112.58, indicating bilaterality. Alcoholics and patients with personality disorders were also classified as bilateral, although at opposite extremes of the category, with scores of 134.24 and 89.94, respectively.

Drawing together these results some reconciliation could be offered by taking recourse to the model offered in Section I. The model would predict rightward movements, indicative of left hemisphere activation, in the acute, remitting, reactive paranoid syndrome and leftward movements in the retarded, poor-prognosis nonparanoid form. The results of Sandel and Alcorn are consistent with this, showing more right hemisphere activation in nonparanoid and depressive patients than in manic–depressives and schizoaffectives, whereas close inspection of Gur's results indicates nonsignificantly higher left hemisphere activation in paranoid patients.

IV. Conclusions

A. Dynamic-Process Asymmetries

In summary, we offer a recapitulation guided by the theoretical framework outlined in Section I. To what extent did the syndromes defined by opposing asymmetries in electrodermal orienting responses, which themselves inextricably involve processes of selective attention and arousal, find a counterpart in other measures of dynamic-process asymmetries? Table 12.2 shows that measures of arousal and attention elicit bidirectional asymmetries in schizophrenia. Measures include EEG rhythms, cortical EPs, the H reflex, lateral eye movements, auditory thresholds, dichotic listening, and somatosensory extinction. Furthermore, syndromes distinguished by the direction of lateralization have some resemblance to those defined by the electrodermal variable. The diversity of measures involved suggests a holistic influence (Boring, 1950) on hemispheric control of dynamic processes, and there may therefore be some truth in notions of global hemispheric arousal (Kinsbourne, 1974).

The auditory studies and the examination of children genetically at risk for schizophrenia imply that the prevailing hemispheric balance is a trait characteristic. Pathological implications apart, this suggests that hemispheric activation differences may be a significant feature of brain function by which individuals can be differentiated (see Gruzelier *et al.*, 1981a). Nevertheless, dynamic-process asymmetry is neither independent of clinical state nor invariant within individuals. A disruption of hemispheric balance accompanied the acute exacerbation of psychotic symptoms found coincidental with hospital admission (Section III,B,1,c). Reversals in lateral asymmetries in electrodermal responses have followed drug treatment (Gruzelier *et al.*, 1981b). Unpublished work of the author and colleagues shows that the shift in lateral advantages in the detection of lexical stimuli presented hemiretinally reverses in students before examinations and corresponds to the one found in anxious patients.

With one exception the relation between syndrome type and direction of asymmetry consistently supports the assumption that when florid symptoms accompany an acute, reactive syndrome this reflects a dominance of left hemisphere activation, whereas the withdrawn, retarded syndrome reflects the dominance of right hemisphere activation (see Table 12.2). Given the different prognostic implications of the syndrome, mechanisms controlling the balance of hemispheric activation may provide a critical influence not only on presenting symptoms but also on the long-term course of the schizophrenic disorder.

The one exception is somatosensory extinction (Section III,A,3). Con-

TABLE 12.2
Evidence of Disparate Syndromes Underpinned by Opposite Imbalances in Dynamic-Process Asymmetries

Process	Measure	Result	Hemispheric functional implication	References
Arousal	Electrodermal orienting response	Larger left hand responses in florid, reactive syndrome; larger right hand responses in retarded syndrome	Neuropsychological interpretations of left hemisphere activation in former and right hemispheric activation in latter, and hemispheres reciprocally related	Gruzelier (1981a), Gruzelier and Manchanda (1982)
	EEG	Left-sided signs in paranoids with active auditory hallucinations; right-sided signs in catatonia	Left hemisphere dysfunction in florid paranoids; right hemisphere dysfunction in catatonia; consistent if syndrome is one of catatonic withdrawal and not excitement	Stevens and Livermore (1982)
		Syndromes with "dominant hemisphere symptoms," left signs; "nondominant hemisphere symptoms," right signs	Left hemisphere activation in former and right hemisphere activation in latter	Coger and Serafetinides (1983)
		Paranoid schizophrenia, left-sided signs compared with low α controls; residual schizophrenia, right-sided signs compared with high α controls	Left hemisphere activation in former and right hemisphere activation in latter	Etevenon *et al.* (1983)
	Cortical EPs	Retarded, anhedonic symptoms correlated with right-sided EPs	Right hemisphere posterior abnormality in retarded syndrome	Rodin *et al.* (1968)
		Nuclear–Schneiderian symptoms in new admissions, left temporal abnormality; hypomanic and situational anxiety in schizophrenia, left occipital abnormality	Loss of left hemisphere inhibition (augmenting pattern) in reactive, florid patients	Connolly *et al.* (1983a,b)
	Hoffman reflex	Right–left suppression in good-prognosis anxiety–depression syndrome; left leg suppression in poor-prognosis, Feighner, withdrawn-retarded syndrome	Left hemispheric dominance in former and right hemisphere dominance in latter	Goode *et al.* (1981)

	Lateral eye movements	More rightward measurements in paranoid than nonparanoid cases (trend)	Left hemisphere activation in paranoids	Gur (1973)
		Left movements in nonparanoids and depressives; fewer leftward movements in manic–depressives and schizo-affectives	Right hemisphere activation in nonparanoids	Sandel and Alcorn (1980)
	Auditory thresholds	Larger right ear advantage in electrodermally nonreactive patients	Dynamics of inhibitory left hemisphere in chronic, nonreactive patients	Gruzelier and Hammond (1979a,b)
Selective attention	Dichotic listening	Paranoids stronger right ear advantage and shift of attention away from right less than nonparanoids	Left hemisphere activated in paranoids compared with nonparanoids	Lerner *et al.* (1977)
		Paranoids stronger right ear advantage despite competing intensities and instructions to direct attention, especially electrodermally reactive ones; shift of attention away from the right less; nonparanoids no right ear bias in free recall and abnormal left ear bias when intensity or focused attention advantages to left	Left hemisphere activation in reactive paranoids and right hemisphere activation in nonparanoids	Gruzelier and Hammond (1979b)
		Positive symptoms	Acute, remitting syndrome associated with left hemisphere activation	Wexler and Heninger (1979)
	Somatosensory extinction	Inattention of right side maximally frequent in younger (good-prognosis?) cases; inattention of left side more frequent in older (poor-prognosis?) cases.	Opposite lateral functional organization associated with age (or prognosis); implications for activation and inhibition unclear	Scarone *et al.* (1981, 1983)

ventionally, this phenomenon is classed with measures of fixed process (Bender, 1952), yet the pattern of results reported here allocates it to the dynamic-process class. Perhaps the nature of the extinction phenomenon requires reconsideration. It is noteworthy that to produce the effect bilateral stimulation is essential because inattention vanishes with unilateral stimulation. Bimanual stimulation appears to evoke an interplay between mutually antagonistic input systems with results analogous to functional occlusions of ipsilateral pathways that release contralateral ones—the neuropsychological rationale for the dichotic listening technique. The fact that the test of somatosensory extinction produced paradoxical results, namely, inattention to the right side of the body in a clinical syndrome, which reveals excessive attention to right ear input, can be accounted for by a number of factors: (*a*) an erroneous inference that subgrouping by age parallels subgrouping by prognosis; (*b*) misalignment of the phenomenon with the dynamic-process class of asymmetries; (*c*) recourse to the inverted-U function of arousal and performance whereby activation of a hemisphere disrupts and immobilizes its functioning (e.g., Gur, 1978; Tomer *et al.*, 1981); and (*d*) anomalies of suppressor mechanisms that control the interplay between ipsilateral and contralateral pathways. At this stage no conclusion can be drawn.

Certainly, the functional roles of ipsilateral and contralateral pathways require elucidation in schizophrenia. Difficulties were revealed in the ability to suppress right ear verbal input in favor of less conspicuous input from the left ear traveling via interhemispheric pathways (Gruzelier and Hammond, 1980). A disruption of normal relations between potentials generated by stimuli traveling via direct and indirect routes and ipsilateral and contralateral pathways was also a persistent theme of the cortical EP studies (Section III,C,2).

Laterality research has revealed the importance of drug influences on cerebral organization in the alteration of dynamic-process asymmetries. This was found in the auditory modality (Section III,B,1,d) and in the divided-visual-field study of Eaton (1979) (Section III,B,3). A relation of visual and auditory processing asymmetries to the H reflex (Section III,C,3) was found only in patients receiving drugs, although it is not clear whether this was due to an alteration in the behavioral or physiological measure or both measures. Psychophysiological evidence from EEG (Goldstein and Stoltzfus, 1973; Serafetinides, 1972, 1973) and electrodermal studies (Gruzelier and Yorkston, 1978; Gruzelier *et al.*, 1981b) is generally consistent with behavioral data showing an increase in left hemispheric activation in patients medicated with neuroleptics, although the opposite reversals have been reported in some patients (Gruzelier *et al.*, 1981b).

B. Fixed-Process Asymmetries

The second premise of the model based on empirical observation was that the bidirectionality in dynamic-process asymmetries would coincide with a homogeneity in asymmetries of fixed structure. Beyond the original observation aligning electrodermal with divided-visual-field asymmetries (Section I) support for this premise is largely indirect because the recording of multiple measures in laterality research is rare, whether with patients or normal subjects. As a compromise recourse can be made to studies clearly documenting a diversity of syndromes or to findings that have been strongly replicated by studies sampling a wide range of patients on aggregate. Samples incorporating a repertoire of syndromes are found only in psychophysiological investigations in which the typically passive nature of the demands on the subject facilitate a cross-sectional approach with large numbers. In these, as documented in the preceding section, bidirectionality has been the predominant finding, but they concern dynamic processes. It is necessary, therefore, to turn to replication.

Replicability is a feature of the divided-visual-field studies in which a disorder in left hemispheric verbal processes is consistently depicted. An impression of a left hemisphere problem recurs in the somesthetic modality, but this will seem more convincing when replications are attempted with standardized procedures. Auditory modality studies afford the most frequent replications, yet here, without exception, the processes delineated are dynamic ones: the left hemisphere temporal decrement, syndrome differences in lateral attentional bias, hemispheric equivalence in acute psychosis and the emergence of lateral preference with remission of acute symptoms, and drug influences in instituting left hemisphere processing advantages. Furthermore, with the possible exception of the left hemisphere temporal decrement, the findings are either directly related to syndrome differences or implicitly so, as in the case of drug influences given that the poor-prognosis, retarded syndrome is refractory to drug treatment. In summary, then, consideration of replicability provides limited but suggestive evidence for a unitary left hemisphere deficit. However, the evidence is more compelling when one draws together the results of the full range of techniques reviewed throughout the chapter.

C. Locus of Dysfunction

As already noted (Section 1,A), the distinction between fixed and dynamic processes is not a mutually exclusive one. Asymmetries of dynamic process may exert a controlling influence over the structural mechanism as exemplified by correlations between measures of the two types of asymmetry (Goode *et al.*, 1980, 1981; Section III,C,3) and in the emergence of left hemisphere preferences in auditory measures of fixed-structure processes when patients remit (Wexler and Heninger, 1979; Johnson and Crocket, 1982; Section III,B,1,c). This interdependence need not necessarily involve separate structures subserving dynamic and fixed processes. Consider the hippocampus. Its involvement in fixed processes of memory storage and retrieval is beyond doubt (Weiskrantz and Warrington, 1975; Butters and Cermack, 1975) to the extent that Milner (1971) has proposed a lawful relation between the extent of hippocampal damage and the extent of memory loss. At the same time it is implicated in dynamic processes, forming the cornerstone of theories of selective attention (Douglas, 1967; Primbram, 1967; Kimble, 1968; Bennett, 1975; Gray, 1982) and assuming a pivotal role in cortical–subcortical arousal systems (Jarrard, 1973).

The example of the hippocampus was not chosen at random. There are references to its involvement in schizophrenia throughout the chapter: in the control of the habituation of the orienting response (Section II,B), which has particular bearing on hemispheric processes since the rate of response habituation correlates with lateral differences in response amplitude (Gruzelier *et al.*, 1981a); in the dynamics of left hemisphere temporal variation in auditory processing (Section III,B,1,a); and in auditory deficits of fixed structure (Section III,B,1,a). Furthermore, to a large extent the structural locus of processes subserving hemispheric specialization revealed by techniques of experimental psychology (Section III,B) and intelligence tests such as the Wechsler (Section III,A,3) resides in temporoparietal regions (Moscovitch, 1979; Milner, 1967). Hippocampal memory and inhibitory functions make this structure a likely candidate for semantic encoding, serial position, and left hemisphere suppression deficits in dichotic listening (Gruzelier and Hammond, 1980; also see Kesner and Novak, 1982).

Finally, the repertoire of symptoms encompassed by the syndromes defined by dynamic-process asymmetries have been shown to accompany organic lesions in the hippocampal system. Bragina (1966; cited in Gruzelier, 1979a) surveyed the cases of 80 people admitted to a neurological hospital with tumors located around the hippocampus and hippocampal gyrus, the amygdaloid nucleus, and adjacent regions including the temporal pole, third and fusiform temporal gyri, and lower horn of the lateral ventricle. Unlike similar patients who had the full gamut of schizophrenic symptoms (Malamud, 1967), Bragina's were free of flagrant signs of psychosis, which otherwise might have masked the motor, emotional, and autonomic signs. Bipolarity was the notable feature of these symptoms she documented. Motor symptoms, for example, took the form of restlessness and impulsiveness as well as rigidity and waxy flexibility. Similarly, emotional symptoms involved agitated depression with constant anxiety, searching movements, or paranoid suspicion, on the one hand, and emotional withdrawal with sluggishness, motor constraint, impassivity of facial expression, ready fatigability, and feelings of weakness and dullness, on the other. Autonomic reactions were also common.

The bipolar nature of the symptoms allows for the possibility that a unilateral lesion in and around the hippocampal system may produce both florid and retarded syndromes. In the survey of Davison and Bagley (Section II,A) florid symptoms as well as blunted affect were associated with organic lesions of the left hemisphere. Presumably, the nature of the syndrome depends on whether processes of excitation or inhibition have the upper hand.

The thalamus also offers intriguing possibilities through its limbic-corticoreticular connections. It is involved in the cortical alerting response and its autonomic sequelae (Lynn, 1966) and influences emotion, motoric arousal, and rate of spontaneous speech (Dimond, 1980), to mention some features which apply to the syndromes listed here. After unilateral ablation or stimulation there are hemisphere specific effects on memory and cognition. It is thought that through its recruiting response the thalamus alerts cortical subregions and thereby influences the balance of activation between subregions (Dimond, 1980; Kinsbourne, 1980).

Thus, from the early organic reports of Flor-Henry, Lishman, and Davison and Bagley (Section II,A) to the investigations of experimental psychology (Section III,B), psychophysiology (Section III,C), and clinical neuropsychology (Section III,A,3), the most common locus of dysfunction has been the posterior temporoparietolimbic regions of the left hemisphere. Disparate clinical syndromes, despite opposite implications for hemispheric functions, could conceivably arise from a unilateral locus in the same region. It would appear that left frontal regions are implicated only when dysfunction is severe (Sections II,A and III,A,3).

The task now becomes one of distinguishing between patients on the basis of the clinical syndromes and delineating the functional effects of overactivation in one syndrome and underactivation in the other on processes of fixed structure, much as Bingley (1958) (Section II,A) did when contrasting patients with tumors and those with epileptic foci. However, this emphasis on left hemisphere functions should not deflect attention from the right hemisphere. Problems in spatial processing or right parietal involvement are referred to throughout this chapter. Verbal processing, at least at the level of comprehension, may also require right hemisphere operations through the default of left hemisphere linguistic functions. The limitations that right hemisphere verbal functions (Searleman, 1977) may impose on cognition may flavor the thought disorder of schizophrenic patients.

The lateral imbalances in dynamic-process asymmetries unraveled in this review appear to be a cardinal issue in brain functional organization in schizophrenia, with implications for diagnosis and treatment. The interplay of dynamic asymmetries with asymmetries of fixed structure becomes a critical issue and one that can be approached only through the integration of techniques of measurement. The concept of a fixed-structure process must not be confused with static notions of function such as those of the strict localizationist school (Boring, 1950), a tendency implicit in current preoccupations with ventricular enlargement in schizophrenia. A leaf could be taken out of Luria's book in conceiving brain organization as the dynamic interaction of complex functional systems (Luria, 1973). Here, the concern with lateral systems has been a small step in this direction.

References

Abbot, C. J. (1982). Laterality deficits in schizophrenia. Middlesex Polytechnic, London, unpublished dissertation.

Abrams, R., and Taylor, M. A. (1979). Laboratory studies in the validation of psychiatric diagnoses. *In* "Hemisphere Asymmetries of Function in Psychopathology" (J. H. Gruzelier and P. Flor-Henry, eds.), pp. 363–372. Elsevier/North Holland, Amsterdam.

Alpert, M., and Martz, M. J. (1977). Cognitive views of schizophrenia in light of recent studies of brain asymmetry. *In* "Psychopathology and Brain Dysfunction" (C. Shagass, G. Gershan, and A. J. Friedhoff, eds.) Raven Press, New York.

Andreasen, N. C., Dermert, J. W., Olsen, S. A., and Damasio, A. R. (1982). Hemisphere asymmetries and schizophrenia. *Am. J. Psychiatry* **139,** 427–430.

Beaumont, J. G., ed. (1982). "Divided Visual Field Studies of Cerebral Organisation." Academic Press, New York.

Beaumont, J. G., and Dimond, S. (1973). Brain disconnection and schizophrenia. *Br. J. Psychiatry* **123,** 661–662.

Bender, M. B. (1952). "Disorders in Perception." Charles C Thomas, Springfield, Illinois.

Bennett, T. L. (1975). The electrical activity of the hippocampus and processes of attention. *In* "The Hippocampus" (R. L. Isaacson and K. H. Pribram, eds.), Vol. 2, pp. 71–100. Plenum, New York.

Bigelow, L. B., Nasrallah, H. A., and Rauscher, F. P. (1983). Corpus callosum thickness in chronic schizophrenia. *Br. J. Psychiatry* **142,** 284, 287.

Bingley, T. (1958). Mental symptoms in temporal lobe epilepsy and temporal lobe gliomas. *Acta Psychiat. Neurol.* **33,** Suppl. 120, 1–151.

Boklage, C. E. (1977). Schizophrenia, brain asymmetry development and twinning: Cellular relationship with etiological and possibly prognostic implication. *Biol. Psychiatry* **12,** 17–35.

Bolin, B. J. (1953). Left-handedness and stuttering as signs diagnostic of epileptics. *J. Ment. Sci.* **99,** 483–487.

Boll, T. J. (1981). The Halstead Reiton Battery. *In* "Handbook of Clinical Neuropsychology" (S. B. Filskov and T. J. Boll, eds.), pp. 577–607. Wiley, New York.

Boring, E. G. (1950). "A History of Experimental Psychology." Appleton, New York.

Bradshaw, J. L., and Nettleton, N. C. (1981). The nature of hemisphere specialisation in man. *Behav. Brain Sci.* **4,** 51–93.

Brown, E. L., and Deffenbacher, K. (1979). "Perception and the Senses." Oxford Univ. Press, London and New York.

Buchsbaum, M. S., Carpenter, W. T., Fedio, P., Goodwin, F. M., Murphy, D. L., and Post, R. M. (1979). Hemispheric differences in evoked potential enhancement by selective attention to hemiretinally presented stimuli in schizophrenic, affective and post-temporal lobetomy patients. *In* "Hemisphere Asymmetries of Function in Psychopathology" (J. H. Gruzelier and P. Flor-Henry, eds.), pp. 317–328. Elsevier/North-Holland, Amsterdam.

Butters, N., and Cermak, L. S. (1975). Some analyses of amnesic syndromes in brain-damaged patients. *In* "The Hippocampus" (R. L. Isaacson and K. H. Pribram, eds.), Vol. 2, pp. 377–410. Plenum, New York.

Butters, N., and Cermak, L. S. (1980). "Alcoholic Korsa Koff's Syndrome." Academic Press, New York.

Carr, S.A. (1980). Interhemispheric transfer of stereognostic information in chronic schizophrenics. *Br. J. Psychiatry* **136,** 53–58.

Chandler, C. M. (1934). Hand, eye and foot preference of two hundred psychiatric patients and two hundred college students. *Psychol. Bull.* **31,** 593–594.

Coger, R. W., and Serafetinides, E. A. (1983). *In* "Laterality and Psychopathology" (P. Flor-Henry and J. H. Gruzelier, eds.), Vol. 2. Elsevier/North-Holland, Amsterdam (in press).

Cohen, G. (1982). Theoretical interpretations of lateral asymmetries. *In* "Divided Visual Field Studies of Cerebral Organization" (J. G. Beaumont, ed.), pp. 87–115. Academic Press, New York.

Colbourn, C. J., and Lishman, W. A. (1979). Lateralisation of function and psychotic illness: A left hemisphere deficit? *In* "Hemisphere Asymmetries of Function in Psychopathology" (J. H. Gruzelier and P. Flor-Henry, eds.), pp. 647–672. Elsevier/North-Holland, Amsterdam.

Connolly, J. F. (1982). Letter. *Br. J. Psychiatry* **140,** 429–430.

Connolly, J. F., Gruzelier, J. H., Kleinman, K. M., and Hirsch, S. R. (1979). Lateralised abnormalities in hemisphere-specific tachistoscopic tasks in psychiatric patients and controls. *In* "Hemisphere Asymmetries of Function in Psychopathology" (J. H. Gruzelier and P. Flor-Henry, eds.), pp. 491–510. Elsevier/North-Holland, Amsterdam.

Connolly, J. F., Gruzelier, J. H., Manchanda, R., and Hirsch, S. R. (1983a). Visual evoked potentials in schizophrenia: Intensity effects and hemispheric asymmetry. *Br. J. Psychiatry* **142,** 152–155.

Connolly, J. F., Gruzelier, J. H., and Manchanda, R. (1983b). Electrocortical and perceptual asymmetries in schizophrenia. *In* "Laterality and Psychopathology" (P. Flor-Henry and J. H. Gruzelier, eds.), Elsevier/North-Holland, Amsterdam (in press).

Connolly, J. F., Gruzelier, J. H., and Hirsch, S. R. (1983c). The auditory event-related potential to lateralised stimuli in schizophrenia patients. (In preparation.)

Corsi, P. M. (1967). The effects of contralateral noise upon the perception and immediate recall of monaurally-presented verbal material. M. A. Thesis, McGill University, Montreal (unpublished).

Crow, T. J. (1980). Molecular pathology of schizophrenia: More than one disease process? *Br. Med. J.* **280,** 66–68.

Davison, K., and Bagley, C. R. (1969). Schizophrenia-like psychoses associated with organic disorders of the central nervous system: A review of the literature. *In* "Current Problems in Neuropsychiatry" (R. N. Herrington, ed.), pp. 113–184. Headley Bros., Ashford, Kent.

Day, M. E. (1964). On eye movement phenomenon relating to attention, thought and anxiety. *Percept. Mot. Skills* **19,** 443–446.

Dimond, S. J. (1976). Depletion of attentional capacity after total commissurotomy in man. *Brain* **99,** 347–356.

Dimond, S. J. (1980). "Neuropsychology." Butterworths, London.

Dimond, S. J., and Beaumont, J. G. (1973). Difference in vigilance performance of the right and left hemisphere. *Cortex* **9,** 259–265.

Dimond, S. J., Scammell, R. E., Pryce, J. Q., Huss, D., and Gray, C. (1979). Callosal transfer and left-hand anomia in schizophrenia. *Biol. Psychiatry* **14,** 735–739.

Dimond, S. J., Scammell, R., Pryce, I. J., Haws, D., and Gray, C. (1980). Some failures of intermanual and cross-lateral transfer in chronic schizophrenia. *J. Abnorm. Psychol.* **89,** 505–509.

Dixon, N. F., and Henley, S. H. A. (1974). Laterality effects in perceptual matching. *Perception* **3,** 99–100.

Douglas, R. J. (1967). The hippocampus and behaviour. *Psychol. Bull.* **67,** 416–442.

Dvirskii, A. E. (1976). Functional asymmetry of the cerebral hemispheres in clinical types of schizophrenia. *Neurosci. Behav. Physiol.* **7,** 236–239.

Dykman, R. A., Reese, W. G., Galbrecht, C. R., Ackerman, P. T., and Sunderman, R. S. (1968). Autonomic responses in psychiatric patients. *Ann. N.Y. Acad. Sci.* **147,** 237–303.

Eaton, E. M. (1977). Intra- and inter-hemispheric processing of visual information in process and reactive schizophrenia. Doctoral dissertation, University of Southern California, Los Angeles (unpublished).

Eaton, E. M. (1979). Hemisphere-related visual information processing in acute schizophrenia before and after neuroleptic treatment. *In* "Hemisphere Asymmetries of Function in Psychopathology" (J. H. Gruzelier and P. Flor-Henry, eds.), pp. 511–527. Elsevier/North-Holland, Amsterdam.

Eaton, E. M., Busk, J., Maloney, M. P., Sloane, R. B., Whipple, K., and White, K. (1979). Hemispheric dysfunction in schizophrenia. *Psychiatry Res.* **1,** 325–332.

Ellenberg, L., and Sperry, R. W. (1979). Capacity for holding sustained attention following commissurotomy. *Cortex* **15,** 421–438.

Epstein, S., and Coleman, P. (1970). Drive theories of schizophrenia. *Psychosom. Med.* **32,** 113–140.

Etevenon, P., Peron-Magnon, P., Campistron, D., Vordeaux, G. and Deniker, P. (1983). Differences in EEG symmetry between patients with schizophrenia. *In* "Laterality and Psychopathology" (P. Flor-Henry and J. H. Gruzelier, eds.), Vol. 2. Elsevier/North-Holland, Amsterdam (in press).

Filskov, S., and Goldstein, S. (1974). Diagnostic validity of Halstend–Reitan Neuropsychological Battery. *J. Consult. Clin. Psychol.* **42,** 382–388.

Fisher, S., and Cleveland, S. E. (1959). Right–left body reactivity problems in disorganised states. *J. Nerv. Ment. Dis.* **128,** 396–400.

Fleminger, J. F., Dalton, R., and Standage, K. F. (1977). Handedness in psychiatric patients. *Brit. J. Psychiat.* **12,** 448–452.

Flor-Henry, P. (1969). Psychoses and temporal lobe epilepsy: A controlled investigation. *Epilepsia* **10,** 363–395.

Flor-Henry, P. (1974). Psychosis, neurosis and epilepsy. *Br. J. Psychiatry* **124,** 144–150.

Flor-Henry, P. (1979). Laterality, shifts of cerebral dominance, sinistrality and psychosis. *In* "Hemisphere Asymmetries of Function in Psychopathology" (J. H. Gruzelier and P. Flor-Henry, eds.), pp. 3–20. Elsevier/North-Holland, Amsterdam.

Flor-Henry, P., and Koles, Z. J. (1982). Statistical quantitative EEG studies of depression, mania, schizophrenia, and normals. *Biol. Psychol.* (in press).

Flor-Henry, P., and Yeudall, L. T. (1979). Neuropsychological investigation of schizophrenia and manic-depressive psychoses. *In* "Hemisphere Asymmetries of Function in Psychopathology" (J. H. Gruzelier and P. Flor-Henry, eds.), pp. 341–362. Elsevier/North-Holland, Amsterdam.

Flor-Henry, P., Koles, Z. J., Howorth, B. G., and Burton, L. (1979). Neurophysiological studies of schizophrenia, mania and depression. In "Hemisphere Asymmetry of Function in Psychopathology" (J. H. Gruzelier and P. Flor-Henry, eds.), pp. 189–236. Elsevier North-Holland Biomedical Press, Amsterdam.

Gazzaniga, M. S. (1970). "The Bisected Brain." Appleton, New York.

Gazzaniga, M. S., and Le Doux, J. F. (1978). "The Integrated Mind." Plenum, New York.

Geschwind, N., and Levitsky, W. (1968). Human brain: Left-right asymmetries in temporal speech region. *Science* **161,** 186–187.

Giannitrapani, D., and Kayton, L. (1974). Schizophrenia and EEG spectral analysis. *Electroencephalogr. Clin. Neurophysiol.* **36,** 377–386.

Golden, C. J., MacInnes, W. D., and Anil, R. M. (1982). Cross-validation of the ability of the Luria–Nebraska Neuropsychological Battery to differentiate chronic schizophrenics with and without ventricular enlargement. *J. Consult. Clin. Psychol.* **50,** 87–95.

Goldstein, L., and Stoltzfus, N. W. (1973). Psychoactive drug-induced changes of interhemispheric EEG amplitude relationships. *Agents Actions* **3,** 124–132.

Goode, D. J., Meltzer, H. Y., Mazura, T. A., and Cryaton, J. W. (1977). Physiologic abnormalities of the neuromuscular system on psychosis. *Schizophrenia Bull.* **3,** 121–130.

Goode, D. J., Meltzer, H. Y., and Mazura, T. A. (1979). Hoffman reflex abnormalities in psychotic patients. *Biol. Psychiatry* **14,** 95–110.

Goode, D. J., Glenn, S., Manning, A. A., and Middleton, J. F. (1980). Lateral asymmetry of the Hoffmann reflex: Relation to cortical laterality. *J. Neurol., Neurosurg. Psychiatry* **43,** 831–835.

Goode, D. J., Manning, A. A., and Middleton, J. F. (1981). Cortical laterality and asymmetry of the Hoffman reflex in psychiatric patients. *Biol. Psychiatry* **16,** 1137–1157.

Gray, J. A. (1964). "Pavlov's Typology." Pergamon, Oxford.

Gray, J. A. (1982). "The Neuropsychology Anxiety." Pergamon, Oxford.

Green, P. (1978). Defective interhemispheric transfer in schizophrenia. *J. Abnorm. Psychol.* **87,** 472–480.

Green, P., and Kotenko, V. (1980). Superior speech comprehension in schizophrenics under monaural versus binaural listening conditions. *J. Abnorm. Psychol.* **89,** 399–408.

Gruzelier, J. H. (1973). Bilateral asymmetry of skin conductance orienting activity and levels in schizophrenia. *J. Biol. Psychol.* **1,** 21–41.

Gruzelier, J. H. (1978). Bimodal states of arousal and lateralised dysfunction in schizophrenia: The effect of chlorpromazine. *In* "The Nature of Schizophrenia: New Approaches to Research and Treatment" (L. Wynne, R. Cromwell, and S. Matthysee, eds.), pp. 167–187. Wiley, New York.

Gruzelier, J. H. (1979a). Lateral asymmetries in electrodermal activity and psychosis. *In* "Hemisphere Asymmetries of Function in Psychopathology" (J. H. Gruzelier and P. Flor-Henry, eds.), pp. 149–168. Elsevier/North-Holland, Amsterdam.

Gruzelier, J. H. (1979b). Synthesis and critical review of the evidence for hemisphere asymmetries of function in psychopathology. *In* "Hemisphere Asymmetries of Function in Psychopathology" (J. H. Gruzelier and P. Flor-Henry, eds.), pp. 647–672. Elsevier/North-Holland, Amsterdam.

Gruzelier, J. H. (1981a). Hemispheric imbalances masquerading as paranoid and non-paranoid syndromes. *Schizophr. Bull.* **7,** 662–673.

Gruzelier, J. H. (1981b). Cerebral laterality and psychopathology: fact and fiction. *Psychol. Med.* **11,** 219–227.

Gruzelier, J. H., and Hammond, N. V. (1976). Schizophrenia: A dominant hemisphere temporal–limbic disorder? *Res. Commun. Psychol., Psychiatry Behav.* **1,** 33–72.

Gruzelier, J. H., and Hammond, N. V. (1978). The effect of chlorpromazine upon psychophysiological endocrine and information processing measures in schizophrenia. *J. Psychiatr. Res.* **14,** 167–182.

Gruzelier, J. H., and Hammond, N. V. (1979a). Gains, losses and lateral differences in the hearing of schizophrenic patients. *Br. J. Psychol.* **70,** 319–330.

Gruzelier, J. H., and Hammond, N. V. (1979b). Lateralised auditory processing in medicated and unmedicated schizophrenic patients. *In* "Hemisphere Asymmetries of Function in Psychopathology" (J. H. Gruzelier and P. Flor-Henry, eds.), pp. 603–638. Elsevier/North-Holland, Amsterdam.

Gruzelier, J. H., and Hammond, N. V. (1980). Lateralised deficits and drug influences on the dichotic listening of schizophrenic patients. *Biol. Psychiatry* **15,** 759–779.

Gruzelier, J. H., and Manchanda, R. (1982). The syndrome of schizophrenia: Relations between electrodermal response, lateral asymmetries and clinical ratings. *Br. J. Psychiatry* **141,** 488–495.

Gruzelier, J. H., and Venables, P. H. (1973). Skin conductance responses to tones with and without attentional significance in schizophrenic and non-schizophrenic patients. *Neuropsychologia* **11,** 221–230.

Gruzelier, J. H., and Venables, P. H. (1974). Bimodality and lateral asymmetry of skin conductance orienting activity in schizophrenics: Replication and evidence of lateral asymmetry in patients with depression and disorders of personality. *Biol. Psychiatry* **8,** 55–73.

Gruzelier, J. H., and Yorkston, N. J. (1978). Propranolol and schizophrenia: Objective evidence of efficacy. *In* "Biological Basis of Schizophrenia" (W. Hemmings and G. Hemmings, eds.), pp. 127–146. M.T.P. Press, Lancaster.

Gruzelier, J. H., Lykken, D. T., and Venables, P. H. (1972). Schizophrenia and arousal revisited: Two-flash threshold and electrodermal activity in activated and non-activated conditions. *Arch. Gen. Psychiatry* **26,** 427–432.

Gruzelier, J. H., Mednick, S., and Schulsinger, F. (1979). Lateralised impairments in the WISC profiles of children at genetic risk for psychopathology. *In* "Hemisphere Asymmetries of Function in Psychopathology" (J. H. Gruzelier and P. Flor-Henry, eds.), pp. 149–168. Elsevier/North-Holland, Amsterdam.

Gruzelier, J. H., Eves, F. F., and Connolly, J. F. (1981a). Habituation and phasic reactivity in the electrodermal system: Reciprocal hemispheric influences. *Physiol. Psychol.* **9,** 313–317.

Gruzelier, J. H., Connolly, J. F., Eves, F. F., Hirsch, S. R., Zaki, S. A., Weller, M. F., and Yorkston, N. J. (1981b). Effect of propanolol and phenothiazines on electrodermal orienting and habituation in schizophrenia. *Psychol. Med.* **11,** 93–108.

Gur, R. E. (1977). Motoric laterality imbalance in schizophrenia: A possible concomitant of left hemisphere dysfunction. *Arch. Gen. Psychiatry* **34,** 33–37.

Gur, R. E. (1978). Left hemisphere dysfunction and left hemisphere overactivation in schizophrenia. *J. Abnorm. Psychol.* **87,** 226–238.

Gur, R. E. (1979). Cognitive concomitants of hemispheric dysfunction in schizophrenia. *Arch. Gen.Psychiat.* **36,** 269–274.

Hammond, N. V., and Gruzelier, J. H. (1978). Laterality, attention and rate effects in the auditory temporal discrimination of chronic schizophrenics: The effect of chlorpromazine. *Q. J. Exp. Psychol.* **30,** 91–103.

Hartlage, L. C., and Garber, J. (1976). Spatial and nonspatial measuring ability in chronic schizophrenics. *J. Clin Psychol.* **32,** 235–237.

Heinburger, R. F., and Reiton, R. M. (1961). Easily administered written test for lateralising brain lesions. *J. Neurosurg.* **18,** 301–312.

Hellige, J. B., Cox, P. J., and Litrae, L. (1979). Information processing in the cerebral hemispheres: Selective hemispheric activation and capacity limitations. *J. Exp. Psychol., Gen.* **108**, 251–279.

Hillsberg, B. (1979). A comparison of visual discrimination performance of the dominant and nondominant hemispheres in schizophrenia. *In* "Hemisphere Asymmetries of Function in Psychopathology" (J. H. Gruzelier and P. Flor-Henry, eds), pp. 527–538. Elsevier/North-Holland, Amsterdam.

Hiscock, M. (1977). Effects of examiners location and subjects anxiety on gaze laterality. *Neuropsychologia* **15,** 409, 411.

Holtzman, P. S., Proctor, L. R., Levey, D. L., Yasillo, N. J., Meltier, H. Y., and Herot, S. W. (1974). Eye-tracking dysfunctions in schizophrenic patients and their relatives. *Arch. Gen. Psychiatry* **31,** 143–151.

Jarrard, L. F. (1973). The hippocampus and motivation. *Psychol. Bull.* **79,** 1–12.

Jerger, J. (1973). Diagnostic audiometry. *In* "Modern Developments in Audiology" (J. Jerger, ed.), 2nd ed. Academic Press, New York.

Jernigan, T. L., Ztaz, L. M., Moses, J. A., and Cardellino, J. P. (1982). Computed tomography in schizophrenics and normal volunteers. II. Cranial asymmetry. *Arch. Gen. Psychiatry* **39,** 771–777.

Johnson, O., and Crockett, D. (1982). Changes in perceptual asymmetries with clinical improvement of depression and schizophrenia. *J. Abnorm. Psychol.* **91,** 45–54.

Jones, G. H., and Millar, J. J. (1981). Functional tests of the corpus callosum in schizophrenia. *Br. J. Psychiatry* **139,** 553–557.

Kameyama, T., Niwa, S., Hiramatsu, K., and Saitoh, O. (1983). Hand preference and eye dominance patterns in schizophrenia and affective disorders. *In* "Laterality and Psychopathology" (P. Flor-Henry and J. H. Gruzelier, eds.), Vol. 2. Elsevier/North-Holland, Amsterdam (in press).

Kesner, R. P., and Novak, J. M. (1982). Serial position curve in rats: Role of dorsal hippocampus. *Science* **218,** 173–175.

Kety, S. S. (1980). The syndromes of schizophrenia: Unresolved questions and opportunities for research. *Br. J. Psychiatry* **136,** 421–436.

Kimble, D. P. (1968). Hippocampus and internal inhibition. *Psychol. Bull.* **79,** 285–295.

Kinsbourne, M. (1970). The cerebral basis of lateral asymmetries in attention. *Acta Psychol.* **33,** 193–201.

Kinsbourne, M. (1973). The control of attention between the cerebral hemispheres. *In* "Attention and Performance IV". (S. Kornblum ed.), pp. 239–256. Academic Press, New York.

Kinsbourne, M. (1974). The mechanism of hemispheric control of the lateral gradient of attention. *In* "Attention and Performance V" (P. M. A. Rabbitt and S. Dornic, eds.), pp. 81–97. Academic Press, London.

Kinsbourne, M. (1980). A model for the ontogeny of cerebral organization in non-right-handers. *In* J. Herron, (ed.), "Neuropsychology of left-handedness." Academic Press, New York.

Kostandov, E. A. (1980). Asymmetry of visual perception and interhemispheric interaction. *Neurosci. Behav. Physiol.* **10,** 36–47.

Kugler, B. T. (1983). Auditory processing in schizophrenic patients. *In* "Laterality and Psychopathology" (P. Flor-Henry and J. H. Gruzelier, eds.), Vol. 2. Elsevier/North-Holland, Amsterdam (in press).

Kugler, B. T., and Caudrey, D. J. (1983). Phoneme discrimination in schizophrenia. *Br. J. Psychiatry* **142,** 53–59.

Kugler, B. T. and Henley, S. H. A. (1979). Laterality effects in the tactile modality in schizophrenia. *In* "Hemisphere Asymmetries of Function in Psychopathology" (J. H. Gruzelier and P. Flor-Henry, eds.), pp. 475–489. Elsevier/North-Holland, Amsterdam.

Kugler, B. T., Caudrey, D. T., and Gruzelier, J. H. (1982). Bilateral auditory acuity of schizophrenic patients: Effects of repeated testing, time of day and medication. *Psychol. Med.* **12,** 775–781.

Lerner, J., Nachshon, I., and Carmon, A. (1977). Responses of paranoid and non-paranoid schizophrenics in a dichotic listening task. *J. Nerv. Ment. Dis.* **164,** 247–252.

Le May, A. (1976). Morphological cerebral asymmetries of modern man, fossil man, and nonhuman primates. *Ann. N.Y. Acad. Sci.* **280,** 349–366.

Lishman, W. A. (1966). Psychiatric disability after head injury: The significance of brain damage. *Proc. R. Soc. Med.* **59,** 261–266.

Lishman, W. A. (1968). Brain damage in relation to psychiatric disability after head injury. *Br. J. Psychiatry* **114,** 373–410.

Lishman, W. A., and McKeekan, E. R. L. (1976). Hand preference in psychiatric patients. *Br. J. Psychiatry* **129,** 158–166.

Lishman, W. A., Toone, B. K., Colbourn, C. J., McMeekan, E. R. L., and Mance, R. M. (1978). Dichotic listening in psychotic patients. *Br. J. Psychiatry* **132,** 333–341.

Luchins, D. J. (1983). Psychopathology and cerebral asymmetries detected by computed tomography. *In* "Laterality and Psychopathology" (P. Flor-Henry and J. H. Gruzelier, eds.), Vol. 2. Elsevier/North-Holland, Amsterdam (in press).

Luchins, D. J., Weinberger, D. R., and Wyatt, R. J. (1979). Schizophrenia: Evidence of a subgroup with reversed cerebral asymmetry. *Arch. Gen. Psychiatry* **36,** 1309–1311.

Luchins, D. J., Pollin, W., and Wyatt, R. J. (1980). Laterality in monozygotic schizophrenic twins: An alternative hypothesis. *Biol. Psychiatry* **15,** 87–94.

Luchins, D. J., Weinberger, D. R., and Wyatt, R. J. (1982). Schizophrenia and cerebral asymmetry detected by computed tomography. *Am. J. Psychiatry* **139,** 753–757.

Luria, A. R. (1973). "The Working Brain." Penguin, Harmondsworth.

Luria, A. R., and Homskaya, E. D. (1963). Letronble du role regulateur du language au course des lesions au lobe frontal. *Neuropsychologia,* **1,** 9–26.

Luria, A. R., and Homskaya, E. D. (1970). Frontal lobe and the regulation of arousal processes. *In* "Attention: Contemporary Theory and Research" (D. Mostofsky, ed.). Appleton, New York.

Lynn, R. (1966). "Attention, Arousal and the Orienting Reactions." Pergamus, London.

Magaro, P. A. (1980). "Cognition in Schizophrenia and Paranoia: The Integration of Cognitive Processes." Erlbaum Associates, Hillsdale, New Jersey.

Malamud, N. (1967). Psychiatric disorders with intracranial tumours of the limbic system. *Arch. Neurol. (Chicago)* **17,** 113–123.

Marin, R. S., and Tucker, G. J. (1981). Psychopathology and hemisphere dysfunction. *J. Nerv. Ment. Dis.* **169,** 546–557.

Mellor, C. S. (1970). First rank symptoms of schizophrenia. *Br. J. Psychiatry* **117,** 15–23.

Milner, B. (1967). Brain mechanisms suggested by studies of the temporal lobes. *In* "Brain Mechanisms Underlying Speech and Language" (C. H. Millikane and F. L. Darley, eds.). Grune & Stratton, New York.

Milner, B. (1971). Interhemispheric differences in the localisation of psychological processes in man. *Br. Med. Bull.* **27,** 272–277.

Moscovitch, M. (1979). Information processing and the cerebral hemispheres. *In* "Handbook of Behavioral Neurobiology" (M. S. Gazzoniga, ed.), Vol. 2, pp. 379–446. Plenum, New York.

Nachson, G. (1980). Hemispheric dysfunctions in schizophrenia. *J. Nerv. Ment. Dis.* **168,** 241–242.

Naeser, M. A., Levine, H. L., Benson, D. F., Stuss, D. T., and Weir, W. S. (1981). Frontal leuctomy size and hemispheric asymmetries on computerised tomographic scars of schizophrenics with variable recovery. *Arch. Neurol. (Chicago)* **38,** 30–37.

Niwa, S., Hiramatsu, K., Makeyama, T., Saitoh, O., and Itoh, K. (1983). Dichotic detection task and schizophrenic attentional deficit. *In* "Laterality and Psychopathology" (P. Flor-Henry and J. H. Gruzelier, eds.), Vol. 2. Elsevier/North-Holland, Amsterdam (in press).

Noffsinger, P. D., and Kurdzicl, S. A. (1979). Assessment of central auditory lesions. *In* "Hearing Assessment" (W. F. Rintelman, ed.), pp. 351–377. University Park Press, Baltimore.

Nyback, H., Wiesel, F. A., Berggren, B. M., and Hindmarsh, T. (1982). Computed tomography of the brain in patients with acute psychosis and in health volunteers. *Acta Psychiatr. Scand.* (in press).

Oddy, H. C., and Lobstein, T. J. (1972). Hand and eye dominance in schizophrenia. *Br. J. Psychiatry* **120,** 331–332.

Overall, J. E., and Gorham, D. R. (1962). *Psychol. Rep.* **10**, 799–812.

Pick, A. K., Magaro, P. A., and Wade, E. A. (1979). Hemispheric functioning in paranoid and nonparanoid schizophrenia. *Biol. Psychiat.* **14,** 891–903.

Pribram, K. H. (1967). The limbic systems, efferent control of neural inhibition and behaviour. *Prog. Brain Res.* **27**.

Pribram, K. H., and McGuinness, D. (1975). Arousal, activation and effort in the control of attention. *Psychol. Rev.* **82,** 116–147.

Rodin, E., Grisell, J., and Gottlieb, J. (1968). Some electrographic differences between chronic schizophrenic patients and normal subjects. *In* "Recent Advances in Biological Psychiatry" (J. Wortis, ed.). Plenum, New York.

Roemer, R. A., Shagass, C., Straumanis, J. J., and Amadeo, M. (1978). Pattern evoked potential measurements suggesting lateralised hemispheric dysfunction in chronic schizophrenics. *Biol. Psychiatry* **13,** 185–192.

Rosenthal, R., and Bigeton, L. B. (1972). Quantitative brain measurement in chronic schizophrenia. *Brit. J. Psychiat.* **121,** 259–264.

Saito, O., Hiramatsu, K-I, Niwa, S-I, Kameyama, T. and Itoh. (1983). Abnormal ERP findings in schizophrenics with special regard to dichotic detection tasks. *In* "Laterality and Psychopathology," Vol. 2. (P. Flor-Henry and J. Gruzelier, eds.) (in press).

Salamy, A. (1978). Commissural transmission: Maturational changes in humans. *Science* **200,** 1409–1411.

Sandel, A., and Alcorn, J. D. (1980). Individual hemisphericity and maladaptive behaviours. *J. Abnorm. Psychol.* **89,** 514–517.

Satz, P. (1980). Incidence of aphasia in lefthanders: A test of some hypothetical models of cerebral speech organisation. *In* "The Neuropsychology of Left-handedness" (J. Herron, ed.), pp. 189–198. Academic Press, New York.

Scarone, S., Garvaglia, P. F., and Gazzulo, C. L. (1981). Further evidence of dominance hemisphere dysfunction in chronic schizophrenia. *Br. J. Psychiatry* **140,** 354–355.

Scarone, S., Gambini, O., and Pieri, E. (1983). Dominant hemisphere dysfunction in chronic schizophrenia: Schwartz Test and Short Aphasia Screening Test. *In* "Laterality and Psychopathology" (P. Flor-Henry and J. H. Gruzelier, eds.), Vol. 2. Elsevier/North-Holland, Amsterdam (in press).

Schwartz, A. S., Marchok, P. L., and Flynn, R. E. (1977). A sensitive test for tactile extinction: Results in patients with parietal and frontal lobe disease. *J. Neurol., Neurosurg. Psychiatry* **40,** 228–233.

Schwartz, A. S., Marchok, P. L., Kreinick, C. J., and Flynn, R. E. (1979). The asymmetric lateralisation of tactile extinction in patients with unilateral cerebral dysfunction. *Brain* **102,** 669–684.

Schweitzer, L. (1979). Differences if cerebral lateralisation among schizophrenic and depressed patients. *Biol. Psychiatry* **14,** 721–733.

Schweitzer, L., Becker, E., and Walsh, H. (1978). Abnormalities of cerebral lateralisation in schizophrenic patients. *Arch. Gen. Psychiatry* **35,** 982–985.

Searleman, A. (1977). A review of right hemisphere linguistic capabilities. *Psychol. Bull.* **84,** 503–528.

Serafetinides, E. A. (1972). Laterality and voltage in the EEG of psychiatric patients. *Dis. Nerv. Syst.* **33,** 422.

Serafetinides, E. A. (1973). Voltage laterality in the EEG of psychiatric patients. *Dis. Nerv. Syst.* **34,** 190–191.

Shagass, C., Roemer, R. A., Straumanis, J. J., and Amadeo, M. (1979). Evoked potential evidence of lateralised hemispheric dysfunction in the psychosis. *In* "Hemisphere Asymmetries of Function in Psychopathology" (J. H. Gruzelier and P. Flor-Henry, eds.), pp. 293–316. Elsevier/North-Holland, Amsterdam.

Shagass, C., Josiassen, R. C., Roemer, R. A., Straumanis, J. J., and Stepner, S. M. (1983). Failure to replicate evoked potential observature suggesting corpus callosum dysfunction in schizophrenia. *Br. J. Psychiatry* **142,** 471–476.

Shaw, J. C., Brooks, S., Colter, N., and O'Connor, K. P. (1979). A comparison of schizophrenic and neurotic patients using EEG power and coherence spectra. *In* "Hemisphere Asymmetries of Function in Psychopathology" (J. H. Gruzelier and P. Flor-Henry, eds.), pp. 257–284. Elsevier/North-Holland, Amsterdam.

Silverstein, M. L. (1983). Neuropsychological dysfunction in the major psychoses. *In* "Laterality and Psychopathology" (P. Flor-Henry and J. H. Gruzelier, eds.), Vol. 2. Elsevier/North Holland, Amsterdam (in press).

Small, J. G., Sharpley, P. H., Milstein, V., and Small, I. F. (1979). Research diagnostic criteria and EEG findings in hospitalised schizophrenic patients. *In* "Biological Psychiatry Today" (J. Obiols, C. Ballus, E. Gonzalezmonelus, and J. Pujol, eds.). Elsevier/North-Holland, Amsterdam.

Sourek, K. (1965). ["The Nervous Control of Skin Potentials in Man."] Praha Nakiadateistvi Cesckoslovenska Akademic Ved.

Sperry, R. W. (1968). Mental unity following surgical disconnection of the cerebral hemispheres. *Harvey Lect.* **62,** 293–323.

Stevens, J. R., and Livermore, A. (1982). Telemetred EEG in schizophrenia spectral analysis during abnormal behaviour episodes. *J. Neurol., Neurosurg. Psychiatry* **45,** 385–395.

Stevens, J. R., Bigelow, L., Denney, D., Lipkin, J., Livermore, A. H., Rausler, F., and Wyatt, R. J. (1979). Telemetred EEG–EOG during psychotic behaviours of schizophrenia. *Arch. Gen. Psychiatry* **36,** 251–262.

Syz, H. C. (1926). Psychogalvanic studies in schizophrenia. *Arch. Neurol. Psychiatry* **14,** 747–760.

Taylor, D. C. (1975). Factors influencing the occurrence of schizophrenia-like psychoses in patients with temporal lobe epilepsy. *Psychol. Med.* **5,** 249–256.

Taylor, P., Dalton, R., Fleminger, J. J., and Lishman, W. A. (1982). Differences between two studies of hand preference in psychiatric patients. *Br. J. Psychiatry* **140,** 166–173.

Tomer, R., Mintz, M., Levy, A., and Myslobodsky, M. (1979). Reactive gaze laterality in schizophrenic patients. *Biol. Psychol.* **9,** 115–122.

Tomer, R., Mintz, M., Levy, A., and Myslobodsky, M. (1981). Smooth pursuit pattern in schizophrenic patients during cognitive tasks. *Biol. Psychiatry* **16,** 131–144.

Tress, K. H., Kugler, B. T., and Caudrey, D. J. (1979). Interhemispheric integration in schizophrenia. *In* "Hemisphere Asymmetries of Function in Psychopathology" (J. H. Gruzelier and P. Flor-Henry, eds.), pp. 449–462. Elsevier/North-Holland, Amsterdam.

Trevarthen, C. (1974). Analysis of cerebral activities that generate and regulate consciousness in commisurotomy patients. *In* "Hemisphere Function in the Human Brain" (S. J. Dimond and J. G. Beaumont, eds.), pp. 235–263. Elek, London.

Venables, P. H. (1977). The electrodermal psychophysiology of schizophrenics and children at risk for schizophrenia: Controversies and developments. *Schizophr. Bull.* **3,** 28–48.

Wahl, O. F. (1976). Handedness in schizophrenia. *Percept. Mot. Skills* **42,** 944–946.

Walker, E., Hoppes, E., and Emory, E. (1981). A reinterpretation of findings on hemispheric dysfunction in schizophrenia. *J. Nerv. Ment. Dis.* **169,** 378–380.

Weinberger, D. R., Luchins, D. J., Morihisa, J. M., and Wyatt, R. J. (1982). Asymmetric volumes of the right and left frontal and occipital regions of the human brain. *Ann. Neurol.* **11,** 97–100.

Weiskrantz, L., and Warrington, E. K. (1975). The problem of the amnesic syndrome in man and animals. *In* "The Hippocampus" (R. L. Isaacson and K. H. Pribram, eds.), Vol. 2, Plenum, New York.

Weller, M., and Kugler, B. T. (1979). Tactile discrimination in schizophrenia and affective psychoses. *In* "Hemisphere Asymmetries of Function in Psychopathology" (J. H. Gruzelier and P. Flor-Henry, eds.), pp. 463–474. Elsevier/North-Holland, Amsterdam.

Weller, M., and Montague, J. H. (1979). Electroencephalographic coherence in schizophrenia: A preliminary study. *In* "Hemisphere Asymmetries of Function in Psychopathology" (J. H. Gruzelier and J. Flor-Henry, eds.), pp. 285–292. Elsevier/North-Holland, Amsterdam.

Wexler, B. F., and Heninger, G. R. (1979). Alterations in cerebral laterality in acute psychotic illness. *Arch. Gen. Psychiatry* **36,** 278–284.

Wing, J. K., Cooper, J. E., and Sartorius, N. (1974). "The Measurement and Classification of Psychiatric Symptoms." Cambridge Univ. Press, London and New York.

World Health Organization Study Group on Schizophrenia (1959). *Am. J. Psychiatry* **115,** 865–872.

Yozawitz, A., Bruder, G., Sutton, S., Sharpe, L., Gurlanx, B., Heiss, J., and Costa, L. (1979). Dichotic perception: Evidence for right hemisphere dysfunction in affective psychosis. *Br. J. Psychiatry* **135,** 224–237.

Zangwill, O. L. (1960). "Cerebral Dominance and its Relation to Psychological Function." Oliver & Boyd, Edinburgh.

13: Temporal and Spatial Dynamics Underlying Two Neuropsychobiological Hemisyndromes: Hysterical and Compulsive Personality Styles

ARNOLD J. MANDELL

Department of Psychiatry
University of California, San Diego
La Jolla, California

I. Dynamic Patterns in Brain Processes 327
II. Relevant Notions from Modern Mathematical Theory 329
III. The Concepts of Dimensionality and Stability 331
IV. Additive versus Multiplicative Information Processing 335
V. Intermittency: Cluster Behavior in the Time Domain 337
VI. A Neurochemical Locus for Spatiotemporal Asymmetries and Hemispheric Disconnection 338
References 342

I. Dynamic Patterns in Brain Processes

For the crest of his knighthood, Niels Bohr chose the Taoist symbol of complementarity, *yin/yang*. This binary example of social arrangement as stability, and therefore as existence itself in complex interactive systems, suggests that emergent cooperative properties "slave" elemental mechanisms to become the macroscopic behavior of multiparticipant ensembles. Topological features of subspaces are independent of the specific coordinates (Alexandroff, 1960), so the cohesive and multidetermined neighborhood qualities representing neurobiological style can be found in cooperative dynamic regions of abstract vector space of transformed experimental data across levels of observation [from brain enzymes, receptors, neurons, and electromagnetic fields to behavior (Mandell *et al.*, 1981, 1982)] and in the phenomenology of our thinking about them as well. Because relating theory to observables is itself a feature of brain function, the patterns formed during comprehension may be portraying

HEMISYNDROMES:
Psychobiology, Neurology,
Psychiatry

ISBN 0-12-512460-0

the dynamics of the knower in the shape of the known. As contrasting approaches to a theory of complex systems (Chandrasekhar, 1943; Haken, 1978), perhaps invariant features of geometric–topological transformation differ from stochastic differential equations in search of specific coefficients in much the same way that hysterical cognitive style contrasts with compulsiveness in configuring an individual's problem-solving modes.

Reich (1945) described the distribution of energy (libido) in the compulsive personality as compact, restrained, stable, and advancing directly toward its object goal. In contrast, the hysterical personality's energetics are diffuse, less restrained, and characterized by unstable specifics that nonetheless evolve stable global patterns of display despite the sequential disorder, often representing a goal symbolically. Gathering together things just as they are, an obsessive–compulsive's "pedantic sense of order" and circumstantial (linear–causal) ruminations contrast with the "pseudologia" and vivid imagination of the hysteric, which portrays emergent solutions in the form of "fantasized experience." The purest form of autistic child, offspring of two "scientifically...cold," obsessional parents, is characterized by an intolerance of any transformation of primary sensory experience, needing everything to stay exactly as originally perceived; human relations and other affective aggregates of symbolic condensation are meaningless (Rimland, 1964).

Hemispheric differences in cognitive style, as studied in split-brain subjects, temporal lobe epileptics, and normal subjects, seem to mirror these two patterns. The left side is sequential, algebraically and verbally, flat affectually, obsessional, logical, and unintuitive; the right side is geometric, characterized by fast relaxations (discontinuities) in cognitive trajectories leading to loss of logical sequence associated with an emergence of new, self-generated dynamic structure, visual, excitable, hysterical, illogical, and intuitive. Evidence of oscillations between these two ways of thinking with periods in minutes and hours comes from time-dependent neuropsychological measures. For example, studies of normal subjects have demonstrated periodic changes in strategy for problem solving between linear–causal and geometrically visual (*gestalt*-like) solutions (see Mandell, 1980, for review).

It is tempting to speculate that this dualism in cognitive and emotional pattern, described by psychoanalysts, is generated by reciprocal bilateral activating–inhibiting neurophysiological mechanisms influencing time-dependent instabilities in the geometric–spatial and analytical–temporal dichotomy of hemispheric function. In favor of an anatomical hypothesis, transcallosal reciprocal activation–inhibition of bihemispheric pairs of caudate neurons has been demonstrated (Hull *et al.*, 1974). In contrast, attempts to find brainstem biogenic amine neuronal networks with long enough spatial correlation lengths to cross the midline and satisfy such a neural mechanism have thus far failed (G. Aghajanian, personal communication). S. D. Glick (personal communication) has demonstrated by studies of rats with large numbers of subjects that the bilateral asymmetries of amine neurotransmitter concentrations consistently favor the left by a small but statistically significant margin, and early evidence for characteristic time-dependent fluctuations in left–right electroencephalographic (EEG) indicators in man has not been rigorously confirmed (P. Flor-Henry, personal communication).

The alternative possibility, to be examined here, is derived from theoretical studies suggesting that these two disparate qualities can unfold in the time dynamics of both Hamiltonian and dissipative systems that manifest homoclinic orbits (Birkhoff, 1927; Kaplan and Yorke, 1979a). The loss through disconnection-related pathologies of the hemisyndromes (Geschwind, 1965) of the time-dependent hemispheric complementarity in neural function will be viewed as a disruption in the normal "intermittency" in laminar–elliptic versus turbulent–chaotic behavior as seen in both dissipative and area-preserving dynamic systems. These features represent distributed (nonlocalizable) dynamic properties of brain function as well as fluctuations in the style of self-mapping in the solipsistic perceptions of the observer. A smoother and/or quasi-periodic flow is conjectured to be consonant with a cognitive pattern represented by a phase-maintaining trajectory, a sequential code. A turbulent flow is speculated to leave only a shape or geometry of an invariant set as its symbolic representation as sequentially coded information is lost in a pattern of phase mixing. Intermittency represents a dynamic pattern of spontaneous alternation between these two time dynamics as seen in "preturbulence" (Kaplan and Yorke, 1979a) and in the "intermittency route" to turbulence (Pomeau and Manneville, 1980) in dissipative systems or in the alternation between elliptic and stochastic behavior among the infinite number of periodic and aperiodic recurrent motions of area-preserving diffeomorphisms in the region of a homoclinic orbit (Birkhoff, 1927; Smale, 1967). In the latter case a helpful image in R^2 may be a two-torus T^2, the winding number of which, m/n, fluctuates between integer and irrational values. The dynamics of synthesis of biogenic amine neurotransmitters and their binding by receptors, distributed throughout the brain, demonstrate both patterns (Knapp *et al.*, 1981; Mandell and Russo, 1981a; Russo and Mandell, 1983; Mandell, 1982).

II. Relevant Notions from Modern Mathematical Theory

Following Poincaré's work in the late nineteenth century, theorists began to see mathematical representations of primary physical mechanisms, ordinary differential equations, in a new way. The iterative crowding of a small set against a limit to trap a specific answer or linearized stability analysis of local behavior began to give way to a search for the asymptotic geometric characteristics of more global solutions, the stable shapes of manifolds on which more variable trajectories play (Lefschetz, 1942). In psychoanalysis these invariant geometries make up personality and character; in music and art, a style. The image changed from one of impressed Newtonian forces in Euclidean space to one of time-dependent spontaneous evolution of point-set topology in abstract vector space. Soon it became apparent that the dynamic behavior of $f(x,\dot{x},t)$ manifested a limited taxonomy that was independent of the specifics; only a few kinds of hyperbolic limit sets and cycles emerged after transients died away (Smale, 1967). Thom's (1975) patterns of emergent discontinuities in bounded gradient systems depended only on the number of independent and dependent variables, that is, on the dimensionality of the dynamic structure. Psychodynamic personality typologies list few modal forms (Fenichel, 1945).

In parallel conceptual developments in physics, experimental observations did not consistently confirm the equilibrium statistical mechanics of Boltzmann, whose ergodic hypothesis suggested that in constant-energy systems a point visits everywhere in phase space. Even at low density, with the imposition of an external gradient, a test particle does not follow Markovian behavior at long times; its second hit is not completely independent of its first. Systems of "independent random events" manifest nonconvergent distributions, long-time autocorrelations, and coupling-related restrictions of motion in phase space (Montroll and Green, 1954). Far-from-equilibrium nonlinearities make characteristic cooperative shapes in both phase and probability space along dissipative and area-preserving flows that are neither ergodic nor completely integrable. As the geometers of dynamic systems are busy documenting, unmitigated randomness in statistical physics has failed.

Prigogine noted that, under equilibrium conditions, statistical fluctuations, $\Delta^2 S$ as Einstein (1926) designated these emergent dynamic structures, would regress because of "compensatory changes" [LeChatelier–Braun's principle of moderation (Prigogine and Defay, 1954)], the system being stabilized by the principle of minimum entropy production. In contrast, a changing curvature of $d\Delta^2 S$ at critical parameter values could lead to the growth of fluctuations and competition among their modes, allowing a few dimensions to emerge and dominate the system (Glansdorff and Prigogine, 1971; Haken, 1978); persistent deviations from expectation self-organized into style. In the language of far-from-equilibrium thermodynamics, then, this theoretical step beyond Onsager's (1931) near-equilibrium linear reciprocity relations deals with the same dichotomy with respect to stability that Poincaré studied by examining the behavior of orbits in the neighborhood of a given periodic orbit at point x, $\phi(x)$. There Poincaré followed the point's behavior on a transverse section, a smooth hypersurface in the phase space passing through x but not tangential to any orbit. In the pattern of returns generated by n iterates of the matrix M representing $\phi(x)$, M^n, if the linear terms of M have an eigenvalue of λ with an eigenvector of y, then $M^n y = \lambda^n y$. Points separated by a vector in the direction of y go away from x if $|\lambda| > 1$ or return to x if $|\lambda| < 1$. (If $|\lambda| = 1$ and $\lambda \neq 1$, they will circle x.) This is local linearized stability theory generalized to the characteristic pattern of separation (beyond diffusion) of two points that enter the system close together, portraying the system's kind of sensitivity to initial conditions.

To place these notions in the context of psychodynamic personality description, we might say that hysterical cognition mixes on a geometrically definable attractor, whereas compulsives think in more laminar flow, maintaining their perception-derived sequence (phase). Thus, we see two different approaches to the same realities in the form of two different kinds of dynamic systems stability. Studies of patients with visual agnosia (F. Benson, personal communication) have shown that those with intact left parietal lobes depend on a numbered sequence of straight lines and turns to find their way home, whereas those with the right side intact use an overall image of the route without remembering the details.

III. The Concepts of Dimensionality and Stability

The generic behavior of the residual set of a dynamic system depends on the number of dimensions of its manifold, which is related to the Lyapounov spectrum (Ladrappier, 1981) from transformed eigenvalues as $D \simeq n[\bar{\lambda}(+),\bar{\lambda}(0)] + [\bar{\lambda}(+)/-\bar{\lambda}(-)]$ (Kaplan and Yorke, 1979b). In integer dimension 2 (R^2) there are only limit points and limit periodic orbits. In R^3 there are limit points, periodic orbits T^1, two-dimensional tori T^2, and limit sets of more irregular (fractional dimensional) structure called strange attractors, the appearance of which is generic for $\dim \geq 3$ (Ruelle and Takens, 1971a,b). As noted, beginning with Euclidean phase space of initial conditions of infinite dimensions, some modes are damped, transients disappear, and a few winning modes come to dominate or "slave" the dynamics (Haken, 1978). A relatively low-dimensional spectrum of characteristic Lyapounov exponents comes to represent a higher dimensional reality (Farmer, 1982) by a process not unlike the growth of our own comprehension. First, the dimensionality of the information-processing system expands through the addition of new quantities as independent probabilities ($A \cup B \cup C$). Then it contracts through the discovery and/or manufacture of underlying arrangements imparting relations among those previously independent coordinates ($A \cap B \cap C$), multiplicative interactions capable of generating a new geometrically symbolic lower dimensional scheme. A group of experimental dimensions reduced by interactions among their common features representing a smaller quotient group can be portrayed in an abstract probabilistic geometry, which can then be parametized.

We have derived a measure on asymptotically invariant geometries of neurobiological states using a measure on the tradeoff of entropy between dimensionality and the average amplitude of fluctuations. Kolmogorov described two classes of solutions to constant-energy systems: (*a*) the nontransitive, countable periodic, weakly mixing (KAM) toroidal flow yielding discrete Fourier spectra (T^1, T^2,...), an amplitude that adds nonmultiplicatively with dimension and may manifest increased occupancy of phase space with increasing dimension; and (*b*) the transitive, uncountable periodic and aperiodic chaotic, multiplicatively mixing flows with evidence of broad-band, continuous, or $1/f$ spectra, which may demonstrate condensation to a compact geometry as a lower dimensional object emerges from many more initial coordinates (Kolmogorov, 1954; Monin and Yaglom, 1965; Farmer *et al.*, 1980). The first has the reality-oriented logic of the "splitter" gathering information into the disjoint neighborhoods of the original categories of collection (compulsives may become depressed when ruminating over their large burdens of unintegrated facts). The second "lumps" it all into an emergent transmuted form, a quotient group scenario from the subgroup of all (perceived) powers of the commonalities (hysterics may become paranoid with a tale symbolizing an underlying theme).

These two classes of dynamic systems manifest different styles of temporal evolution. Represented by the generalized differential equation $\dot{x}=F\mu(x)$, where $x=x_1, x_2, \ldots$ and μ is a parameter, if attracting, the first has a stationary solution given by $x = x_0$. As $\mu > \mu_c$, x_0 may lose its attraction and become a separatrix generating a periodic solution via a Hopf bifurcation with more dependence by amplitude than frequency on $(\mu - \mu_c)^{1/2}$ (Marsden and McCracken, 1976). As μ is increased still further, $x(t) = f(\omega_1 t, \omega_2 t, \ldots, \omega_n t)$, where f is periodic of 2π in each argument and $\omega_1 t$, $\omega_2 t$,... are independent frequencies. Perturbation of the initial conditions, $\Delta x_0=\alpha$, replaces $\omega_1 t$ by $\omega_1 t+\alpha$ and $\omega_2 t$ by $\omega_2 t+\alpha$ and, if α is small, $\Delta x(t)$ continues to ride the rational integer torus, retaining the topological relation of adjacency (maintained phase information) in a system relatively insensitive to initial conditions. As $N \geqq 3$, however, it can become unstable under small changes of $F\mu(x)$. The second general class of attractor as an asymptotic locus of solutions to $\dot{x} = F\mu(x)$ responds to perturbation of the initial condition Δx_0 by an exponential divergence in $\Delta x(t)$, that is, loss of phase information through mixing, seen as increased sensitivity to initial conditions.

In the language of Lyapounov characteristic exponents, in Hamiltonian multiplicative chaos (div = 0), points are both separating ($\overline{\lambda}[+]$) and coming together ($\bar{\lambda}[-]$) in an interactive homogenization of specifics that often "outlines" a lower-dimensional conceptual geometry more quickly than if complete phase-dependent evolution of the specific trajectories in all of the dimensions were required for perception. The strange attractors of dissipative dynamic systems display a similar mixed spectrum of Lyapounov numbers $\bar{\lambda}(+,-,0)$ (Froehling *et al.*, 1981). A positive Lyapounov exponent quantifying the average asymptotic rate of divergence, the process of amplification of initial measurement uncertainty, also describes the rate of emergence of new geometric structure (Shaw, 1981). A study of the characteristics of forced dissipative motion in an anharmonic oscillator over period-doubling regimes suggests different kinds of stability at the two extremes of the bifurcation gap caused by the noise driving: a regime with a narrow range of potential new behavior and maintenance of sequence; a chaotic regime of emergent (turbulent) structure, the stability of which is more geometric and statistical (Crutchfield and Huberman, 1980). Shaw (1981) has suggested that the time it takes for a dynamic system to lose its initial (sequentially coded) information is $\bar{t} = H_{iN} |\bar{\lambda}|$, where H_{iN} is the amount of initial data and $|\bar{\lambda}|$ represents the absolute Lyapounov value. This kind of stability is fragile because in systems that bifurcate to quasi periodicity in dim $\geqq 3$, sequence-dependent indices of dimensionality labeled by discrete frequencies (f_1, f_2. . .) can be altered by small changes. Obsessionals suffer from the confusion of information overload, an unreduced dimensionality. The other kind of dynamic stability, a mixing flow on a geometrically defined attractor, is not dependent on the maintenance of phase, it loses (initial) informational stability but gains symbolic representation through the emergence of a new cooperative structure accompanying the dimensional reduction. Initial specific information lost, the adaptive functioning of hysterics may suffer from judgments based on unrealistic geometric and statistical solutions.

An estimate of dimensionality in a stationary, sequence-dependent system can be obtained from the independent frequencies of its Fourier spectrum. For more chaotic, sequence-independent systems the dimension can be derived from the system by using its texture, the quality of "roughness" in the sense of Anosov (1962). Sequence-independent variational frequency, that is, nonperiodic recurrence, can be viewed as the reciprocal of durations (λ) between successive equalizations (zero crossings) with a finite expectation: $E\lambda = \Sigma(\lambda_1, \lambda_2, \ldots, \lambda_K)/K$. The behavior of this stochastic frequency of variation ($E\lambda^{-1}$) around the mean linear or nonlinear behavior is intimately linked to the number of and degrees of independence among contributing degrees of freedom, the dimensionality of the system. Changes in dimensionality can be seen in the distribution function and its higher moments (if translationally invariant even when unbounded) as approximate quantities (Feller, 1950). As a limiting example a coherent cooperative organization of elements yielding a sine wave leads to a dimensional reduction in description, toroidal periodicity T^1, with all the probability mass in the tails. Systems capable of turbulent dynamics often manifest an inverse relationship between the widths of the frequency and probability distributions (Monin and Yaglom, 1965). Boltzmann's energy–probability transform describes the convergence of the tail of probability density function (p.d.f.) as $d^{-\epsilon/kT}$ (Feynman *et al.*, 1963). That may be analogous to e^{-x^D}, in which D is the dimensionality (see later). This elision of the quantities energy, entropy, and contributing dimensionality leads to the interpretation of a smoother function such as a sine wave as resulting from entropy loss through increased cooperativity among the elements, that is, a reduction in the dimensionality of the system, and to our conjecture that $E\lambda$ varies as D^{-1}. This dimension-dependent relationship between recurrence time wavelength and the distribution function is analogous to theorems demonstrating that, in dim ≤ 3, the mean first passage time of a fluctuating process to boundary β scales as β^D $(1 \leq D \leq 2)$, in which D $(D \simeq \mu)$ also describes the essential exponential quality of the characteristic function of a Levy process, $\phi(|k|) \simeq \exp(-|k|^\mu)$, in which $\mu = 1$ in a nonconvergent Cauchy distribution and 2 in a gaussian distribution (Seshadri and West, 1982). Vertically integrated phenomena across several levels of neurobiological data as infinitely divisible, self-similar processes can be characterized as probability-determined dynamics with sequence-independent frequency as a stable, textured quantity. The intermittent catalytic and binding actions of "breathing" brain enzymes and receptors, intermittent "bursting" solutions to the Hodgkin–Huxley membrane equations (Carpenter, 1981), "parabolic" bursting in single neurons (Selverston, 1980), second-order variations in EEG frequency bands, and temporal–spatial patterns of behavior in animals and humans exemplify an integrated hierarchy of cooperative neural dynamics (Fig. 13.1; Abraham and Shaw, 1983). Intermittency versus ergodicity in time is well suited for qualitative dis-

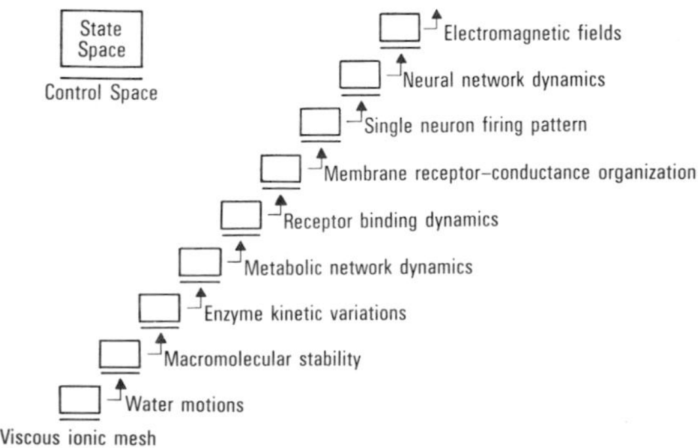

FIG. 13.1. Schematic for an integrated hierarchy of cooperative neural dynamics.

crimination using the noninteger fractal dimension D reflecting characteristics of these infinitely divisible processes that may be self-similar across scale (Mandelbrot, 1974, 1977), $1 \leqq D \leqq 2$.

As noted earlier, whereas the Fourier spectrum serves to identify the dimensionality of a superimpositional system through the number of independent frequencies, a sensitive and reliable index of dimensionality in a multiplicatively mixing system with the potential for a more uncountable spectrum can be derived from the roughness of the surface of the function treated as a geometric object, a Jordan curve (Mandelbrot, 1967). The relationship between the roughness of a dynamic geometry and its underlying dimensionality (the number of independent coordinates projecting information onto a one-dimensional manifold) can be analogized from the following argument (Manin, 1981). Removing the middle 90% of a line of unit length (dim = 1) leaves 10% at the "surface" of the two ends; removing a circle of diameter 0.9 from the unit disc (dim = 2) leaves about 20% at the surface; in dim = 3 the removal of a concentric ball of diameter 0.9 from the unit sphere leaves about 28% at the surface. In the limit, the internal volume of a geometric object of diameter 0.9 and dimension D, 0.9^D, goes to 0 as $D \rightarrow \infty$. In the geometry of multidimensional volumes, the higher the dimensionality, the greater the arc length of the perimeter relative to its volume. The minimum number of arbitrarily fine unit coverings required increases with an increase in integer dimensionality as $D + 1$ (Alexandroff, 1960).

As with the Fourier spectra of sequence-dependent systems in which power is partitioned among frequencies, here also an exchange of entropy between dimensionality and variance (Misra *et al.*, 1979) requires that the two aspects of the dynamics be considered together. A relationship observed in some systems can be understood intuitively by analogy to the transformation of a C shaped arrangement of points on a plane (dim = 2) to one on a line (dim = 1) (Shepard, 1962). With dimensional reduction from dim = 2 to dim = 1, the points at either end move farther apart and the ones in the middle move closer together. In cooperative dynamic systems, a reduction in the dimension of the manifold may increase the variance in the distances between points (Alexandroff, 1960).

IV. Additive versus Multiplicative Information Processing

From our studies of the variational dynamics of multiple neurobiological systems, determinations of roughness-derived dimensionality (D) and average amplitude of deviation from a linear mean function, variance (Var), reflect two different patterns of relation. In the information-processing schematic on the left in Fig. 13.2 the quantities A, B, and C

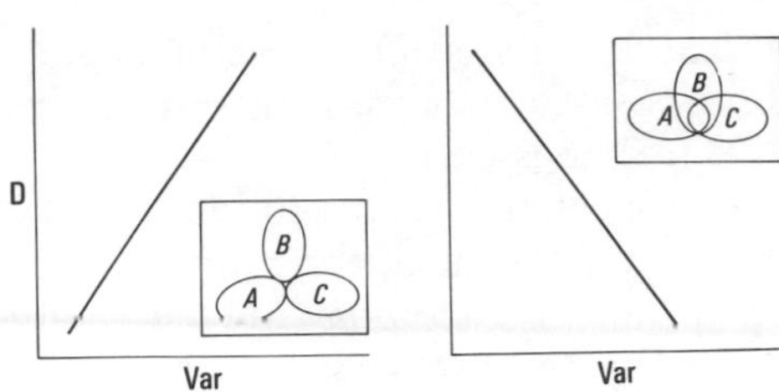

FIG. 13.2. Dimensional and Lebesque-measure relationships in additive versus multiplicative interactions of brain systems.

add independently (noncooperatively), as would a sequence of independent random events, and the occupancy of phase space increases with dimensionality. The set theoretic process of the "additive noise" (inset) is one of union, $\cup_{ABC}$, allowing the continued identification of contributing trajectories as in a weakly mixing system on KAM tori. The spectral bands in such systems are discrete; the open set of spectral frequencies has a theoretical topological dimension of zero. In the system on the right the informational dimensions are multiplied as $\cap_{ABC}$ ("multiplicative noise") and, depending on the parameter values, the moments can diverge [in this context D can be regarded as a "fractal moment" (Mandelbrot, 1977)]. The set theoretic process is one of intersection, and the cooperative dynamics in the shared neighborhood may lead to reduced occupancy of phase space by either a laminar limit cycle or a geometrically defined chaotic attractor (Ruelle and Takens, 1971a,b). The identifiability of the contributing sets is lost, and a new lower-dimensional geometric object emerges in the multiplicatively mixing system $\cap_{ABC}$, which, depending on the region in phase space, may be characterized by a more continuous spectrum (the closure of the set of spectral frequencies has a theoretical topological dimension of 1).

Complementary sequencing of the two kinds of dynamic systems, one gathering information with dimensional expansion and the other making a lower dimensional interpretive dynamic structure from it, would not be difficult to defend as the way in which we grow in understanding and might be responsible for the periodically changing characteristics of cognition and behavior attributed to left–right hemispheric oscillations in many psychophysiological and psychophysical studies (Gruzelier and Flor-Henry, 1979). As noted earlier, transitions between these two generic behaviors can occur in generalized dynamic systems in small zones of parameter (μ) space with time, not anatomical region, subserving their distinctness (Lorenz, 1980). The Landau (1944) route to turbulence over increasing μ via an infinite number of bifurcations has been generally rejected in favor of several other scenarios, for example, a transition via three Hopf bifurcations through quasi periodicity (f_1, f_2, f_3) as independent frequencies (Ruelle and Takens, 1971a,b; Curry and Yorke, 1978), finite "jump" transitions (Collet and Eckmann, 1980), and period-doubling bifurcations (Grossmann and Thomae, 1977; Coullet and Tresser, 1978; Feigenbaum, 1979; Geisel and Nierwetberg, 1982).

V. Intermittency: Cluster Behavior in the Time Domain

Because of the intermittent pattern of activity in many neurobiological systems and the quasi-regular oscillations between sequential time-dependent and geometric time-independent cognitive states in man (a pattern of instability between instabilities), the intermittency route to turbulence of Pomeau and Manneville (1980) is of greatest interest to us here. The discontinuities are derived from saddle-node bifurcations (Abraham and Marsden, 1978) in which unstable fixed points (the saddle nodes) and sinks annihilate one another to become complex fixed points at a critical value of μ. Using a one-parameter family of iterated maps, $x_{N+1} = f\mu(x_N)$, $f\mu(x) = 1-\mu x^2$ ($\mu \in [0,z]$; $x \in [-1,1]$), Collet and Eckmann (1980) found that $f^3\mu$ manifests a stable periodic orbit of three in a small interval near $\mu = 1.75$ and maps chaotically above that. In the critical region, regular periodic oscillations are interrupted intermittently by temporal patches of irregularity, as in Fig. 13.3 (after Eckmann, 1981). "Intermittency," that is, cluster behavior in the time domain, is a common feature of hydrodynamic, solid-state, astrophysical, and informational systems as well as the brain at several disciplinary levels. Trajectories alternate between a phase-maintaining rotation around an unstable periodic orbit and intermittent departures from it in more chaotic mixing patterns. As intermittent turbulent behavior alternates with periods of laminar flow with statistically average durations, the amount of time in the laminar state (a recurrence time $E\lambda$) scales as $(\mu-\mu_c)^{-1/2}$ and in the presence of noise (σ is standard deviation of the fluctuations) as $(\mu-\mu_c)^{-1/2}\, T[\sigma/(\mu-\mu_c)^{3/4}]$. This transition to turbulence through intermittency [Eckmann, 1981] may be a model for how fluctuating changes in cognitive style can

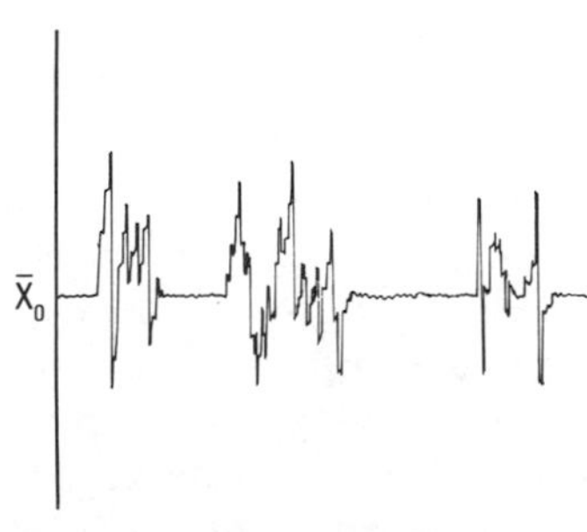

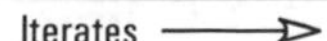

FIG. 13.3. Intermittency, a common dynamic of neuropsychobiological mechanisms.

be a time-dependent, anatomically distributed phenomenon. Alternations between two kinds of statistical context periodically interchange conditions favoring the characteristic behavior of one hemispheric style over the other. A primitive example of neurobiological intermittency is represented in single cells by bacterial behavior that fluctuates irregularly between laminar and chaotic motion (Koshland, 1980). In sleeping man the alternations between smooth slow waves and the more rapidly changing ("alphoid") EEG oscillations in dreaming sleep may be a comparable example (Dement, 1955).

Another mechanism for intermittent behavior in addition to the evolution of an intrinsic pattern of intermittency might be μ fluctuating in a range of values that would select one and then the other of the two contrasting behaviors. Indeed, Shaw (1981) has shown that the relationship between μ and the Lyapounov characteristic exponents $\overline{\lambda}(-)$ versus $\overline{\lambda}(+)$ is a widely varying function across small differences in a large range of μ in general systems of nonlinear difference equations.

VI. A Neurochemical Locus for Spatiotemporal Asymmetries and Hemispheric Disconnection

The dopaminergic system in the brain serves as a locus for both anatomical–spatial and dynamic–temporal mechanisms for oscillation in cognitive style and the disconnections of the hemisyndromes. A drug-sensitive hemispheric asymmetry in dopamine concentration has been well documented (Glick *et al.*, 1977; see also Chapter 2), as have autonomous reciprocal bilateral oscillations in nigrostriatal dopamine biosynthesis rates *in vivo*, with periods in minutes (Nieoullon *et al.*, 1978). Differential suppression of hemispheric style by pathologically asymmetric concentrations of biogenic amine inhibitors of cell discharge rates provides a chemical–anatomical hypothesis for the hemisyndromes. With respect to cognitive style, EEG and neuropsychological studies have suggested that defects in left hemisphere inhibitory regulation of the right hemisphere are correlated with increased prominence ("release") of hysterical traits, including the characteristic frigidity (Flor-Henry, 1979, 1980; Flor-Henry *et al.*, 1981). As a hemisyndrome of space (Mandell *et al.*, 1983), a maintained fixation in either a hysterical or a compulsive personality style might be explained by a limit-cycle lockup into a periodically driving "ectopic focus" in one hemisphere, beginning with brainstem biogenic amine asymmetry "releasing" a hemisphere from below and progressing to (additional) transcallosal inhibition of cell discharge on the other side by the already advantaged hemisphere (Hull *et al.*, 1974). Kindling, permanently decreasing the threshold for a neurobiological event through repetitions, might explain its persistence (Goddard *et al.*, 1969).

With respect to time, we have seen that, in a generalized representation of the evolution of a one-parameter family of maps, the value of parameter μ could determine the degree of intermittency between sequential laminar (compulsive) and multiplicative mixing (hysterical) styles. The nigrostriatal dopamine-synthesizing system in rat brain may have such a parameter in the far-from-equilibrium (with respect to enzyme kinetics) concentrations of tetrahydrobiopterin, the hydroxylase cofactor BH_4 (Mandell and Russo, 1981b). Using a kinetic scattering paradigm, we sample sequentially the initial rate behavior of aliquots from closed, partially enriched homogenates of rat brain tyrosine hydroxylase, graining the intervals of observation in minutes to be consistent with the periods of the slow, soliton-like (Jardetsky and King, 1983) autonomous motions characteristic of globular proteins in solution (Mandell and Russo, 1981a; Russo, 1982; Russo and Mandell, 1983). Each globular protein in solution is viewed as an ensemble of interconverting structures, the trajectories of which through sequential states manifest ligand sensitivity in both the time distribution among the multiple forms and the phasing within the population. Plotting the median values of triplicate determinations of enzyme product concentrations (Fig. 13.4A) and varying the concentration of BH_4 as the kinetic scattering parameter μ, we examined the morphology of the Fourier spectra $Gx(f)$, the autocorrelation graph $Rx(\tau)$, and di-

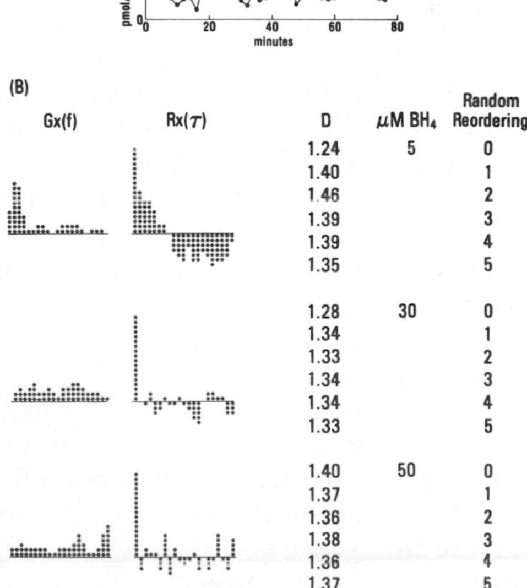

FIG. 13.4. (A) Representative plot of median values of triplicate determinations of tyrosine hydroxylase product concentrations. (B) Power (frequency) spectra $Gx(f)$, autocorrelation graphs $Rx(\tau)$, and dimensionality D at three levels of BH_4 cofactor as assayed (zero reordering) and after five independent random reorderings. Note that the higher D values are relatively more resistant to the random reordering in this examination of the dependency of the index of dimensionality on the maintenance of phase information.

mensionality D by methods published elsewhere (Mandell and Russo, 1981a). A fourth technique involved the use of a random perturbation group g to examine the dependency of the index of dimensionality on the stability of the sequence, that is, on the maintenance of phase information:

$$\begin{array}{ccc} D & \xrightarrow{f} & D' \\ g \downarrow & & \downarrow g \\ D'' & \xrightarrow{f'} & D''' \end{array}$$

Here, f and f' represent two similar but not identical conditions of the scattering parameter BH_4, and g represents the random reordering group (g being *one-to-one, onto,* and bijective with respect to D). We conjectured that the equivalence g would preserve the dimensional index of the dynamic structure of f and f' in the phaseless mixing system ($gf = f'g$) and fail to do so ($gf \neq f'g$) in the sequence-dependent periodic and quasi-periodic regimes.

Figure 13.4A shows a typical data set, the medians of triplicate determinations across time. A value of μ, BH_4 at 5 μM, elicits a periodic limit cycle and autocorrelation graph and a dimensional exponent that is sensitive to g. With BH_4 at 50 μM a chaotic spectrum and aperiodic autocorrelation graph are consonant with a higher index of dimensionality, which is relatively resistant to the random reordering group g. Features of both appear at 30 μM BH_4. Amphetamine, a unique drug with respect to its capacity to decrease brain BH_4 levels (Mandell and Russo, 1981b), may lead to limit-cycle, sequence-dependent periodicities in the behavior of brain enzyme, receptors, single nigrostriatal neurons, electrical fields, and behavior in animals and man (Mandell *et al.*, 1981) via its effect on the temporal pattern of diffusely distributed dopamine synthesis (Fig. 13.4B, 5 μM BH_4). "Speed" cognition is composed of compulsively repetitious and detailed sequencing in speaking, writing, and art. The behavior of a child with the hyperactivity syndrome is more ordered, more sequential, following the administration of amphetamine (Wender, 1971). In contrast, high BH_4 levels generate a phaseless mixing condition in the measures of kinetic scattering (Russo and Mandell, 1983). We speculate that BH_4 could be μ in Pomeau–Manneville intermittency, with the distance from the critical value $(\mu - \mu_c)^{-1/2}$ determining the temporal interval between laminar and turbulent states (Fig. 13.3), *turbulent* here meaning phase mixing on an emergent geometric structure. We demonstrated in rats that, like high doses of amphetamine (Mandell *et al.*, 1980), life-threatening stress reduced brain BH_4 levels to within the critical range (Mandell and Russo, 1981b), suggesting that $(\mu - \mu_c)^{-1/2}$ may be involved in the emergence of fear-induced monotonic delusion (paranoia) often attributed to malfunction of the brain dopaminergic system (Mandell *et al.*,

1981); a similar dynamic systems approach has been taken to the role of dopamine dynamics and their bifurcation in the syndromes of schizophrenia (King *et al.*, 1981).

Wiener (1958) decomposed the resting, alert, "meditative" rhythm (10 Hz) of the EEG spectrum heterodyned with a central frequency into a quasi-stable compromise of antithetical pulls by positive and negative (time-reversal) frequencies (θ = 4–6 Hz and β = 14–40 Hz) as well as a superimposition of the "gathering" frequency with nearby linear and nonlinear modes. We can argue analogously that ideal cognition is a compromise of pulls between a logical, sequential, information-gathering laminar flow and an emergent cooperative process out of which new laminar and geometric–chaotic images grow. If the EEG is viewed as the dynamic surface of a multidimensional volume, β rhythm would reflect the higher dimensionality of the disjoint addition of independent frequencies (a high β-rhythm density is seen in perceptual arousal and as a chronic state in compulsive people); θ rhythm would reflect the reduced dimensionality of multiple interactions specifying a more compact geometry [a high θ rhythm is more characteristic of hysterical personalities and individuals with strong visual imagery (Walter, 1953)]. As Wiener suggested, the α rhythm is a fragile compromise. In evoked potential studies, patients with multiple personalities demonstrated, upon suitable suggestion, amplitudes and latencies characteristically identified with both obsessive–compulsiveness and hysterical personality (Putnam, 1982). This finding is consonant with our abstraction of these qualities as dynamic states of brain as well as syndromes in individuals.

Multiplicative mixing in Hamiltonian systems may be more consonant than dissipative dynamics with emergent brain processes at both global and molecular levels in that whole brain energy utilization does not change in clinical psychiatric extremes (Kety, 1950; Sokoloff *et al.*, 1981), and instability-dependent motion in enzymes and receptors requires no energy in addition to the potential for motion imparted by innate macromolecular instability and thermodynamic bombardment by the surrounding water molecules at body temperature (Gurd and Rothgeb, 1979). In such organizations, topological invariants such as dimension (Hurewicz and Wallman, 1941) may offer more generalizable tools of description than contrived mechanistic energetics mapped as a geodesic flow on a one-dimensional potential gradient.

Some studies have demonstrated a "phasing" effect (Fig. 13.2, right) of tricyclic antidepressants (which facilitate the emergence of manic–depressive cycles) and a "dephasing" influence (Fig. 13.2, left) of lithium (which prevents their emergence) across many neuropsychobiological levels (Knapp *et al.*, 1981; Mandell *et al.*, 1982). From the duality in dynamic processes conjectured to underlie man's two fluctuating cognitive styles, a prediction followed that imipramine (a tricyclic) would facilitate

TABLE 13.1
Effect of Imipramine and Lithium Treatment on Cognitive Styles[a]

Task	Direction of change ($p <$)	
	Imipramine (N = 20)	Lithium (N = 16)
Cognitive processing	↑ (0.02)	↓ (0.037)
Pair associate learning	↑ (0.047)	↓ (0.05)
Minnesota clerical task	↑ (0.001)	↓ (0.05)
Proteus maze	↓ (0.017)	No change
Trail making	↓ (0.02)	No change

[a] After Judd *et al.* (1977, 1981) and Squire *et al.* (1980).

sequential processing and that lithium-induced mixing on a geometric attractor (Mandell *et al.*, 1982), although impairing those functions, would leave spatial tasks intact. Table 13.1 summarizes the findings of Judd *et al.* (1977, 1981) and Squire *et al.* (1980) in normal volunteers taking one of the two agents daily for 2 to 3 weeks. The hypothesis was supported. Imipramine facilitated the first three tasks, which emphasized sequential and/or analytical cognition, and impaired the two that depended more on the use of geometric patterns; lithium treatment did the opposite.

A major contribution of classical psychoanalytical research is the classification of "defense" or coping styles with obsessive–compulsive and hysterical modes representing the extremes of a descriptive continuum (Fenichel, 1945). The global analysis of the behavior of complex interactive neurobiological systems may show that those patterns exist at every disciplinary level.

Acknowledgments

This theoretical development was supported by a grant from the W. M. Keck Foundation and United States Public Health Service Grant DA-00265–11. Appreciation is expressed to E. Ben-Jacob, J. Crutchfield, D. Farmer, G. Feher, A. Garfinkel, H. Haken, A. Iberall, S. Knapp, D. Koshland, B. Mandelbrot, P. Russo, M. Weissman, and B. West for valuable conversations.

References

Abraham, R., and Marsden, J. E. (1978). "Foundations of Mechanics." Benjamin/Cummings, Reading, Massachusetts.

Abraham, R., and Shaw, C. (1983). Dynamics—a visual introduction. *In* Self-Organizing Systems: The Emergence of Order" (F. E. Yates, ed.). Plenum, New York.

Alexandroff, P. S. (1960). "Elementary Concepts of Topology," pp. 11–55. Dover, New York.

Anosov, D. V. (1962). Roughness of geodesic flows on compact Riemannian manifolds of negative curvature. *Sov. Math. (Engl. Transl.)* **3**, 1068–1070.

Birkhoff, G. D. (1927). On the periodic motions of dynamical systems. *Acta Math.* **50**, 359–379.

Carpenter, G. A. (1981). Normal and abnormal signal patterns in nerve cells. *SIAM-AMS Proc.* **13**, 49–90.

Chandrasekhar, S. (1943). Stochastic problems in physics and astronomy. *Rev. Mod. Phys.* **15**, 1–89.

Collet, P., and Eckmann, J.-P.(1980). "Iterated Maps on the Interval as Dynamical Systems," pp. 107–121. Birkhaeuser, Basel.

Coullet, P., and Tressor, J. (1978). Iterations d'endomorphismes et groupe de renormalisation. *J. Phys. (Orsay, Fr.)* **C5**, 25–34.

Crutchfield, J. P., and Huberman, B. A. (1980). Fluctuations and the onset of chaos. *Phys. Lett. A* **77A,** 407–410.

Curry, J. Y., and Yorke, J. A. (1978). A transition from Hopf bifurcation to chaos: Computer experiments with maps on R^2. *Lect. Notes Math.* **668**, 131–148.

Dement, W. (1955). Dream recall and eye movements during sleep in schizophrenics and normals. *J. Nerv. Ment. Dis.* **122**, 263–269.

Eckmann, J.-P. (1981). Roads to turbulence in dissipative dynamical systems. *Rev. Mod. Phys.* **53**, 643–654.

Einstein, A. (1926). "Investigations on the Theory of the Brownian Movement, " pp. 19–35. Methuen, London.

Farmer, J. D. (1982). Chaotic attractors of an infinite-dimensional dynamical system. *Physica D* **4D**, 366–393.

Farmer, J. D., Crutchfield, J., Froehling, H., Packard, N., and Shaw, R. (1980). Power spectra and mixing properties of strange attractors. *Ann. N. Y. Acad. Sci.* **357**, 453–472.

Feigenbaum, M. (1979). Quantitative universality for a class of nonlinear transformations. *J. Stat. Phys.* **21**, 669–706.

Feller, W. (1950). "An Introduction to Probability Theory and Its Applications," Vol. I, pp. 303–341. Wiley, New York.

Fenichel, O. (1945). "The Psychoanalytic Theory of Neurosis," pp. 463–540. Norton, New York.

Feynman, R. P., Leighton, R. B., and Sands, M. (1963). "The Feynman Lectures on Physics," Vol. I, Addison-Wesley, Reading, MA., pp. 1–6.

Flor-Henry, P. (1979). On certain aspects of the localization of the cerebral systems regulating and determining emotion. *Biol. Psychiatry* **14**, 677–698.

Flor-Henry, P. (1980). Cerebral aspects of the orgasmic response: Normal and deviational. *In* "Medical Sexology" (R. Forleo and W. Pasini, eds.), pp. 256–262. Elsevier, Amsterdam.

Flor-Henry, P., Fromm-Auch, D., Tapper, M., and Schopflocher, D. (1981). A neuropsychological study of the stable syndrome of hysteria. *Biol. Psychiatry* **16**, 601–626.

Froehling, H., Crutchfield, J. P., Farmer, D., Packard, N. H., and Shaw, R. (1981). On determining the dimension of chaotic flows. *Physica D* **3D**, 605–617.

Geisel, T., and Nierwetberg, J. (1982). Onset of diffusion and universal scaling in chaotic systems. *Phys. Rev. Lett.* **48**, 7–10.

Geschwind, N. (1965). Disconnexion syndromes in animals and man. Parts I and II. *Brain* **88**, 237–294, 585–664.

Glansdorff, P., and Prigogine, I. (1971). "Thermodynamic Theory of Structure, Stability and Fluctuations." Wiley (Interscience), New York.

Glick, S. D., Jerussi, T. P., and Zimmerberg, B. (1977). Behavioral and neuropharmacological correlates of nigrostriatal asymmetry in rats. *In* "Lateralization in the Nervous System" (S. Harnad, L. Goldstein, R. W. Doty, J. Jaynes, and G. Krauthamer, eds.), pp. 213–251. Academic Press, New York.

Goddard, G. V., McIntyre, D. C., and Leech, C. K. (1969). A permanent change in brain function resulting from daily electrical stimulation. *Exp. Neurol.* **25**, 295–330.
Grossmann, S., and Thomae, S. (1977). Invariant distributions and stationary correlation functions of one-dimensional discrete processes. *Z. Naturforsch. A* **32A**, 1353–1363.
Gruzelier, J. H., and Flor-Henry, P., eds. (1979). "Hemisphere Asymmetries of Function in Psychopathology." Elsevier/North-Holland, Amsterdam.
Gurd, F. R. N., and Rothgeb, T. M. (1979). Motions in proteins. *Adv. Protein Chem.* **33**, 73–165.
Haken, H. (1978). "Synergetics," pp. 69–224. Springer-Verlag, New York.
Hull, C. D., Levine, M. S., Buchwald, N. A., Heller, A., and Browning, R. A. (1974). The spontaneous firing patterns of forebrain neurons. *Brain Res.* **73**, 241–262.
Hurewicz, W., and Wallman, H. (1941). "Dimension Theory," pp. 208–146. Princeton Univ. Press, Princeton, New Jersey.
Jardetsky, O., and King, R. (1983). Soliton theory of protein dynamics. *Ciba Found. Symp.* **93**, (in press).
Judd, L. L., Hubbard, R. B., Huey, L. Y., Attewell, P. A., Janowsky, D. S., and Takahashi, K. I. (1977). Lithium carbonate and ethanol induced "highs" in normal subjects. *Arch. Gen. Psychiatry* **34**, 463–467.
Judd, L. L., Rausch, J. L., Janowsk, D. S., and Huey, L. Y. (1981). Effect of imipramine on cognition in normals. *Am. Psychiat. Assoc. New Res. Abstracts,* NR 166.
Kaplan, J. L., and Yorke, J. A. (1979a). Preturbulence: A regime observed in a fluid flow model of Lorenz. *Commun. Math. Phys.* **67**, 93–108.
Kaplan, J. L., and Yorke, J. A. (1979b). Functional differential equations and approximation of fixed points. *Lect. Notes Math.* **730**, 204–228.
Kety, S. S. (1950). Circulation and metabolism of the human brain in health and disease. *Am. J. Med.* **8**, 205–217.
King, R., Raese, J. D., and Barchas, J. D. (1981). A mathematical model of central dopaminergic transmission and the dopamine hypothesis of schizophrenia. *In* "Function and Regulation of Monoamine Enzymes: Basic and Clinical Aspects" (E. Usdin, N. Weiner, and M. Youdim, eds.), pp. 399–408. Macmillan, New York.
Knapp, S., Ehlers, C., Russo, P. V., and Mandell, A. J. (1981). A cross-disciplinary approach to the action of lithium; a vertical integration. *In* "Basic Mechanisms in the Action of Lithium" (H. M. Emrich, J. B. Aldenhoff, and H. D. Lux, eds.), pp. 102–119. Excerpta Medica, Amsterdam.
Kolmogorov, A. N. (1954). The general theory of dynamical systems and classical mechanics. *In* "Foundations of Mechanics" (R. Abraham and J. E. Marsden, eds.), pp. 263–280. Benjamin, New York, 1967.
Koshland, D. E., Jr. (1980), Bacterial chemotaxis in relation to neurobiology. *Annu. Rev. Neurosci.* **3**, 43–75.
Ladrappier, F. (1981). Some relations between dimension and Lyapounov exponents. *Commun. Math. Phys.* **81**, 229–238.
Landau, C. D. (1944). Turbulence. *Dokl. Akad. Nauk SSSR* **44**, 339–342.
Lefschetz, S. (1942). "Algebraic Topology." American Mathematical Society, New York.
Lorenz, E. N. (1980). Noisy periodicity and reverse bifurcation. *Ann. N.Y. Acad. Sci.* **357**, 282–291.
Mandelbrot, B. B. (1967). How long is the coast of Britain? Statistical self-similarity and fractional dimension. *Science* **155**, 636–638.
Mandelbrot, B. B. (1974). Intermittent turbulence in self-similar cascades: divergence of high moments and dimension of the carrier. *J. Fluid Mech.* **62**, 331–358.
Mandelbrot, B. B. (1977). "Fractals: Form, Chance, and Dimension," pp. 95–108. Freeman, San Francisco, California.
Mandell, A. J. (1980). Toward a psychobiology of transcendence: God in the brain. *In* "The

Psychobiology of Consciousness" (J. M. Davidson and R. J. Davidson, eds.), pp. 379–464. Plenum, New York.

Mandell, A. J. (1982). The influence of a centrally active peptide on receptor macromolecular dynamics: Toward a neuropharmacology of phase. *Ann. N. Y. Acad. Sci.* **398,** 191–206.

Mandell, A. J., and Russo, P. V. (1981a). Striatal tyrosine hydroxylase activity: Multiple conformational kinetic oscillators and product concentration frequencies. *J. Neurosci.* **1**, 380–389.

Mandell, A. J., and Russo, P. V. (1981b). Short-term regulation of hydroxylase cofactor in rat brain. *J. Neurochem.* **37**, 1573–1578.

Mandell, A. J., Bullard, W. P., Russo, P. V., and Yellin, J. B. (1980). The influence of D-amphetamine on rat brain striatal reduced biopterin concentrations. *J. Pharmacol. Exp. Ther.* **213**, 569–574.

Mandell, A. J., Stewart, K. D., and Russo, P. V. (1981). The Sunday syndrome: From kinetics to altered consciousness. *Fed. Proc., Fed. Am. Soc. Exp. Biol.* **40**, 2693–2698.

Mandell, A. J., Russo, P. V., and Knapp, S. (1982). Strange stability in hierarchically coupled neurobiological systems. *In* "Evolution of Chaos and Order in Physics, Chemistry, and Biology" (H. Haken, ed.). pp. 270–286. Springer-Verlag, New York (in press).

Mandell, A. J., Knapp, S., Ehlers, C. L., and Russo, P. V. (1983). The stability of constrained randomness: Lithium prophylaxis at several neurobiological levels. *In* "The Neurobiology of the Mood Disorders" (R. M. Post and J. C. Ballenger, eds.). Williams & Wilkins, Baltimore, Maryland.

Manin, Y. I. (1981). "Mathematics and Physics," pp. 35–51. Birkhaueser, Basel.

Marsden, J. E., and McCracken, M. (1976). "The Hopf Bifurcation and Its Applications," pp. 63–84. Springer-Verlag, New York.

Misra, B., Prigogine, I., and Courbage, M. (1979). From deterministic dynamics to probabilistic descriptions. *Proc. Natl. Acad. Sci. U.S.A.* **76**, 3607–3611.

Monin, A. S., and Yaglom, A. M. (1965), "Statistical Fluid Mechanics: Mechanics of Turbulence," pp. 222–256. MIT Press, Cambridge, Massachusetts.

Montroll, E. W., and Green, M. (1954). The statistical mechanics of transport and non-equilibrium processes. *Annu. Rev. Phys. Chem.* **5**, 449–571.

Nieoullon, A., Cheramy, A., and Glowinski, J. (1978). Release of dopamine evoked by electrical stimulation of the motor and visual areas of the cerebral cortex in both caudate nuclei and in the substantia nigra in the cat. *Brain Res.* **145**, 69–83.

Onsager, L. (1931). Reciprocal relations in irreversible processes. II. *Phys. Rev.* **38**, 2265–2279.

Pomeau, Y., and Manneville, P. (1980). Intermittent transition to turbulence in dissipative dynamical systems. *Commun. Math. Phys.* **74**, 189–197.

Prigogine, I., and Defay, R. (1954). "Chemical Thermodynamics," pp. 26–50. Langmans, Green, New York.

Putnam, F. W. (1982). The three brains of Eve: EEG data. *Sci. News* **121**, 356.

Reich, W. (1945). "Character Analysis," pp. 204–224. Simon & Schuster, New York.

Rimland, B. (1964). "Infantile Autism: The Syndrome and Its Implications for a Neural Theory of Behavior." Appleton, New York.

Ruelle, D., and Takens, F. (1971a). On the nature of turbulence. *Commun. Math. Phys.* **20**, 167–192.

Ruelle, D., and Takens, F. (1971b). *Commun. Math. Phys.* **23**, 343–344.

Russo, P. V. (1982). A mathematical model for the effects of tetrahydrobiopterin level on tyrosine hydroxylase kinetic fluctuations. *Psychopharmacol. Bull.* **18,** 36–39.

Russo, P. V., and Mandell, A. J. (1983). A kinetic scattering approach to the nonlinear instability of a rat brain tyrosine hydroxylase system at several levels of tetrahydrobiopterin cofactor. *Brain Res.* (submitted for publication).

Selverston, A. I. (1980). Are central pattern generators understandable? *Behav. Brain Sci.* **3**, 535–571.

Seshadri, V., and West, B. J. (1982). Fractal dimensionality of a Levy process. *Proc. Natl. Acad. Sci. U.S.A.* **79**, 4501–4505.

Shaw, R. (1981). Strange attractors, chaotic behavior, and information flow. *Z. Naturforsch. A* **36A**, 80–112.

Shepard, R. N. (1962). The analysis of proximities: Multidimensional scaling with an unknown distance function. *Psychometrika* **27**, 125–140.

Smale, S. (1967). Differentiable dynamical systems. *Bull. Am. Math. Soc.* **73**, 747–817.

Sokoloff, L., Bunney, W., Kuhl, D., Buchsbaum, M., Chase, T., Rapoport, S., Rush, A. J., and Farkas, T. (1981). Positron emission tomography and cortical utilization: Clinical studies in psychiatry and neurology. *Annu. Mtg. Am. Coll. Neuropsychopharmacol., 1981.*

Squire, L. R., Judd, L. L., Janowsky, D. S., and Huey, L. Y. (1980). Effects of lithium carbonate on memory and other cognitive functions. *Am. J. Psychiatry* **137**, 1042–1046.

Thom, R. (1975). "Structural Stability and Morphogenesis." Benjamin, Reading, Massachusetts.

Walter, W. G. (1953). "The Living Brain," pp. 197–254. Norton, New York.

Wender, P. H. (1971). "Minimal Brain Dysfunction in Children," pp. 163–192. Wiley (Interscience), New York.

Wiener, N. (1958). "Nonlinear Problems in Random Theory," pp. 67–77. M.I.T. Press, Cambridge, Massachusetts.

14: Neuroleptic Effects and the Site of Abnormality in Schizophrenia

MICHAEL S. MYSLOBODSKY, MATTI MINTZ, and RACHEL TOMER

Psychobiology Research Unit
Department of Psychology
Tel-Aviv University
Ramat-Aviv, Israel

I. Introduction 347
II. Lateral Eye Movements: An Index of Abnormal Hemisphere Balance in Schizophrenia or Neuroleptic Effects? 348
III. Neuroleptic-Induced Asymmetry of Visual Evoked Potentials 350
IV. Attention-Induced Changes of $\dot{P}_{300}$ 360
V. Who Is the "Nonresponder"? 364
VI. Who Is the Blinker? 368
VII. Is the Deficit in Schizophrenia Left-sided, Right-sided, or of Callosal Transfer Origin? 371
VIII. Epilogue: Diagnosis *ex Juvantibus* 377
References 379

I. Introduction

Although *hyperdopaminergia* is assumed to be the dominant pathophysiological mechanism of schizophrenia, a limited attempt has been made to employ the dopamine (DA) hypothesis in the context of concepts relating schizophrenia to aberrant hemisphere balance (Flor-Henry, 1969; see also Chapter 7).

In line with Flor-Henry's hypothesis (1969), schizophrenia came to be regarded by an increasing number of writers as involving left hemisphere dysfunction, and some attempts were made to adjust old data and theories to this new mode of reasoning. The assumed abnormality of the left hemisphere and therapeutic ramifications of the DA hypothesis may suggest that it is reasonable to expect signs of hyperdopaminergia of the left hemisphere. The left hemisphere is believed to be responsible for con

HEMISYNDROMES:
Psychobiology, Neurology,
Psychiatry

ISBN 0-12-512460-0

scious wakefulness (Serafetinides *et al.*, 1965), and schizophrenia can be defined as a disease of consciousness (Frith, 1979). A simple syllogism might therefore be that the hyperfunction of the dopaminergic machinery in the left hemisphere (Gruzelier, 1979; Gur, 1979a; Myslobodsky *et al.*, 1979) is solely responsible for the dominant features of the disease, including hyperalertness, fragmentation and instability of attention, and overinclusive thinking (McGhie and Chapman, 1961; Kornetsky and Mirsky, 1966; Venables, 1966; Mirsky, 1969).

The hypothesis of left hemisphere hyperactivity in schizophrenia might predict that the therapeutic potency of neuroleptic drugs is directly related to their capacity to restore normal hemispheric balance via relative suppression of left hemisphere hyperalertness. Specifically, one would anticipate treatment-related enhancement of left-sided lateral eye movements, alterations of electroencephalographic (EEG) and evoked potentials over the left hemisphere, and a higher incidence of contralateral (right-sided) extrapyramidal symptoms.

However, there is a measure of uncertainty, if not confusion, as to whether different methods of laterality assessment examine the same aspects of hemisphere imbalance and whether, by exploring laterality in medicated patients, we learn something about the pathophysiology of schizophrenia. This chapter attempts to bring into focus some factors affecting the assessment of laterality patterns.

II. Lateral Eye Movements: An Index of Abnormal Hemisphere Balance in Schizophrenia or Neuroleptic Effects?

Attempts to assess brain laterality in schizophrenic patients using the lateral eye movement (LEM) technique (Table 14.1) are hindered by a lack of understanding as to how neuroleptic treatment, given in the majority of studies, interferes with LEM directionality. Given that medication may differentially affect the right and left hemispheres (Myslobodsky and Weiner, 1976), the directionality of LEMs may be confounded by the intrinsic asymmetry of the drug uptake, causing another type or variety of imbalance similar to the lateralized neuroleptic-induced extrapyramidal syndrome (Waziri, 1980).

In order to identify the drug-sensitive component of the LEM technique, we compared the directionality of reflective LEMs in drug-free and neuroleptic-treated, right-handed schizophrenic patients (see Table 14.2 for clinical summary). To determine LEM asymmetry the procedure used by Tomer *et al.* (1979) was employed.

The major LEM findings are summarized in Table 14.3. As the table

TABLE 14.1
Previous LEM Findings in Schizophrenic Patients

Number of patients	Medication	Findings	Reference
48	All on phenothiazines	Patients display more right LEMs than normal subjects	Gur (1978)
29	Nine drug free, 20 medicated (not specified)	Patients show more right LEMs than normal subjects; no effect of medication	Schweitzer *et al.* (1978)
13	All on phenothiazines	Schizophrenics show more right LEMs than controls	Schweitzer (1979)
29	No data given	Patients show more right LEMs than normal controls	Schweitzer and Chacko (1980)
20	Four drug free	Schizophrenics mostly right movers; normal subjects mostly left movers	Tomer *et al.* (1979)

TABLE 14.2
Clinical Characteristics of Subjects in LEM and VEP Studies

Characteristic	Patients LEM study ($N = 35$)	Patients VEP study ($N = 38$)	Controls VEP study ($N = 34$)
Sex (male/female)	10/25	13/25	8/26
Age (years ± *SD*)	22 ± 4.6	21.5 ± 4.6	24.6 ± 6.4
Education (years ± *SD*)	10.6 ± 1.8	10.5 ± 1.8	12.8 ± 1.03
Drug-free/medicated	7/28	9/29	
In patient/out patient	17/18	20/18	
Chronic/acute	18/17	18/20	
Number of hospitalizations			
Chronic (mean ± *SD*)	2.9 ± 3.0	3.2 ± 3.3	
Acute (mean ± *SD*)	1.2 ± 0.5	1.2 ± 0.5	
Duration of illness			
Chronic (years ± *SD*)	7.2 ± 3.6	7.4 ± 3.5	
Acute (months ± *SD*)	8.2 ± 2.8	7.1 ± 5.6	

shows there was a large number of nonresponders,* all of whom were medicated patients. Among responders the mean LEM asymmetry index (AI, the number of rightward LEMs minus the number of leftward LEMs divided by the higher LEM score) of medicated patients did not differ significantly from that of nonmedicated patients. However, when the type

*Subjects who demonstrated LEMs in at least 25% of the trials were defined as "responders" in the LEM paradigm. These patients should not be confused with "responders–nonresponders" in the EDA paradigm (see Section V).

TABLE 14.3
LEM Findings in Medicated and Nonmedicated Schizophrenics

Patients	Percentage of nonresponders		LEM AI[a] in responders (mean ± *SD*)	
Medicated				
Piperazine ($N = 20$)	55		$+0.38 \pm 0.56$ ($N = 9$)	$p < 0.05$[b]
Nonpiperazine ($N = 8$)	50		-0.35 ± 0.39 ($N = 4$)	
Total ($N = 28$)	53	$p < 0.006$[c]	$+0.16 \pm 0.61$ ($N = 13$)	not significant
Nonmedicated ($N = 7$)	0		-0.01 ± 0.66 ($N = 7$)	

[a] AI is the number of rightward LEMs minus the number of leftward LEMs divided by the higher LEM score.
[b] $t(11) = 2.21$.
[c] Test for the significance of differences between proportions.

of medication was also taken into consideration, a different result emerged. The medicated sample was divided into patients receiving drugs with piperazine derivatives, alone or in combination with other neuroleptics, and patients receiving neuroleptics with aliphatic, piperidine, or thioxanthine derivatives. This subdivision did not change the relative number of nonresponders, who were similarly distributed in the two treatment groups (Table 14.3). However, comparison of the LEM AI revealed a clear difference. Whereas the piperazine-treated patients were mostly right movers, the patients who received nonpiperazine drugs were left movers ($p < 0.05$). No differences in AI directionality were found between actue and chronic patients or between male and female patients.

These results indicate that the findings reported in the literature, including a report from our laboratory (Tomer *et al.*, 1979), may have been considerably confounded by neuroleptic medication. The possibility that some neuroleptics (piperazine derivatives) may produce hemispheric asymmetries of their own cannot be ruled out.

III. Neuroleptic-Induced Asymmetry of Visual Evoked Potentials

To examine this conjecture further we compared bilaterally recorded visual evoked potentials (VEPs) in nonmedicated schizophrenics, patients treated with neuroleptics of different classes, and control individuals (Table 14.2). The techniques employed were as described elsewhere (Mintz *et al.*, 1982a; see also Table 14.4 for scoring of VEP components).

TABLE 14.4

Amplitudes of VEP Components in Control Subjects, Schizophrenic Patients, and Patients Regrouped as Nontreated and Medicated by Different Subtypes of Neuroleptics[a]

	P_{100}		P_{300}		VEP_{max}	
	L	R	L	R	L	R
Patients ($N = 38$)	17.5[b] ± 10.0	19.1 ± 8.7	30.6[c] ± 13.2	31.4 ± 13.8	33.8[d] ± 13.2	34.0 ± 13.9
Piperazine-treated ($N = 18$)	17.9 ± 12.1	21.4 ± 10.9	32.3 ± 14.2	35.3 ± 15.0	35.0[e] ± 13.9	38.1 ± 14.8
Nonpiperazine-treated ($N = 11$)	15.8 ± 7.5	15.2 ± 4.4	32.9 ± 14.2	31.6 ± 14.3	34.6 ± 14.5	33.2 ± 15.1
Nontreated ($N = 9$)	18.4 ± 8.6	19.1 ± 6.7	24.6 ± 7.9	23.2 ± 5.7	30.2[f] ± 10.9	26.9 ± 6.8
Controls ($N = 34$)	15.8 ± 8.3	17.7 ± 7.6	24.1 ± 8.8	23.3 ± 7.5	25.8 ± 9.9	24.7 ± 8.3

[a] In this and following tables L and R stand for left and right hemispheres, respectively. Amplitudes (in microvolts; means ± SD) of VEP components were determined by measuring the vertical distance between adjacent positive (P_{100} and P_{300}) and negative (N_{130} and N_{400}) peaks and troughs. The VEP_{max} is the maximal amplitude of the secondary components [the most positive component of Seales (1973)]. It represents the vertical distance from P_{300} or P_{200} (whichever is maximal) to N_{400}.

[b] Comparison between patient and control groups: hemisphere effect, $F(1,61) = 4.98$, $p < 0.03$.

[c] Comparison between patient and control groups: group effect, $F(1,70) = 7.92$, $p < 0.007$.

[d] Comparison between patient and control groups: group effect, $F(1,70) = 10.15$, $p < 0.003$.

[e] Comparison within the patient group: hemisphere-by-category-of-medication interaction (piperazine, nonpiperazine, and nontreated), $F(2,35) = 5.25$, $p < 0.01$.

[f] Comparison within the patient group: hemisphere-by-treatment interaction (treated versus nontreated), $F(1,36) = 4.91$, $p < 0.033$.

The N_{130} component was significantly delayed in schizophrenics as compared with normal subjects ($N < 0.05$). Amplitude analysis revealed that late components were bilaterally facilitated in schizophrenics as compared with VEPs of controls ($p < 0.003$ for VEP_{max} and $p < 0.007$ for P_{300}; Table 14.4). Further analylsis showed that later components were bilaterally enhanced in chronic patients as compared with actue patients ($p < 0.005$ for VEP_{max} and $p < 0.043$ for P_{300}). This result suggests that the previously mentioned enhancement of later components in schizophrenia (above control values) can be attributed to the chronic patients.

A comparison of VEPs in drug-free and medicated patients revealed that mean latency values did not differ significantly between the two subgroups of patients. However, the amplitude of late components was higher over the right hemisphere in treated patients, whereas reversed asymmetry was observed in patients free of medication ($p < 0.033$).

Looking next for individual differences in patients responding to drugs, we plotted the AI of the VEP_{max} as a function of daily dosage of neuroleptic treatment [expressed as chlorpromazine (CPZ) equivalent]. The AI was computed as the difference between the VEP amplitudes (right minus left) over the higher amplitude. The scattergram (Fig. 14.1) shows that the AI of VEP_{max} changes from negative to positive values with increasing doses up to 500 mg CPZ equivalence ($r = 0.48$, $p < 0.01$). It also shows that positive AI values were contributed to largely by patients treated with piperazine alone or in combination with other drugs. The bilateral VEP values of the piperazine-treated group were compared with those recorded from patients medicated with "other" neuroleptics (aliphatic, piperidine, and thioxanthene) and with nonmedicated patients. This analysis revealed a relative enhancement of VEP_{max} over the right hemisphere in piperazine-treated patients ($p < 0.01$; see Table 14.4). A similar trend was observed for P_{300} values.

In order to rule out the possibility that the effect of the class of medication was confounded by the duration of illness, another analysis of variance was performed to test the interaction of duration of illness by treatment category by hemisphere. This demonstrated that the significant effect of piperazine holds for both chronic and acute patients ($p < 0.015$).

These findings again emphasize that neuroleptics do not necessarily reduce interhemispheric asymmetry. On the contrary, medication may have caused a new asymmetry, as evidenced by the enhanced VEP components over the right hemisphere in patients treated with piperazine derivatives. To complicate matters piperazine seems to affect predominantly the hemisphere that has not been assumed to be hyperactive in schizophrenia. Homolateral EEG power increase, especially in θ–δ bands, paralleled right hemisphere VEP enhancement (Mintz, 1982, unpublished) suggesting that the right hemisphere was relatively more "se-

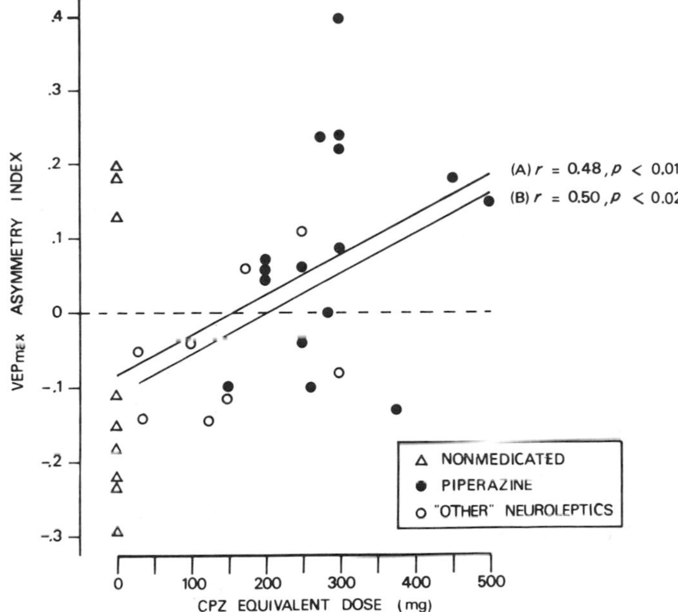

FIG. 14.1. Correlation scattergram between scores of VEP_{max} asymmetry index (the net difference between VEP amplitudes, right minus left, over the maximal amplitude) and the CPZ equivalent daily dose of neuroleptics (in milligrams). The scattergram also includes data for nontreated patients (CPZ dose, 0 mg). In (A) the correlation was computed for all (medicated and nonmedicated) patients; in (B) the correlation was based on data for medicated patients only. Key: △, nonmedicated; •, piperazine; o, "other" neuroleptics. Adapted from Mintz (1982a).

dated," in a dose-dependent fashion. Koukkou *et al.* (1979) noted that on the tenth day of medication with clozapine there was significantly higher hypersynchronous activity on the right temporal region than on the left. The similarity between the mechanisms of sedation and paroxysmal EEG ("fragments of sleep") has been discussed elsewhere (Myslobodsky, 1976).

There are two major mechanisms whereby the drug may preferentially alter the activity of one hemisphere: *(a)* sharpening or altering an intrinsic imbalance of certain neurotransmitter systems and *(b)* affecting the delivery rate of the chemical compound due to an asymmetry of blood flow (Myslobodsky and Weiner, 1976).

If the two hemispheres were neurochemically and structurally identical, the right-sided VEP alteration might be related to a higher activity of the right hemisphere in schizophrenia. Then the activity-related blood flow would increase the drug availability, leading to earlier development of neuroleptic-induced VEP alterations over the right hemisphere (Myslobodsky and Weiner, 1976). The likelihood of this possibility can be gleaned from the intrinsic asymmetry in blood volume in normal subjects, there being higher values for the right hemisphere (Carmon *et al.*, 1972). In addition, however, the two hemispheres are hardly symmetrical neurochemically (see Chapter 17).

Especially relevant to an understanding of the present findings is an interesting asymmetry of the globus pallidus, which is larger in the right hemisphere (Orthner and Sendler, 1975). Given that the globus pallidus is the major outflow of fibers containing γ-aminobutyric acid (GABA) (Kim *et al.*, 1971) and considering the role of GABA in the feedback regulation of DA activity (Hökfelt *et al.*, 1977), one might conjecture a state of DA hyperregulation in the right hemisphere. Correspondingly, DA blockade caused by chronic neuroleptic treatment would be expected to be achieved sooner in the right dopaminergic system. Although this explanation implicating the right hemisphere in the therapeutic action of the piperazine derivatives seems attractive, it is not clear why other neuroleptics do not show asymmetric distribution.*

One possibility is that piperazine derivatives mimic the DA conformation accurately and are more potent clinically than other neuroleptics, especially those with alkylamino side chains (Snyder, 1976). Correspondingly, they affect sensory transmission and motor activity in the form of Parkinson's syndrome or tardive dyskinesia more frequently (Leuscherer *et al.*, 1980) than do other neuroleptics. Figure 14.1 suggests, however, that the involvement of the right hemisphere is dose dependent, and the effect might have been the same had other neuroleptics been given in higher doses.

These considerations bring us back to the controversial issue of associating the lateralized action of neuroleptics at DA receptors and the assumed site of abnormality in schizophrenia. A more pronounced antidopaminergic effect in the right hemisphere should cause relative activation of the left hemisphere, which is therapeutically undesirable, according to the dominant laterality concepts in schizophrenia (Chapter 7).

It is known that piperazine derivatives have a clear activating effect (Itil, 1978; Janke, 1980), which is in line with the present explanation that the left hemisphere release is due to a relative suppressant effect of piperazine in the right hemisphere.

It is important to note that effective pharmacotherapy requires doses of neuroleptics that are higher than 300 mg/day (Davis, 1976). As Fig. 14.1 demonstrates, right hemisphere VEP enhancement was observed when

*Of course, the role of GABA is more complex. Increased availability of GABA in the descending output system of the striatum may produce amphetamine-like effects in rats (Scheel-Krüger *et al.*, 1981). GABA-related "hyperdopaminergia" permits one to reinterpret the asymmetry of the globus palladus as suggesting that the right hemisphere is endogenously the more active side of the brain. The role of the right hemisphere in the arousal control discussed in subsequent sections seems to add some support to this conjecture.

doses of neuroleptics were within the range 200–500mg suggesting that the positive values of VEP AI may reflect a therapeutically favorable change of hemisphere activity balance produced by neuroleptic treatment. It is of interest that CPZ treatment also caused dose-related improvement of left hemisphere processing; patients receiving high doses tended to exhibit better left hemisphere performance than patients receiving lower doses (Hammond and Gruzelier, 1978).

In view of this evidence, the concept of left hemisphere hyperalertness in schizophrenia may seem insufficient. Three explanations are suggested.

1. *The right hemisphere may be decompensated by the schizophrenic process.* The deterioration of right hemisphere functions in schizophrenia has been noted by some writers (Hartlage and Garber, 1976; Flor-Henry and Yeudall, 1979; Venables, 1981). There is a striking similarity between hemineglect after right hemisphere lesioning and some aspects of schizophrenia. Both conditions share disorientation for place and date; both show denial of illness, or anosognosia. Schizophrenic speech abnormality and Wernicke aphasia have many features in common. However, whereas the awareness of deviant speech production in schizophrenia is limited (Lecours and Vanier-Clement, 1976), the awareness of abnormality can be easily detected in Wernicke aphasia (Critchley, 1979). Also, anosognosic patients acknowledge their disease while they are in the hospital and readily accept treatment against the denied condition (Weinstein and Kahn, 1955).

As in schizophrenia, in the denial syndrome mood changes from apathy and withdrawal with akinetic mutism, to euphoria, hypersexuality, and paranoid attitudes (Weinstein and Kahn, 1955). Also, the denial syndrome develops in patients with a premorbid tendency toward withdrawal, pain asymbolia, symbols of death, and violence (Weinstein and Kahn, 1955). Finally, like anosognosic patients schizophrenics may have the altered "corporeal awareness" of Critchley (1979) or wrong body image as suggested by reportedly successful therapeutic efforts in the direction of "ego building" or ego strengthening (Goertzel *et al.*, 1965).

2. *The simplistic "balance" model may not be adequate because the left hemisphere actually requires the right-sided machinery for its activation.* It is generally accepted that the left hemisphere is specialized for analytical, sequential processing, whereas the right hemisphere is involved largely in the parallel, *gestalt* evaluation of information. It is further assumed that dominance of one or the other mode leads to a suppression of the neighboring hemisphere via callosal pathways.

Some time ago Kok (1967) noted that visuoperceptive as well as visuoconstructive performance is affected either by left or by right brain damage. Contrary to the widely circulated idea that the right hemisphere is the major mechanism of holistic analysis, she reasoned that the left hemisphere would be unable to secure an adequate symbolic representation of the world acting only as a complex "feature detector." For the understanding of a letter, a word, or a sentence irrespective of the style in which it is written, spoken, or sung, a high order of abstraction and holistic performance is required. Martin (1979) showed that the local aspects of the stimulus were more efficiently processed in the left hemisphere. However, when attention was directed to global processing, no signs of either hemisphere advantage were found. In other words, the left hemisphere would not "reject" information directed from the right hemisphere on the basis of its being "incompetent" and, since the flow of this information is not gated, the left hemisphere may be easily flooded.

When one is engaged in a motor task that requires accurate or fast performance, its execution may be impaired if one must deal with a concurrent spatial or verbal message. On the basis of Kinsbourne's model one can predict a symmetric pattern of the task "collision"-related alterations in motor performance. Verbal tasks would selectively interfere with the right but not left hand motor activity, whereas a need to accommodate spatial information would affect largely left but not right hand activity (see Kinsbourne and Cook, 1971). However, this symmetry is not perfect, and right hand performance declines more than left hand performance under the pressure of concurrent tasks (Hicks *et al.*, 1975). This finding suggests (although indirectly) that the left hemisphere has a lower resistance to overload and is more vulnerable than the right. Some writers (Hellige and Cox, 1976; Hellige *et al.*, 1979) theorize that the verbal hemisphere has a limited processing capacity and, when required to do too much processing, its performance should suffer in comparison with right hemisphere performance.

In 1964 Serafetinides and associates reported that patients undergoing intracarotid amobarbital administration more often showed signs of impaired consciousness when the drug was injected into the left carotid. According to Schwartz (1967) 38 of 46 patients with stroke of the left hemisphere experienced loss of consciousness, in contrast to 3 of 54 with a similar ischemic lesion of the right hemisphere. Electrical stimulation of the hippocampus of the dominant side also appears to lead to amnestic confusional phenomena resembling transient global amnesia more often than does stimulation of the nondominant hippocampus (Serafetinides *et al.*, 1975). These findings are believed to suggest that a "selective arousal mechanism exists that preferentially alerts the left hemisphere with the means for making more rapid time judgments [Albert *et al.*, 1976, p. 454]." Although the left hemisphere may be neurochemically equipped to generate a greater amount of "focal" arousal, the possibility that a source of generalized arousal would normally "reside" in the right hemisphere cannot be ruled out (see Chapters 8, 10).

Idelson (1966) demonstrated bilateral EEG suppression when his subjects manipulated objects with the left hand. Right hand manipulation caused more localized contralateral EEG suppression. This effect was not related to the complexity of the task since object recognition was accomplished more successfully by the nonpreferred hand. Heilman and Van Den Abell (1979) reported that the EEG of the left parietal lobe is desynchronized predominantly by lateralized right visual field stimuli; right parietal lobe activation was noted after either right or left hemifield stimulation. These findings may also suggest that the left hemisphere elaborates bilateral electrophysiological arousal. However, Myslobodsky (1976) noted that EEG α and VEP α afterdischarge were symmetrically suppressed during a visuospatial task, whereas there was rather consistent EEG and VEP suppression over the left occiput in most subjects during a verbal–numerical task.

A neuropsychological "vigilance" study conducted by Dimond (1979) in patients with complete or partial commissurotomy showed that it may be the right hemisphere that controls sustained attention. Performance based on left hemisphere mechanisms showed a phenomenon of "gaps of attention," often lasting many seconds. Ellenberg and Sperry (1979) subsequently retested most of the patients examined by Dimond, but none of them seemed to display the anticipated "black holes of consciousness." Although the failure to replicate these findings was puzzling, the results of Dimond cannot be easily dismissed because the right hemisphere does have an important and probably crucial share in attention control. Deisenhammer (1981) reported that wave–spike discharges in the right temporal area lead to a typical attack of transient global amnesia.

3. *Neuroleptic treatment causes a hemisphere disconnection syndrome.* The idea of disconnection in schizophrenia is not novel. Since Rosenthal and Bigelow (1972) showed a considerable enlargement of the corpus callosum in schizophrenic patients, several studies have attempted to make neuropsychological or electrophysiological sense of this observation. Beaumont and Dimond (1973) were probably the first to hypothesize that the performance of schizophrenics is somewhat similar to that of human subjects with disconnected hemispheres. Although callosal enlargement would better fit the "hyperconnection" (Laitinen, 1972; Randall, 1980) rather than "disconnection" mode of interhemispheric activity, subsequent studies largely confirmed that on a number of neuropsychological tests, validated in commissurotomized patients, the interhemispheric communication in schizophrenia is deficient and dormant (see Table 14.5). The willingness with which scientists cling to the disconnection idea is striking since at the London symposium devoted to hemisphere asymmetry of functions and psychopathology, where the disconnection hypothesis was actively debated, some contradictory evidence was mentioned. Laitinen (1972) demonstrated that in 11 patients (7 of whom were diagnosed as schizophrenics) sectioning the corpus cal-

losum produced a striking alleviation of anxiety, tension, and, in one case, hallucinations. Although joining the advocates of the interhemispheric transfer hypothesis, Butler (1979) did not seem to be impressed by the split-brain model of schizophrenia: "A lack of interhemispheric communication cannot be the *cause* of schizophrenia. Split-brain patients suffer none of the key features of this disorder; they do not experience hallucinations or delusions, nor do they display paranoid or catatonic signs. The loss of interhemispheric transfer in schizophrenia is therefore secondary to some other fault [p. 49]."

Indeed, the disruption of interhemispheric communication by tumors of the corpus callosum was associated mainly with symptoms of depression and dementia (Nasrallah and McChesney, 1981). Depression is not uncommon in unmedicated schizophrenia, but it is much more often encountered in patients receiving high doses of neuroleptics or in those who show extrapyramidal side effects (Johnson, 1981).

In addition, a comprehensive analysis of cognitive functions in a large sample of patients with callosal agenesis reported by Chiarello (1980) showed no indication whatsoever of schizophrenic symptoms. Moreover, these patients, as well as a single patient studied by Sadowsky and Reeves (1975), although showing impaired performance on some tests, did not display the classic split-brain syndrome. From a more general perspective it has yet to be proved that having all cerebral commissures in order is of indispensable benefit for cognitive functions. It is of interest that the massa intermedia connecting the thalami of the two hemispheres is often absent (Ajmone-Marsan, 1965). Its presence seemed to be correlated with a relative deterioration of nonverbal (but not verbal) skills in men, but there was no such effect in women (Lansdell and Davie, 1972). Given this evidence the allusion of Butler (1979) to some "other factors" leading to brain disconnection is well justified.

The juxtaposition of LEM and VEP findings suggests that neuroleptic medication may be this "other factor" leading to the brain disconnection syndrome. Table 14.5 demonstrates that a number of studies in which the disconnection symptoms were salient were based on patients who were receiving neuroleptic medication. Green (1978), who provided the strongest neuropsychological evidence of poor interhemispheric communication in schizophrenics, specifically mentioned that his patients were deliberately "stabilized" for at least 2 months by the administration of phenothiazines with a piperazine side chain. Thus, the interesting hypothesis regarding the role of hemisphere disconnection in schizophrenia must be rejected because disconnection may be a "side effect" (in the pathophysiological but not necessarily the therapeutic sense) of neuroleptic medication. This effect of neuroleptics has been ignored until now because of a widely shared conviction that the mechanisms responsible for hemispheric balance are not altered as long as schizophrenics remain

TABLE 14.5
Findings of Hemispheric Disconnection in Schizophrenia

Number of patients	Authors' conclusion	Medication[a]	Reference
12	"The two cerebral hemispheres are partially disconnected [p. 662]."	No details	Beaumont and Dimond (1973)
10 (chronic)	"Defective interhemispheric communication accompanies schizophrenia [p. 56]."	Stabilized on PTZ at least 3 months	Carr (1980)
24 (chronic)	"Split-brain symptoms . . . in schizophrenia [p. 45]"	Medicated (no details)	Dimond (1979)
24 (chronic)	"Noisy communication channel which cannot always be relied upon to convey the correct message [p. 738]"	Medicated (no details)	Dimond *et al.* (1979)
20	"Schizophrenics suffer from something like split-brain syndrome [p. 479]."	Stabilized on PTZ for at least 2 months	Green (1978)
20	"Evidence of defective interhemispheric transfer of auditory information [p. 407]"	Stabilized on PTZ at least 2 months	Green and Kotenko (1980)
18 (acute)	"Disruption of the interhemispheric relationships [p. 15]"	No details	Goldstein (1981)
12	"Deficiencies in interhemispheric interaction and integration [p. 488]"	Eleven on PTZ; 1 nonmedicated	Kugler and Henley (1979)
15	"An abnormality in the interhemispheric commissures [p. 339]"	All on PTZ	Lishman *et al.* (1978)
6	"Nonparanoid schizophrenics may experience difficulties only when required to integrate the processing of right and left hemispheres [p. 902]"	All medicated	Pic'l *et al.* (1979)
12	"Lower interhemisphere coherence . . . suggests greater independence of the two hemispheres and may relate to the impairment of function in the corpus callosum [p. 283]."	All on PTZ	Shaw *et al.* (1979)
16 (chronic)	"Compatible with abnormality of corpus callosum in schizophrenia [p. 392]"	Fifteen on PTZ; 1 nonmedicated	Tress *et al.*, (1979)
60	"The hypothesis of defective interhemispheric transfer seems to offer the most parsimonious explanation [p. 380]."	All medicated; CPZ or haloperidol	Walker *et al.* (1981) [reinterpretation of Lerner *et al.* (1977)
40	"Difficulties in the transfer of information across the hemispheres [p. 472]"	Most on PTZ; some drug free	Weller and Kugler (1979)
6	"Disordered interhemispheric communication [p. 290]"	All medicated	Weller and Montagu (1979)
8	"Breakdown of interhemispheric inhibition during illness [p. 283]"	Some on PTZ; some drug free[b]	Wexler and Heninger (1979)

[a] PTZ, phenothiazines.
[b] Washout period of 7–14 days.

"severely disabled despite medication [Dimond, 1979, p. 41]." Moreover, R. E. Gur (1978) stated that "there is no reason to expect that medication would have a differential effect on the two hemispheres [p. 236]."

IV. Attention-Induced Changes of P_{300}

The dose-related enhancement of VEP_{max} and P_{300} over the right hemisphere in schizophrenics receiving neuroleptic medication was taken as an index of the inhibitory state of the neocortex. However, the amplitude of VEP components has long been suggested to reflect both excitatory and inhibitory changes in cortical neurons. Because of this it seemed desirable to examine VEP alterations during the performance of a simple cognitive task.

This section discusses the effects of an attention-demanding task (for a detailed description of the procedure, see Mintz *et al.*, 1982b) on bilateral VEP and the related assumption that abnormal changes of P_{300} and VEP_{max} in this situation support the hypothesis of neuroleptic-induced suppression of the right hemisphere and hemispheric disconnection in schizophrenia.

Component P_{300}, a surface positive potential with a latency of about 300 msec, is known to be sensitive to the psychological context of the experimental environment. Attention to target stimuli enhances P_{300} (for review, see Donchin and Smith, 1970). Table 14.6 shows that, unlike normal subjects showing the anticipated task-related facilitation of secondary VEP potentials (VEP_{max}), schizophrenics reacted with bilaterally reduced P_{300} and VEP_{max} ($p < 0.031$). Moreover, the suppression in the schizophrenic sample ($p < 0.005$) seemed to be stronger than the facilitation of this component in normal subjects.

We reasoned that a lack of attention (as reflected in the number of errors in the estimation of lights presented) may be responsible for VEP suppression. Indeed, this conjecture was supported for normal subjects; facilitation was noted in subjects making less than 5% of errors ($p < 0.025$ and $p < 0.05$ for VEP_{max} and P_{300}, respectively, in the χ^2 test). However, in schizophrenics a later reduction in VEP components did not depend on the accuracy of performance.

When the VEPs of patients receiving neuroleptics and nonmedicated patients were compared, another important finding emerged. Nontreated patients, like controls, showed slight task-induced P_{300} and VEP_{max} enhancement over the right hemisphere. The suppression of these components in a task condition seems to be a neuroleptic-related effect, especially pronounced in piperazine-treated patients, over the right hemisphere. These effects are presented in Fig. 14.2, where P_{300} values during task performance are expressed as the percentage of change from the rest-

TABLE 14.6

Mean Amplitude[a] of Selected VEP Components during Relaxation and Task Sessions in Schizophrenic and Control Subjects

	P_{100}		P_{300}[b]		VEP_{max}[c]	
	L	R	L	R	L	R
Patients (N = 21)						
Relaxation	18.3[d] ± 11.1	15.8 ± 7.8	27.6[e] ± 8.5	28.6 ± 9.6	28.3[f] ± 8.6	28.8 ± 9.7
Task	15.3 ± 14.2	16.9 ± 12.9	23.6 ± 9.9	22.6 ± 9.9	24.1 ± 9.7	23.5 ± 7.7
Controls (N = 22)						
Relaxation	17.6 ± 9.5	19.4 ± 7.7	26.1 ± 7.1	24.8 ± 7.2	27.3 ± 9.9	25.6 ± 8.9
Task	16.3 ± 8.4	18.9 ± 7.5	25.4 ± 10.9	25.0 ± 9.9	28.0 ± 12.3	26.4 ± 10.3

[a] In microvolts (mean ± SD).

[b] Comparison between groups: task-by-group interaction, $F(1,41) = 3.79$, $p < 0.058$.

[c] Comparison between groups: task-by-group interaction, $F(1,41) = 4.99$, $p < 0.031$.

[d] Comparison within the patient group: task-by-hemisphere interaction, $F(1,16) = 7.23$, $p < 0.02$.

[e] Comparison within the patient group: task effect, $F(1,20) = 11.29$, $p < 0.003$.

[f] Comparison within the patient group: task effect, $F(1,20) = 9.87$, $p < 0.005$.

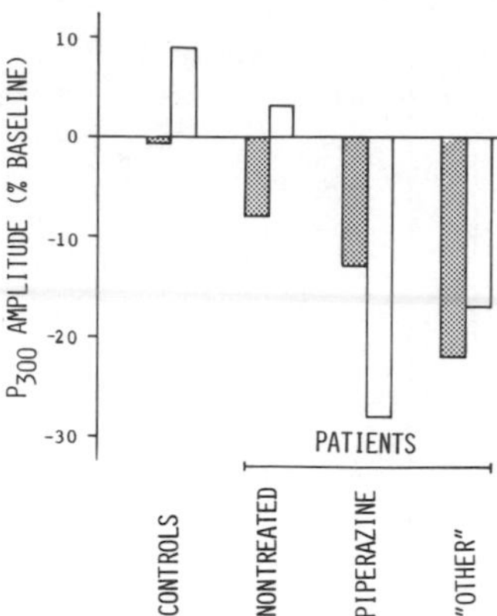

FIG. 14.2. Task-related change of P_{300} amplitude (expressed as percentage of change from relaxation session values) over the left (L – H, stipled bars) and right (R – H, plain bars) hemispheres. Data are shown for control subjects (N = 22) and patients [nontreated (N = 5), treated with piperazine derivatives (N = 9), and treated with "other" neuroleptics (N = 7)]. Analysis of variance performed on the raw data of patients regrouped according to the treatment condition indicated significant task-by-treatment-by-hemisphere interaction for the P_{300} component [$F(2, 18) = 4.67$, $p < 0.023$], whereas marginal significance was obtained for VEP_{max} values [$F(2,18) = 3.39$, $p < 0.056$].

ing session values. The significance of relative unilateral suppression of P_{300}, which is believed to be a bilaterally symmetric wave, is uncertain.

Given that P_{300} is regarded as the index of sensory processing, perception of signal relevance, or perception of novelty, that is, functions requiring a sufficient capacity of arousal mechanisms, the reduction of P_{300} may be related to the realm of attention deficiency, maladaptive arousal, sensory overload, poor filtering, lack of surprise, etc. Roth *et al.* (1980), who observed the reduction of the "P3" wave of auditory evoked potentials (AEP) in schizophrenia, believe that this phenomenon reflects a lack of surprise toward unexpected stimuli. The present attentional situation was deliberately simplified in order not to carry an enhanced novelty or surprise load for accurate performance. Since no reliable deterioration of performance was observed in schizophrenic patients, the P_{300} suppression cannot be related to a diminished accuracy of signal processing.

One aspect of these findings is noteworthy. Although P_{300} reduction is considered to be related to schizophrenia, neither Roth *et al.* (1980) in AEP nor Josiassen *et al.* (1981) in somatosensory evoked potentials (SEP) seem to have found drug-related effects on P_{300} (P_{400}) amplitude. The present findings are at variance with their conclusions, because they demonstrate that nontreated patients did not consistently generate bilaterally depressed P_{300}.

It would be instructive if P_{300} metamorphosis was interpreted neurophysiologically. Unfortunately, however, in a search for functions rather than mechanisms, the analysis of human VEPs in general and P_{300} in particular is reduced to the level of reaction time techniques. The reason for this temperance is understandable; the origin of VEP components remains obscure. Beck *et al.* (1980) have summarized the state of the art: "The trend in analyzing the P_{300} complex has been mainly in the direction of detailed psychological correlates of the response, with only cavalier concern regarding the neural mechanisms involved [p. 539]." A review of the P_{300} mechanisms by Desmedt and Debecker (1979) practically refrains from discussing the neural origin of this wave. It is hardly surprising that Purpura (1978) predicts that it may be 10 or 15 years before we learn which synaptic system is responsible for P_{300}.

It is encouraging, however, that there are features common to human VEPs and the far better understood brain reaction in animals (Creutzfeldt and Kuhnt, 1967; Myslobodsky, 1976). These might be employed to analyze the data. Naturally, a discussion of the neurophysiological mechanism of P_{300} amplitude changes could be only conjectural at this point.

It is well known that evoked potentials reflect postsynaptic potentials in neuronal aggregates with minor contribution from cellular action potentials (Purpura, 1959; Creutzfeldt and Kuhnt, 1967; Humphrey, 1968). Superficially located scalp electrodes largely "see" potentials synchronously developing in pyramidally shaped neurons with long apical dendrites, which extend upward to ramify in the superficial layers. This cellular arrangement may be viewed as a powerful dipole layer with the axis perpendicular to the surface of the scalp. Potentials developing in the oblique and horizontal dipoles as well as pyramids that do not project their apical dendrites to the cortical surface would thus add little to the voltage "seen" at the surface.

Surface positive VEP components in experimental animals are recognized as representing deep excitatory potentials, that is, excitatory postsynaptic potentials (EPSPs) largely developing in pyramidal cells displaying strong dipole properties. Let us consider, even if tentatively, that P_{300} belongs to the same category of events. It should be recalled that enhanced surface positive potentials do not necessarily reflect heightened neocortical excitability. In fact, faster EPSPs cause the excited cells to reach firing levels sooner and are then terminated by action potentials. As a result the surface positivity is reduced. Clearly, a situation can be envisaged in which the amplitude of the VEP and its positive components would increase with decreased excitability (Amassian *et al.*, 1964). The reduction of P_{300} after neuroleptic treatment in schizophrenic patients might therefore be related to enhanced firing of DA-sensitive cells rendered supersensitive under chronic neuroleptic medication and responding more actively to the task-induced increment of the neurotransmitter. Alternatively, enhanced neocortical responding may be related to the neuroleptic-induced increase of excitability of presynaptic dopaminergic terminals (Groves *et al.*, 1981). These explanations, although rather consistent with experimental evidence, imply that P_{300} enhancement in normal individuals reflects a relative inhibitory state of the cortical cells. Arousal-related inhibitory effects in the neocortex are not uncommon (Oshima, 1981), and their significance for information transmission and selective attention has been suggested (Pittman and Feeney, 1974). However, the relevance of this evidence for P_{300} enhancement is obscure and has not been explored to any extent.

The other uncertainty is associated with the fact that any VEP component might change with a shift in the generator's location along the vertical axis. If, according to the simplistic "sliding apical synapse" logic (Humphrey, 1968), EPSPs leading to the surface positive components develop closer to the recording electrode, that is, on the somata of the more superficially located pyramids, then their proximity to the electrode would reduce the amplitude of the P_{300} and even complicate its form. Although highly speculative, such vertical redistribution of activity is not unlikely due to the peculiar pattern of monoaminergic innervation of the neocortex. The heaviest DA innervation in the frontal and prefrontal areas has been shown to be predominantly in the depth of the cortex (layers V–VI) (Berger *et al.*, 1974; Lindvall *et al.*, 1974). If neuroleptics block dopaminergic neurotransmission in the lower cortical layers, then attention-related VEP changes should involve an alternative neurotransmitter circuitry implicated in arousal. Indeed, the superficial-layers (I–III), and especially the outer molecular layer, receive a prominent norepinephrinergic projection (Fuxe *et al.*, 1968; Levitt and Moore, 1978). Neuroleptics and especially piperazine derivatives probably block DA effects in the lower layers while having a lesser influence on cells sensitive to norepinephrine (NE) (Bunney, 1979). It is tempting to conjecture that the task-related reduction of later VEP components in schizophrenia is a reflection of the NE component of attentional response in the presence of a relatively more profound DA blockade of the lower layers.

Finally, transcallosal fibers are unevenly distributed in different cortical layers. After the removal of the contralateral cortex, areas 18 and 19 show a remarkable sparsity of degenerating material in the upper layers. The largest amount of degenerating fibers is concentrated in the deep layers (Jacobson and Trojanowski, 1974; Pines and Maiman, 1939; Szentágothai, 1969). In other words, if neuroleptics preferentially block DA-mediated activity in the lower layers of the neocortex, this effect, among other things, may lead to a reduction of traffic carrying DA-triggered messages across the corpus callosum.

V. Who Is the "Nonresponder"?

Gruzelier and associates (Gruzelier, 1973; Gruzelier and Venables, 1974), assessing electrodermal activity (EDA) in schizophrenia, made two major observations: *(a)* schizophrenics show a high incidence of nonresponding or underresponding; and *(b)* patients have a larger amount of EDA on the right hand than on the left hand. Subsequent studies replicated these findings and further demonstrated that neuroleptic medication can reduce (Gruzelier and Hammond, 1976) or reverse (Gruzelier and Hammond, 1978) this laterality.

Findings from our laboratory (summarized in the previous sections) have shown that some laterality effects in schizophrenia may be caused rather than reduced by neuroleptics. Given this evidence, we examined bilateral EDA in a group of nonmedicated and medicated schizophrenic patients. The techniques employed were similar to those described elsewhere (Myslobodsky and Rattok, 1977). Reactive EDA was recorded in two conditions: during "relaxation," in response to nonsignal photic stimuli, and during the performance of a task that required the patients to attend to the stimuli (for a detailed description of the task procedure, see Mintz *et al.*, 1982b). We subdivided the sample into the following two subgroups: (*a*) "nonresponders," who failed to produce any EDA orienting response or were unresponsive in the initial three trials of each experimental session; and (*b*) "responders," who produced consistent EDA orienting response or became habituated after three or more trials. On the basis of these criteria, 12 (52%) patients were defined as nonresponders. Eight were found to be nonresponders during relaxation and task sessions, whereas 4 patients could be defined as "fast habituators" (Patterson and Venables, 1978) during relaxation and "nonresponders" during task performance. Among 11 (48%) responders, only 1 failed to react during the relaxation session and, in the case of another, data for the relaxation session were not available.

Table 14.7 compares responders and nonresponders in relation to selected clinical and psychophysiological variables. The most interesting result was the significant higher dose of neuroleptics administered to nonresponders. Also, nonresponders seemed to have a slightly longer duration of illness.

Given that neuroleptics lead to Parkinsonism and that DA deficit in the right hemisphere correlates with EDA nonresponding in hemi-Parkinson patients (Chapter 10), one may ask whether EDA nonresponding is related to the selective involvement of the right hemisphere. The analysis of Table 14.7 does not support this conjecture, since LEM findings are suggestive of a rather balanced hemispheric activity, whereas VEP (P_{300}) amplitude is significantly shifted toward left hemisphere predominance during task performance. Moreover, three of the six nonmedicated patients in the present sample were EDA nonresponders.

Nonresponders were found among "high-risk" subjects (Venables, 1977) and asymptomatic individuals with Huntington's chorea (Lawson, 1981). Therefore, if right hemisphere involvement is suggested for medicated patients, the possibility should be considered that a special category of

TABLE 14.7
Clinical and Psychophysiological Correlates of Responders and Nonresponders on EDA[a]

	Responders ($N = 11$)	Nonresponders ($N = 12$)
Age (years ± *SD*)	17.9 ± 2.1	18.4 ± 2.0
Sex (male/female)	6/5	7/5
Education (years ± *SD*)	10.3 ± 1.5	10.6 ± 1.3
Family history (%)	2	3
Age at first admission (years ± *SD*)	17.5 ± 1.9	17.6 ± 1.6
Illness duration (months ± *SD*)	14.2 ± 19.9	24.6 ± 23.2
Neuroleptic daily dose[b] (CPZ equivalent, mean ± *SD*)	236 ± 165 ($N = 8$)	886 ± 780 ($N = 9$), $p < 0.05$
EDA (left/right hand, mean ± *SD*)		
Relaxation	233 ± 213/279 ± 323	—
Task	141 ± 118/186 ± 179	—
Blinking (% of normal ± *SD*)	118 ± 66 ($N = 8$)	72 ± 66 ($N = 8$), n.s.[c]
LEM AI (± *SD*)	+0.20 ± 0.47 ($N = 4$)	+0.08 ± 0.71 ($N = 5$), n.s.[c]
Task		
VEP_{max} AI (± *SD*)	+0.10 ± 0.24 ($N = 10$)	−0.14 ± 0.16 ($N = 10$), $p < 0.05$
P_{300} AI (± *SD*)	+0.09 ± 0.21 ($N = 10$)	−0.14 ± 0.16 ($N = 10$), $p < 0.02$

[a] A response was defined as a resistance decrement that started up to 5 sec after stimulus presentation and the amplitude of which resulted in at least 20 counts of the EDA counter. Twenty counts were equal to 330 Ω per 5 sec of resistance decrement.
[b] In each group three patients were drug free.
[c] n.s., not significant.

patients and at-risk individuals show a selective DA deficit in the right hemisphere.

Given that neuroleptics may have affected EDA in responding patients, the mean EDA values obtained during the relaxation and task periods were correlated with the neuroleptic dose (CPZ equivalent) for the right and left hand, separately. The results proved that EDA responding increases as a function of the CPZ dose during both relaxation and task conditions, the effect being more pronounced for the right hand (Fig. 14.3A).

Bilateral EDA changes computed as an AI (Fig. 14.3B) further demonstrate the change in EDA asymmetry as a function of CPZ dose; EDA was higher on the left hand with small doses, and this asymmetry was reversed in patients treated with higher doses of neuroleptics. If we imagine that, in contrast to neuroleptics in the nonresponding group, neuroleptics in responders predominantly blocked DA receptors in the left hemisphere, the similarity to the responding profile in hemi-Parkinsonism with left hemideficit is difficult to overlook. In both cases there is a relative decrease in the homolateral (left hand) EDA and an increase

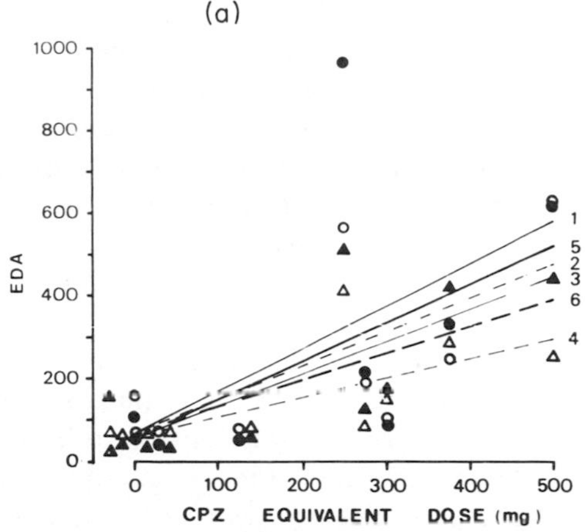

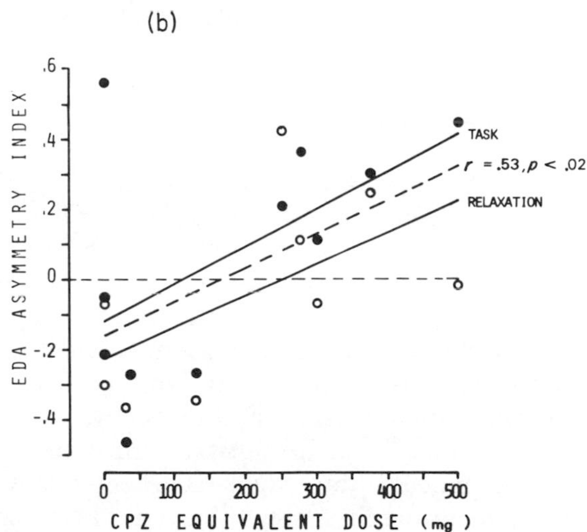

FIG. 14.3. (a) Bilateral EDA recorded during relaxation (left, ○; right, •) and attention task (left, △; right, ▲) sessions as a function of CPZ equivalent daily dose (in milligrams). The individual mean EDA values are based on responses to the first 20 stimuli presented in each session. Regression lines are plotted separately for the right hand (solid lines) and the left hand (dashed lines) for each experimental session and for data pooled across sessions. Relaxation: 1, right hand (not significant); 2, left hand ($p < 0.05$). Attention task: 3, right hand ($p < 0.01$); 4, left hand ($p < 0.02$). Pooled across sessions: 5, right hand ($p < 0.01$); 6, left hand ($p < 0.01$). (b) EDA asymmetry index [net difference of bilateral EDA (right minus left) over the higher EDA value] computed for relaxation (○) and task (•) sessions as a function of CPZ equivalent daily dose (in milligrams). Positive values of AI indicate predominance of EDA over the right hand. Circles represent individual values of AI. Regression lines are plotted separately for relaxation and task sessions (solid lines) and for data pooled across both experimental sessions (dashed line).

in the contralateral EDA (see Table 14.7 for the schizophrenic sample and Chapter 10 for the hemi-Parkinson sample). In line with Gruzelier *et al.* (1981), this pattern of responding may be interpreted as suggesting a relative disinhibition of the right hemisphere. Table 14.7 supports this impression; responders showed consistent positive values of VEP amplitude AI during task performance, that is a response pattern typical of normal individuals and unmedicated patients (Fig. 14.2). However, unlike VEP findings, EDA asymmetry did not reach significance.

In summary, an answer to the question of the section title is not available. However, the results suggest that neuroleptics distributed asymmetrically toward either the right or the left hemisphere DA circuitry may cause different patterns of bilateral EDA responding, nonresponding, and underresponding. The abundance of nonresponders among the at-risk population allows the conjecture that responders and nonresponders have dissimilar pathophysiology (predominantly left versus right hemisphere abnormality), which may be detected before medication, and underlines the asymmetry of drug distribution (Chapter 17).

VI. Who Is the Blinker?

Asymmetries of LEMs and saccades during smooth pursuit have become a recognized "soft" neurological sign of aberrant laterality. Another prominent "soft" neurological sign of psychosis, increased spontaneous blinking (Brezinova and Kendell, 1977; Stevens, 1978; Karson *et al.*, 1981), has never been on the agenda of laterality research. Nevertheless, it is not unlikely that an aberrant laterality pattern contributes to spontaneous blinking or paroxysms of blinking. Blinking is often associated with other oculomotor symptoms (Cegalis and Sweeney, 1979; Pivik, 1979; Tomer *et al.*, 1979), which tend to show asymmetric patterns. Also, blinking as well as other oculomotor signs have been related to abnormal functioning of the dopaminergic system (Stevens, 1978). In rats, which have an intrinsically asymmetric nigrostriatal system (Glick *et al.*, 1976), unilateral blinking is not an uncommon component of the interictal or postictal state (Myslobodsky, 1981). Stevens and Livermore (1978) speculated that blinking is an equivalent of a waking REM episode. Some writers believe that REM is strongly associated with the right hemisphere (Bakan, 1978). In view of this evidence it would be interesting to examine whether in schizophrenic patients displaying an abnormally high blinking rate there is a specific laterality pattern, as assessed by LEM or VEP technique.

Blinking during the resting period and during the performance of a cognitive task was measured in a group of 36 schizophrenic patients, as well as in 50 normal control subjects. Four periods of 15 sec each were rated, and the average number of blinks was taken as the score for each subject. In 4 patients periods of paroxysmal blinking were noted, whereas the others had a relatively constant rate. Blinking ranged from an average of 5.5 per 15 sec for the normal group to 9.1 per 15 sec for the patients ($p < 0.02$). We then assessed the relationship between blinking rate and the *absolute* LEM AI in a group of 46 normal subjects and 21 schizophrenics (who were responders in the LEM paradigm). An inverse relationship between blinking and the degree of LEM asymmetry was noted for both groups ($p < 0.05$ for the patients and $p < 0.02$ for normal subjects). In other words, the inverse relationship between blinking and LEM asymmetry suggests that LEMs should be symmetric for blinks to be maximally pronounced.

Blinking is often regarded as a symptom of anxiety or fear (Harris *et al.*, 1966). Psychologically, it can be regarded as a device for "screening out" disagreeable experiences and securing "perceptual defense" (Spence, 1967). Volkmann *et al.* (1979) reported that blinking increases visual threshold, as do saccades. Given the role of the right hemisphere in the elaboration of emotional responses (Flor-Henry, 1979; Chapter 7; Gainotti, 1972) and in accord with Kinsbourne's model (1972), the anxiety hypothesis requires a predominantly leftward LEM deviation. Visual–emotional processing is reportedly associated with a predominance of leftward LEMs (Schwartz *et al.*, 1975). However, experiments of Tucker *et al.* (1978) demonstrated that stressful experience may actually increase the number of right-directed LEMs along with nonlateralized responses (stares and vertical eye movements).*

Some reports (see Table 14.1), including those from our laboratory (Tomer *et al.*, 1979), demonstrate that schizophrenics as a group generate predominately rightward LEMs. About 70% of the patients in our sample were designated as "blinkers." Therefore, the present finding of symmetric LEMs in some of the patients stands in contrast to the previously described results. This symmetry has probably been overlooked in previous studies due to predominantly rightward LEMs, which can be attributed to nonblinkers. When schizophrenics were separated into blinkers and nonblinkers, the higher incidence of right-directed LEMs among nonblinkers became noticeable (AI being +0.33 in nonblinkers versus −0.09 in blinkers; not significant).

*These results point to some relationship between lateral asymmetry and blinking. However, a report of increased blinking following cerebellectomy (Freed *et al.*, 1981), as well as studies relating cerebellar pathology to schizophrenia (Heath *et al.*, 1979; Weinberger *et al.*, 1979; Kutty *et al.*, 1981), perhaps suggest that there may be some cerebellar influence on blinking in schizophrenia or interaction between cerebellar functioning and laterality.

Since symmetric LEMs can be interpreted as a "no-win" hemisphere confrontation, one might anticipate that a perfect balance of the hemispheres in a typical blinker would be corroborated by symmetric VEP values. However, correlating the *absolute* AI of P_{300} (recorded during relaxation) with the blinking rate showed a positive relationship ($p < 0.05$). This result can be understood if, unlike LEMs, VEPs are asymmetric in blinkers. In fact, when the *relative* AI of P_{300} was correlated with the blinking rate, it showed a relative enhancement of positive values of VEP AI as a function of blinking ($r = +0.33$; not significant). This result, although short of statistical significance, merits special attention because it suggests that in a large proportion of patients showing symmetric LEMs accompanied by a high rate of blinking, P_{300} should be slightly enhanced over the right hemisphere. In other words, the results of two laterality measures may not necessarily march in step. When the highest rate of blinking in those patients was considered, the correlation between VEP AI and blinking rate became significant ($r = +0.473$, $p < 0.05$).

An enhanced P_{300} in the baseline condition was correlated with increased EEG power in the δ–θ range (M. Mintz, 1982, unpublished). This finding casts doubt on the likelihood that P_{300} facilitation in the resting condition can be attributed to attention enhancement. Also, enhanced attention is known to decrease the rate of spontaneous blinking (Mecacci and Pasquali, 1980). Therefore, again, we are inclined to relate the relative facilitation of P_{300} in the right hemisphere to relative suppression of this hemisphere by neuroleptic treatment.

There are some reasons for believing that right hemisphere "sedation" may cause bilateral disruption of certain functions. A lesion of the right hemisphere was often correlated with one of the most generalized epileptiform rhythms, 3 cycle per second wave–spike discharges of petit mal epilepsy (Myslobodsky, 1976). Wave–spike discharges are most commonly provoked by "centrasthenic," that is, arousal-reducing, conditions or lesions in the reticular formation (Myslobodsky, 1976), suggesting intimate involvement of the right hemisphere in generalized arousal-related EEG control. In fact, wave–spike discharges are often provoked by photic stimulation. It has been demonstrated that right hemisphere (left visual field) stimulation more often induces bilateral photoconvulsive EEG response than stimuli delivered in the right visual field (Wilkins *et al.*, 1981).

A careful study by Howes and Boller (1975) demonstrated that lesions of the right hemisphere produce far greater impairment of simple reaction time than do lesions of the left hemisphere. The examination of brain scan images suggested that there are two major locations of lesion leading to increased reaction times: basal ganglia or posterior parietal area.

Lesions in the parietal area produce a profound deficit in behaviors dealing with orientation and detection of visual and nonvisual stimuli

(Weinstein and Friedland, 1977). Although these locations do not explain the findings by Howes and Boller, they emphasize the fact that the right hemisphere may control orientation and locomotion in the homolateral visual space to a greater extent than the left hemisphere. As Heilman and Valenstein (1978) stated:

> . . . each hemisphere can mediate its own attention-arousal response and the right hemisphere can mediate this response for the left hemisphere better than the left hemisphere can mediate an attention-arousal response for the right hemisphere. Left hemisphere lesions would then produce less neglect than right hemisphere lesions since the right hemisphere would be capable of mediating an attention-arousal response via the left hemisphere. Right hemisphere lesions would produce a bilateral (although asymmetrical) defect because the left hemisphere would be incapable of mediating an attention-arousal response for the right hemisphere and also because left hemisphere arousal would be reduced on account of the right hemisphere damage [p. 169].

Given this evidence, we believe that reduced LEM asymmetry is related to neuroleptic-induced partial suppression of the right hemisphere mechanisms.

VII. Is the Deficit in Schizophrenia Left-sided, Right-sided, or of Callosal Transfer Origin?

At the time that Buchsbaum *et al.* (1979) posed this question, almost all theoretically possible answers had been proposed. As Table 14.8 shows there are advocates of left hemisphere dysfunction in the form of hyperarousal, right hemisphere abnormality, and deficits of callosal transmission in the form of disconnection and hyperconnection. Finally, there are some who failed to find any laterality changes in schizophrenia.

A liberal view would be that schizophrenia is so multifarious that one could find enough evidence to illustrate almost any point. In addition, human individuals are enormously variable, even those who share a common diagnostic label. This liberalism is probably the most disturbing aspect of schizophrenia research. A theory is not easily abandoned even when facts militate against it. Since we are always told that schizophrenics are not a "monolithic" group, we are content when at least some results agree with the specified predictions. Decades of extensive research efforts provided no reliable techniques with which to differentiate even between mendacious organic syndromes in "schizophrenic attires" and typical schizophrenia. This state of the art is unlikely to change in the near future. Therefore, we intend to summarize our position in the search for the "locus" of schizophrenia, avoiding the dispute of its heterogeneity.

TABLE 14.8
Lateral Abnormalities in Schizophrenia: Summary of Major Hypotheses[a]

Abnormality	References
Interhemispheric relationships	Beaumont and Dimond (1973),[b] Carr (1980),[c] Dimond (1979),[c] Dimond *et al.* (1979),[c] Green (1978),[c] Green and Kotenko (1980),[c] Goldstein (1981),[b] Kugler and Henley (1979),[d] Lishman *et al.* (1978),[c] Pic'l *et al.* (1979),[c] Shaw *et al.* (1979),[c] Tress *et al.* (1979),[d] Walker *et al.* (1981),[c] Weller and Kugler (1979),[d] Weller and Montagu (1979),[d] Wexler and Heninger (1979)[d]
Left hemisphere involvement	Abrams and Taylor (1979, 1980),[d] Bazhin *et al.* (1975),[b] Caudrey and Kirk (1979),[c] Caudrey *et al.* (1980),[c] Coger *et al.* (1979),[e] Connolly *et al.* (1979),[c] Etevenon *et al.* (1979),[d] Flor-Henry *et al.* (1979),[d] Golden *et al.* (1981),[b] Gruzelier and Venables (1974),[c] Gruzelier and Hammond (1979),[c,e] Gur (1978, 1979b),[c] Hays (1977),[b] Hillsberg (1979),[b] Nachshon (1980),[c] Rochford *et al.* (1976),[b] Roemer *et al.* (1978, 1979),[e] Scarone *et al.* (1981),[b] Schweitzer (1979),[c] Shagass *et al.* (1980),[c] Tomer *et al.* (1979)[d]
Right hemisphere involvement	Hartlage and Garber (1976),[b] Mathew *et al.* (1981),[e] Sandel and Alcorn (1980)[b]
Left- and/or right-hemisphere involvement with other lateral abnormalities	Eaton *et al.* (1979),[c] Serafetinides *et al.* (1981),[e] Shaw *et al.* (1979),[c] Taylor and Fleminger (1981)[c]
No evidence for asymmetric involvement	Bernstein *et al.* (1981),[d] Bull and Venables (1974),[b] Clooney and Murray (1977),[c] Domino *et al.* (1979),[e] Iacono (1982),[b] Toone *et al.* (1981),[e] Yosawitz *et al.* (1979)[d]

[a] Studies were classified as supporting one hypothesis or another according to the authors' conclusion rather than our interpretation of the data.
[b] No details concerning medication status of the patients.
[c] All patients on neuroleptics.
[d] Some patients medicated and some drug free, but results are not reported separately.
[e] Washout period varying from 1 week to 60 days, except for Domino *et al.* (1979), whose patients were nonmedicated for 6 months.

We failed to find the "common laterality denominator" of schizophrenia that we were searching for at the incipiency of this study. One can question whether a truly integrated picture of any psychosis can be portrayed by EEG, electrooculographic (EOG), VEP, or EDA records in which data by necessity are meager, partial, or missing and bear a heavy "treatment imprint." In dealing with such a nebulous pathological condition as schizophrenia, this right–left polarization, although heuristically useful, may be insufficient. No single laterality measure should be taken as indicating the "laterality vector." When several measures are compared, the directionality of their imbalance may not march in step, suggesting that there are a multitude of mechanisms with individual asymmetries of their own, which together may not produce unbalanced hemispheric reactivity. In short, the major gain in knowledge at this point can best be summarized by paraphrasing Elliot Valenstein: laterality is not located on the surface of our electrodes.

Most writers consider aberrant laterality in schizophrenia to be the enhancement of a normally existing pattern, that is, left hemisphere hyperactivity. Much to our surprise, nonmedicated schizophrenics did not show systematic laterality biases when assessed by electrophysiological methods (EOG, EEG, VEP, and EDA). Although this finding may be related to the small size of the sample of nonmedicated patients examined, this is certainly not the only reason for this failure. In fact, clear signs of laterality were encountered with increasing doses of neuroleptics. Does this mean that the asymmetry in schizophrenia is a man-made phenomenon of no pathophysiological significance?

There is no simple answer to this question, and the possibility that we shall eventually prove the long-neglected pharmacological asymmetry of the brain (Myslobodsky and Weiner, 1976; Chapter 17, this volume) rather than "schizophrenia's hemisyndrome" remains very strong. At least for studies based on treated samples one can give any answer to the question posed by Buchsbaum *et al.* (1979), depending on the dose, type, and duration of neuroleptic medication.

We interpreted our findings as suggesting right hemisphere "sedation" by the drugs. It is of interest that there are some preliminary signs that neuroleptic-induced extrapyramidal symptoms more often develop on the left side (McEntee and Newman, 1981; P. Taylor, personal communication). Affective disorders have been reported to be more frequent among patients with tardive dyskinetic symptoms (Rush *et al.*, 1982). We further proposed that the imbalance induced by neuroleptics may be therapeutically desirable because it disrupts the callosal traffic directed to the left hemisphere. Table 14.5 demonstrates that signs of hemisphere disconnection were detected predominantly by writers who examined medicated patients.

A study by Shaw *et al.* (1979) showed that schizophrenics tend to have higher intrahemisphere and lower interhemisphere EEG coherence values than neurotics and normal subjects. It is of interest that right and left intrahemisphere coherence was high during both spatial imagery and mental arithmetic tasks, suggesting a reduced specificity of hemisphere reaction. Interhemispheric coherence was minimal during the spatial task and enhanced during mental arithmetic tasks. In other words, only the interhemispheric traffic directed to the left hemisphere seems to be selectively reduced. This result may be related to neuroleptic treatment, which was not discontinued during Shaw *et al.*'s study.

To summarize, left (verbal) hemisphere arousal, which is believed to represent the hallmarks of schizophrenic psychosis, is treated by this conjecture as a secondary feature developing subsequently to the primary right hemisphere abnormality. This conjecture is consistent with the suggestion of Weller and Montagu (1979) that schizophrenia may be associated, at least in part, with an "initial predominantly right hemisphere dysfunction which eventually leads to disruption of left hemisphere function [p. 291]." As we pointed out in preceding sections, the involvement of the right hemisphere in the mediation of bilateral effects reduces the visibility of its abnormality, whereas dramatic thought disorders and pronounced difficulties with language suggest that verbal hemisphere dysfunction is associated with schizophrenia. It has not been ruled out, however, that "right hemisphere abnormality in schizophrenia" is a special, pathophysiologically distinct subtype that can be distinguished on the basis of EDA nonresponding.

Unfortunately, this conjecture, although attractive, has several shortcomings. First, there is no explanation for the primary right hemisphere abnormality and its hyperexcitability (see, however, the footnote on p. 354). Second, hemisphere "hyperconnection" cannot be logically derived from the suggested model. Third, emotional changes and abnormalities of the visual sphere are rather meager, compared with primary (and supposedly early) left hemisphere dysfunction. In addition, it remains to be proved whether right hemisphere sedation and correspondingly relative left hemisphere disinhibition develop in the course of lasting medication and whether these changes are therapeutically desirable.

These difficulties invite a more parsimonious hypothesis that links primary schizophrenia abnormalities with early left hemisphere pathology. No findings from the present study support such a contention. However, one may refer to the pronounced tendency to shift cerebral dominance, as evidenced by cases of nondextrality so often reported among schizophrenics and their families (Lishman and McMeekan, 1976; see, however, Taylor *et al.*, 1980).

Moreover, left hemisphere damage is supported by a loss of cerebral density, especially in the anterior part of the left half of the brain (Golden *et al.*, 1981). The patients in the preceding sample were rather young (22–44 years), suggesting that the disorder should have developed fairly early to have attained the described degree of prominence. A higher incidence of epileptiform discharges over the left temporal lobe of schizophrenic patients (Abrams and Taylor, 1979) may also be interpreted as being related to the structural brain deficit reported by Golden *et al.* (1981), inasmuch as the EEG abnormalities they described were predominantly in the form of more "organic" slow-wave activity.

One might have realized that from here on we have to reaffirm the role of the right hemisphere mechanisms. In fact, left hemisphere dysfunction at an early age, if severe enough, may lead to a bilateral representation of language (Hécaen and Albert, 1978), which explains the likelihood of right hemisphere involvement in left hemisphere activities. Similarly, it explains why schizophrenics may have a deficit not only in verbal but in spatial reasoning abilities (Hartlage and Garber, 1976) and abnormalities in stereognosis and right–left identification (Walker, 1981).

The compensatory mechanisms that might operate in association with right hemisphere interference have yet to be explored. So far, only the widened corpus callosum has been shown to facilitate anatomically the increment of traffic directed toward the left hemisphere.

One might still argue that epileptogenicity, postulated to alter the process of normal lateralization of language, is not a typical finding in schizophrenia. Colony (1956) noted only about 5% of abnormal EEG records among 1000 schizophrenics.

According to French (Igert and Lairy, 1962) and Russian (Feigenberg, 1964) writers, epileptiform activity dominates in benign recurrent psychoses, whereas desynchronized ("choppy") EEGs are seen in malignant process schizophrenia. Some writers saw "surprisingly normal" EEGs (Matousek, 1965) in chronic and/or severe psychosis (Stevens, 1958; Small and Small, 1965). Landolt (1958) found that patients with temporal lobe epilepsy also showed "supernormal" EEG patterns when they developed alternating psychotic reactions. Abnormalities in the EEG would build up with the spontaneous or postmedication improvement of behavior.

A similarity between some symptoms of psychosis in temporal lobe epilepsy and schizophrenia has long been suggested (see Chapter 7), although earlier writers had failed to observe any laterality effects (Slater *et al*., 1963). Flor-Henry (1969) emphasized, however, that it is left hemisphere involvement which increases the risk of psychotic episodes. He later demonstrated that schizophrenics have significantly more power in the 20- to 30-Hz band over the left temporal lobe (Flor-Henry, 1976). This parallel between the "forced normalization" of Landolt and left hemisphere hyperarousal may be more than accidental. The suppression of EEG over the left may still be interpreted as a chronic state of supernormality due to the operation of factors that tend to suppress epileptiform activity, at the cost of provoking psychotic behavior.

It is known that attention mobilization, orienting behavior, nonspecific generalized arousal, and REM sleep tend to suppress some forms of hypersynchronous epileptiform rhythmicity. In contrast, reduced alertness was shown to act as a potentially proconvulsive factor (Myslobodsky, 1976). Catecholamines in general and DA in particular have been implicated in epilepsy (Maynert *et al.*, 1975). Can it be that early-developing epileptogenic activity in the left hemisphere promotes the growth of right hemisphere axons toward hyperactive sites? Parenthetically, it should be noted that monoaminergic cell groups are among the first generated during ontogeny (Nicholson *et al.*, 1973), and they are believed to control the development of the corresponding target central nervous system regions by modulating the levels of nucleotide secondary messengers in these innervated neurons (McMahon, 1974). Interhemispheric connections are redundant at early stages of development. With maturation, juvenile callosal neurons lose their callosal axons and form permanent connections ipsilaterally (Innocenti, 1981). Therefore, an early focus in the left hemisphere might prevent the process of gradual disappearance of the superabundant connections. This process can be likened to the sprouting of axons in a severed peripheral nerve, which, although a compensatory response, may be a mixed blessing, leading to a loss of function in the form of spasticity. Similarly, a special role of the right hemisphere in carrying out arousal and limbic-related functions initially used as an antiepileptic, homeostatic, compensating device may lead eventually to a nonadaptive general hyperalertness and hyperarousal of schizophrenia.

The modest boost of left hemisphere arousal thus caused may sharpen normal hemispheric balance and increase the ability to cope in an attention-demanding environment. Some features of schizophrenia, if mild, may be of certain benefit for survival. Jarvik and Deckard (1977) argued that the schizoid–paranoid personality ("Odyssean personality") is inherently more capable of sensing early and responding effectively to potentially hazardous social situations. In an aggressive environment this quality is bound to be lifesaving and gives the Odyssean a better chance than others of leaving viable progeny.

A severe left hemisphere hyperactivity may totally disrupt behavior and require pharmacological, and perhaps even surgical, hemisphere disconnection. The symptoms of malignant hyperattention in the form of obsessive–compulsive syndromes (similar to those developing in patients with Gilles de la Tourette syndrome) were relieved after right- but not left-sided coagulation of the intralaminar thalamic nuclei. In very few cases was it necessary to extend the coagulation into the left hemisphere. This hyperalertness may be likened to an interesting phenomenon of global hemihyperattentiveness and pseudointentional acts involving complex adversive phenomena with loud emotional utterance elicited by stimulation of the pallidum and its efferent and afferent connections (Hassler, 1980).

This speculation is supported by the findings of Pritzel and Huston (Chapter 3) of a "postlesion increase in interhemispheric organization" due to the predominant activation of dormant contralateral pathways originating in the nondamaged hemisphere. Moreover, Pritzel and Huston showed that this phenomenon is associated with, and may lead to, a reduction in postlesion motor imbalance (circling). Taking this observation a step farther, one might suggest a compensatory postlesion increase in interhemispheric organization, reducing the disparity in hemisphere reactivity in schizophrenia similar to that observed in hemi-Parkinsonism (Chapter 10) or in developmental abnormalities (Rhodes *et al.*, 1969). However, the asymmetry may be limited to the pharmacological sensitivity of the lesioned system. Indeed, rotation of rats with a lesion in the nigrostriatal system may be reinstated by stress or the administration of dopamine agonists or antagonists.

VIII. Epilogue: Diagnosis *ex Juvantibus*

At this stage of the study we see no advantage in relating schizophrenia as a whole to either a left or a right hemisyndrome. Undoubtedly, there are patients who have some symptoms that might be conceptualized as predominantly associated with either right or left hemisphere deficits. Gruzelier (Chapter 12) believes that there are two subcategories of psychoses with different degrees of involvement of the verbal versus nonverbal hemisphere. It may be desirable to separate these two groups using biologically based diagnostic procedures, as recommended by Buchsbaum and Haier (1978). However, since laterality patterns become increasingly complicated and confusing with every new experimental step, one might be tempted to diagnose schizophrenia subtypes on the basis of individual responses to different types of neuroleptics. Even though most neuroleptics, when given in equivalent doses, seem to have a limited specificity in their antipsychotic profile, it is widely recognized that a patient refractory to one drug may do well on another. In the context of the present study it is worth considering that some unrecognized properties of drugs differentially affect lateralized dopaminergic circuits. Specifically, it would seem important to examine whether the two types of schizophrenics would respond differently to the more sedating, low-potency neuroleptics, such as CPZ, and to the more energizing, high-potency neuroleptics, such as fluphenazine—in other words, whether the accompanying side effects (sedative versus activating) would act as factors that self-facilitated or self-inhibited the DA blockade at lateralized targets (see Chapter 17). Parenthetically, it should be recalled that sedative and activating neuroleptics are often combined, although no rationale for such a combination is typically given. Advocates of polypharmacy also use combinations of neuroleptics and antidepressants. Most of these combinations have no pathophysiological justification.

In effect, this question is equivalent to an attempt to diagnose the subcategory of psychosis on the basis of the treatment outcome. Among the various types of diagnostic paradigms there is an oblivious one, called diagnosis *ex juvantibus*. Dorland's Illustrated Medical Dictionary (1974) defines it as "a diagnosis based on the results of treatment". Such an approach is valid only when very specific substances acting on a narrow range of pathophysiological mechanisms are employed. Paracelsus believed that there was a specific remedy for each disease and that an effort had to be made to find it. As soon as specific remedies are discovered, even the most complicated diagnosis may resemble a chemical analysis in which a variety of drugs are tried until a successful "drug–disease reaction" is achieved. In a search for specific remedies, the founder of homeopathy, Hahnemann, guided by Paracelsus's ideas, looked for so-called signatures, the shapes or colors of seeds resembling those of the diseased organ. This ancient approach has been shown to be relevant today by the attested effectiveness of psychotropic drugs and their more specific interaction with aberrant behavior, sleep, and alertness than the battery of "specifics" known to Oliver Wendell Holmes.

There are some encouraging signs, indeed, that it is possible to differentiate pathological conditions by means of pharmacotherapy. Myslobodsky (1976) used a group of antiepileptic compounds to select *ex juvantibus* the electrophysiological model of petit mal epilepsy. The latter was described as a state responding to anti-petit mal drugs. Buchsbaum and Haier (1978) suggested that lithium therapy may be used to differentiate affective disorders and schizophrenia. They observed that this approach may change the entire structure of diagnostic procedure so that, whereas the practitioner "might write 'affective disorder' in the chart, the implied diagnosis is really 'lithium-sensitive behavioral syndrome' [p. 474]."

Edelstein *et al.* (1981) also noted that a subcategory of psychosis that bears biological resemblance to mania can be differentiated therapeutically by lithium-induced changes of symptoms. Claridge (1972) argued that predisposition to schizophrenia consists of a special nervous typological organization that might be uncovered by certain drugs, such as LSD-25.

Our findings suggest that diagnosis *ex juvantibus* should be given another chance in the pharmacotherapy of schizophrenia. So far, attempts to define schizophrenic subtypes on the basis of their specific responses to drugs have not been successful (Hollister, 1974). Of course, neuroleptics have multiple sites of action and are often called "dirty" drugs. At the same time, schizophrenia cannot be described as a disease "cured" by neuroleptic drugs (Barchas *et al.*, 1978). However, a part of the problem may be caused by different laterality patterns and a lack of an individualized approach to pharmacotherapy, so that neuroleptics have not necessarily been targeted to the most appropriate circuits, at the most appropriate time, in the company of the most appropriate drugs.

We have to learn, among other things, whether the individual management of the patient, on the basis of the laterality profile, is of any benefit, whether the rate of improvement or deterioration covaries with laterality shifts, whether the fluid symptoms are accompanied by changes in laterality measures, whether some differences in laterality can be detected between treated patients and those who improve spontaneously, whether laterality patterns can be used as predictors of the management outcome, whether the type of neuroleptics being administered should be changed with a change in the direction of the laterality balance, and whether neuroleptic-induced depression is associated with a particular pattern of laterality. We believe that an *ex juvantibus* approach, controlled by techniques allowing one to visualize the effects of drug distribution, would help to elucidate the role of aberrant laterality in the pathophysiology of schizophrenia.

References

Abrams, R., and Taylor, M. A. (1979). Differential EEG patterns in affective disorder and schizophrenia. *Arch. Gen. Psychiatry* **36,** 1355–1358.

Abrams, R., and Taylor, M. A. (1980). Psychopathology and the electroencephalogram. *Biol. Psychiatry* **15,** 871–878.

Ajmone-Marsan, C. (1965). The thalamus. Data on its functional anatomy and on some aspects of thalamo-cortical integration. *Arch. Ital. Biol.* **103,** 847–882.

Albert, L. M., Silverberg, R., Reches, A., and Berman, M. (1976). Cerebral dominance for consciousness. *Arch. Neurol. (Chicago)* **33,** 453–662.

Amassian, V. E., Waller, H. J., and Macy, J., Jr. (1964). Neural mechanism of the primary somatosensory evoked potential. *Ann. N. Y. Acad. Sci.* **112,** 5–32.

Bakan, D. (1975). Dreaming, REM sleep and the right hemisphere: A theoretical integration. *J. Altered States of Consciousness* **3,** 285–307.

Barchas, J. D., Berger, P. A., Matthysse, S., and Wyatt, R. J. (1978). The biochemistry of affective disorders and schizophrenia. *In* "Principles of Psychopharmacology" (W. G. Clark and J. del Giudice, eds.), pp. 105–131. Academic Press, New York.

Bazhin, E. F., Wasserman, L. I., and Tonkonogii, I. M. (1975). Auditory hallucinations and left temporal lobe pathology. *Neuropsychologia* **13,** 481–487.

Beaumont, J. G., and Dimond, S. J. (1973). Brain disconnection and schizophrenia. *Br. J. Psychiatry* **123,** 661–662.

Beck, E. C., Swanson, C., and Dustman, R. E. (1980). Long latency components of the visually evoked potential in man: Effects of aging. *Exp. Aging Res.* **6,** 523–545.

Berger, B., Tassin, J. P., Blanc, R., Moyne, M. A., and Thierry, A. M. (1974). Histochemical confirmation for dopaminergic innervation of the rat cerebral cortex after destruction of the noradrenergic ascending pathways. *Brain Res.* **84,** 332–337.

Bernstein, A., Taylor, K., Starkey, P., Juni, S., Lubowsky, J., and Paley, H. (1981). Initial responsiveness and the effect of prolonged stimulus repetition on SCR, FPV & EEG response in schizophrenics and controls. *Psychophysiology* **18,** 203–204.

Brezinova, V., and Kendell, R. E. (1977). Smooth pursuit eye movements of schizophrenics and normal people under stress. *Br. J. Psychiatry* **130,** 59–63.

Buchsbaum, M. S., and Haier, R. J. (1978). Biological homogeneity, symptom heterogeneity and the diagnosis of schizphrenia. *Schizophr. Bull* **4,** 473–475.

Buchsbaum, M. S., Carpenter, W. T., Fedio, P., Goodwin, F. K., Murphy, D. L., and Post, R.

M. (1979). Hemispheric differences in evoked potential enhancement by selective attention to hemi-retinally presented stimuli in schizophrenic, affective and post-temporal lobectomy patients. *In* "Hemisphere Asymmetries of Function in Psychopathology" (J. H. Gruzelier and P. Flor-Henry, eds.), pp. 317–328. Elsevier/North-Holland, Amsterdam.

Bull, H. C., and Venables, P. H. (1974). Speech perception in schizophrenia. *Br. J. Psychiatry* **125,** 350–354.

Bunney, B. S. (1979). The electrophysiological pharmacology of midbrain dopaminergic systems. *In* "The Neurobiology of Dopamine" (A. S. Horn and B. H. C. Westerink, eds.), pp. 417–452. Academic Press, New York.

Butler, S. (1979). Interhemispheric relations in schizophrenia. *In* "Hemisphere Asymmetries of Function in Psychopathology" (J. H. Gruzelier and P. Flor-Henry, eds.), pp. 47–64. Elsevier/North-Holland, Amsterdam.

Carmon, A., Harishanu, Y., Lowinger, E., and Lavy, S. (1972). Asymmetries in hemispheric blood volume and cerebral dominance. *Behav. Biol.* **7,** 853–859.

Carr, S. A. (1980). Interhemispheric transfer of stereognostic information in chronic schizophrenics. *Br. J. Psychiatry* **136,** 53–58.

Caudrey, D. J., and Kirk, K. (1979). The perception of speech in schizophrenia and affective disorders. *In* "Hemisphere Asymmetries of Function in Psychopathology" (J. H. Gruzelier and P. Flor-Henry, eds.), pp. 581–601. Elsevier/North-Holland, Amsterdam.

Caudrey, D. J., Kirk, K., Thomas, P. C., and Ng, K. O. (1980). Perceptual deficit in schizophrenia: A defect in redundancy utilization, filtering or scanning? *Br. J. Psychiatry* **137,** 352–360.

Cegalis, J. A., and Sweeney, J. A. (1979). Eye movements in schizophrenia: A qualitative analysis. *Biol. Psychiatry* **14,** 13–26.

Chiarello, C. (1980). A house divided? Cognitive functioning with callosal agenesis. *Brain Lang.* **11,** 128–158.

Claridge, G. S. (1972). The schizophrenics as nervous types. *Br. J. Psychiatry* **121,** 1–17.

Clooney, J. L., and Murray, D. J. (1977). Same–different judgement in paranoid and nonparanoid patients: A laterality study. *J. Abnorm. Psychol.* **86,** 655–658.

Coger, R. W., Dymond, A. M., and Serafetinides, E. A. (1979). EEG similarities between chronic alcoholics and chronic, nonparanoid schizophrenics. *Arch. Gen. Psychiatry* **36,** 91–94.

Colony, H. S. (1956). EEG studies of 1000 schizophrenic patients. *Am. J. Psychiatry* **113,** 163–169.

Connolly, J. F., Gruzelier, J. H., Kleinman, K. M., and Hirsch, S. R. (1979). Lateralized abnormalities in hemisphere-specific tachistoscopic tasks in psychiatric patients and controls. *In* "Hemisphere Asymmetries of Function in Psychopathology" (J. H. Gruzelier and P. Flor-Henry, eds.), pp. 491–509. Elsevier/North-Holland, Amsterdam.

Creutzfeldt, O. D., and Kuhnt, U. (1967). The visual evoked potential: Physiological, developmental and clinical aspects. *Electroencephalogr. Clin. Neurophysiol., Suppl.* **26,** 29–41.

Critchley, M. (1979). "The Divine Banquet of the Brain and Other Essays." Raven Press, New York.

Davis, J. M. (1976). Recent developments in the drug treatment of schizophrenia. *Am. J. Psychiatry* **133,** 208–214.

Deisenhammer, E. (1981). Transient global amnesia as an epileptic manifestation. *J. Neurol.* **225,** 289–292.

Desmedt, J. E., and Debecker, J. (1979). Wave form and neural mechanism of the decision P350 elicited without pre-stimulus CNV or readiness potential in random sequences of near-threshold auditory clicks and finger stimuli. *Electroencephalogr. Clin. Neurophysiol.* **47,** 648–670.

Dimond, S. J. (1979). Disconnection and psychopathology. *In* "Hemisphere Asymmetries of Function and Psychopathology" (J. H. Gruzelier and P. Flor-Henry, eds.), pp. 35–46. Elsevier/North-Holland, Amsterdam.

Dimond, S. J., Scammel, R. E., Pryce, I. G., Huws, D., and Gray, C. (1979). Callosal transfer and left-hand anomia in schizophrenia. *Biol. Psychiatry* **14,** 735–739.

Domino, E. F., Demetriou, S., Tuttle, T., and Klinge, V. (1979). Comparison of the visually evoked response in drug-free schizophrenic patients and normal controls. *Electroencephalogr. Clin. Neurophysiol.* **46,** 123–137.

Donchin, E., and Smith, D. B. D. (1970). The contingent negative variation and the late positive wave of the average evoked potential. *Electroencephalogr. Clin. Neurophysiol.* **29,** 201–203.

Dorland's Illustrated Medical Dictionary (1974). 25th ed. Saunders, Philadelphia, Pennsylvania.

Eaton, E. M., Busk, J., Maloney, M. P., Sloane, R. B., Whipple, K., and White, K. (1979). Hemispheric dysfunction in schizophrenia: Assessment by visual perception tasks. *Psychiatry Res.* **1,** 325–332.

Edelstein, P., Schultz, J. R., Hirschowitz, J., Kanter, D. R., and Garver, D. L. (1981). Physostigmine and lithium response in the schizophrenics. *Am. J. Psychiatry* **138,** 1078–1081.

Ellenberg, L., and Sperry, R. W. (1979). Capacity for holding sustained attention following commissurotomy. *Cortex* **15,** 421–438.

Etevenon, P., Pidoux, B., Rioux, P., Peron-Magnan, P., Verdeaux, G., and Deniker, P. (1979). Intra- and interhemispheric EEG differences quantified by spectral analysis. Comparative study of 2 groups of schizophrenics and a control group. *Acta Psychiatr. Scand.* **60,** 57–68.

Feigenberg, I. M. (1964). Comparative electroencephalographic characteristics of various clinical groups of schizophrenic patients. *Z. Neuropatol. Psikhiatr.* **64,** 567–574.

Flor-Henry, P. (1969). Psychosis and temporal lobe epilepsy: A controlled investigation. *Epilepsia* **110,** 363–395.

Flor-Henry, P. (1976). Lateralized temporal–limbic dysfunction and psychopathology. *Ann. N.Y. Acad. Sci.* **280,** 777–795.

Flor-Henry, P. (1979). On certain aspects of the localization of the cerebral systems regulating and determining emotion. *Biol. Psychiatry* **14,** 677–698.

Flor-Henry, P., and Yeudall, L. T. (1979). Neuropsychological investigation of schizophrenia and manic–depressive psychoses. *In* "Hemisphere Asymmetries of Function in Psychopathology" (J. H. Gruzelier and P. Flor-Henry, eds.), pp. 341–362. Elsevier/North-Holland, Amsterdam.

Flor-Henry, P., Koles, Z. J., Howarth, B. G., and Burton, L. (1979). Neurophysiological studies of schizophrenia, mania and depression. *In* "Hemisphere Asymmetries of Function in Psychopathology" (J. H. Gruzelier and P. Flor-Henry, eds.), pp. 189–222. Elsevier/North-Holland, Amsterdam.

Freed, W. J., Karson, C. N., Kleinman, J. E., and Wyatt, R. J. (1981). Increased spontaneous eye blinks in cerebellectomized rats. *Biol. Psychiatry* **16,** 789–792.

Frith, C. D. (1979). Consciousness, information processing and schizophrenia. *Br. J. Psychiatry* **134,** 225–235.

Fuxe, K, Hamberger, B., and Hökfelt, T. (1968). Distribution of noradrenaline terminals in cortical areas of the rat. *Brain Res.* **8,** 125–131.

Gainotti, G. (1972). Emotional behavior and hemispheric side of the lesion. *Cortex* **8,** 41–55.

Glick, S. D., Jerussi, T. P., and Fleisher, L. N. (1976). Turning in circles: The neuropharmacology of rotation. *Life Sci.* **18,** 889–896.

Goertzel, V., May, P. R. A., Salkin, J., and Schoop, T. (1965). Body–ego technique: An approach to the schizophrenic patient. *J. Nerv. Ment. Dis.*, **141,** 53–60.

Golden, C. J., Graber, B., Coffman, J., Berg, R. A., Newlin, D., and Bloch, S. (1981). Structural brain deficits in schizophrenia. *Arch. Gen. Psychiatry* **38,** 1014–1017.

Goldstein, L. (1981). Statistical organizational features of the computerized EEG under various behavioral states. *Adv. Biol. Psychiatry* **6,** 12–16.

Green, P. (1978). Defective interhemispheric transfer in schizophrenia. *J. Abnor. Psychol.* **87,** 472–480.

Green, P., and Kotenko, V. (1980). Superior speech comprehension in schizophrenics under monaural vs binaural listening conditions. *J. Abnorm. Psychol.* **89,** 399–408.

Groves, P. M., Fenster, G. A., Tepper, J. M., Nakamura, S., and Young, S. J. (1981). Changes in dopaminergic terminal excitability induced by amphetamine and haloperidol. *Brain Res.* **221,** 425–431.

Gruzelier, J. H. (1973). Bilateral asymmetry of skin conductance orienting and levels in schizophrenics. *Biol. Psychol.* **1,** 21–41.

Gruzelier, J. H. (1979). Synthesis and critical review of the evidence for hemisphere asymmetries of function in psychopathology. *In* "Hemisphere Asymmetries of Function in Psychopathology" (J. H. Gruzelier and P. Flor-Henry, eds.), pp. 647–672. Elsevier/North-Holland, Amsterdam.

Gruzelier, J. H., and Hammond, N. V. (1976). Schizophrenia: A dominant hemisphere temporal-lobe disorder? *Res. Commun. Psychol., Psychiatry Behav.* **1,** 33–72.

Gruzelier, J. H., and Hammond, N. V. (1978). The effect of CPZ upon psychophysiological, endocrine and information processing measures in schizophrenia. *J. Psychiatr. Res.* **14,** 167–182.

Gruzelier, J. H., and Hammond, N. V. (1979). Gains, losses and lateral differences in the hearing of schizophrenic patients. *Br. J. Psychol.* **70,** 319–330.

Gruzelier, J. H., and Venables, P. (1974). Bimodality and lateral asymmetry of skin conductance orienting activity in schizophrenia: Replication and evidence of lateral asymmetry in patients with depression and disorders of personality. *Biol. Psychiatry* **8,** 55–73.

Gruzelier, J. H., Connolly, J. F., and Hirsch, S. R. (1981). Altered brain functional organization in psychosis: Brain–behaviour relationships. *Adv. Biol. Psychiatry* **6,** 54–59.

Gur, R. E. (1978). Left hemisphere dysfunction and left hemisphere overactivation in schizophrenia. *J. Abnorm. Psychol.* **87,** 226–238.

Gur, R. E. (1979a). Hemispheric overactivation in schizophrenia. *In* "Hemisphere Asymmetries of Function in Psychopathology" (J. H. Gruzelier and P. Flor-Henry, eds.), pp. 113–124. Elsevier/North-Holland, Amsterdam.

Gur, R. E. (1979b). Cognitive concomitants of hemispheric dysfunction in schizophrenia. *Arch. Gen. Psychiatry* **36,** 269–274.

Hammond, N. V., and Gruzelier, J. H. (1978). Laterality, attention and rate effects in the auditory temporal discrimination of chronic schizophrenics: The effect of treatment with chlorpromazine. *Q. J. Exp. Psychol.* **30,** 91–103.

Harris, C. S., Thackray, R. I., and Shoenberger, R. W. (1966). Blink rate as a function of induced muscular tension and manifest anxiety. *Percept. Mot. Skills* **22,** 155–160.

Hartlage, L. C., and Garber, J. (1976). Spatial vs. nonspatial reasoning ability in chronic schizophrenics. *J. Clin. Psychol.* **32,** 235–237.

Hassler, R. (1980). Brain mechanisms of intention and attention with introductory remarks on other volitional processes. *Prog. Brain Res.* **54,** 585–614.

Hays, P. (1977). Electroencephalographic variants and genetic predisposition to schizophrenia. *J. Neurol., Neurosurg. Psychiatry* **40,** 753–755.

Heath, R. G., Franklin, D. E., and Shraberg, D. (1979). Gross pathology of the cerebellum in patients diagnosed and treated as functional psychiatric disorders. *J. Nerv. Ment. Dis.* **167,** 585–592.

Hécaen, H., and Albert, M. L. (1978). "Human Neuropsychology." Wiley, New York.

Heilman, K. M., and Valenstein, E. A. (1978). Mechanisms underlying hemispatial neglect. *Ann. Neurol.* **5,** 166–170.

Heilman, K. M., and Van Den Abell, T. (1979). Right hemisphere dominance for mediating cerebral activation. *Neuropsychologia* **17,** 315–321.

Hellige, J. B., and Cox, P. J. (1976). Effects of concurrent verbal memory on recognition of stimuli from the left and right visual fields. *J. Exp. Psychol. Hum. Percept. Perform.* **2,** 210–221.

Hellige, J. B., Cox, P. J., and Litvac, L. (1979). Information processing in the cerebral hemispheres: Selective hemispheric activation and capacity limitations. *J. Exp. Psychol. Gen.* **108,** 251–279.

Hicks, R. E., Provenzano, F. J., and Rybstein, E. D. (1975). Generalized and lateralized effects of concurrent verbal rehearsal upon performance of sequential movements of the fingers by the left and right hands. *Acta Psychol.* **39,** 119–130.

Hillsberg, B. (1979). A comparison of visual discrimination performance of the dominant hemisphere in schizophrenia. *In* "Hemisphere Asymmetries of Function in Psychopathology" (J. H. Gruzelier and P. Flor-Henry, eds.), pp. 527–538. Elsevier/North-Holland, Amsterdam.

Hökfelt, T., Lungdahl, A., Fuxe, K., Johansson, O., Perez de la Mora, M., and Agrati, L. (1977). Some attempts to explore central GABAergic mechanisms with special reference to control of dopamine neurons. *In* "Neuroregulators and Psychiatric Disorders" (E. Usdin, D. A. Hamburg, and J. D. Barchas, eds.), pp. 358. Oxford Univ. Press, New York

Hollister, L. E. (1974). Clinical differences among phenothiazines in schizophrenia. *In* "The Phenothiazines and Structurally Related Drugs" (I. S. Forrest, C. J. Carr, and E. Usdin, eds.), pp. 667–673. Raven Press, New York.

Howes, D., and Boller, F. (1975). Simple reaction time: Evidence for focal impairment from lesions of the right hemisphere. *Brain* **98,** 317–332.

Humphrey, D. R. (1968). Re-analysis of the antidromic cortical response. II. On the contribution of cell discharge and PSPs to the evoked potentials. *Electroencephalogr. Clin. Neurophysiol.* **25,** 421–442.

Iacono, W. G. (1982). Bilateral electrodermal habituation–dishabituation and resting EEG in remitted schizophrenics. *J. Nerv. Ment. Dis.* **170,** 91–101.

Idelson, A. V. (1966). Cited in Lomov (1966).

Igert, C., and Lairy, G. C. (1962). Prognostic value of EEG in the development of schizophrenics. *Electroencephalogr. Clin. Neurophysiol.* **14,** 183–190.

Innocenti, G. M. (1981). The development of interhemispheric connections. *Trends Neurosci.* **4,** 142–144.

Itil, T. M. (1978). Effects of psychotropic drugs in qualitatively and quantitatively analyzed human EEG. *In* "Principles of Psychopharmacology" (W. G. Clark and J. del Giudice, eds.), pp. 261–277. Academic Press, New York.

Jacobson, S., and Trojanowski, J. Q. (1974). The cells of origin of the corpus callosum in rat, cat, and rhesus monkey. *Brain Res.* **74,** 149–155.

Janke, W. (1980). Psychometric and psychophysiological actions of antipsychotics in man. *In* "Psychotropic Agents " (F. Hoffmeister and G. Stille, eds.), Part I, pp. 305–336. Springer-Verlag, Berlin and New York.

Jarvik, L. F., and Deckard, B. S. (1977). The Odyssean personality. A survival advantage for carriers of genes predisposing to schizophrenia? *Neuropsychobiology* **3,** 179–191.

Johnson, D. A. W. (1981). Studies of depressive symptoms in schizophrenia. *Br. J. Psychiatry* **139,** 89–101.

Josiassen, R. C., Shagass, C., Roemer, R. A., and Straumanis, J. J. (1981). The attention-related somatosensory evoked potential late positive wave in psychiatric patients. *Psychiatry Res.* **5,** 147–155.

Karson, C., Freed, W. J., Kleinman, J. E., Bigelow, L. B., and Wyatt, R. J. (1981). Neuroleptics decrease blinking in schizophrenic subjects. *Biol. Psychiatry* **16,** 679–682.

Kim, J. S., Bak, I. J., Hassler, R., and Okada, Y. (1971). Role of γ- aminobutyric acid (GABA) in the extrapyramidal motor system. 2. Some evidence for the existence of a type of GABA-rich strionigral neurons. *Exp. Brain Res.* **14,** 95–104.

Kinsbourne, M. (1972). Eye and head turning indicates cerebral lateralization. *Science* **176,** 539–541.

Kinsbourne, M., and Cook, J. (1971). Generalized and lateralized effect of concurrent verbalization on a unimanual skill. *Q. J. Exp. Psychol.* **23,** 341–345.

Kok, E. (1967). "Visual Agnosias." Medizine, Leningrad (in Russian).

Kornetsky, C., and Mirsky, A. F. (1966). On certain psychopharmacological and physiological differences between schizophrenic and normal persons. *Psychopharmacologia* **8,** 309–318.

Koukkou, M., Angst, J., and Zimmer, D. (1979). Paroxysmal EEG activity and psychopathology during the treatment with clozapine. *Pharmakopsychiatr./Neuro-Psychopharmakol.* **12,** 173–183.

Kugler, B. T., and Henley, S. H. A. (1979). Laterality effects in the tactile modality in schizophrenia. *In* "Hemisphere Asymmetries of Function in Psychopathology" (J. H. Gruzelier and P. Flor-Henry, eds.), pp. 475–489. Elsevier/North-Holland, Amsterdam.

Kutty, I. N., and Prendes, J. L. (1981). Psychosis and cerebellar degeneration. *J. Nerv. Ment. Dis.* **169,** 390–391.

Laitinen, L. V. (1972). Stereotactic lesions in the knee of the corpus callosum in the treatment of emotional disorders. *Lancet* **1,** 472–475.

Landolt, H. (1958). Serial electroencephalographic investigation during psychotic episodes in epileptic patients and during schizophrenic attacks. *In* "Lectures on Epilepsy" (A. M. Lorentz de Haas, ed.), pp. 91–133. Elsevier/North-Holland, Amsterdam.

Lansdell, H., and Davie, C. (1972). Massa intermedia: Possible relation to intelligence. *Neuropsychologia* **10,** 207–210.

Lawson, E. A. (1981). Skin conductance responses in Huntington's chorea progeny. *Psychophysiology* **18,** 32–35.

Lecours, A. R., and Vanier-Clement, M. (1976). Schizophrenia and jargonaphasia. *Brain Lang.* **3,** 516–565.

Lerner, J., Nachshon, I., and Carmon, A. (1977). Responses of paranoid and nonparanoid schizophrenics in a dichotic listening task. *J. Nerv. Ment. Dis.* **164,** 247–252.

Leuscherer, F., Newman, W., and Hempel, R. (1980). Toxicology of antipsychotic agents. *In* "Psychotropic Agents" (F. Hoffmeister and G. Stille, eds.), Part I, pp. 305–336. Springer-Verlag, Berlin and New York.

Levitt, P., and Moore, R. Y. (1978). Noradrenaline neuron innervation of the neocortex in the rat. *Brain Res.* **139,** 219–232.

Lindvall, O., Björklund, A., Moore, R. Y., and Stenevi, U. (1974). Mesencephalic dopamine neurons projecting to neocortex. *Brain Res.* **81,** 325–331.

Lishman, W. A., and McMeekan, E. R. L. (1976). Hand preference patterns in psychiatric patients. *Br. J. Psychiatry* **129,** 158–166.

Lishman, W. A., Toone, B. K., Colbourn, C. J., McMeekan, E. R. L., and Mance, R. M. (1978). Dichotic listening in psychotic patients. *Br. J. Psychiatry* **132,** 333–341.

Lomov, B. F. (1966). Manual interaction in the process of tactile perception. *In* "Psychological Research in the USSR" (A. Leontyev, A. Luriya, and A. Smirnov, eds.), p. 267. Progress Publishers, Moscow.

McEntee, W. J., and Newman, G. C. (1981). A case report of tardive hemidyskinesia. *Am. J. Psychiatry* **138,** 1380–1381.

McGhie, A., and Chapman, J. (1961). Disorders of attention and perception in early schizophrenia. *Br. J. Med. Psychol.* **34,** 103–116.

McMahon, D. (1974). Chemical messengers in development: A hypothesis. *Science* **185,** 1012–1021.

Martin, M. (1979). Hemispheric specialization for local and global processing. *Neuropsychologia* **17,** 33–40.

Mathew, R. J., Meyer, J. S., Francis, D. J., Schoolar, J. C., Weinman, M., and Mortel, K. F. (1981). rCBF in schizophrenia: A preliminary report. *Am. J. Psychiatry* **138,** 112–113.

Matousek, M. (1965). Variability of the EEG and its clinical significance. *Act. Nerv. Super.* **7,** 51–54.

Maynert, E. W., Marczynski, T. J., and Browning, R. A. (1975). The role of the neurotransmitters in the epilepsies. *Adv. Neur.* **13,** 79–147.

Mecacci, L., and Pasquali, E. (1980). Eyeblink, evoked potentials and visual attention. *Percept. Mot. Skills* **51,** 891–895.

Mintz, M., Tomer, R., and Myslobodsky, M. S. (1982a). Neuroleptic- induced lateral asymmetry of visual evoked potentials in schizophrenia. *Biol. Psychiatry* **17,** 815–828.

Mintz, M., Tomer, R., Radwan, H., and Myslobodsky, M. S. (1982b). A comparison of levodopa treatment and task demands on visual evoked potentials in hemi-Parkinsonism. *Psychiatry Res.* **6,** 245–251.

Mirsky, A. F. (1969). Neuropsychological bases of schizophrenia. *Ann. Rev. Psychol.* **20,** 321–348.

Myslobodsky, M. S. (1976). "Petit Mal Epilepsy: A Search for the Precursors of Wave–Spike Discharges." Academic Press, New York.

Myslobodsky, M. S. (1981). Animal brain laterality: Functional lateralization or a right–left excitability gradient? *Behav. Brain Sci.* **4,** 31–32.

Myslobodsky, M. S., and Rattok, J. (1977). Bilateral electrodermal activity in waking man. *Acta Psychol.* **41,** 273–282.

Myslobodsky, M. S., and Weiner, M. (1976). Pharmacologic implications of hemispheric asymmetry. *Life Sci.* **19,** 1467–1478.

Myslobodsky, M. S., Mintz, M., and Tomer, R. (1979). Asymmetric reactivity of the brain and components of hemispheric imbalance. *In* "Hemisphere Asymmetries of Function in Psychopathology" (J. H. Gruzelier and P. Flor-Henry, eds.), pp. 125–148. Elsevier/North-Holland, Amsterdam.

Nachshon, I. (1980). Hemispheric dysfunction in schizophrenia. *J. Nerv. Ment. Dis.* **168,** 241–242.

Nasrallah, H. A., and McChesney, M. (1981). Psychopathology of corpus callosum tumors. *Biol. Psychiatry* **16,** 633–669.

Nicholson, J., Lauder, J., and Bloom, F. E. (1973). Cell differentiation and synaptogenesis in the locus coeruleus, raphe nuclei and substantia nigra of the rat. *Anat. Rec.* **175,** 398–399.

Orthner, H., and Sendler, W. (1975). Planimetrische volumetrie an menschlichen gehirnen. *Fortschr. Neurol., Psychiatr. Ihrer Grenzgeb.* **43,** 191–209.

Oshima, T. (1981). Cortical neurones in arousal. *Jpn. J. EEG EMG, Suppl.* pp. 73–78.

Patterson, T., and Venables, P. H. (1978). Bilateral skin conductance and skin potential in schizophrenic and normal subjects: The identification of the fast habituator group of schizophrenics. *Psychophysiology* **15,** 556–560.

Pic'l, A. K., Magaro, P. A., and Wade, E. A. (1979). Hemispheric functioning in paranoid and nonparanoid schizophrenia. *Biol. Psychiatry* **14,** 891–903.

Pines, L. J., and Maiman, R. M. (1939). Cells of origin of fibers of corpus callosum. *Arch. Neurol. Psychiatry* **42,** 1076–1082.

Pittman, J. C., and Feeney, D. M. (1974). Modulation of recurrent inhibition in cat association cortex by reticulocortical arousal. *Exp. Neurol.* **44,** 160–170.

Pivik, R. T. (1979). Smooth pursuit eye movements and attention in psychiatric patients. *Biol. Psychiatry* **14,** 859–879.

Poon, L. W., Thompson, L. W., and Marsh, G. R. (1973). Averaged evoked potential changes as a function of processing complexity. *Psychophysiology* **13,** 43–49.
Purpura, D. P. (1959). Nature of electrocortical potentials and synaptic organization in cerebral and cerebellar cortex. *Int. Rev. Neurobiol.* **1,** 47–163.
Purpura, D. P. (1978). Discussion. *In* "Event-Related Brain Potentials in Man" (E. Callaway, P. Tueting, and S. H. Koslow, eds.), pp. 346–347. Academic Press, New York.
Randall, P. L. (1980). A neuroanatomical theory on the aetiology of schizophrenia. *Med. Hypotheses* **6,** 645–658.
Rhodes, L. E., Dustman, R. E., and Beck, E. C. (1969). The visual evoked response. A comparison of bright and dull children. *Electroencephalogr. Clin. Neurophysiol.* **27,** 364–372.
Rochford, J. M., Swartzburg, M., Chowdhrey, S. M., and Goldstein, L. (1976). Some quantitative EEG correlates of psychopathology. *Res. Commun. Psychol., Psychiatry Behav.* **1,** 211–226.
Roemer, R. A., Shagass, C., Straumanis, J. J., and Amadeo, M. (1978). Pattern evoked potential measurements suggesting lateralized hemispheric dysfunction in chronic schizophrenia. *Biol. Psychiatry* **13,** 185–202.
Roemer, R. A., Shagass, C., Straumanis, J. J., and Amadeo, M. (1979). Somatosensory and auditory evoked potential studies of functional differences between the cerebral hemispheres in psychosis. *Biol. Psychiatry* **14,** 357–373.
Rosenthal, R., and Bigelow, L. B. (1972). Quantitative brain measurements in chronic schizophrenia. *Br. J. Psychiatry* **121,** 259–264.
Roth, W. T., Pfefferbaum, A., Horvath, T. B., Berger, P. A., and Kopell, B. S. (1980). P3 reduction in auditory evoked potentials of schizophrenics. *Electroencephalogr. Clin. Neurophysiol.* **49,** 497–505.
Rush, M., Diamond, F., and Alpert, M. (1982). Depression as a risk factor in tardive dyskinesia. *Biol Psychiatry* **17,** 387–392.
Sadowsky, C., and Reeves, A. G. (1975). Agenesis of the corpus callosum with hypothermia. *Arch. Neurol. (Chicago)* **32,** 774–776.
Sandel, A., and Alcorn, J. D. (1980). Individual hemisphericity and maladaptive behaviors. *J. Abnorm. Psychol.* **89,** 514–517.
Scarone, S., Garavagl, P. F., and Cazzullo, C. L. (1981). Further evidence of dominant hemisphere dysfunction in chronic schizophrenia. *Br. J. Psychiatry* **138,** 354–355.
Scheel-Krüger, J., Magelund, G., and Olianas, M. (1981). The role of GABA in the basal ganglia and limbic system for behaviour. *In* "Amino Acid Neurotransmitters" (F. V. DeFeudis and P. Mandel, eds.), pp. 23–36. Raven Press, New York.
Schwartz, B. (1967). Hemispheric dominance and consciousness. *Acta Neurol. Scand.* **43,** 513–525.
Schwartz, G. E., Davidson, R. J., and Maer, F. (1975). Right hemisphere lateralization for emotion in the human brain: Interaction with cognition. *Science* **190,** 286–288.
Schweitzer, L. (1979). Differences of cerebral lateralization among schizophrenic and depressed patients. *Biol. Psychiatry* **14,** 721–733.
Schweitzer, L., and Chacko, R. (1980). Cerebral lateralization: Relation to subject's sex. *Cortex* **16,** 559–566.
Schweitzer, L., Becker, E., and Welsh, H. (1978). Abnormalities of cerebral lateralization in schizophrenic patients. *Arch. Gen. Psychiatry* **35,** 982–985.
Seales, D. M. (1973). Cited in Poon *et al.* (1973).
Serafetinides, E. A., Hoare, R. D., and Driver, M. V. (1964). Modification of intracarotid amylobarbitone test—findings about speech and consciousness. *Lancet* **1,** 249–250.
Serafetinides, E. A., Hoare, R. D., and Driver, M. V. (1965). Intracarotid sodium amylobarbitone and cerebral dominance for speech and consciousness. *Brain* **88,** 107–130.
Serafetinides, E. A., Walter, R. D., and Cherlow, D. G. (1975). Amnestic confusional phe-

nomena, hippocampal stimulation and laterality factors. *In* "The Hippocampus" (R. L. Isaacson and K. M. Pribram, eds.), Vol. 2, pp. 363–375. Raven Press, New York.

Serafetinides, E. A., Coger, R. W., Martin, J., and Dymond, A. M. (1981). Schizophrenic symptomatology and cerebral dominance patterns: A comparison of EEG, AER and BPRS measures. *Compr. Psychiatry* **22,** 218–225.

Shagass, C., Roemer, R. A., and Straumanis, J. J. (1980). Deviant topography of sensory evoked potentials in psychosis. *Adv. Biol Psychiatry* **4,** 94–101.

Shaw, J. C., Brooks, S., Cotler, N., and O'Connor, K. P. (1979). A comparison of schizophrenic and neurotic patients using EEG power and coherence spectra. *In* "Hemisphere Asymmetries of Function in Psychopathology" (J. H. Gruzelier and P. Flor-Henry, eds.), pp. 257–284. Elsevier/North-Holland, Amsterdam.

Slater, E., Beard, A. W., and Glithero, E. (1963). The schizophrenia-like psychoses of epilepsy. *Br. J. Psychiatry* **109,** 95–150.

Small, J. G., and Small, I. F. (1965). Reevaluation of clinical EEG findings in schizophrenia. *Dis. Nerv. Syst.* **26,** 345–349.

Snyder, S. H. (1976). The dopamine hypothesis of schizophrenia: Focus on the dopamine receptor. *Am. J. Psychiatry* **133,** 197–202.

Spence, D. P. (1967). Subliminal perception and perceptual defence. *Behav. Sci.* **12,** 183–193.

Stevens, J. M., and Derbishire, A. J. (1958). Shifts along the alert–repose continuum during remission of catatonic stupor with amobarbital. *Psychosom. Med.* **20,** 99–107.

Stevens, J. R. (1978). Disturbances of ocular movements and blinking in schizophrenia. *J. Neurol., Neurosurg. Psychiatry* **42,** 1024–1030.

Stevens, J. R., and Livermore, A. (1978). Eye blinking and rapid eye movement: Pulsed photic stimulation of the brain. *Exp. Neurol.* **60,** 541–556.

Szentágothai, J. (1969). Architecture of the central cortex. *In* "Basic Mechanisms of the Epilepsies" (H. H. Jasper, A. A. Ward, and A. Pope, eds.), pp. 13–28. Little, Brown, Boston, Massachusetts.

Taylor, P. J., and Fleminger, J. J. (1981). The lateralization of symptoms in schizophrenia. *Br. J. Med. Psychol.* **51,** 59–65.

Taylor, P. J., Dalton, R., and Fleminger, J. J. (1980). Handedness in schizophrenia. *Br. J. Psychiatry* **136,** 375–383.

Tomer, R., Mintz, M., Levy, A., and Myslobodsky, M. S. (1979). Reactive gaze laterality in schizophrenic patients. *Biol. Psychol.* **9,** 115–127.

Toone, B. K., Cooke, E., and Lader, M. H. (1981). EDA in the affective disorders and schizophrenia. *Psychol. Med.* **11,** 497–508.

Tress, K. H., Kugler, B. T., and Caudrey, D. J. (1979). Interhemispheric integration in schizophrenia. *In* "Hemisphere Asymmetries of Function in Psychopathology" (J. H. Gruzelier and P. Flor-Henry, eds.), pp. 449–462. Elsevier/North-Holland, Amsterdam.

Tucker, D. M., Antes, J. R., Stenslie, C. E., and Barnhardt, T. M. (1978). Anxiety and lateral cerebral function. *J. Abnorm. Psychol.* **87,** 380–383.

Venables, P. H. (1966). The psychophysiological aspects of schizophrenia. *Br. J. Med. Psychol.* **39,** 289–297.

Venables, P. H. (1977). The electrodermal psychophysiology of schizophrenics and children at risk for schizophrenia: Controversies and developments. *Schizophr. Bull.* **3,** 28–48.

Venables, P. H. (1981). Psychophysiology of abnormal behaviour. *Br. Med. J.* **37,** 199–203.

Volkmann, F. C., Riggs, L. A., and Moore, R. K. (1979). A comparison of saccades and blinks in suppression of vision. *Invest. Opthalmol. Visual Sci.* **18,** April Suppl., 140P.

Walker, E. (1981). Attentional and neuromotor functions of schizophrenics, schizoaffectives, and patients with other affective disorders. *Arch. Gen. Psychiatry* **38,** 1355–1358.

Walker, E., Hoppes, E., and Emory, E. (1981). A reinterpretation of findings on hemispheric dysfunction in schizophrenia. *J. Nerv. Ment. Dis.* **169,** 378–380.

Waziri, R. (1980). Lateralization of neuroleptic-induced dyskinesia indicates pharmacologic asymmetry in the brain. *Psychopharmacology* **68,** 51–53.

Weinberger, D. R., Torsey, E. F., and Wyatt, R. J. (1979). Cerebellar atrophy in chronic schizophrenia. *Lancet* **1,** 718–719.

Weinstein, E. A., and Friedland, R. P. (1977). Behavioral disorders associated with hemi-inattention. *In* "Hemi-inattention and Hemisphere Specialization" (E. A. Weinstein and R. P. Friedland, eds.), pp. 51–62. Raven Press, New York.

Weinstein, E. A., and Kahn, R. L. (1955). "Denial of Illness: Symbolic and Physiological Aspects." Thomas, Springfield, Illinois.

Weller, M., and Kugler, B. T. (1979). Tactile discrimination in schizophrenic and affective psychoses. *In* "Hemisphere Asymmetries of Function in Psychopathology" (J. H. Gruzelier and P. Flor-Henry, eds.), pp. 463–474. Elsevier/North-Holland, Amsterdam.

Weller, M., and Montagu, J. D. (1979). Electroencephalographic coherence in schizophrenia: A preliminary study. *In* "Hemisphere Asymmetries of Function in Psychopathology" (J. H. Gruzelier and P. Flor-Henry, eds.), pp. 285–292. Elsevier/North-Holland, Amsterdam.

Wexler, B. E., and Heninger, G. R. (1979). Alterations in cerebral laterality during acute psychotic illness. *Arch. Gen. Psychiatry* **36,** 278–284.

Wilkins, A. J., Binnie, C. D., and Darby, C. E. (1981). Interhemispheric differences in photosensitive epilepsy. I. Pattern sensitivity thresholds. *Electroencephalogr. Clin. Neurophysiol.* **52,** 461–468.

Yosawitz, A., Bruder, G., Sutton, S., Sharpe, L., Gurland, B., Fleiss, J., and Costa, L. (1979). Dichotic perception: Evidence for right hemisphere dysfunction in psychosis. *Br. J. Psychiatry* **135,** 224–237.

15: Hemisphere Dysfunction in Psychopathy and Behavior Disorders

ISRAEL NACHSHON

Department of Criminology
Bar-Ilan University
Ramat Gan, Israel

I. Historical Antecedents 389
II. Performance > Verbal Pattern 390
III. Clinical Evidence 394
IV. Experimental Evidence 397
A. Electrodermal Responsivity 397
B. Visual Field Differences 399
C. Lateral Preferences 399
V. Summary and Conclusions 403
VI. Theoretical Speculations and Applications 404
References 406

I. Historical Antecedents

Psychopathy and behavior disorders are the subject matter of psychopathology as well as criminology. In criminology the scientific study of criminal behavior is usually associated with the so-called positive school. In contradistinction to the classical and the neoclassical schools, "the positive school represents the first formulations and applications to the field of criminology of the point of view, methodology, and logic of the natural sciences to the study of human behavior [Vold, 1979, pp. 18–19]." Consequently, in looking for the causes of crime this school focuses on the personal characteristics of the individual criminal rather than on the properties of the criminal act.

Among the theoretical orientations conceived within the framework of the positive school, Lombroso's (1874) criminal anthropology is one of the best known. According to this theory the criminal's inadequacy and

HEMISYNDROMES:
Psychobiology, Neurology,
Psychiatry

ISBN 0-12-512460-0

degeneracy are manifested by specific physical characteristics, or stigmata. Two of these stigmata have to do with lateral asymmetries: abnormal asymmetry of the face and imbalance of the cerebral hemispheres. Hemisphere dysfunctions in criminals were subsequently reported by Talbot (1898), who identified seven types of brain deformations, three of which had to do with lateral abnormalities: atypical asymmetries of the bulk and gyral development of the cerebral hemispheres and defective development of the great interhemispheric commissures. These asymmetries of the criminal's skull were later attributed to overdevelopment of specific regions in the cortex at the expense of other regions (Lamb, 1903). Finally, cranial asymmetries among violent criminals were repeatedly reported by Lydston (1904).

Underlying these findings were the phrenological assumptions that structure determines function and that the exterior of the skull conforms to the interior and the shape of the brain (Vold, 1979, pp. 51, 53). Cranial asymmetry therefore represents hemispheric asymmetry. Hence, criminals who show atypical cranial asymmetry suffer from hemisphere dysfunction.

With the fall of phrenology as a scientific discipline due to a lack of empirical support (Fink, 1962, p. 19; Vold, 1979, p. 55), the notion that physical abnormalities can be consistently related to legally and sociologically defined criminal behavior disappeared (Vold, 1979, p. 73), and by 1910 the hypothesis of the "criminal brain" had been generally abandoned (Fink, 1962, p. 113).

However, with the accumulation of new evidence, psychobiological theories in criminology have been enjoying a revival (Nachshon, 1982), and, among the variety of biological factors of criminal behavior, hemisphere dysfunction has drawn considerable attention. As Nachshon (1982) pointed out, the scientific *Zeitgeists* in criminology very much correspond to the dominant *Zeitgeists* in psychopathology. The shifts from biological to sociological and eventually to psychobiosocial causation of normal and abnormal behavior took place in these two fields of research at about the same time. No wonder, then, that the interest in the hemispheric etiology of criminal behavior originally emerged within the context of studies on hemisphere dysfunctions in psychopathology (Flor-Henry, 1973, 1974; Flor-Henry and Yeudall, 1973). Therefore, in the following discussion there are numerous references to psychopathological literature.

II. Performance > Verbal Pattern

Early attempts to relate hemisphere dysfunctions to behavior disorders go back to Wechsler (1958), the creator of the Wechsler Adult Intelligence Scale (WAIS). Ever since their inception the WAIS and related scales [the

Wechsler Intelligence Scale for Children (WISC) and the Wechsler–Bellevue Scale] have been continuously used, not only as measures of intellectual potential, which is their primary purpose, but also as indices of brain damage in general and of hemisphere dysfunction in particular.

The 11 tests of the WAIS are divided into verbal (V) and performance (P) subscales. It was argued that, since the left hemisphere normally processes verbal stimuli and the right hemisphere normally processes spatial stimuli (Kimura, 1967; Atkinson and Egeth, 1973; Nachshon, 1973; Nachshon and Carmon, 1975; Bryden, 1976; Moskovitch, 1979), the differential performance on the two subscales could be used as an index of hemispheric asymmetry. A higher score on the verbal subscale (V > P) might thus indicate left hemisphere dominance for processing verbal stimuli, whereas a higher score on the performance subscale (P > V) might indicate right hemisphere dominance for processing spatial stimuli.

In pathological conditions a unilateral hemisphere dysfunction may result in lower scores on tests that tap functions which are normally processed in that hemisphere. In severe cases the decrease in scores may even lead to a reversal of the V–P pattern. Thus, a left hemisphere dysfunction may be reflected by a P > V pattern, whereas a right hemisphere dysfunction may be reflected by a V > P pattern.

In testing this assumption, a few studies (Smith, 1966a,b; McIntyre *et al.*, 1976) failed to lend experimental support, but many others (Anderson, 1951; Reitan, 1955; Milner, 1958; Kløve, 1959; Balthazar and Morrison, 1961; McFie, 1961; Fitzhugh *et al.*, 1962; Dennerl, 1964a,b; Fitzhugh and Fitzhugh, 1964; Mathews and Reitan, 1964; Guertin *et al.*, 1966; Fedio and Mirsky, 1969; Parsons *et al.*, 1969; Uzzell *et al.*, 1979) revealed that in performance on the WAIS, patients with left hemisphere damage show the P > V pattern, whereas patients with right hemisphere damage show the V > P pattern (see also Hutt, 1976).

For example, in reviewing seven studies, Woods (1980) found that a total of 128 patients with left hemisphere lesions achieved mean scores of 87.1 and 91.4 on the verbal and performance scales, respectively; the corresponding mean scores for 204 patients with right hemisphere lesions were 97.2 and 85.4. Similar ratios were obtained in six studies conducted on 211 children, except for those who sustained the brain damage at a very young age (Woods and Teuber, 1973; Woods, 1980).

The hypothesis that patterns of V–P score ratios are associated with hemisphere function and dysfunction is further supported by three lines of evidence. First, studying sex differences in these patterns, McGlone (1977, 1978) found that the side of a lesion affects the V–P ratio in males only; in females the side of a lesion has no differential effect. This sex difference corresponds to sex differences in cerebral organization, which are characterized by a more pronounced hemispheric specialization among males than among females (Kimura, 1969; Harshman *et al.*, 1976;

Levy and Reid, 1976; Bryden, 1979; Levy and Gur, 1980; McGlone, 1980). Second, left-handed individuals, who, like females, have more bilateral hemispheric representation than right-handed individuals (Nachshon, 1978; Gur and Gur, 1980; Levy and Gur, 1980; Witelson, 1980), differ from the latter in patterns of V–P ratios, although sometimes their full IQ scores are not significantly different from each other (Levy, 1969; Bradshaw *et al.*, 1981). Finally, young children who had sustained brain damage before the hemispheric specialization was firmly established also failed to show a relationship between locus of lesion and V–P pattern (Woods and Teuber, 1973; Woods, 1980).

Regarding behavior disorders Wechsler himself suggested that, in responding to the WAIS, adolescent male psychopaths show the P>V pattern (Wechsler, 1958). This pattern was subsequently found among delinquents (Altus and Clarke, 1949; Clarke and Moore, 1950; Diller, 1952; Blank, 1958; Manne *et al.*, 1962; Andrew, 1974a,b), sociopaths (Wiens *et al.*, 1959), acting-out juveniles (Corotto, 1961), offenders (Andrew, 1978b), and recidivist criminals (Yeudall and Wardell, 1978). Three authors, however, failed to find the P>V pattern among sociopaths, people with character disorders, criminals, and delinquents (Foster, 1959; Field, 1960; Kahn, 1968). Two additional studies were concerned with the appearance of the P>V pattern among female delinquents; one found it (Bernstein and Corsini, 1953), and the other did not (Camp, 1966).

Reviewing 24 independent studies, Prentice and Kelly (1963) concluded that delinquents did not differ from nondelinquents in performance scores but that they did in verbal scores; scores were lower for the former than for the latter. This finding was corroborated by Flor-Henry and Yeudall (1973). Significantly, reduced verbal ability among delinquents, as reflected in their characteristic P>V pattern, appeared across samples despite variations in age, sex, race, setting, form of Wechsler scale administered, and substantial differences in criteria for delinquency (Prentice and Kelly, 1963).

Although these findings are generally accepted, their interpretation has been somewhat controversial. The reduced verbal relative to performance ability in subjects with behavior disorders has been attributed to a number of factors. Whereas some authors have attributed it to immaturity (Andrew, 1974a,b) or to situational variables (Manne *et al.*, 1962; Camp, 1966) many researchers have maintained that the P>V pattern is related to learning difficulties (in particular, reading disability) rather than to delinquency. The reasoning behind this hypothesis is as follows. Subjects who suffer from learning or reading difficulties do better on performance than on verbal tests, because verbal scores are more greatly affected by learning achievement than are performance scores. Now, since learning difficulties are a frequent concomitant of delinquency, it is obvious why many delinquents show the P>V pattern, but this pattern has nothing to do with delinquency as such (Glueck and Glueck, 1950; Graham, 1952; Vane and Eisen, 1954; Graham and Kamano, 1959).

Telegdy (1973), however, failed to find a relationship between reading ability and the P>V pattern. Beyond that, as has been shown earlier, the appearance of the P>V pattern in a variety of pathological populations is associated with left hemisphere dysfunction. Furthermore, it has been found that, regardless of criminality, whenever reading disability comes together with P>V pattern, left hemisphere dysfunction is involved (Muehl *et al.*, 1965; Zurif and Carson, 1970). Hence, both the P>V pattern and reading disability are presumably caused by left hemisphere dysfunctions.

Finally, Yeudall and Wardell (1978) showed that, regardless of reading ability, recidivist criminals performed poorly on both tests of left hemisphere functions and the verbal tests of the WAIS, but not on tests of right hemisphere functions and the performance tests of the WAIS. Similarly, testing habitual criminals, Yeudall *et al.* (1981) found that psychopaths and other violent criminals who had been diagnosed as having (exclusively or mainly) left hemisphere dysfunctions showed the P>V pattern on the WAIS, whereas depressive patients who had been diagnosed as having (exclusively or mainly) right hemisphere dysfunctions showed the V>P pattern (Table 15.1).

Group differences appeared only in the V–P pattern but not in the full IQ score. In full scores both groups were similarly inferior to the normal controls, who showed no significant differences between the scores obtained on the verbal and on the performance subscales.

TABLE 15.1
Frequency of Lateralized Neuropsychological Impairments and WAIS IQ Scores for Psychopathic and Depressive Groups

		Neuropsychological lateralization (frequency)			WAIS		
Group	*N*	Left	Right	Normal	Full	Verbal	Performance
Psychopaths	25	15	4	6	97.0	93.4	102.2[a]
Homicide	33	21	10	2	98.2	97.9	100.7
Rape	20	15	5	0	94.8	91.8	99.2[a]
Physical assault	37	23	10	4	95.9	93.3	99.9[a]
Total	115	74	29	12	96.5	94.1	98.8
Periodic–affective	25	0	22	3	95.4	99.8	90.8[a]
Personality disorder	25	8	15	2	95.7	98.3	93.0
Total	50	8	37	5	95.5	99.0	91.9
Normal subjects	25	0	0	25	110.9	108.9	112.4

[a] Correlated *t* test between verbal IQ and performance IQ are significant at $p < 0.001$. Adapted from Yeudall *et al.* (1981).

Since there is no reason to assume that different groups of habitual criminals systematically differ among themselves in their reading ability, the reading ability hypothesis regarding the etiology of the P>V pattern among psychopaths and subjects with behavior disorders must be rejected. Instead, it is proposed that the abnormal P>V pattern shown by these criminals is indicative of left hemisphere dysfunction. Flor-Henry (1976, 1978) pointed out that the correlation between left hemisphere dysfunction and the P>V pattern does not necessarily imply that the former causes the latter. Rather, he suggested, both are reflections of an underlying lateral cerebral organization, the nature of which, however, he left unspecified.

Yet regardless of the specific causal relations between V–P patterns and hemisphere dysfunction, the very acceptance of an association between the two may have far-reaching implications. For example, it may be assumed that alcoholics who show the V>P pattern (Miglioli *et al.*, 1979), which is due mainly to poor performance scores (Wechsler, 1941; Teicher and Singer, 1946) suffer, as some have suggested (Jones and Parsons, 1971; Parsons *et al.*, 1972), from a right hemisphere dysfunction.

III. Clinical Evidence

The more recent search for correlations between deviant behavior and hemisphere dysfunction began about a decade ago, when Flor-Henry and Yeudall (Flor-Henry, 1973, 1974; Flor-Henry and Yeudall, 1973), who were looking for a neurological model of psychiatric syndromes, advanced the hypothesis that schizophrenia is associated with left hemisphere dysfunction, whereas affective psychoses are associated with right hemisphere dysfunction. Although still controversial, this hypothesis has received a considerable amount of support (for reviews, see Flor-Henry and Yeudall, 1979; Wexler, 1980; Marin and Tucker, 1981; Merrin, 1981; Newlin *et al.*, 1981). For example, it was found that schizophrenics show the P>V pattern, whereas manic–depressive patients show the reverse, V>P pattern (Flor-Henry, 1976; Gruzelier and Hammond, 1976; Abrams *et al.*, 1981).

Flor-Henry (1973) and Flor-Henry and Yeudall (1973) further hypothesized that psychopathy, like schizophrenia, is associated with left hemisphere dysfunction. This hypothesis was based on Serafetinides' (1965) finding of overt physical aggressiveness in 36 of 100 consecutive temporal lobe epileptics, most of whom had a left temporal lobe focus. These findings were subsequently corroborated by Lishman (1966) and Falconer and Taylor (1970). Similarly, Taylor (1969, 1972) found an association between psychopathy and operations on the left side of the brain.

To investigate the relationship between hemisphere dysfunction and behavior disorders further, Yeudall and associates (see Yeudall and

Fromm-Auch, 1979) have developed a 32-item test battery, which has been administered to subjects of various pathological groups. The results are summarized in Table 15.2, which shows, first, that at least 73% (in most cases, over 85%) of those in the pathological groups manifested signs of neuropsychological abnormalities. In contrast, a control group of 25 normal subjects showed no abnormal signs.

Furthermore, considering lateralized hemisphere dysfunctions, Table 15.2 shows that predominantly left hemisphere dysfunctions were evi-

TABLE 15.2
Abnormal Neuropsychological Profile Ratings[a]

Group	*N*	Percentage of abnormal profiles	Percentage of lateralized hemisphere dysfunction	
			Left	Right
Psychopaths				
Mixed group	25	76	79	21
Homicide	33	94	68	32
Rape	20	100	75	25
Physical assault	37	89	70	30
Alcoholics	30	97	66	34
Alcoholics with personality disorders (nonaffective)	67	100	66	34
Alcoholics with affective psychiatric disorders	37	86	29	71
Male violent criminals	75	89	72	28
Depressive psychiatric patients	25	88	0	100
Individuals with personality disorders, affective	25	92	35	65
Mentally handicapped adults with behavioral disorders	46	100	85	15
Sex offenders	24	96	70	30
Female violent criminals	11	73	50	50
Male adolescents with severe conduct disturbances	28	93	73	27
Female adolescents with conduct disturbances	26	80	52	48
Male juvenile delinquents				
Violent	23	78	44	56
Nonviolent	41	85	46	54
Female juvenile delinquents				
Violent	14	86	34	66
Nonviolent	21	86	28	72
Controls				
Juvenile delinquents	46	11	50	50
Individuals with learning disabilities	65	14	50	50

[a] Adapted from Yeudall and Fromm-Auch (1979).

dent among psychopaths, alcoholics with personality disorders, male adolescents with severe conduct disturbances, mentally handicapped adults with behavioral disorders, sex offenders, and male violent criminals. Predominantly right hemisphere dysfunctions were evident among depressive patients, patients with affective personality disorders, female juvenile delinquents, and alcoholics with affective disorders. Finally, no lateralized dysfunctions were found among male juvenile delinquents, female adolescents with conduct disturbances, female violent criminals, and control subjects.

It thus appears that psychopathic, violent behavior is associated with left hemisphere dysfunctions, whereas affective disorders are associated with right hemisphere dysfunctions. This conclusion was corroborated by a study of 98 violent criminals and 99 persistent, but nonviolent criminals (Yeudall, 1979), which revealed that, among the subjects showing neuropsychological impairments, 72% of the violent criminals had left hemisphere dysfunctions, whereas 79% of the nonviolent criminals had right hemisphere dysfunctions. These findings are in line with Yeudall and Wardell's (1978) report of poorer performance on verbal tests (greater $P > V$ pattern) among violent than among nonviolent recidivist criminals.

Corroborating electroencephalographic (EEG) data were provided by Yeudall and Wardell (1978), who took EEG measurements of their violent and nonviolent subjects while performing various tasks. Power spectral analyses of their data showed that, during the processing of verbal stimuli, the violent subjects failed to show the normal activation pattern, particularly in the frontal and temporal regions of the left hemisphere. They also had significantly more α frequencies in the left parietal regions when the eyes were closed, and significantly more power in the α and β frequencies during the processing of the verbal stimuli, indicating a dysfunction of the left hemisphere. Overall, the electrophysiological data showed that 91% of the violent criminals had significant signs of neurological impairment, 73% of whom with greater deficits in the left than in the right hemisphere.

An interesting finding that emerged from this series of studies is the difference between adult criminals and juvenile delinquents. Whereas the former had predominantly left hemisphere dysfunctions, the latter had predominantly right hemisphere dysfunctions (among males this tendency was not significant). These findings were corroborated by Yeudall (1979) in a study of 99 juvenile delinquents. The subjects showed a rate of neuropsychological impairment (84%) similar to that of adult psychopaths but, in contrast to their adult counterparts, 60% of the impairments were associated with right rather than left hemisphere dysfunctions. This rate was similar to that found among criminals with affective disturbances and among nonviolent offenders. The juvenile delinquents' records, in fact, showed that more than 90% of them had committed nonviolent crimes. Moreover, examination of the violent juveniles showed that they suffered from depression, which is associated with right hemisphere dysfunction (Yeudall *et al.*, 1982).

To the extent that juvenile delinquency is characterized by impulsive behavior, these data are in line with McIntyre *et al.*'s (1976) finding of an association between right hemisphere dysfunction and impulsiveness. Furthermore, the idea that juvenile and adult criminality are differentially associated with unilateral right and left hemisphere dysfunctions, respectively, is in line with similar findings among schizophrenics, who show signs of right hemisphere dysfunction in childhood and of left hemisphere dysfunction in adulthood (Venables, 1980). However, the finding that schizophrenics and criminals who have right hemisphere dysfunctions when they are young might have left hemisphere dysfunctions when they are adults seems to imply that schizophrenic children and juvenile delinquents who grow up to become adult schizophrenics and criminals may undergo a lateral shift of hemisphere dysfunction from left to right. This means that at a certain time the hitherto functioning left hemisphere begins to dysfunction, and at the same time the dysfunctioning right hemisphere recovers.

This hypothesis may make sense, however, as long as cortical dysfunctions do not imply underlying structural damage, as maintained by Venables (1980), because if hemisphere dysfunctions are correlated with structural deficits, as has been suggested (Ratcliffe *et al.*, 1980; Golden *et al.*, 1981) this hypothesis would imply a shift of a structural deficit as a function of age, a highly unlikely event. The "shift hypothesis" therefore requires further clarification before it can be seriously considered.

IV. Experimental Evidence

A. Electrodermal Responsivity

Abnormal electrodermal lateral asymmetries among psychotics have been used as indices of unilateral hemisphere dysfunctions. In line with other indices, electrodermal data have consistently shown that schizophrenia and depression are differentially associated with left and right hemisphere dysfunctions, respectively (for review, see Gruzelier, 1979).

The single attempt so far to study lateral asymmetries in electrodermal responses among psychopaths was made by Hare (1978). Delivering 1000-Hz tones to 69 inmates, he found that psychopaths gave larger electrodermal responses in their left hand when the rise time of the tones was slow, whereas the nonpsychopaths gave larger responses in the same hand when the rise time was fast. This finding was left uninterpreted.

In addition, Hare (1978) found that psychopaths showed slower electrodermal recovery time than nonpsychopaths to more intense tones, but only in the left hand and when the stimulus rise time was fast. This finding corroborates Venables's (1976, cited in Hare, 1978) data showing that children with criminal or psychopathic parents have longer electrodermal recovery times than normal children, but only in the left hand.

The consistency of electrodermal data notwithstanding, their interpretation is problematic. That is because Gruzelier (1973, 1978) and Gruzelier and Venables (1974) have argued that, unlike the cortical control of other lateral responses, cortical control of electrodermal responses is ipsilateral rather than contralateral. This argument is based on two studies implying the existence of ipsilateral pathways for electrodermal responsivity: Luria and Homskaya's (1963) report of a patient suffering from a left frontal tumor who failed to show phasic responses to incidental stimuli in the left hand and Sourek's (1965) finding of postoperative reduction in electrodermal responsivity in the extremities ipsilateral to the side of the operation.

If, indeed, cortical control of electrodermal activity is ipsilateral, Hare's (1978) data seem to show a left hemisphere dysfunction in psychopaths, since nonresponding on the left hand may indicate a reduction of left side influences (Gruzelier, 1978). Sourek (1965) himself, however, was the first to note that his data were amenable to an alternative interpretation in terms of a contralateral increase (rather than an ipsilateral decrease) in electrodermal responsivity, which is caused, in turn, by the loss of inhibitory effects of the operated (ipsilateral) hemisphere. Thus, as Gruzelier (1979) pointed out, reduced responsivity on the hand ipsilateral to a lesion could reflect either reduced excitation mediated ipsilaterally or reduced inhibition mediated contralaterally or the coexistence of both possibilities.

Accumulating evidence shows that electrodermal activity is controlled contralaterally (Holloway and Parsons, 1969; Dawson *et al.*, 1977; Myslobodsky and Horesh, 1978; La Croix and Comper, 1979; Smith *et al.*, 1980). For example, Myslobodsky and Horesh (1978) and Smith *et al.* (1980) interpreted higher and lower electrodermal responsivity on a given hand as indicating greater excitation and inhibition, respectively, in the contralateral hemisphere. Finally, even one of the proponents of the "ipsilateral control" hypothesis has admitted that "the views previously expressed concerning the ipsilaterality of electrodermal mechanisms are probably incorrect, and, in line with general data on pathways in the nervous system, contralaterality of connections is probably the correct view to adopt [Venables, 1980, p. 251]."

Hence, Hare's (1978) findings do not lend support to the notion that psychopathy is associated with left hemisphere dysfunction. Since lateral electrodermal asymmetries were obtained in Hare's (1978) experiment under very specific conditions, more data are needed before any conclusion can be reached concerning the relationship between these asymmetries and hemisphere dysfunctions in psychopaths.

In accumulating electrodermal data, one should be aware of some serious methodological considerations, which may have a bearing on the interpretation of the data. In particular, one should be aware of the need to distinguish between signal and nonsignal stimuli, between specific and nonspecific responses, and between phasic and background electrodermal activities (Gruzelier, 1979).

B. Visual Field Differences

Visual field differences in stimulus identification are customarily associated with hemispheric asymmetry, since stimuli projected to either the left or the right visual field are processed in the contralateral hemisphere (for review, see White, 1969). Hence, verbal material, which is normally processed in the left hemisphere, is better recognized from the right visual field, whereas spatial material, which is normally processed in the right hemisphere, is better recognized from the left visual field (White, 1969). Deviation from this pattern may thus indicate hemisphere dysfunction. For example, the finding that schizophrenics identify both verbal and spatial stimuli better from the right than from the left visual field was attributed by Gur (1978) to a left hemisphere dysfunction.

Testing groups of psychopaths and nonpsychopath controls, Hare (1979) presented his subjects with three-letter words, which were projected to either the left or the right visual field. A variety of scoring criteria and analyses failed to reveal any group differences in right visual field superiority for stimulus identification. However, when this study was later replicated with stimuli that required more complex semantic processing (Hare and Frazelle, 1981), psychopaths failed to show a visual field superiority effect.

This finding, together with a similar finding from a dichotic listening study (no ear superiority for psychopaths), may indicate, according to Hare and Frazelle (1981), that psychopaths suffer from a lack of hemispheric lateralization rather than from a left hemisphere dysfunction. However, an alternative interpretation could conceivably be that the nonlateralized performance was due to a decrease in the right visual field superiority as a function of a left hemisphere dysfunction. Further experimentation is clearly needed before any association between patterns of visual field identifications and psychopathy can be established.

C. Lateral Preferences

An outstanding feature of human paired parts is their functional asymmetry. Testing 962 subjects, Porac *et al.* (1980a) found that most people show right (as opposed to left) hand (92.3%), eye (71.0%), and foot preferences (90.5%). More recently, examining data of 7364 subjects, Nachshon *et al.* (1983) found similar figures (except for eye preference; the right eye was preferred over the left by only about 55% of the subjects).

However, in certain pathological conditions associated with left hemisphere dysfunction, such as schizophrenia, epilepsy, mental retardation, and dyslexia, increased rates of left side preferences usually appear (Hécaen and Ajuriaguerra, 1964; Wold, 1968; Walker and Birch, 1970; Oddy and Lobstein, 1972; Satz, 1972, 1973, 1979; Dvirskii, 1976; Lishman and McMeekan, 1976; Boklage, 1977; Colby and Parkinson, 1977; Gur, 1977; Flor-Henry, 1979; Luchins *et al.,* 1980). In particular, it was suggested that whenever a left hand preference is not congruent with the direction of other lateral preferences, it might be due to the effects of birth stress rather than to heredity (Gur and Gur, 1974). This suggestion is based on Satz's model (Satz, 1972, 1973, 1979; Silva and Satz, 1979), which postulates that early damage to a given hemisphere can result in a reduced function of the contralateral hand. If that is the preferred hand, the person may then switch preferences and become a "pathological left hander" or a "pathological right hander." Since natural (genetic) left-handedness is less frequent than natural right-handedness, the absolute number of left handers becoming pathological right handers following brain damage to the right hemisphere is smaller than the number of natural right handers becoming pathological left handers following damage to the left hemisphere. Assuming that brain damage is about equally distributed between the two hemispheres, the relatively large number of pathological left handers in a brain-damaged population can increase the rate of manifest left-handedness considerably.

This model, originally conceived to explain left-handedness, can also be applied to the other lateral preferences (Porac and Coren, 1976; Levy and Gur, 1980). Hence, a high incidence of any left side preference may indicate left hemisphere damage.

Given that a high incidence of left side preference among schizophrenics are related to left hemisphere dysfunctions (Gur, 1977) and assuming that psychopathy and related behavioral disorders share common etiological factors with schizophrenia (Flor-Henry, 1974, 1976), it is reasonable to expect a high incidence of left side preference among psychopaths and subjects with behavior disorders as well.

In 1963 Palmer found that undifferentiated handedness was associated with maladjustment. More recently, Fitzhugh (1973) found that 32% of a group of juvenile delinquents were left handed. Using writing as a criterion for hand preference, Andrew (1978a) found that 13 of 70 (18.6%) male offenders, preferred the left over the right hand. However, in another study she found (Andrew, 1980) that left-handed offenders were less violent than right-handed offenders. More recently, Wardell and Yeudall (1980) found that, among psychopaths in whom left hemisphere dysfunctions were established by both neuropsychological tests and psychophysiological measurements, 14% were left handers.

Considering lateral eye and foot preferences as well as hand preference, Krynicki (1978) found that assaultive patients, who performed poorly on a short-term memory test—an indication of left hemisphere dysfunction—were ambidextrous in all three preferences, to an extent similar to that previously established for psychiatric patients (Walker and Birch, 1970; Lishman and McMeekan, 1976). However, Hare (1979) failed to find differences between psychopaths and nonpsychopaths in handedness and in an overall index of lateral preference (hand, eye, and foot).

In an attempt to correlate measurements of lateral preferences (taken in 1972) with delinquent behavior (ascertained in 1978), Gabrielli and Mednick (1980) found that delinquents showed significant left preferences of hand and foot, but not of eye. For example, considering hand preference, 64.7% of the left handers but only 29.5% of the right handers had been arrested at least once. Furthermore, among offenders committing multiple crimes, 33% were left handers; among offenders committing single crimes, 11% were left handers; and among nonoffender controls, only 7% were left handers. Finally, Gabrielli and Mednick (1980) argued that thefts and traffic offenses could be predicted from similar patterns of hand preference.

In line with the interpretation of similar patterns of lateral preferences found in schizophrenics (Gur, 1977), Gabrielli and Mednick (1980) interpreted their findings as showing an association of left hand and foot preferences with left hemisphere dysfunctions among delinquents. Eye preference was not similarly associated with hemisphere functions, since, given bilateral control of each eye by the two hemispheres, it was believed that there is no reason for assuming a hemisphere–eye relationship (Porac and Coren, 1976).

Different findings, however, were reported by Nachshon and Denno (1983). They also correlated measurements of lateral preferences (taken between 1959 and 1962) with patterns of criminal behavior (ascertained in 1981). However, instead of recording the number of arrests, as did Gabrielli and Mednick (1980), they used offense type as the dependent variable. Their sample included 1066 subjects, 313 of whom were juvenile delinquents with police contacts for one or more of the following offenses: violent crimes, acts of vandalism, thefts, and nonindex offenses. The other 753 subjects were nonoffender controls. Data analysis showed no significant group differences in incidence of right preferences for hand and foot—the distributions resembled those obtained on a sample of over 7000 subjects (Nachshon *et al.*, 1983)—but showed significant intergroup differences for eye preference. Except for the very violent subjects (murderers, rapists, and very assaultive people) and the vandals (people convicted for causing property damage without personal injury), all groups were divided between about 60% of the subjects who showed right eye preference and about 40% who showed left eye preference. The very violent subjects showed exactly the reverse pattern of eye preference (60% left and 40% right), whereas 76.5% of the vandals showed right eye preference, and only 23.5% showed left eye preference. Distribution of eye preference among the vandals resembles that (71.0%) obtained by Porac *et al.* (1980a) and may therefore be considered within the normal range. However, the high incidence of left eye preference among the very violent subjects may indicate a left hemisphere dysfunction and thus support Yeudall's (1979) finding of a left hemisphere dysfunction among violent as opposed to nonviolent criminals.

This conclusion makes sense, of course, provided that eye preference is related to cerebral dominance. Recall that Porac and Coren (1976) concluded that there is no anatomical basis for a hemisphere–eye association. New electrophysiological data seem to imply, however, that a hemisphere–eye association may exist, since there is hemispheric control of the contralateral eye (Seyal *et al.*, 1981). Seyal and associates were able to record (from three locations) higher amplitudes from the dominant than from the nondominant eye in right-eye-dominant subjects. A similar trend was also observed in the left-eye-dominant subjects but in only one of the three recording locations (amplitude asymmetry was not related to handedness). Seyal and associates (1981) interpreted these findings as providing electrophysiological evidence for eye lateralization in the nervous system, since "a demonstration of asymmetry in visual evoked potentials, obtained by stimulating the dominant or non-dominant eye, would imply the presence of a morphological or physiological substrate in the visual cortex that generates the asymmetric response [p. 424]."

These as well as other findings support the conclusion that eye preference may be at least partially related to laterality (Gur, 1977; Porac *et al.*, 1980b; Nachshon *et al.*, 1983). Therefore, the different lateral preferences are expected to correspond to each other, but only partially, either because they measure different aspects of laterality (Gur, 1977) or because they are differentially affected by environmental stimuli (Nachshon *et al.*, 1983). As Nachshon *et al.* (1983) found, that is indeed the case. It is therefore conceivable that under various conditions different patterns of lateral preference would appear. Gabrielli and Mednick's (1980) study differs from that of Nachshon and Denno (1983) in terms of subjects' characteristics, lateral measures, delinquency records, scoring criteria, and data analyses. All these might have contributed to the differences between the results of the two studies. Taken together, however, the two studies show that certain features of criminal behavior may be associated with left hemisphere dysfunction, as indicated by specific patterns of lateral preferences. More research is needed, however, to delineate the intricacies of these associations, in particular the relations between different patterns of lateral preferences and specific types, or extent, of criminal behavior.

V. Summary and Conclusions

The systematic study of the relationship between psychopathological manifestations and hemisphere dysfunction began about a decade ago with Flor-Henry's (1973) and Flor-Henry and Yeudall's (1973) pioneering work in this area. It is noticeable that one of the first two articles (Flor-Henry, 1973) was concerned with "*psychiatric syndromes* considered as manifestations of lateralized temporal–limbic dysfunction [emphasis mine]," whereas the other article (Flor-Henry and Yeudall, 1973) was concerned with "lateralized cerebral dysfunction in depression and in *aggressive criminal psychopathy* [emphasis mine]." Yet, whereas psychotic disorders have gained considerable attention in this respect (for reviews, see Wexler, 1980; Marin and Tucker, 1981; Merrin, 1981; Newlin *et al.*, 1981), there has been a paucity of research on psychopathy and behavior disorders.

This chapter is an attempt to describe the state of the art concerning the relationship between hemisphere dysfunction and psychopathy and behavior disorders. Flor-Henry's and Yeudall's speculations are based, in part, on earlier attempts to infer dysfunctions of the left hemisphere in subjects with behavior disorders from their patterns of performance on the WAIS. In particular, it has been found that higher scores on the performance relative to the verbal subscales (the P>V pattern), an index of left hemisphere dysfunction, are characteristic of various delinquent and criminal groups. Claims that the P>V pattern can be attributed to learning difficulties have been refuted, and so it seems that this pattern, a frequent concomitant of schizophrenia as well as psychopathy and behavior disturbances, may indicate an association between these disorders and left hemisphere dysfunction.

Clinical evidence has been marshaled by Yeudall and associates (see Yeudall and Fromm-Auch, 1979). A battery of 32 neuropsychological tests was employed, sometimes in conjunction with electrophysiological measures, to find neuropsychological dysfunctions in hundreds of psychiatric patients, psychopaths, and subjects with behavior disorders, as well as in normal controls. In most cases over 85% of those in the pathological groups showed signs of neuropsychological abnormalities. These signs were lateralized in the left hemisphere among violent subjects and in the right hemisphere among subjects showing affective disorders, such as juvenile delinquents. A possible implication of these findings is that some juvenile delinquents who later become adult criminals undergo a shift of hemisphere dysfunction from right to left, a highly improbable event, considering that behavioral dysfunctions may be correlated with structural damages (Ratcliff *et al.*, 1980; Golden *et al.*, 1981).

Beyond that, one wonders to what extent Yeudall *et al.*'s findings can be generalized, since their samples consisted of clinical patients, most of whom suffered from neuropsychological abnormalities. Possibly, different data would be obtained from nonclinical populations (see Hare, 1979, 1981). However, experimental evidence from nonclinical populations is scarce and so far somewhat inconsistent. Electrodermal and visual field studies failed to support the hypothesis that psychopathy is associated with left hemisphere dysfunction (Hare, 1978, 1979). Two studies (Gabrielli and Mednick, 1980; Nachshon and Denno, 1983) apparently demonstrated a relationship between lateral preferences and behavior disorders, but the specific patterns of lateral preferences differed in the two studies. It therefore seems that, whereas theoretical considerations, related findings, and clinical evidence may support the notion that behavior disturbances, like psychotic disorders, are associated with unilateral hemisphere dysfunctions, this association requires further experimental support.

Finally, two authors (Yeudall, 1977; Schalling, 1978) have presumably found signs of interhemispheric disconnection, rather than of intrahemisphere dysfunction, among psychopaths. Since similar arguments have been raised with regard to the cause of psychotic disorders (for review, see Newlin *et al.*, 1981; Mintz *et al.*, 1982; see also Chapter 14), this hypothesis seems to warrant further consideration by students of deviant behavior.

VI. Theoretical Speculations and Applications

As pointed out in Section I a pivotal point in the Lombrosian phrenological approach was that cranial abnormalities indicate underlying brain abnormalities. Hence, abnormal asymmetries in the skull imply similar asymmetries in the brain. With the fall of phrenology this idea was discarded. However, new evidence (LeMay, 1977) seems to show a relationship between the shape of the brain and the shape of the skull. If this finding is corroborated, one may wonder to what extent hemisphere dysfunctions, which are apparently correlated with structural deficits (Ratcliff *et al.*, 1980; Golden *et al.*, 1981) are reflected in corresponding abnormal asymmetries in the skull. Such a correspondence would imply, as Boring (1957) and LeMay (1977) have pointed out, that phrenological notions of localization of function were wrong in details but not in principle.

To many researchers this suggestion would certainly seem to be neo-Lombrosianism, since it allegedly implies that a person may be "born criminal" (see Moran, 1978; Jeffrey, 1979). When a related issue concerning the association between genetic factors and criminal behavior arose, Wolfgang (1975) took pains to show that "crime is not in our genes [p. 461]." Therefore, in line with many others (Bach-y-Rita, 1975; Moyer, 1976; Christiansen, 1977; Yeudall, 1977; Jeffrey, 1978; Addad, 1980; Yeudall *et al.*, 1981, 1982; Nachshon, 1982), it must be reemphasized that, by itself, no biological factor, normal or abnormal, predetermines behavior. Rather, overt behavior is a product of interacting biological and environmental factors.

The most intriguing problem is therefore not the existence, but the nature, of the biosocial interaction. In this respect views differ widely. Some suggest that biological factors have a major effect on the behavior of those 6.3% or so of a given birth cohort who, according to Wolfgang and associates (1972; Wolfgang, 1975), commit 52% of all offenses leading to a police record (Mark and Ervin, 1970; Monroe *et al.*, 1977; Yeudall, 1980; Yeudall *et al.*, 1982). Others consider the interaction of biological factors with socioeconomic status. Contradictory conclusions have been reached, however, by authors who attribute a relatively larger role to biological factors in affecting criminal behavior among members of high (Christiansen, 1977; Mednick, 1980) or of low (Yeudall, 1977; Yeudall *et al.*, 1981) socioeconomic status. In spite of the differences, however, these authors agree that biological factors explain behaviors that are difficult to account for by social factors. In formulating this idea somewhat differently, Yeudall (1979) suggested that, in accounting for criminal behavior, biological factors must first be ruled out before psychosocial factors are considered.

Clearly, then, to the extent that hemisphere dysfunction affects violent behavior, it is (*a*) never the sole factor; (*b*) a major factor in accounting for the behavior of only a few, recidivist violent people; and (*c*) a factor affecting "impulsive" (innate) but not "instrumental" (learned) aggression (see Moyer, 1980). For these people control of aggressive behavior may be best achieved by medical means (Monroe *et al.*, 1977), perhaps along the lines suggested by Yeudall and associates (Yeudall *et al.*, 1981).

Finally, the basic question of why hemisphere dysfunctions should be associated at all with behavior disorders ought to be addressed. So far this problem has not been thoroughly discussed in the literature, and therefore only guidelines for a tentative solution can be offered. Considering the right hemisphere first, it may be speculated that, since it normally mediates emotional behavior (Carmon and Nachshon, 1973; Schwartz *et al.*, 1975; Ley and Bryden, 1981), when it malfunctions it may bring about mood disturbances (for reviews, see Flor-Henry, 1976; Ley, 1979; Flor-

Henry and Yeudall, 1979; Gainotti, 1979), some of which might lead to disorderly behavior (Yeudall, 1980). More specifically, the right hemisphere, by virtue of its undifferentiated, diffuse mode of orienting responses (for review see Myslobodsky and Rattok, 1977 and Chapter 10), is suitable for mediating "fight or flight" reactions. Aggressive behavior may therefore result from an inappropriate control of these reactions due to a malfunctioning right hemisphere.

In contrast, the left hemisphere is distinguished by a differentiated, stimulus-specific mode of orienting responses (Myslobodsky and Rattok, 1977). Under threatening conditions a malfunctioning left hemisphere might cope with the stimuli in an inappropriate manner, for example, by facilitating aggressive responses. If this speculation is correct, it follows that aggression resulting from a left hemisphere dysfunction is qualitatively different from that resulting from a right hemisphere dysfunction. Whereas the former constitutes an inappropriate goal-directed response, the latter constitutes an impulsive emotional outburst. As speculated earlier, the ill-controlled, left-hemisphere-mediated aggression presumably characterizes the behavior of adult criminals, whereas the impulsive, right-hemisphere-mediated aggression presumably characterizes the behavior of juvenile delinquents.

Evidently, these conclusions are based on the underlying assumption that hemispheric representation is dichotomized between the two hemispheres. However, this assumption has been challenged by authors (Luria, 1966; Bradshaw and Nettleton, 1981; Myslobodsky *et al.*, 1982; see also Chapter 10) who have forcefully argued for a functional continuum or interdependence between the two hemispheres. The data on the relationship between hemisphere dysfunction and behavior disorders, as currently presented in the literature, do not readily lend themselves to reexamination and reinterpretation from these new perspectives. However, if additional findings lend empirical support to the new outlooks, the newly gained insights might critically challenge existing theories of the functioning and dysfunctioning cerebral hemispheres.

References

Abrams, R., Redfield, J., and Taylor, M. A. (1981). Cognitive dysfunction in schizophrenia, affective disorder and organic brain disease. *Br. J. Psychiatry* **139,** 190–194.

Addad, M. (1980). Violence from an integrative point of view. *Crime Soc. Deviance* **8,** 5–24 (in Hebrew).

Altus, W. D., and Clarke, J. H. (1949). Subtest variation of the Wechsler–Bellevue for two institutionalized behavior problem groups. *J. Consult. Psychol.* **13,** 444–447.

Anderson, A. L. (1951). The effect of laterality localization of focal brain lesions on the Wechsler–Bellevue subtests. *J. Clin. Psychol.* **7,** 149–153.

Andrew, J. M. (1974a). Delinquency, the Wechsler P > V sign, and the I-level system. *J. Clin. Psychol.* **30,** 331–335.

Andrew, J. M. (1974b). Immaturity, delinquency and the Wechsler P>V sign. *J. Abnorm. Child Psychol.* **2,** 245–251.

Andrew, J. M. (1978a). Laterality on the tapping test among legal offenders. *J. Clin. Child Psychol.* **7,** 149–150.

Andrew, J. M. (1978b). The classic Wechsler P>V sign and violent crime. *Crime Justice* **6,** 246–248.

Andrew, J. M. (1980). Are left handers less violent? *J. Youth Adolescence* **9,** 1–10.

Atkinson, J., and Egeth, H. (1973). Right hemisphere superiority in visual orientation matching. *Can. J. Psychol.* **27,** 152–158.

Bach-y-Rita, G. (1975). Biological basis of aggressive behavior: Clinical aspects. *In* "Human Behavior and Brain Function" (H. J. Widroe, ed.), pp. 24–35. Charles C Thomas, Springfield, Illinois.

Balthazar, E. E., and Morrison, D. H. (1961). The use of Wechsler intelligence scales as diagnostic indicators of predominant left–right and intermediate unilateral brain damage. *J. Clin. Psychol.* **17,** 161–165.

Bernstein, R., and Corsini, R. J. (1953). Wechsler–Bellevue patterns of female delinquents. *J. Clin. Psychol.* **9,** 176–179.

Blank, L. (1958). The intellectual functioning of delinquents. *J. Soc. Psychol.* **47,** 9–14.

Boklage, C. E. (1977). Schizophrenia, brain asymmetry development, and twinning: Cellular relationship with etiological and possible prognostic implications. *Biol. Psychiatry* **12,** 19–35.

Boring, E. G. (1957). "A History of Experimental Psychology." Appleton, New York.

Bradshaw, J. L., and Nettleton, N. C. (1981). The nature of hemispheric specialization in man. *Behav. Brain Sci.* **4,** 51–91.

Bradshaw, J. L., Nettleton, N. C., and Taylor, M. J. (1981). Right hemisphere language and cognitive deficit in sinistrals? *Neuropsychologia* **19,** 113–132.

Bryden, M. P. (1976). Response bias and hemispheric differences in dot localization. *Percept. Psychophys.* **19,** 23–28.

Bryden, M. P. (1979). Evidence for sex-related differences in cerebral organization. *In* "Sex-Related Differences in Cognitive Functioning" (M. Wittig and A. C. Peterson, eds.), pp. 121–143. Academic Press, New York.

Camp, B. W. (1966). WISC performance in acting out and delinquent children with and without EEG abnormality. *J. Consult. Psychol.* **30,** 350–353.

Carmon, A., and Nachshon, I. (1973). Ear asymmetry in perception of emotional nonverbal stimuli. *Acta Psychol.* **37,** 351–357.

Christiansen, K. O. (1977). A review of studies of criminality among twins. *In* "Biosocial Bases of Criminal Behavior" (S. A. Mednick and K. O. Christiansen, eds.), pp. 45–88. Gardner Press, New York.

Clarke, J. H., and Moore, J. H. (1950). The relationship of Wechsler–Bellevue patterns to psychiatric diagnosis of army and air force prisoners. *J. Consult. Psychol.* **14,** 493–495.

Colby, K. M., and Parkinson, C. (1977). Handedness in autistic children. *J. Autism Child. Schizophr.* **7,** 3–9.

Corotto, L. V. (1961). The relation of performance to verbal IQ in acting-out juveniles. *J. Psychol. Stud.* **12,** 162–166.

Dawson, M. E., Schell, A. M., and Catania, J. J. (1977). Autonomic correlates of depression and clinical improvement following electroconvulsive shock therapy. *Psychophysiology* **14,** 569–578.

Dennerl, R. D. (1964a). Cognitive deficits and lateral brain dysfunction in temporal lobe epilepsy. *Epilepsia* **5,** 177–191.

Dennerl, R. D. (1964b). Prediction of unilateral brain dysfunction using Wechsler test scores. *J. Consult. Psychol.* **28,** 278–284.

Diller, L. (1952). A comparison of the test performances of delinquent and nondelinquent girls. *J. Genet. Psychol.* **81,** 167–183.

Dvirskii, A. E. (1976). Functional asymmetry of the cerebral hemispheres in clinical types of schizophrenia. *Neurosci. Behav. Physiol.* **7,** 236–239.

Falconer, M. A., and Taylor, D. C. (1970). Temporal lobe epilepsy: Clinical features, pathology diagnosis and treatment. *In* "Modern Trends in Psychological Medicine" (J. H. Price, ed.), pp. 346–373. Butterworth, London.

Fedio, P., and Mirsky, A. F. (1969). Selective intellectual deficits in children with temporal lobe or centrencephalic epilepsy. *Neuropsychologia* **7,** 287–300.

Field, J. G. (1960). The performance–verbal IQ discrepancy in a group of sociopaths. *J. Clin. Psychol.* **16,** 321–322.

Fink, A. E. (1962). "Causes of Crime: Biological Theories in the United States 1800–1915." Barnes, New York. (Originally published, 1938.)

Fitzhugh, K. B. (1973). Some neuropsychological features of delinquent subjects. *Percept. Mot. Skills* **36,** 494.

Fitzhugh, K. B., Fitzhugh, L. C., and Reitan, R. M. (1962). Wechsler–Bellevue comparisons in groups with "chronic" and "current" lateralized and diffuse brain lesions. *J. Consult. Psychol.* **26,** 306–310.

Fitzhugh, L. C., and Fitzhugh, K. B. (1964). Relationship between Wechsler–Bellevue form I and WAIS performances of subjects with longstanding cerebral dysfunction. *Percept. Mot. Skills* **19,** 539–543.

Flor-Henry, P. (1973). Psychiatric syndromes considered as manifestations of lateralized temporal–limbic dysfunction. *In* "Surgical Approaches in Psychiatry" (L. V. Latimer and K. E. Livingston, eds.), pp. 22–26. Med. Tech. Publ. Co. Ltd., Lancaster, England.

Flor-Henry, P. (1974). Psychosis, neurosis and epilepsy: Developmental and gender-related effects, and their etiological contribution. *Br. J. Psychiatry* **124,** 144–150.

Flor-Henry, P. (1976). Lateralized temporal–limbic dysfunction and psychopathology. *Ann. N. Y. Acad. Sci.* **280,** 777–795.

Flor-Henry, P. (1978). Gender, hemispheric specialization and psychopathology. *Soc. Sci. Med.* **123,** 155–162.

Flor-Henry, P. (1979). On certain aspects of the localization of the cerebral systems regulating and determining emotion. *Biol. Psychiatry* **14,** 677–698.

Flor-Henry, P., and Yeudall, L. T. (1973). Lateralized cerebral dysfunction in depression and in aggressive criminal psychopathy: Further observations. *Int. Res. Commun. Syst.* July, p. 31.

Flor-Henry, P., and Yeudall, L. T. (1979). Neuropsychological investigation of schizophrenia and manic–depressive psychoses. *In* "Hemisphere Asymmetries of Function in Psychopathology" (J. H. Gruzelier and P. Flor-Henry, eds.), pp. 341–362. Elsevier/North-Holland, Amsterdam.

Foster, A. L. (1959). A note concerning the intelligence of delinquents. *J. Clin. Psychol.* **15,** 78–79.

Gabrielli, W. F., and Mednick, S. A. (1980). Sinistrality and delinquency. *J. Abnorm. Psychol.* **89,** 654–661.

Gainotti, G. (1979). The relationships between emotions and cerebral dominance: A review of clinical and experimental evidence. *In* "Hemisphere Asymmetries of Function in Psychopathology" (J. H. Gruzelier and P. Flor-Henry, eds.), pp. 21–34. Elsevier/North-Holland, Amsterdam.

Glueck, S., and Glueck, E. (1950). "Unravelling Juvenile Delinquency." Commonwealth Fund, New York.

Golden, C. J., Graber, B., Coffman, J., Berg, R. A., Newlin, D. B., and Bloch, S. (1981). Structural brain deficits in schizophrenia. *Arch. Gen. Psychiatry* **38,** 1014–1017.

Graham, E. E. (1952). Wechsler–Bellevue and WISC scattergrams of unsuccessful readers. *J. Consult. Psychol.* **16,** 268–271.

Graham, E. E., and Kamano, D. (1959). Reading failure as a factor in the WAIS subtest patterns of youthful offenders. *J. Clin. Psychol.* **14,** 302–305.

Gruzelier, J. H. (1973). Bilateral asymmetry of skin conductance orienting activity and levels in schizophrenics. *Biol. Psychol.* **1,** 21–41.

Gruzelier, J. H. (1978). Bimodal states of arousal and lateralized dysfunction in schizophrenia: Effects of chlorpromazine. *In* "The Nature of Schizophrenia" (L. C. Wynne, R. Cromwell, and S. Matthysse, pp. 167–187. Wiley, New York.

Gruzelier, J. H. (1979). Lateral asymmetries in electrodermal activity and psychosis. *In* "Hemisphere Asymmetries of Function in Psychopathology" (J. H. Gruzelier and P. Flor-Henry, eds.), pp. 149–168. Elsevier/North-Holland, Amsterdam.

Gruzelier, J. H., and Hammond, N. (1976). Schizophrenia: A dominant hemisphere temporal–limbic disorder? *Res. Commun. Psychol., Psychiatry Behav.* **1,** 33–72.

Gruzelier, J. H., and Venables, P. H. (1974). Bimodality and lateral asymmetry of skin conductance orienting activity in schizophrenics: Replication and evidence of lateral asymmetry in patients with depression and disorders of personality. *Biol. Psychiatry* **8,** 55–73.

Guertin, W. H., Ladd, C. E., Frank, G. H., Rabin, A. I., and Hiester, D. S. (1966). Research with the Wechsler Intelligence Scale for Adults: 1960–1965. *Psychol. Bull.* **66,** 385–409.

Gur, R. C., and Gur, R. E. (1974). Handedness, sex, and eyedness as moderating variables in the relation between hypnotic susceptibility and functional brain asymmetry. *J. Abnorm. Psychol.* **83,** 635–643.

Gur, R. C., and Gur, R. E. (1980). Handedness and individual differences in hemispheric activation. *In* "Neuropsychology of Left-Handedness" (J. Herron, ed.), pp. 211–232. Academic Press, New York.

Gur, R. E. (1977). Motoric laterality imbalance in schizophrenia: A possible concomitant of left hemisphere dysfunction. *Arch. Gen. Psychiatry* **34,** 33–37.

Gur, R. E. (1978). Left hemisphere dysfunction and left hemisphere overactivation in schizophrenia. *J. Abnorm. Psychol.* **87,** 226–238.

Hare, R. D. (1978). Psychopathy and electrodermal responses to nonsignal stimulation. *Biol. Psychol.* **6,** 237–246.

Hare, R. D. (1979). Psychopathy and laterality of cerebral function. *J. Abnorm. Psychol.* **88,** 605–610.

Hare, R. D. (1981). Psychopathy and violence. *In* "Violence and the Violent Individual" (J. R. Hays, T. K. Roberts, and K. S. Solway, eds.), pp. 53–74. Spectrum Publ., Jamaica, New York.

Hare, R. D., and Frazelle, J. (1981). Psychobiological correlates of criminal psychopathy. Paper presented at a symposium on biosocial correlates of crime and delinquency. *Ann. Meet. Amer. Soc. Crim.*

Harshman, R. A., Remington, R., and Krashen, S. D. (1976). Sex, language and the brain: Adult sex differences in lateralization. *In* "Conference on Human Brain Function" (D. O. Walter, L. Rogers, and J. M. Finzi-Fried, eds.), pp. 27–30. Brain Information Service Publication Office, Los Angeles, California.

Hécaen, H., and Ajuriaguerra, J. (1964). "Left Handedness." Grune & Stratton, New York.

Holloway, F. A., and Parsons, O. A. (1969). Unilateral brain damage and bilateral skin conductance levels in humans. *Psychophysiology* **6,** 138–148.

Hutt, S. J. (1976). Cognitive development and cerebral dysfunction. *In* "The Development of Cognitive Processes" (V. Hamilton and M. D. Vernon, eds.), pp. 591–643. Academic Press, New York.

Jeffrey, C. R. (1978). Criminology as an interdisciplinary behavioral science. *Criminology* **16,** 149–169.

Jeffrey, C. R. (1979). Biology and crime. *In* "Biology and Crime" (C. R. Jeffrey, ed.), pp. 7–18. Sage, Beverly Hills, California.

Jones, B. M., and Parsons, O. A. (1971). Impaired abstracting ability in chronic alcoholics. *Arch. Gen. Psychiatry* **24,** 71–75.

Kahn, M. W. (1968). Superior performance IQ of murderers as a function of overt act or diagnosis. *J. Soc. Psychol.* **76,** 113–116.
Kimura, D. (1967). Functional asymmetry of the brain in dichotic listening. *Cortex* **3,** 163–178.
Kimura, D. (1969). Spatial localization in left and right visual fields. *Can. J. Psychol.,* **23,** 445–448.
Kløve, H. (1959). Relationship of differential electroencephalic patterns to distribution of Wechsler–Bellevue scores. *Neurology* **9,** 871–876.
Krynicki, V. E. (1978). Cerebral dysfunction in repetitively assaultive adolescents. *J. Nerv. Ment. Dis.* **166,** 59–67.
La Croix, J. M., and Comper, P. (1979). Lateralization in the electrodermal system as a function of cognitive/hemispheric manipulations. *Psychophysiology* **16,** 116–129.
Lamb, R. B. (1903). The mind of the criminal. *Proc. Am. Medico-Psychol. Assoc.* **10,** 260, cited in Fink (1962).
LeMay, M. (1977). Asymmetries of the skull and handedness: phrenology revisited. *J. Neurol. Sci.* **32,** 243–253.
Levy, J. (1969). Possible basis for the evolution of lateral specialization of the human brain. *Nature (London)* **224,** 614–615.
Levy, J., and Gur, R. C. (1980). Individual differences in psychoneurological organization. *In* "Neuropsychology of Left-Handedness" (J. Herron, ed.), pp. 199–210. Academic Press, New York.
Levy, J., and Reid, M. (1976). Variations in writing posture and cerebral organization. *Science* **194,** 337–339.
Ley, R. G. (1979). Cerebral asymmetries, emotional experience, and imagery: Implications for psychotherapy. *In* "The Potentials of Fantasy and Imagination" (A. A. Sheikh and J. T. Schaffer, eds.), pp. 41–65. Random House, New York.
Ley, R. G., and Bryden, M. P. (1981). Consciousness, emotion, and the right hemisphere. *In* "Aspects of Consciousness" (G. Underwood and R. Stevens, eds.), Vol. 2, pp. 215–240. Academic Press, New York.
Liberman, A. M. (1974). The specialization of the language hemisphere. *In* "The Neurosciences: Third Study Program" (F. O. Schmidt and F. O. Worden, eds.), pp. 43–56. MIT Press, Cambridge, Massachusetts.
Lishman, W. A. (1966). Brain damage in relation to psychiatric disability after head injury. *Br. J. Psychiatry* **114,** 373–410.
Lishman, W. A., and McMeekan, E. R. L. (1976). Hand preference patterns in psychiatric patients. *Br. J. Psychiatry* **129,** 158–166.
Lombroso, C. (1874). "L'Uomo Delinquente." *Bocca, Torino.*
Luchins, D., Pollin, W., and Wyatt, R. J. (1980). Laterality in monozygotic schizophrenic twins: An alternative hypothesis. *Biol. Psychiatry* **15,** 87–93.
Luria, A. L., and Homskaya, E. G. (1963). Le trouble du role régulateur du langage au cours des lésions du lobe frontal. *Neuropsychologia* **1,** 9–26.
Luria, A. R. (1966). "Higher Cortical Functions in Man." Basic Books, New York.
Lydston, G. F. (1904). "The Disease of Society." Lippincott, Philadelphia, Pennsylvania.
McFie, J. (1961). Intellectual impairment in children with localized postinfantile cerebral lesions. *J. Neurol. Neurosurg. Psychiatry* **24,** 361–365.
McGlone, J. (1977). Sex differences in the cerebral organization of verbal functions in patients with unilateral brain lesions. *Brain* **100,** 775–793.
McGlone, J. (1978). Sex differences in functional brain asymmetry. *Cortex* **14,** 122–128.
McGlone, J. (1980). Sex differences in human brain asymmetry: A critical survey. *Behav. Brain Sci.* **3,** 215–263.
McIntyre, M., Pritchard, P. B., III, and Lombroso, C. T. (1976). Left and right temporal lobe epileptics: A controlled investigation of some psychological differences. *Epilepsia* **17,** 377–386.

Manne, S. H., Kandel, A., and Rosenthal, D. (1962). Differences between performance IQ and verbal IQ in a severely sociopathic population. *J. Clin. Psychol.* **18,** 73–77.

Marin, R. S., and Tucker, G. J. (1981). Psychopathology and hemispheric dysfunction: A review. *J. Nerv. Ment. Dis.* **169,** 546–557.

Mark, V. H. and Ervin, F. R. (1970). "Violence and the Brain." Harper, New York.

Mathews, C. G., and Reitan, R. M. (1964). Correlations of Wechsler–Bellevue rank orders of subtest means in lateralized and non-lateralized brain damaged groups. *Percept. Mot. Skills* **19,** 391–399.

Mednick, S. A. (1980). Human Nature, crime and society: Keynote address. *Ann. N. Y. Acad. Sci.* **347,** 335–348.

Merrin, E. L. (1981). Schizophrenia and brain asymmetry: An evaluation of evidence for dominant lobe dysfunction. *J. Nerv. Ment. Dis.* **169,** 405–416.

Miglioli, M., Buchtel, H. A., Campanini, T., and De Risio, C. (1979). Cerebral hemispheric lateralization of cognitive deficits due to alcoholism. *J. Nerv. Ment. Dis.* **167,** 212–217.

Milner, B. (1958). Psychological effects produced by temporal lobe excision. *Res. Publ.—Assoc. Res. Nerv. Ment. Dis.* **36,** 244–257.

Mintz, M., Tomer, R., and Myslobodsky, M. S. (1982). Neuroleptic-induced lateral asymmetry of visual evoked potentials in schizophrenia. *Biol. Psychiatry* **17,** 815–828.

Monroe, R. R., Hulfish, B., Balis, G., Lion, J., Rubin, J., McDonald, M., and Barick, J. D. (1977). Neurologic findings in recidivist aggressors. *In* "Psychopathology and Brain Dysfunction" (C. Shagass, S. Gershon, and A. J. Friedhoff, eds.), pp. 241–253. Raven Press, New York.

Moran, R. (1978). Biomedical research and the politics of crime control: A historical perspective. *Contemp. Crises* **2,** 335–357.

Moskovitch, M. (1979). Information processing and the cerebral hemispheres. *In* "Handbook of Behavioral Neurobiology" (M. S. Grazzaniga, ed.), Vol. 2, pp. 379–446. Plenum, New York.

Moyer, K. E. (1976). "The Psychobiology of Aggression." Harper, New York.

Moyer, K. E. (1980). Brain mechanisms and crime. *In* "Anatomy of Criminal Justice" (C. H. Foust and D. R. Webster, eds.), pp. 33–52. Lexington Books, Lexington, Kentucky.

Muehl, S., Knott, J. R., and Benton, A. L. (1965). EEG abnormality and psychological test performance in reading disability. *Cortex* **1,** 434–440.

Myslobodsky, M., and Horesh, N. (1978). Bilateral electrodermal activity in depressive patients. *Biol. Psychiatry* **6,** 111–120.

Myslobodsky, M. S., and Rattok, J. (1977). Bilateral electrodermal activity in waking man. *Acta Psychol.* **41,** 273–282.

Myslobodsky, M., Mintz, M., Ben-Mayor, V., and Radwan, H. (1982). Unilateral dopamine deficit and lateral EEG asymmetry: Sleep abnormalities in hemi-Parkinson's patients. *Electroencephalogr. Clin. Neurophysiol.* **54,** 227–231.

Nachshon, I. (1973). Effects of cerebral dominance and attention on dichotic listening. *J. Life Sci.* **3,** 107–114.

Nachshon, I. (1978). Handedness and dichotic listening to nonverbal features of speech. *Percept. Mot. Skills* **48,** 1111–1114.

Nachshon, I. (1982). Toward biosocial approaches in criminology. *J. Soc. Biol. Struc.* **5,** 1–9.

Nachshon, I., and Carmon, A. (1975). Hand preference in sequential and spatial discrimination tasks. *Cortex* **11,** 123–131.

Nachshon, I., and Denno, D. (1983). Violent behavior and hemisphere function. *In* "Biosocial Bases of Antisocial Behavior" (S. A. Mednick, ed.) Kluwer Niejoff, Boston. (in press).

Nachshon, I., Denno, D., and Aurand, S. (1983). Lateral preferences of hand, eye and foot: Relation to cerebral dominance. *Int. J. Neurosci.* **18,** 1–10.

Newlin, D. B., Carpenter, B., and Golden, C. J. (1981). Hemispheric asymmetries in schizophrenia. *Biol. Psychiatry* **16,** 561–582.

Oddy, H. C., and Lobstein, T. J. (1972). Hand and eye dominance in schizophrenia. *Br. J. Psychiatry* **120,** 331–332.

Palmer, R. D. (1963). Hand differentiation and psychological functioning. *J. Personality* **31,** 445–461.

Parsons, O. A., Tarter, R., and Edelberg, R. (1972). Altered motor control in chronic alcoholics. *J. Abnorm. Psychol.* **72,** 308–314.

Parsons, O. A., Vega, A., Jr., and Burn, J. (1969). Different psychological effects of lateralized brain damage. *J. Consult. Clin. Psychol.* **33,** 551–557.

Porac, C., and Coren, S. (1976). The dominant eye. *Psychol. Bull.* **83,** 880–897.

Porac, C., Coren, S., and Duncan, P. (1980a). Life-span age trends in laterality. *J. Gerontol.* **35,** 715–721.

Porac, C., Coren, S., Steiger, J. H., and Duncan, P. (1980b). Human laterality: A multidimensional approach. *Can. J. Psychol.* **34,** 91–96.

Prentice, W., and Kelly, F. J. (1963). Intelligence and delinquency: A reconsideration. *J. Soc. Psychol.* **60,** 327–337.

Ratcliff, G., Dila, C., Taylor, L., and Milner, B. (1980). The morphological asymmetry of the hemispheres and cerebral dominance for speech: A possible relationship. *Brain Lang.* **11,** 87–98.

Reitan, R. M. (1955). Certain differential effects of left and right cerebral lesions in human adults. *J. Comp. Physiol. Psychol.* **48,** 474–477.

Satz, P. (1972). Pathological left handedness: An explanatory model. *Cortex* **8,** 121–135.

Satz, P. (1973). Left handedness and early brain insult: An explanation. *Neuropsychologia* **11,** 115–117.

Satz, P. (1979). Pathological left handedness: Cross-cultural tests of a model. *Neuropsychologia* **17,** 77–81.

Schalling, D. (1978). Psychopathy—A partial interhemispheric disconnection syndrome? A neuropsychological analysis. *Symp. Psychophysiol. Neuropsychol. Psychopathic Antisoc. Behav.*

Schwartz, G. E., Davidson, R. J., and Maer, F. (1975). Right hemisphere lateralization for emotion in the human brain: Interaction with cognition. *Science* **190,** 286–288.

Serafetinides, F. A. (1965). Aggressiveness in temporal lobe epileptics and its relation to cerebral dysfunction and environmental factors. *Epilepsia* **6,** 33–42.

Seyal, M., Sato, S., White, B. G., and Porter, R. J. (1981). Visual evoked potentials and eye dominance. *Electroencephalogr. Clin. Neurophysiol.* **52,** 424–428.

Silva, D. A., and Satz, P. (1979). Pathological left handedness: Evaluation of a model. *Brain Lang.* **7,** 8–16.

Smith, A. (1966a). Certain hypothesized hemispheric differences in language and visual functions in human adults. *Cortex* **2,** 109–126.

Smith, A. (1966b). Verbal and nonverbal test performances on patients with "acute" lateralized brain lesions (tumors). *J. Nerv. Ment. Dis.* **141,** 517–523.

Smith, B. D., Ketterer, M. W., and Concannon, M. (1980). Hemispheric variables in bilateral electrodermal activity. *Psychophysiology* **17,** 305.

Sourek, K. (1965). "The Nervous Control of Skin Potential in Man." Nakladatelstvi Ceskoslovenska Akademic Ved., Prague. (cited in Gruzelier, 1973.)

Talbot, E. S. (1898). A study of the stigmata of degeneracy among the American criminal Youth. *JAMA, J. Am. Med. Assoc.* **30,** 849–856.

Taylor, D. C. (1969). Aggression and epilepsy. *J. Psychosom. Res.* **13,** 229–236.

Taylor, D. C. (1972). Mental state and temporal lobe epilepsy: A correlative account of 100 patients treated surgically. *Epilepsia* **13,** 727–765.

Teicher, M., and Singer, E. (1946). A report on the use of the Wechsler–Bellevue scale in an overseas general population. *Am. J. Psychiatry* **103,** 91–93.

Telegdy, G. A. (1973). The relationship between sociometric status and patterns of WISC scores in children with learning disabilities. *Psychol. in Sch.* **10,** 426–430.

Uzzell, B. P., Zimmerman, R. A., Dolinskas, C. A., and Obrist, W. D. (1979). Lateralized psychological impairment associated with CT lesions in head injured patients. *Cortex* **15,** 391–401.

Vane, J. R., and Eisen, V. W. (1954). Wechsler–Bellevue performance of delinquent and non-delinquent girls. *J. Consult. Psychol.* **18,** 221–225.

Venables, P. H. (1980). Primary dysfunction and cortical lateralization in schizophrenia. *In* "Functional States of the Brain: Their Determinants" (M. Koukkou, D. Lehmann, and J. Angst, eds.), pp. 243–264. Elsevier/North-Holland Biomedical Press, Amsterdam.

Vold, G. B. (1979). "Theoretical Criminology" (2nd ed. prepared by T. J. Bernard). Oxford Univ. Press, New York (Originally published in 1958.)

Walker, H. A., and Birch, H. G. (1970). Lateral preference and right–left awareness in schizophrenic children. *J. Nerv. Ment. Dis.* **151,** 341–351.

Wardell, D., and Yeudall, L. T. (1980). A multidimensional approach to criminal disorders: The assessment of impulsivity and its relation to crime. *Adv. Behav. Res. Ther.* **2,** 159–177.

Wechsler, D. (1941). The effects of alcohol on mental activity. *Q. J. Study Alcohol* **2,** 479–485.

Wechsler, D. (1958). "The Measurement and Appraisal of Adult Intelligence," 4th ed. Williams & Wilkins, Baltimore, Maryland (1st ed., 1939).

Wexler, B. E. (1980). Cerebral laterality and psychiatry: A review of the literature. *Am. J. Psychiatry* **137,** 279–291.

White, M. (1969). Laterality differences in perception: A review. *Psychol. Bull.* **72,** 387–405.

Wiens, A. N., Matarazzo, J. D., and Gver, R. D. (1959). Performance and verbal IQ in a group of sociopaths. *J. Clin. Psychol.* **15,** 191–193.

Witelson, S. F. (1980). Neuroanatomical asymmetry of left handers: A review and implications for functional asymmetry. *In* "Neuropsychology of Left Handedness" (J. Herron, ed.), pp. 79–114. Academic Press, New York.

Wold, R. M. (1968). Dominance—fact or fantasy: Its significance in learning disabilities. *J. Am. Optom. Assoc.* **39,** 908–916.

Wolfgang, M. E. (1975). Delinquency and violence from the viewpoint of criminology. *In* "Neural Bases of Violence and Aggression" (W. S. Field and W. A. Sweet, eds.), pp. 456–489. Warren H. Green, St. Louis, Missouri.

Wolfgang, M. E., Figlio, R. M., and Sellin, T. (1972). "Delinquency in a Birth Cohort." Univ. of Chicago Press, Chicago, Illinois.

Woods, B. T. (1980). The restricted effects of right-hemisphere lesions after age one: Wechsler test data. *Neuropsychologia* **18,** 65–70.

Woods, B. T., and Teuber, H.-L. (1973). Early onset of complementary specialization of cerebral hemispheres in man. *Trans. Am. Neurol. Assoc.* **98,** 113–117.

Yeudall, L. T. (1977). Neuropsychological assessment of forensic disorders. *Can. Ment. Health* **25,** 7–16.

Yeudall, L. T. (1979). Neuropsychological concomitants of persistent criminal behavior. *Annu. Meet. Ont. Psychol. Assoc.*

Yeudall, L. T. (1980). A neuropsychological perspective of persistent juvenile delinquency and criminal behavior: Discussion. *Ann. N. Y. Acad. Sci.* **347,** 349–355.

Yeudall, L. T., and Fromm-Auch, D. (1979). Neuropsychological impairments in various psychopathological populations. *In* "Hemisphere Asymmetries of Function in Psychopathology" (J. H. Gruzelier and P. Flor-Henry, eds.), pp. 401–428. Elsevier/North-Holland, Amsterdam.

Yeudall, L. T., and Wardell, D. M. (1978). Neuropsychological correlates of criminal psychopathy. Part II. Discrimination and prediction of dangerous and recidivistic offenders. *In* "Human Aggression and its Dangerousness" (L. Beliveau, C. Canepa, and

D. Szabo, eds.), Pinel Institute, Montreal.

Yeudall, L. T., Fedora, O., Fedora, S., and Wardell, D. (1981). Neurosocial perspective on the assessment and etiology of persistent criminality. *Aust. J. Forensic Sci.* **13,** 131–159, **14,** 20–44.

Yeudall, L. T., Fromm-Auch, D., and Davies, P. (1982). Neuropsychological impairment in persistent delinquency. *J. Nerv. Ment. Dis.* **170,** 257–265.

Zurif, E. B., and Carson, G. (1970). Dyslexia in relation to cerebral dominance and temporal analysis. *Neuropsychologia* **8,** 351–361.

16: Psychogenic Somatic Symptoms on the Left Side: Review and Interpretation

DONNEL B. STERN

Department of Psychology
City College of the City University of New York
New York, New York

I. Introduction 415
II. Evidence for Symptom Lateralization 416
A. Clinical Observations, 1859 to the Present 416
B. Early Research Findings 417
C. Galin's [1974] Hypothesis 423
D. Recent Research Findings 423
E. Overview of the Data 426
III. Explanations for Symptom Lateralization 428
A. Alternatives to Hemispheric Specialization 428
B. Hemispheric Specialization and Symptom Lateralization 432
References 441

I. Introduction

In the past few years a number of investigators have reported that psychogenic somatic symptoms occur with a higher frequency on the left side of the body than on the right (Section II, D). It is less widely known that there also exists a substantial body of early literature, including both clinical impressions (Section II, A) and quantitative observations (Section II, B), documenting the same phenomenon. This chapter is, in part, a review of all these findings, including methodologies and statistical evaluations. In the case of the early reports the aim is to make a relatively obscure literature more widely known. Taken as a whole, the data establish the finding on a firmer level of certainty than is usually the case for generalizations regarding psychiatric symptoms. In Section III explanatory hypotheses are considered. The finding that psychogenic somatic

HEMISYNDROMES:
Psychobiology, Neurology,
Psychiatry

ISBN 0-12-512460-0

symptoms occur more frequently on the left side might be sufficient by itself, because of the crossing of the sensorimotor fibers, to raise the question of particular right hemisphere involvement. The case is strengthened by findings that two phenomena closely related to psychogenic somatic symptoms, emotion and hypnosis, are linked to right hemisphere functioning.

II. Evidence for Symptom Lateralization

A. Clinical Observations, 1859 to the Present

As early as 1859 Briquet reported that conversion symptoms occur three times more frequently on the left side of the body than on the right, and similar observations have been made over and over again since then. Pitres (1891) and Gilles de la Tourette (1891) both described a greater frequency on the left side. In 1909 Dubois wrote, "It is striking to see so many hysterics avow that they feel less on the left side [p. 179; quoted in Ley, 1980]." Schilder (1950) wrote that Pötzl, in a 1919 volume entitled *Zur Klinik und Anatomie der Worttaubheit* (complete reference not given), claimed that the right cerebral hemisphere has a special influence on the "vegetative functions." Schilder also stated that Hirschl developed this idea further, although no reference is offered. In 1924 Purves-Stewart wrote in his clinical text that hysterical hyperesthesia often occurs in "little islands of skin" and that these tender points, "when not in the middle line, are generally left-sided [p. 626]." Discussing hysterical anesthesia, the same writer observed, "Its commonest distribution is a hemianesthesia. This is usually left-sided [p. 628]." Sandor Ferenczi, a psychoanalyst, made the same observation in 1926 about hysterical stigmata and went on to write, "It is possible that—in right-handed people—the sensational sphere for the left side shows from the first a certain predisposition for unconscious impulses [p. 115]." Fenichel (1945) cited Ferenczi and added his own corroboration. Schilder (1950), discussing nonperception of one-half of the body, which he believed could be either psychological or organic in origin, observed that "in the majority of cases, the left side of the body is affected." He went on, "One might assume that only centres in the right hemisphere have a sufficiently close relation to central emotional activities [p. 37]." Engel (1970) commented in a clinical text that psychogenic hemisensory disturbances more often occur on the left side than on the right. I have come across only one dissenting clinical impression: Weintraub (1977) wrote that, in hysteria, "hemisensory loss to all modalities" is "usually on the dominant side for the patient [p. 12]," that is, usually on the right side.

Perhaps the most interesting of these clinical comments, because of its matter-of-fact tone, comes from Magee's (1962) article: "Various theories have been advanced to explain the predominant occurrence of psychiatric symptoms on the left side of the body. They need not be repeated here since they are readily available in psychiatric texts [p. 345]." One wishes that he *had* repeated them, or at least offered references! It is likely that a search of older texts would unearth more clinical observations in the same vein and explanatory hypotheses as well. At any rate, it does seem abundantly clear that an awareness of a predominance of left-sided psychiatric symptoms has been part of clinical lore for many years.

B. Early Research Findings

A number of quantitative studies of the lateralization of psychogenic symptoms also appeared before interest developed in hemispheric specialization. Some of these studies, scattered among books and journals of various academic areas, have been rediscovered and referenced, one or two at a time, by several authors, but the results have not been reviewed in detail and have not been available in one place. It might be added that more studies may be available in the early literature, because those that have been discovered report only incidentally their data on the lateral distribution of symptoms. A study qualified for inclusion in this chapter if it contained data on the lateral distribution of any kind of somatic symptom that was psychologically determined.

In order to simplify the task of comparison, standard statistical tests were carried out for all studies, even those recent ones that reported their own statistics. Each test was a bidirectional evaluation of the departure of the data from the distribution expected by chance, that is, 50% left-sided, 50% right-sided. Whenever the information was available, the age distribution of the patients and body part affected were reported in the text. Data on sex and handedness are reviewed in Section II,E.

The earliest available data are those from Halliday's (1937) study of 21 consecutive cases of "psychosomatic rheumatism." Halliday found no evidence of organic disease in these patients, who complained of what they called rheumatism (i.e., pain in muscles, joints, and tissues) in neck, shoulders, and arms. Each patient had encountered "one or more disturbing psychological factors" before the development of the symptom, to which the response had been "an emotional reaction which merged into a psychoneurotic anxiety state [p. 264]." Each patient also had many other symptoms.

The chief complaint was pain or stiffness, but there were also numbness, prickling sensations, and sudden attacks of loss of power. The duration of the incapacity ranged from a few weeks to over a year, and several patients had recurrent episodes. Among the patients with lateralized symptoms, mean male age ($N=7$) was 40.29 years, with a range of 22 to 56. Mean female age ($N=7$) was 33.14 years, with a range of 17 to 53 years. Symptoms were concentrated in the limbs. Of the 14 patients with lateralized symptoms, 13 had them predominantly on the left side (χ^2 = 10.28, $p<0.01$).

Boland and Corr (1943) studied 50 cases of "pure psychogenic rheumatism" (states in which symptoms such as pain, stiffness, subjective sense of swelling, or limitation of motion are presented "in the complete absence of structural joint or muscle abnormalities"). Of 16 patients showing laterality of symptoms, 9 showed left side involvement and 7 showed right side involvement. All 50 patients were military servicemen, and most had received diagnoses of "psychoneurosis" before entering the military. Forty-six had "definite associated psychoneurotic symptoms" in addition to the rheumatic complaints.

Edmonds (1947) selected from his general medical practice the 183 patients whom he had diagnosed as neurotic and then investigated the 87 patients who had pain with no discernible organic origin. These 87 patients had other psychosomatic symptoms. The pain was distributed in the chest, lumbar region, neck, and limbs. The pain was predominantly unilateral in 51 cases, and in 44 of these it was mainly left-sided ($\chi^2=26.84$, $p < 0.001$).

Edmonds noted Halliday's (1941) explanation of the left side phenomenon as an expression of the symbolism of "left." In folklore, myth, superstition, and dreams, Halliday had said, the left is associated with grief, disaster, and evil. Edmonds accepted this symbolic association but suggested that both the symbolic association and the predominance of left-sided symptoms were due to the asymmetry of function of the cerebral hemispheres. Edmonds's prescient hypothesis, which bears a close resemblance to certain modern theorizing regarding emotionality (e.g., Gainotti, 1972; Galin, 1974), was that, because of left hemisphere dominance for linguistic functions in right-handed persons, the emotional ("thalamic") impulses directed to the dominant side of the body (the right side) were under "cortical restraint." However, the right hemisphere could provide no such restraint, and "the merely thalamic expression of emotion," therefore, had more access to the left side of the body (p. 47).

Noting that conversion reactions such as blindness, deafness, and motor loss in an extremity were becoming increasingly rare, Magee (1962) asserted that a particular kind of conversion symptom, paralysis and loss of sensation on one whole half of the body, was being recognized with greater frequency. Magee's article is a clear and sophisticated summary of the differential diagnosis of this syndrome and the various neurological conditions for which it might be mistaken. It is claimed that "paresis or paralysis develops on one side of the body, usually on the left side. Associated with the paralysis is a diminution or loss of all types of sensation, including the special senses, on the involved side of the body [p. 340]." These diminished functions may include vision, hearing, taste, olfaction, touch, surface pain, deep pain, vibration sense, kinesthesis, and stereognosis. At the end of the article Magee writes that "this syndrome was present on the right side of the body in only three of more than 50 cases I have observed [p. 344]."

Spear's M.D. thesis (1964) has been cited in various publications, but the results relevant here have not yet appeared in the literature in detail. The present summary is based on the account by Merskey and Spear (1967).

Spear examined 132 English psychiatric patients (inpatients, day patients, and outpatients) who had pain. It was found that pain was significantly associated with a history of surgical operations, overt anxiety, the presence of other somatic symptoms, and, in men, low socioeconomic status. Most of the patients were diagnosed as depressed or anxious–hysterical. The information about pain was gathered while the patients were followed "for varying periods." The 132 patients described 222 pains; most had either one pain (72 patients) or two pains (42 patients). Of the total 222 pains, 188 were located in the head and trunk. There were 92 lateralized pains, of which 65 occurred on the left side ($\chi^2 = 15.7$, $p < 0.001$). Unfortunately, there is no way to convert these data to the number of patients with right- and left-sided pains. However, since the 18 patients with more than two pains accounted for only 66 of the total number of pains, it is unlikely that the right–left disparity is due to a small number of patients who had many pains, all on the left side.

Kenyon (1964) attempted to evaluate whether there exists a condition of primary, or essential, hypochondriasis. All the subjects of the study were patients who had received a diagnosis of hypochondriasis at the Bethlehem Royal and Maudsley Hospitals (London) from 1951 to 1960. Of the 512 patients selected for study, 295 were inpatients and 217 were outpatients. The primary hypochondriasis group (301 cases) consisted of patients with a primary or sole diagnosis of hypochondriasis. In the secondary hypochondriasis group (211 cases) the diagnosis of hypochondriasis was secondary to some other diagnosis. The two groups were compared on many variables, and it was concluded that they did not differ in any meaningful way. Kenyon reported, as an incidental finding, that 18.9% of the patients in the primary group had definite unilateral symptoms and that 65.5% of these patients experienced their symptoms on the left side. In the secondary group 12.3% had unilateral hypochondriacal complaints, and 80.7% of these patients experienced their symptoms on the left side. Converting these percentages to raw data and collapsing the primary and secondary groups, we find that 58 of 83 patients (70%) with unilateral symptoms experienced their symptoms on the left side ($\chi^2 = 13.12$, $p < 0.001$).

Merskey (1965) examined 100 psychiatric patients with persistent pain. These patients were a consecutive series and met the following criteria:

(*a*) pain was present continuously or intermittently for more than 3 months; (*b*) pain was spontaneously mentioned as a major complaint; and (*c*) pain was *prima facie* not due to organic disease.

In 48 patients pain was bilateral and symmetric. Pain was entirely right-sided in 4 patients and entirely left-sided in 3 patients. In 27 patients pain was bilateral but greater on the left, and in 18 patients pain was bilateral but greater on the right. Collapsing the patients with unilateral pain and those reporting asymmetric bilateral pain, there were 30 patients with left-sided predominance and 22 with right-sided predominance. This result does not reach statistical significance.

Morgenstern (1970) studied factors that play a role in maintaining a state of chronic, severe pain after amputation. He suspected that psychological and psychiatric aspects would be significant. Subjects were chosen by a random process from lists of several thousand British patients who attended a limb-fitting center and a special clinic for intractable postamputation pain. All prospective subjects had been operated on at least 2 years before the study. Eventually, 164 patients were selected. According to carefully quantified clinical criteria, these patients were separated into groups characterized by high pain ($N=55$), intermediate pain ($N=68$), and no pain ($N=41$). The high-pain group was considered the experimental group, and the no-pain group the control or comparison group. The following is a selection of the pertinent findings:

1. There was no association between chronic pain and the final state of the stump, suggesting that organic factors at the amputation site were not significant in pain maintenance.
2. Chronic pain was associated with areas of anesthesia on the stump. It was not associated with hyperesthesias. The mechanism here is unknown, but it is at least possible that these anesthesias were a variety of conversion symptom.
3. The incidence of "recurrent depressive illness" was significantly higher in the high-pain than in the no-pain group. It was not possible to determine whether the depressions occurred for the first time before the amputation or after it. However, Morgenstern commented that pain was relieved without the depressive mood changing in some cases, and in others the depressive mood lifted although the pain was not affected.
4. Patients with chronic, severe pain had undergone significantly more surgery for other, unrelated conditions than patients with no pain. The additional surgery in the high-pain group tended to consist of operations in which pressure from the patient may influence the course of treatment—for example, ulcer, hernia, and hemorrhoids.
5. High-pain patients scored significantly higher than no-pain patients

on the neuroticism scale of the Eysenck Personality Inventory (Eysenck, 1964).

6. On the Cornell Medical Index (Brodman *et al.*, 1951) high-pain patients scored significantly higher than no-pain patients on the neuroticism scale, the psychosomatic scale, and the symptoms scale. That is, despite their generally similar medical histories, the high-pain group reported many more symptoms of medical disorders.

Of course, these findings are correlations. There is no way of knowing whether they might be the cause of the high pain or the result of it. On the other hand, it is well known that postamputation pain may persist after all afferent pathways from the site of the amputation have been severed. Morgenstern's findings seem to point toward a minimal peripheral organic factor and a major psychological factor in the maintenance of severe, chronic postamputation pain.

Other work by Morgenstern (1964), in which he successfully used a distraction procedure to reduce postamputation pain, points in the same direction. In fact, in the pain-modification study Morgenstern described patients who behaved in a manner suggesting that they were reluctant to receive treatment for their pain, even though they knew that there were no dangers and that there was a good chance of obtaining some relief. These patients seemed to manifest resistance to the loss of pain.

The finding directly relevant to this chapter is the proportion of patients with severe, chronic pain who had had left-sided and right-sided amputations. Among the 51 unilateral amputees with severe pain, 34 (67%) had had left-sided amputations, and 17 (33%) had had right-sided amputations. This left-sided predominance departs significantly from chance ($\chi^2 = 5.67, p < 0.02$). The finding would be meaningless, of course, if most amputees with no pain had also had left-sided operations. This was not the case, however. There was a significant difference ($\chi^2 = 7.01$, $p < 0.01$) between the proportion of left-sided amputees who developed high pain (34 of 76, or 45%) and the proportion of right-sided amputees who developed high pain (17 of 71, or 24%).

Morgenstern did not report age and sex separately for right- and left-sided amputees, but he did show that age is significantly positively related to high pain and that sex is not related. Most of the 164 patients (146, or 89%) were men.

Morgenstern's data on the sidedness of pain are particularly important because they suggest that, even given equal trauma on the two sides of the body, the left side is more likely to develop cortically mediated symptoms.

Fallik and Sigal (1971) reported the only statistically significant contradictory findings available. They studied 40 inpatient cases of "sensory–motor conversive symptoms," which included monoparesis, hemiparesis, paraparesis, ptosis, anesthesia, hyperesthesia, torticollis, stiff-man syndrome, blindness, deafness, and mutism. All patients had been referred because ambulatory treatment had not resulted in symptom relief. Excluded from consideration were patients with paroxysmal hysterical attacks, conversion symptoms in the autonomic nervous system, organic syndromes, and "psychotic reactions masked by hysterical symptoms [p. 311]." The age of 85% of the patients was less than 30 years, and 90% of the patients were men. Both figures are notable; most of the studies summarized here reported a majority of women of older age. In most patients (85%) the writers found that "the hysterical symptom occurred as the result of interpersonal conflict [p. 312]," and the symptom was generally accompanied by secondary gain. The aim of the study was to investigate choice of symptom site. The findings were as follows: (*a*) 65% of the patients had had a previous lesion in the limb or area in which the conversion symptom appeared; (*b*) 20% of the patients developed conversion reactions after or during hospitalizations on orthopedic or neurological wards (iatrogenic suggestion); (*c*) Of the 33 patients with unilateral symptoms, 25 (76%) had them on the right side, and 8 (24%) had them on the left side. These proportions deviate significantly from chance ($\chi^2 = 8.76$, $p < 0.01$).

Agnew and Merskey (1976) studied the type of pain descriptions used by patients with chronic severe pain of organic versus psychiatric origin. Pain had existed for at least 3 months and usually for more than 6 months. The psychiatric group consisted of 21 men (mean age 41 years) and 42 women (mean age 41 years). Of these 63 patients, 46 had headache, and a larger number had left-sided than right-sided pain. Overall, 42 patients had lateralized pain, and 27 (64%) had the pain on the left side. This proportion approaches significance ($\chi^2 = 3.43$, $p < 0.10$). It is worth noting that, among 40 patients with lateralized organic pain, a larger proportion (24, or 60%) also had left-sided pain than right-sided pain (16, or 40%).

Stephánsson *et al.* (1976) reported on 64 patients with conversion symptoms; these patients were seen in Iceland or Monroe County, New York, from 1960 to 1969. In 56% of the cases the psychiatric diagnosis was accompanied by an organic diagnosis unrelated to the conversion symptoms. Mean age for the 25 men was 42.7 years; mean age for the 39 women was 31.9 years. Sensory symptoms such as pain, anesthesia, hyperesthesia, paresthesia, and pruritis were the most common type, followed by motor symptoms such as paralysis, tics, weakness, and spasm. Pain was the most frequent symptom, appearing in 44 cases (69%). Abdominal pain was most frequent, followed by headache and pain in the chest. Breathing difficulties appeared in 18 cases (28%); anesthesias or paresthesias were reported by 18 patients (28%); 13 patients (20%) had paralysis or weakness. Of the 31 symptoms (the unit of analysis here was the symptom, not the patient) that could be clearly lateralized, 19 (61%) were, in agreement with Fallik and Sigal (1971), on the right side. The finding is not statistically significant.

C. Galin's [1974] Hypothesis

Edmonds (1947), Halliday (1949), Schilder (1950), Kenyon (1964), and Morgenstern (1970) all speculated that the left-sided predominance of the symptoms they studied suggested a special role for the right hemisphere, but none of these proposals seems to have generated much interest. Perhaps this is because the psychiatric *Zeitgeist* was at the time more receptive to psychological than physiological explanations. Today, of course, the situation has changed. Repudiating simple dichotomies such as "major" hemisphere and "minor" hemisphere, Galin (1974, 1976, 1977) has presented creative notions regarding possible links between psychiatry and hemispheric asymmetry of function. On the basis of the seeming dissociation of the experience of the two cerebral hemispheres after commissurotomy, Galin (1974) presented the provocative proposal that "in normal, intact people events in the right hemisphere can become disconnected functionally from the left hemisphere (by inhibition of neuronal transmission across the corpus callosum and other cerebral commissures), and can continue a life of their own [This and subsequent quotes from Galin, 1974, are reprinted from Galin, D. Implications for psychiatry of left and right cerebral specialization. *Arch. Gen. Psychiatry* **31**, 572–583. Copyright 1974, American Medical Association. pp. 574–575]." In other words, Galin conjectured, perhaps repression is actually a disconnection of certain psychic material in the right hemisphere from the language centers in the left hemisphere. Perhaps the right hemisphere is the "locus for the unconscious mental contents [p. 575]."

On the basis of this general hypothesis, Galin made a number of specific proposals, one of which is that "somatic representations, psychosomatic disorders, and somatic delusions" should occur primarily on the left side of the body (because of the crossing of the sensorimotor fibers).

D. Recent Research Findings

All the studies reviewed in this section, unlike the studies reviewed in Section II,B, were conducted with the express purpose of evaluating the hypothesis that psychogenic somatic symptoms occur more frequently on the left side of the body than on the right. All seem to have been directly or indirectly stimulated by Galin's (1974) hypothesis.

Stern (1977) studied the hospital charts of all patients who had received a diagnosis of "hysterical reaction, conversion type" at the university hospitals of the University of Iowa between 1966 and 1976. To qualify for inclusion in the study, patients had to have received a firm diagnosis of conversion reaction in the form of muscular weakness or paralysis, or numbness or anesthesia. Of the patients selected, there were 140 females (mean age 34.6 years) and 51 males (mean age 35.5 years). The results were tabulated separately for muscular weakness or paralysis and for numbness or anesthesia. In order to be counted as a unilateral patient and tabulated in the lateralization findings, a patient had to have had entirely unilateral symptoms (i.e., not bilateral with greater intensity on one side), and all unilateral symptoms in the past had to have occurred on the same side of the body.

Symptoms were located in arms, hands, and legs. A small proportion were limited to the head. A large proportion of the patients (69, or 36%) described unilateral symptoms of both types, and all but three had them on the same side.

Of the 114 patients with unilateral sensory symptoms, 78 (68%) had them on the left ($\chi^2 = 15.47, p < 0.001$). Of the 81 patients with unilateral motor symptoms, 52 (64%) had them on the left ($\chi^2 = 6.53, p < 0.02$).

Galin *et al.* (1977) began by selecting for review the charts of all patients from the university hospitals of the University of California, San Francisco, who had received a primary or secondary discharge diagnosis, between 1963 and 1974, of hysterical neurosis, hysterical personality, conversion neurosis, or psychophysiological reaction of the musculoskeletal system or the central nervous system. The charts selected also contained adequate documentation of physical, laboratory, and psychiatric evaluation. From the 195 charts selected 52 were chosen for study on the basis of the following stringent criteria:

1. The patient must have had at least one unilateral symptom.
2. If different symptoms occurred during different hospitalizations, all unilateral symptoms must have been on the same side.
3. The patient must have met all diagnostic criteria described by Engel (1970) for conversion.
4. There must have been no indication in the history of brain disease or trauma.
5. There must have been no trauma to or surgery performed on the symptomatic area unless the symptom existed before the trauma or surgery.
6. There must have been no prominent workmen's compensation suits pending.
7. All three of the authors must have agreed, on the basis of independent reviews of charts from which information regarding symptom lateralization was removed, that all the preceding criteria had been met.

This careful subject selection procedure seems to have had two purposes. It ensured that the diagnosis was valid, and it attempted to exclude cases that might have been explained on any basis other than special involvement of the right hemisphere.

The overall mean age was 34.3 years, with a range from 7 to 63 years. Most patients (36, or 69%) had both sensory and motor symptoms, and 64% of these patients had both on the left side. Eleven had only sensory symptoms, and five had only motor symptoms.

Of the 52 patients, 33 (63%) experienced their symptoms on the left side, a finding that approaches significance ($\chi^2 = 3.77$, $p < 0.10$). Wishing to exclude any factors that would compromise their hypothesis of right hemisphere involvement, Galin *et al.* discarded data from three left-handed patients who otherwise seem to have qualified for study. All three had left-sided symptoms. If these patients are reintroduced to the sample, increasing N to 55, the proportion of patients with left-sided symptoms rises to 65.5% (36 of 55), a statistically significant finding ($\chi^2 = 5.25$, $p < 0.05$).

Bishop *et al.* (1978) studied 22 cases of hysterical neurosis (conversion type), hysterical personality, conversion neurosis, and psychophysiological musculoskeletal or central nervous system reaction seen at the Eugene Talmadge Memorial Hospital (Atlanta, Georgia) between 1966 and 1976. The criteria for subject selection were approximately the same as those used by Galin *et al.* (1977; Section II,C). There were 11 men (mean age 45.09 years) and 11 women (mean age 31.27 years) in the sample. Seven men and 5 women (55%) had left-sided symptoms, a result that did not reach statistical significance.

Axelrod *et al.* (1980) investigated cases drawn from the psychiatric literature, from the late 1800s to the present, that met the following criteria: (*a*) the patient was individually described, and the symptom was diagnosed as indicating psychogenicity; and (*b*) all symptoms so diagnosed were unilateral. This procedure resulted in the compilation of 150 cases, of which 40 (20 left-sided, 20 right-sided) showed possible "organic bias" (previous surgery, trauma, or disease on the site of the symptom). An additional 16 patients (7 left-sided, 9 right-sided) showed possible "psychological bias" (a nonorganic factor that might have influenced symptom site, such as a relative with a symptom in the same location). Of the total 150 patients, 82 (55%) had left-sided symptoms ($\chi^2 = 1.13$, not significant). The same proportion (55%) of the total number of symptoms ($N = 260$) were left-sided ($\chi^2 = 2.6$, not significant). When all cases of possible "bias" were excluded (cases that might have diluted a right hemisphere factor in symptom location), 58.5% (55 of 94) of the remaining patients had left-sided symptoms ($\chi^2 = 2.72$, $0.05 < p < 0.10$). A majority of the 260 symptoms (61%) were sensory (e.g., pain, anesthesia), whereas the minority were motor (e.g., tremor, paralysis).

Seven of the cases (3 left-sided, 4 right-sided) in this study were collected from case illustrations in the article by Fallik and Sigal (1971; Section II,B). In addition, Axelrod *et al.* collected cases from one source (Janet, 1907) that was also used in an archival study by Ley (1980; Section II,C). In order to eliminate overlap in the present review, these cases (3 left-sided, 7 right-sided), as well as the cases of Fallik and Sigal (1971), have been removed, lowering N to 133. The subtraction of these 17 cases (6 left-sided, 11 right-sided) changes the overall proportion of left-sided cases from 55 to 57% ($\chi^2 = 2.71$, $p = 0.10$).

Ley (1980) also carried out an archival study, but in contrast to Axelrod *et al.* (1980), most of whose cases came from literature published after 1930, Ley concentrated on case histories by earlier writers (e.g., Breuer and Freud, Charcot, and Janet). The criteria for the selection of cases were: (*a*) diagnosis of hysteria or hysterical, (*b*) at least one unilateral symptom, and (*c*) identification of the patient's sex. As in most other contemporary studies, patients in whom there were lateralized symptoms on each side of the body, either simultaneously or over time, were not counted as unilateral patients. Differential lateral intensity of bilateral symptoms was not counted as unilateral. Of the 100 cases selected, 66 (66%) had left-sided symptoms, a significant finding ($\chi^2 = 10.24$, $p < 0.01$).

Fleminger *et al.* (1980) examined lateralized psychogenic somatic symptoms by conducting interviews with 106 female psychiatric outpatients ("neurotic and personality disorder") at Guy's Hospital, London. Patients were excluded if they had histories of psychosis, epilepsy, brain damage, deafness, or electroconvulsive therapy (ECT) (within the year before the study). Age was restricted to 49 years or less. The age of the subjects ranged from 18 to 48 years, with a mean of 29.1 years. Interviews were supplemented by a review of case notes. Eighteen of the 24 patients (75%) with clearly lateralized sensory symptoms had them on the left side ($x^2 = 6.00$, $p < 0.02$). Nine of the 14 patients (64.5%) with unilateral motor symptoms had them on the left ($\chi^2 = 1.14$, not significant).

E. Overview of the Data

Psychogenic somatic symptoms occur more frequently on the left side than they occur on the right side. Of the 10 studies with statistically significant results, 9 reported the left-sided predominance. The results of 2 more studies with results in the same direction approached significance. Overall, 15 of the 17 studies (88%) reported findings favoring the left side, a proportion that significantly ($p < 0.01$) exceeds the 50% expected by chance.

The circumstances under which the finding has appeared are diverse. It has been described by French, German, English, and American clinicians for over 100 years. It has appeared as an incidental finding in studies originally conducted for other purposes and in studies in which it was predicted; in studies with differing subject selection procedures, ranging from the careful criteria of Galin *et al.* (1977) to the inclusion of every "rheumatic" patient whose complaints could not be explained on an organic basis; in studies of hospital records and studies of private practice patients; in widely scattered rural and urban areas; and, in support of clinical wisdom, past and present, in studies of contemporary patients and studies of patients who had their symptoms over half a century ago. Perhaps most interesting, the finding appears in studies of several different types of symptom: psychiatric pain, psychogenic sensory loss, psychogenic motor loss, psychogenic rheumatism, hypochondriasis, and chronic, severe postamputation pain. The sidedness of positive psychogenic motor symptoms (e.g., tics and tremors) and the sidedness of psychogenic somatic symptoms in non-Western cultures have not been separately investigated, but the hypothesis for these studies, which should be carried out, seems clear.

The consistency of the findings makes it all the more interesting why Fallik and Sigal (1971; Section II,B) registered a significant predominance of right-sided symptoms. One finding that may provide a hint is that the symptoms of 65% of the patients in the Fallik and Sigal study developed at the time of an injury in the same area and then either continued after the organic recovery was complete or returned some time later. Presumably, since most of the conversion symptoms were right-sided, most of the injuries occurred on the right side. On this basis, perhaps the laterality data were skewed by an unusual degree of what Axelrod *et al.* (1980; Section II,D) referred to as "organic bias."

1. SEX AND SYMPTOM LATERALIZATION

In none of the seven studies that reported sex by laterality of symptoms (Halliday, 1937; Agnew and Merskey, 1976; Stern, 1977; Galin *et al.*, 1977 ; Bishop *et al.*, 1978; Axelrod *et al.*, 1980; Ley, 1980) was there a significant interaction between sex and symptom sidedness. Axelrod *et al.* (1980) calculated a significant interaction ($p < 0.05$) in the data of Galin *et al.* In my estimation, however, this effect only approaches significance ($\chi^2 = 2.71$, $p < 0.10$). The reason for this difference lies in the inclusion, in this chapter, of the three non-right-handed patients whom Galin *et al.* discarded in the original presentation of the data (see Section II,D). All three of these patients had left-sided symptoms. Two were female, and one was male.

2. HANDEDNESS AND SYMPTOM LATERALIZATION

In clinical and early research reports, there seemed to be an association between handedness and lateralization of psychogenic symptoms. Ferenczi (1926) and Purves-Stewart (1924) each suggested that the laterality of these symptoms is reversed (i.e., right-sided) in sinistrals. The one right-sided patient reported by Halliday (1937; Section II,B) was ambidextrous, and Edmonds (1947; Section II,B) reported that two of his seven patients with right-sided pains were left-handed. Magee (1962; Section II,B) stated that one of his three patients with right-sided hemianesthesia and/or hemiplegia was left-handed, although at least one other left-handed individual in his series had left-sided symptoms.

However, these writers presented their data in the form of single case examples of non-right-handed individuals with right-sided symptoms. It seemed to have been thought that sinistrals with right-sided symptoms were particularly worthy of notice. It was not until somewhat later that the distribution of unilateral psychogenic somatic symptoms was presented for non-right-handed individuals as a group. In fact, in the four studies in which data are available on handedness and symptom sidedness (Fallik and Sigal, 1971; Stern, 1977; Galin *et al.*, 1977; Fleminger *et al.*, 1980), a greater proportion of non-right-handed patients had left-sided symptoms. The greater symptom lateralization reaches significance only for the data of Fallik and Sigal. This one significant result is not convincing, however, because it is due to atypical symptom distribution among right-handed patients. Nevertheless, across all studies the difference is there and, if the same pattern were obtained with a larger group of non-right-handed individuals, the finding would eventually reach statistical significance.

However, all that can be concluded on the basis of the data presently available is that non-right-handed patients, like right-handed patients, show a strong predominance of left-sided symptoms.

III. Explanations for Symptom Lateralization

There are several hypotheses that might explain the predominance of left-sided symptoms. Three of these—the hypothesis of "silent" right hemisphere lesions, the organic bias hypothesis, and the symbolism hypothesis—are not explicitly concerned with hemispheric specialization. Each of these ideas is examined before hypotheses based on lateralization of function are considered.

A. Alternatives to Hemispheric Specialization

1. "SILENT" CORTICAL LESIONS IN THE RIGHT HEMISPHERE

A growing body of literature (Slater, 1965; Slater and Glithero, 1965; Whitlock, 1967; Merskey and Buhrich, 1975; Merskey and Trimble, 1979; Roy, 1977, 1979) suggests that a large proportion of patients with conversion symptoms also have, or have had, organic brain disorder. In Whitlock's (1967) careful study, for instance, 62.5% of patients with diagnoses of conversion symptoms or dissociative reactions showed evidence of preceding or coexisting organic brain disorder, compared with an incidence of 5.3% in a control group of psychiatric patients with other diagnoses. For many of these patients the brain disorder was acute (e.g., concussion) and seemed to pass, serving more as a psychological precipitant than as an organic one. Nevertheless, these data require that we consider the possibility that a certain proportion of left-sided psychiatric symptoms (a large enough proportion to erase the left-sided predominance) are symptoms of disorder or disease of the right hemisphere. Because of the sparing of linguistic performance and general intellectual functioning, subtle right hemisphere lesions probably go undetected more often than equally subtle disease of the left hemisphere. According to the "silent" lesion hypothesis, some of these otherwise unnoticed right hemisphere lesions may cause sensory or motor deficits, which are then misinterpreted as psychogenic symptoms. This possibility is illustrated by Ross's (Ross and Mesulam, 1979; Ross, 1981; Ross *et al.*, 1981) descriptions of a group of patients with right hemisphere lesions who show no intellectual deficit and may present with only left-sided sensory and motor loss and lack of emotional expressiveness. It is easy to imagine these patients being misdiagnosed.

However, there are several reasons for doubting the "silent" lesion hypothesis. First, of course, is the fact that psychogenic sensory loss is, by definition, distributed according to the patient's *idea* of the nervous system (e.g., glove and stocking anesthesia), not according to actual anatomical distribution (Magee, 1962; Weintraub, 1977). The sensory and motor loss is untrue to the facts of neurology in other ways as well, clinical examples of which are numerous in Magee's (1962) paper on differential diagnosis.

Second, most of the papers discussed earlier mention that the symptoms appeared after one or more psychological precipitants.

Third, in careful diagnostic studies in which all cases in which there was even a hint of prior or coexisting brain disorder were excluded (Stern, 1977; Galin *et al.*, 1977), the left-sided predominance was still observed.

Fourth, it has been shown that the left-sided predominance (and even approximately the same proportions) holds for psychogenic pain as well as for psychogenic sensory and motor loss. However, to explain both of these symptoms on the basis of "silent" right hemisphere lesions would seem to require the positing of two separate lesions. Lesions of the thalamus are the most common hemispheric cause of pain, and this pain, it is true, is often referred to the opposite side of the body. Sensory loss usually accompanies this pain but is characterized by "thalamic overreaction," a form of hyperpathia in which, although sensory thresholds are raised, suprathreshold stimuli arouse intense sensations of peculiar and distinctive discomfort (Bannister, 1973). Overreaction is not characteristic of psychogenic sensory loss. Furthermore, pain is not a symptom of the kind of cortical damage that might cause uncomplicated sensory loss. To account for psychogenic pain and sensory loss as consequences of "silent" lesions would seem to require subtle thalamic lesions that cause pain but no sensory loss, an improbable event, and, at the same time, subtle lesions in the cortex. Given the similarities between psychogenic pain and psychogenic sensory loss (the evidence for psychological precipitation, the similar left-sided proportions, and the nonanatomical distributions), it is highly unlikely that an explanation of this complexity is necessary. If unilateral lesions seem an improbable explanation, then the data linking brain damage and conversion reactions is probably not relevant to an understanding of the left-sided predominance of psychogenic symptoms. Thus, the left side phenomenon does not seem to be a manifestation of definable central nervous system disorder.

2. ORGANIC BIAS HYPOTHESIS

In case studies it is emphasized again and again that a psychogenic somatic symptom may develop on the site of a previous organic symptom. In the data of Fallik and Sigal (1971) organic bias seemed to play a part in symptom location for 65% of the patients. If the left side of the body more often becomes injured or diseased than the right side, organic bias might be responsible for the predominance of psychogenic somatic symptoms. One piece of suggestive evidence for this position comes from the data of Agnew and Merskey (1976; Section II,B), who studied both organic pain and psychiatric pain and found the same left-sided predominance for both types (although only the findings for psychiatric pain approached significance).

Axelrod *et al.* (1980), citing these data, tested the organic bias hypothesis in two ways. First, making extensive use of a survey by Schnall and Smith (1974), they described the organic pathologies and developmental anomalies that show asymmetric distribution on the two sides of the body. Those that occur more often on the left and those that occur more often on the right were approximately equal in number. Second, the writers studied 4247 consecutive admissions to a hospital emergency room and ascertained that 1021 cases involved unilateral complaints. There was no difference between the proportion of left-sided and right-sided complaints. The incidence of trauma was the same on the two sides of the body, and there was also no lateral difference for any of the 38 diagnoses employed in the emergency room. Axelrod *et al.* concluded that organic bias is not the cause of the predominance of left-sided symptoms.

A possible second source of evidence comes from Morgenstern (1970; Section II,B), who reported that chronic severe pain after amputation is more common in left-sided cases than right-sided ones. Like much pain of this nature these symptoms had no demonstrable organic basis. If replicated, this finding would be excellent grounds on which to reject the organic bias hypothesis, for it shows that symmetric distribution of trauma still results in the same asymmetric distribution of psychogenic pain.

3. SYMBOLISM HYPOTHESIS

The hypothesis that the predominance of left-sided psychogenic symptoms is due to the symbolism of left and right is more difficult to dismiss. It probably does, in fact, play a part in choice of symptom site. One woman in Stern's (1977) study, for instance, spontaneously reported to her physician that she had dreamed, the night before she developed left-sided hemiparalysis and hemianesthesia, that she had been sexually attacked and "hurt" on the left side of her body. Ferenczi (1926) presented a case in which he correlated left-sided hysterical hemianesthesia with a nightmare in which the patient felt a mouse running into his throat. Upon awakening, the patient found that, representing the mouse, his own left hand was stuffed into his mouth, while the right hand was desperately trying to pull it out. [The similarity of this case to certain emotion-laden "battles" of one hand with the other in cases of commissurotomized patients (Gazzaniga, 1970) is striking.] The patient was unable for a few moments after awakening to distinguish his left hand from the mouse.

Ferenczi's explanation was that, because the right side of the body is more "skillful" and "active" (in right-handed individuals), it is less vulnerable to being adapted to the representation of unconscious impulses. It is interesting that, reminiscent of Axelrod *et al.* (1980), Ferenczi distinguished between the left-sided symptoms that occur because of "physical predisposition" (previous trauma) in the area and the left-sided symptoms that occur, as Edmonds (1947) and Galin (1974) conjectured, because of a "purely physiological disposition of the affected parts of the body [p. 115]."

The symbolism of left as bad, mysterious, and dirty and right as good, rational, and clean has been well documented in cultures all over the world. There seems to be no record, in fact, of a culture in which these meanings are reversed (Blau, 1946; Hertz, 1960). Domhoff (1969–1970) showed that these meanings are of more than anthropological significance. After reviewing examples from widely scattered cultures and from psychoanalytical case studies, he went on to demonstrate, using Osgood's (Osgood *et al.*, 1957) semantic differential, that present-day American college students show approximately the same associations with left and right that have been reported in other eras and cultures.

Most writers, even those who have correlated conversion symptoms and cerebral disease (e.g., Whitlock, 1967), agree that psychogenic somatic symptoms often occur after psychological precipitation. By definition, the precipitants involve unpleasant affects. If we take one more step and say that what is being expressed by the symptoms are thoughts or feelings that in some way are unacceptable to the patient, then expressing them on the side of the body felt to be bad, weak, etc., would be natural.

There are several ways to test the symbolism hypothesis. Axelrod *et al.* (1980) suggested that, if the symbolism hypothesis is accurate, the proportion of left-sided symptoms should be even higher in cultural groups, such as those of Muslims and Hindus, in which the association between left and bad, dirty, and so forth, is even more extreme than it is in the West. Another test would involve the study of unilateral hysterical blindness or impaired vision. Since the visual field of each eye is subserved by both cerebral hemispheres, one could not make a hypothesis about the sidedness of unilateral blindness on the basis of hemispheric specialization. However, the symbolism hypothesis would predict that the left eye would be more often affected than the right. A third test would be an adaptation of Domhoff's semantic differential technique. If symbolism is a major determinant of the predominance of left-sided symptoms, then patients with left-sided symptoms might be expected to rate "left" in more unfavorable ways than patients with right-sided symptoms.

However, even if the symbolism hypothesis is supported, there is no reason why it cannot coexist with hypotheses based on hemispheric specialization. In fact, the very ubiquity of the left-right associations suggests that the symbolism may itself be derived from some universal factor, perhaps some aspect of human biology. It may very well be based on the phenomenon of handedness or perhaps on the accessibility of the left side to emotional expression (Sackeim and Gur, 1978; Sackeim *et al.*, 1978) and thus on hemispheric specialization (Edmonds, 1947; Corballis, 1980).

B. Hemispheric Specialization and Symptom Lateralization

In this era of increasing awareness of hemispheric specialization, one thinks immediately of the functional asymmetry of the brain when confronted with a hemisyndrome. In the case of psychogenic somatic symptoms, however, there are also other reasons to suspect a special role for the right hemisphere. Two phenomena closely related to these symptoms, emotion and hypnosis, have been linked to the functioning of the right hemisphere.

1. EMOTION AND THE RIGHT HEMISPHERE

The right hemisphere plays the leading role in the production, expression, and perhaps reception (or understanding) of emotion. The burgeoning literature supporting this conclusion is too extensive to summarize here (for review, see Chapter 8). It is enough for the present purpose to indicate that the hypothesis of a link between emotion and the right hemisphere is based on data from several sources: experimental data from both normal subjects and certain psychiatric groups, clinical psychiatric data, and clinical and experimental studies of the effects of brain damage. Since we can certainly say that psychogenic somatic symptoms are an affective phenomenon, the leading role of the right hemisphere in the mediation of emotion is consistent with the idea that the right hemisphere also has a special role in the left-sided distribution of these symptoms.

One of the explanations offered for the role of the right hemisphere in emotion is particularly relevant to the subject at hand. Gainotti (1972) presented, as a statement of his own speculative explanation, one of the conclusions of a study by Hécaen and Angelergues (1963) on visual agnosia: "In the dominant hemisphere sensory data undergo a complex conceptual elaboration by means of language, while in the minor hemisphere, where language is not represented, they are *processed in a more primitive way, so that they retain their immediateness and rich affective value* [p. 53]." There is a close relationship between this notion and the ideas of Edmonds (1947), Galin (1974), Bogen (1969), and Bear and Fedio (1977), all of whom focus on the absence of language in the right hemisphere as an important ingredient in that hemisphere's leading role in emotion. In the case of psychogenic somatic symptoms we are dealing with symptoms that are clearly based on sensory data with "rich affective value" and that, considering that their connection to psychological precipitants is almost always, perhaps inevitably, unknown to the patient, have also been denied "complex conceptual elaboration by means of language." Gainotti's ideas, originally intended to explain certain anomalies of emotion in neurological patients, seem to fit very well these psychiatric symptoms.

A second hypothesis (Dimond *et al.*, 1976; Dimond and Farrington, 1977; Sackeim and Gur, 1978) is that the two hemispheres play different roles in emotional experience. Broadly speaking, the left hemisphere is said to subserve "positive" or pleasant emotion, and the right hemisphere, "negative" or unpleasant emotion. Since the affect contained in or related to psychogenic somatic symptoms is uniformly unpleasant, the dual-hemisphere view is as congruent as Gainotti's view with the hypothesis that the right hemisphere is especially involved in the production of these symptoms.

2. HYPNOSIS, PSYCHOGENIC SOMATIC SYMPTOMS, AND THE RIGHT HEMISPHERE

Hypnosis and psychogenic somatic symptoms have shared a long history, both becoming topics of clinical speculation during Mesmer's era, generating increasing interest through the time of Charcot, Bernheim, Janet, and early Freud, and then waning in clinical significance with the decline in frequency of conversion reactions and the replacement of hypnosis by free association as the accepted form of psychotherapy (Ellenberger, 1970). For all those years hypnosis was the primary method of treating psychogenic somatic symptoms, and it remains today a most effective way of obtaining symptomatic relief in these cases (e.g., Kampmann and Kuha, 1975; Frankel, 1978; Winer, 1978). Furthermore, the reverse is also true; only with hypnosis is it possible to create symptoms that are indistinguishable from psychogenic somatic symptoms (e.g., Hilgard *et al.*, 1975; Frankel, 1978). Many clinicians, including Janet (1901, 1907), Charcot (Ellenberger, 1970), and Breuer, Freud's early collaborator (Breuer and Freud, 1893–1895), thought that there was an intimate connection between hypnosis and hysteria—hysteria in this context meaning the psychopathological state of which conversion reactions were the symptoms. In the modern era Hilgard (1977) and Frankel (1978) revived the ideas of Janet, suggesting that the same capacity for dissociation underlies the ability to be hypnotized and the development, under stress, of certain psychopathological symptoms, including somatic reactions. Other writers as well, differing at some points in theory but concurring in their observations of the links between the two phenomena, have concluded that hypnosis and conversion reactions are manifestations of the same underlying psychological organization (James, 1890; Gill and Brenman, 1959; Chertok, 1975).

What makes this association between hypnosis and psychogenic somatic symptoms relevant to the present discussion are two sets of findings: (*a*) a study on hypnotically induced somatic symptoms and (*b*) a more complex body of data correlating the hypnotic state and hypnotizability (the ability to be hypnotized) with the functioning of the right hemisphere.

Fleminger *et al.* (1980) administered individual hypnotic inductions to 100 female nurses and 106 female nonpsychotic psychiatric patients and then gave suggestions of increased sensation in the hands. Eventually, according to the instructions, tingling would begin in one of the hands. The hand to be affected was not specified. When tingling occurred, the subject was to raise the hand in which it was felt. Nearly 60% of each group raised the left hand, a finding that approaches statistical significance. Handedness had no effect.

Many of the patients in the study had experienced unilateral psychogenic somatic symptoms. Of the 12 with left-sided sensory symptoms, 11 raised the left hand; of the 7 patients with unilateral motor symptoms on the left side, 5 raised the left hand. By contrast, only 1 of 4 patients with right-sided sensory symptoms and 2 of 4 patients with right-sided motor symptoms raised the left hand. Combining groups, 16 of the 19 patients with left-sided symptoms raised the left hand, a highly significant finding. The interaction (side of symptom by side of raised hand), which was not tested by the investigators, is also significant.

The left hand seems to be more amenable to hypnotic somatic suggestion than the right hand, and this effect is strongest among patients with left-sided psychogenic symptoms. The finding supports the claim that hypnosis and psychogenic somatic symptoms are derived from the same kind of psychological organization. One might speculate, since both hypnotic and psychiatric symptoms show a left-sided predominance, that the commonality in their derivation is based on the activity of the right hemisphere. The following findings are consistent with this notion.

Teitelbaum (1954) and Day (1964, 1967) made the clinical observation that, when asked a question requiring reflective thought, people tend to break eye contact and move their eyes to one side or the other. The direction of these conjugate lateral eye movements is consistent within individuals (Bakan and Strayer, 1973), allowing a typology of "left movers" and "right movers" to be established. The finding was substantiated in the laboratory by Duke (1968) and Bakan and Svorad (1969). Bakan (1969, 1971), reflecting that lateral eye movement is under the control of the hemisphere contralateral to the direction of movement, hypothesized that hypnotizability, which he felt was a capacity subserved by the right hemisphere, would be higher among left movers (i.e., those whose eye movements indicate "activation" of the right hemisphere) than among right movers. Bakan did, indeed, find a statistically significant association, and other investigators (Bakan and Svorad, 1969; Morgan *et al.*, 1971; Gur and Gur, 1974) have replicated it.

A number of studies have demonstrated that total electroencephalographic production is significantly related to hypnotizability (Nowlis and Rhead, 1968; London *et al.*, 1968, 1974). Morgan and coworkers (1971, 1974) went on to show that, under a variety of conditions, the right hemisphere consistently generates more α activity than the left hemisphere. One speculative interpretation here is that the predominance of right hemisphere activity is responsible for the relationship between hypnotizability and total α activity. However, it was not found, as might have been expected, that the proportion of right hemisphere α activity (i.e., right hemisphere α activity/total α activity) is higher in highly hypnotizable subjects than in those with little hypnotic ability.

Linking the work on conjugate lateral eye movements and α activity, Bakan and Svorad (1969) showed that each of these variables is related positively to hypnotizability and to each other.

Finally, using a standard dichotic listening procedure, Frumkin *et al.* (1978) measured right ear (left hemisphere) advantage before, during, and after hypnosis. The right ear advantage was significantly lower during hypnosis than it was during trials before and after hypnosis. The authors concluded that the right hemisphere is especially involved in hypnosis. Because hypnosis is so often associated with heightened emotionality, both in clinical work (Breuer and Freud, 1893–1895; Janet, 1901; Brenman and Gill, 1947; Gill and Brenman, 1959; Ellenberger, 1970) and in research settings (Luria, 1932; Bobbit, 1958; Reyher, 1967; Sommerschield and Reyher, 1973; Levitt and Chapman, 1979), the particular involvement of the right hemisphere in emotionality may have something to do with the link between hypnosis and the right hemisphere.

3. A SPECIFIC HYPOTHESIS: RIGHT HEMISPHERE MECHANISM FOR THE PRODUCTION OF PSYCHOGENIC SOMATIC SYMPTOMS

Psychogenic somatic symptoms, hypnotically induced somatic symptoms, the hypnotic state per se, and emotion are intimately and repeatedly interrelated on psychological grounds and perhaps on neurological grounds as well. This accumulated evidence, however, although it does strengthen the case for a particular involvement of the right hemisphere in the mediation of unilateral psychogenic somatic symptoms, does not indicate the particular mechanism involved.

There is Galin's (1974) suggestion that the primary process and the unconscious mental contents are located in the right hemisphere, predisposing the left side of the body, but this hypothesis has shortcomings. One is the widespread disavowal in modern psychoanalysis of those biological concepts that Freud devised as general psychological principles, or "metapsychology." Many modern Freudian psychoanalysts (Gill and Holzman, 1976; Klein, 1976; Schafer, 1976) are interested in jettisoning these aspects of the theory (e.g., the primary process) and consolidating psychoanalysis around the data and ideas that arise directly from clinical material. For many other psychoanalysts, who would describe their orientation as interpersonal or existential, the rejection of metapsychology is so intrinsic that it is no longer considered remarkable enough to require explicit statement (e.g., Sullivan, 1940, 1953; Fromm, 1941, 1947; May *et al.*, 1958; Fromm-Reichmann, 1959; Binswanger, 1963; Thompson, 1964; Farber, 1966; Levenson, 1972, 1979; Wolstein, 1981). This is not to say that the idea of the primary process, for example, is not useful, but it is an idea, not a fact, and not even an idea that psychoanalysts themselves agree on. Moreover, even if the primary process is accepted as an idea, it is an unacceptable reification to suggest that it has a physical location, and, of course, this reification does not specify the mechanism involved. How does the right hemisphere carry out its task?

It is probably wise to keep specific psychoanalytical propositions and neuropsychology separate for the time being. The task for psychoanalysis is to identify those conditions of experience and motivation under which particular neurological mechanisms come into play. The understanding of that twilight in which the self somehow sets off neural events (Popper and Eccles, 1977) awaits a future day.

Although a neuropsychological description of etiology may not be possible, there does seem to be enough evidence to offer a speculative neuropsychological hypothesis of mechanism. The hypothesis is presented in two parts: (*a*) a hypothesis specific to psychogenic somatic symptoms and (*b*) a general hypothesis, of which the specific one is a part.

The specific hypothesis is derived from an observation familiar in the psychiatric literature. Fetterman (1940), describing psychosomatic problems of the back, stated it lucidly:

> In all diseases, symptoms are more than the expression of a pathologic process, they represent the mental elaboration of sensations bombarding the brain. The mind may filter out some of the sensations, ignore them, or set them aside. Or, the mind is capable of selecting certain impulses and, by attention to them, increasing their significance tremendously. Symptoms become important to the degree to which they reach the foreground of consciousness and according to the interpretation which the mind places on them. A fundamental characteristic of neurotic illness is the tendency to concentrate upon internal processes and to interpret such processes in an unhappy, often magnified manner. Introspection interposes a distorting lens on the mind's eye, which is capable of enlarging sensations manifoldly (Reprinted by permission of the publisher from Fetterman, J. L. (1940). Vertebral neuroses. *Psychosom. Med.* **2**, 265–275. Copyright 1940 by the American Psychosomatic Society, Inc. p. 268].

Very simply, the specific hypothesis states that sensations reaching the right hemisphere—those from the left side of the body—are more likely to be interpreted in an "unhappy" or "magnified" way than sensations reaching the left hemisphere. In Fetterman's terms it is the right hemisphere that "interposes a distorting lens on the mind's eye." On the basis of the hypothesis that weakness, paralysis, tics, and tremors are due to distortion of proprioceptive input (Whitlock, 1967), this same "distortion" account can be applied to motor symptoms. Loss of sensory function, too, is meant to fall under the rubric of *distortion of input*. One might describe the emotional influence in these cases more as a "muffling" effect than as an "embroidery," as in pain.

The key word in this hypothesis is *interpretation*. The idea specifically excludes dysfunction of the right hemisphere and leaves open the possibility of there being unconscious meaning in the production of psychogenic somatic symptoms. As the general hypothesis clarifies, the production of these symptoms is conceptualized as the adaptation of a normal and automatic neuropsychological mechanism to the service of (unspecified) psychological purposes.

One immediate prediction from this hypothesis would be that, despite the subjective absence of function, cortical responses to stimulation should remain unaffected in individuals with psychogenic somatic symptoms. Whitlock (1967) has reviewed evidence indicating that, in hysterical anesthesia, cortical evoked potentials in most instances do remain unchanged. A second prediction would be that, since the symptom is a matter of interpretation of input and not lack of capacity, there might be conditions under which it could be shown that capacity is intact. Clinically, such evidence is commonplace, the psychogenically blind patient who consistently avoids obstacles in his path, for example. Moreover, in the laboratory, Sackeim *et al.* (1979) have been collecting evidence that, in the case of psychogenic blindness, visual processing can occur independently of awareness of visual representation. That unimpaired underlying capacity can coexist with impaired functioning without necessarily implying malingering is another clinical commonplace, but Sackeim's program of research constitutes the beginning of an experimentally based understanding of how this can be so.

4. A GENERAL HYPOTHESIS: EMOTIONAL INFLUENCE ON SOMATIC INPUT FROM THE LEFT SIDE

Part of Whitlock's (1967) neuropsychiatric theory of hysteria and those of other writers as well (Kennedy, 1940; Kretschmer, 1960; Henderson and Batchelor, 1962; Jaspers, 1963) is that the tendency to develop psychogenic somatic symptoms is an exaggeration of mechanisms that we all have. Whitlock presents Jaspers's point of view that "the hysterical mechanism" is present in all people to one degree or another. It may be dominant in one person's adaptation to stress, whereas in others it appears only at times of the greatest stress or organic dysfunction. Whitlock (1967) himself wrote, "If this view is correct, one would need to consider the possibility that the hysterical symptom is a behavior pattern based upon some inherent quality of structure and function of the central nervous system [This and subsequent quotes from Whitlock, 1967, are reprinted from Whitlock, F. A. The aetiology of hysteria. *Acta Psychiatr. Scand.* **43**, 144–162. Copyright © 1967 Munksgaard International Publishers Ltd., Copenhagen, Denmark. p. 146]."

The general hypothesis to be put forward here is a speculation about this "inherent quality." The proposition is that, in all of us, because the right hemisphere has a special role in emotionality, the *experience* of somatic input reaching the right hemisphere is likely to be affected by moods and feelings. The experience of somatic input reaching the left hemisphere is less likely to be affected in this way. In this view, the predominance of left-sided psychogenic somatic symptoms is a particularly dramatic manifestation of a more pervasive phenomenon.

If emotional influence on somatic input from the left side is a general phenomenon as well as a psychiatric one, it ought to be observable in normal subjects, and in some way in patients with brain damage. There do exist suggestive data for both these groups that are at least consistent with this line of speculation.

One piece of evidence (Fleminger *et al.,* 1980; Section III,B) is that, in normal subjects, the left side is particularly amenable to the development of hypnotically induced somatic symptoms. If we say, as the researchers and practitioners cited earlier have said, that hypnosis is an affect-laden procedure, then it is not a long jump to the conclusion that hypnotically induced symptoms are emotionally mediated. Furthermore, as might be expected on the basis of the present hypothesis, psychiatric patients with left-sided psychogenic symptoms (i.e., those patients posited to be especially prone to affective coloring of left side sensation) show the most consistent left-sided hypnotic response.

A second piece of suggestive evidence is an incidental finding in a study by Wolff and Jarvik (1964) that correlations between pain thresholds were consistently lower in the left hand than in the right hand. That is, in the left hand the relation of stimulus to pain was more variable. (The difference between the correlations was nearly the same for all the pain-inducing techniques but reached statistical significance for only the technique for which *N* was large.)

One interpretation here is that, in the right hand (left hemisphere), the experience of pain is closely related to the actual information arriving on the afferent nerves, and so correlations between various pain thresholds are relatively high. In the left hand, however, the relationship between the experience of pain and the information encoded in the neural impulse is mediated by the current emotional state, resulting in lower correlations between thresholds. Of course, Wolff and Jarvik's finding, particularly because of its incidental nature, is merely suggestive, as is this interpretation of it, but the finding does suggest a direction for future research. If pain thresholds were taken in both hands before and after an unpleasant emotional experience, the correlation between the two thresholds should be higher in the right hand than in the left. Such a finding would support the notion of an ongoing, everyday role for right hemisphere emotionality in the experience of somatic sensation.

Morgenstern's (1964) data on chronic, severe pain in unilateral amputees, otherwise somewhat mysterious, might be understood according to the distortion hypothesis. All of his subjects had experienced severe physical and emotional trauma, but it was primarily those with left-sided amputations who experienced chronic, severe pain. The findings might be conceptualized as follows. Chronic, severe postamputation pain with no organic basis is a neurotic coping reaction to the loss of a limb. The success of Morgenstern's (1964) distraction technique in eliminating pain, his descriptions of some patients' seeming reluctance to lose their pain, and the general high level of neuroticism among the high-pain patients are all consistent with this notion. Those with left-sided amputations were most able (or prone) to adopt this solution, magnifying or distorting the left-sided sensations. Those neurotic patients with right-sided amputations were more likely to be forced to find other ways of adapting themselves to the trauma.

Among brain-damaged patients the phenomenon that may be related to the hypothesis under discussion is the clinical neurological symptom of *anosognosia*, or denial of illness. Patients with this symptom show dramatic denial of paresis and paralysis, among other disabilities, and take the classic hysterical attitude of *la belle indifference* to their incapacity. If asked to raise the paralyzed arm, for instance, they may cheerfully raise the nonparalyzed arm, feeling that they have accomplished the task and sensing no contradiction. Anosognosia is more common in patients with right hemisphere damage than in patients with damage restricted to the left hemisphere (Babinski, 1914; Critchley, 1953; Weinstein and Kahn, 1955; Weinstein *et al.*, 1964; Weinstein and Friedland, 1977; Cutting, 1978).

Goldstein (1939), Sandifer (1946), Schilder (1950), and Weinstein and Kahn (1955) emphasized a motivational component in anosognosia—the wish to deny the physical impairment—and also stressed the continuity of this defensive posture with the mechanism of denial seen in normal people. Assuredly, paralysis, like amputation, is an emotionally traumatic event of the first order. If the right hemisphere is damaged, perhaps its "language of emotion" can be disinhibited, leading to a kind of "fluent aphasia" of feeling. If this were to happen, the tendency of the right hemisphere to influence the experience of somatic sensation according to the current emotional state might be exaggerated even more than in patients with psychogenic somatic symptoms. The input from the limb, rather than being merely influenced, might actually be invented.

The proposal of right hemisphere emotional influence on left-sided somatic sensation coincides with most earlier conceptualizations. It suggests, with Gainotti (1972; see also Chapter 8), that sensation in the right hemisphere "retains . . . rich affective value." However, whereas Gainotti suggests that sensation is laden with affect in its "pristine" state, losing it through conceptual elaboration, the present account emphasizes the role of the right hemisphere in *adding* affective meaning to sensations. Like Edmonds' (1947) view, the distortion account agrees (metaphorically, if not anatomically) that "the merely thalamic expression of emotion has more access to the left side [p. 47]." The hypothesis also coincides with Galin (1974), substituting emotionality for primary process but retaining an important role for psychological events occurring outside awareness. Finally, the hypothesis is consistent with clinical description, and it links, on a neurological level, phenomena that have long been thought to be psychologically related. As Frankel (1978) wrote regarding the high degree of hypnotizability of several patients with psychogenic somatic symptoms:

> It is difficult to ignore the strong likelihood that the mental mechanism underlying this ability is involved in the development and maintenance of

> their symptoms, which [like their experience under hypnosis] comprised essentially altered or distorted perceptions of bodily sensations, . . . a fixed preoccupation from time to time with those perceptions, and inability to register or disregard any contradicting logic [p. 667].

Perhaps this description captures, in exaggerated form, a right hemisphere process common to us all. Who has not had the experience, even if momentary, of exaggerating and focusing attention on a physical discomfort that is clearly insignificant in retrospect?

References

Agnew, D. C., and Merskey, H. (1976). Words of chronic pain. *Pain* **2**, 73–81.

Axelrod, S., Noonan, M., and Atanacio, B. (1980). On the laterality of psychogenic somatic symptoms. *J. Nerv. Ment. Dis.* **168**, 517–525.

Babinski, J. (1914). Contribution à l'étude des troubles mentaux dans l'hémiplégie organique cérébrale (Anosognosie). *Rev. Neurol.* **27**, 845–848.

Bakan, P. (1969). Hypnotizability, laterality of eye movement, and functional brain asymmetry. *Percept. Mot. Skills* **28**, 927–932.

Bakan, P. (1971). The eyes have it. *Psychol. Today* **4**, 64.

Bakan, P., and Strayer, F. E. (1973). On the reliability of conjugate lateral eye movements. *Percept. Mot. Skills* **36**, 429–430.

Bakan, P., and Svorad, D. (1969). Resting EEG alpha and asymmetry of reflective lateral eye movements. *Nature (London)* **223**, 975–976.

Bannister, R. (1973). "Brain's Clinical Neurology," 4th ed. Oxford Univ. Press, London.

Bear, D. M., and Fedio, P. (1977). Quantitative analysis of interictal behavior in temporal lobe epilepsy. *Arch. Neurol. (Chicago)* **34**, 454–467.

Binswanger, L. (1963). "Being-in-the-World: Selected Papers." Basic Books, New York.

Bishop, E. R., Mobley, M. C., and Farr, W. F. (1978). Lateralization of conversion symptoms. *Compr. Psychiatry* **19**, 393–396.

Blau, A. (1946). The master hand. *Am. J. Orthopsychiatr. Assoc. Monogr.* **5**.

Bobbit, R. A. (1958). The repression hypothesis studied in a situation of hypnotically induced conflict. *J. Abnorm. Soc. Psychol.* **56**, 204–212.

Bogen, J. E. (1969). The other side of the brain. II. An appositional mind. *Bull. Los Angeles Neurol. Soc.* **34**, 135–162.

Boland, E. W., and Corr, W. P. (1943). Psychogenic rheumatism. *JAMA, J. Am. Med. Assoc.* **123**, 805–809.

Brenman, M., and Gill, M. M. (1947). "Hypnotherapy: A Survey of the Literature." International Universities Press, New York.

Breuer, J., and Freud, S. (1893–1895). Studies in hysteria. *In* "Standard Edition of the Complete Psychological Works of Sigmund Freud" (J. Strachey, ed.), Vol. II. Hogarth Press, London, 1955.

Briquet, P. (1859). "Traité clinique de thérapeutique de l'hystérie." Ballière et Fils, Paris.

Brodman, K., Erdmann, A. J., Lorge, I., Wolff, H. G., and Broadbent, T. H. (1951). The CMI-health questionnaire. *JAMA, J. Am. Med. Assoc.* **145**, 152.

Chertok, L. (1975). Hysteria, hypnosis, psychopathology. *J. Nerv. Ment. Dis.* **161**, 367–378.

Corballis, M. C. (1980). Laterality and myth. *Am. Psychol.* **35**, 284–295.

Critchley, M. (1953). "The Parietal Lobes." Arnold, London.

Cutting, J. (1978). A cognitive approach to Korsakoff's syndrome. *Cortex* **14**, 485–495.

Day, M. E. (1964). An eye movement phenomenon relating to attention, thought, and anxiety. *Percept. Mot. Skills* **19**, 443–446.

Day, M. E. (1967). An eye-movement indicator of individual differences in the physiological organization of attentional processes and anxiety. *J. Psychol.* **66**, 51–62.

Dimond, S. J., and Farrington, L. (1977). Emotional response to films shown to the right or left hemisphere of the brain measured by heart rate. *Acta Psychol.* **41**, 255–260.

Dimond, S. J., Farrington, L., and Johnson, P. (1976). Differing emotional responses from right and left hemisphere. *Nature (London)* **261**, 690–692.

Domhoff, G. W. (1969–1970). But why did they sit on the king's right in the first place? *Psychoanal. Rev.* **56**, 586–596.

Dubois, P. (1909). "The Psychic Treatment of Mental Disorders." Funk & Wagnalls, New York.

Duke, J. (1968). Lateral eye-movement behavior. *J. Gen. Psychol.* **78**, 189–195.

Edmonds, E. P. (1947). Psychosomatic non-articular rheumatism. *Ann. Rheum. Dis.* **6**, 36–49.

Ellenberger, H. F. (1970). "The Discovery of the Unconscious." Basic Books, New York.

Engel, G. (1970). Conversion symptoms. *In* "Signs and Symptoms: Applied Pathologic Physiology and Clinical Interpretation" (C. M. MacBryde and R. S. Blacklow, eds.), pp. 650–658. Lippincott, Philadelphia, Pennsylvania.

Eysenck, H. J. (1964). Eysenck Personality Inventory: The measurement of personality: A new inventory. *J. Indian Acad. Psychol.* **1**, 1.

Fallik, A., and Sigal, M. (1971). Hysteria—the choice of symptom site. *Psychother. Psychosom.* **19**, 310–318.

Farber, L. H. (1966). "The Ways of the Will: Essays toward a Psychology and Psychopathology of Will." Basic Books, New York.

Fenichel, O. (1945). "The Psychoanalytic Theory of Neurosis." Norton, New York.

Ferenczi, S. (1926). "Further Contributions to the Theory and Technique of Psychoanalysis." Brunner/Mazel, New York, 1980.

Fetterman, J. L. (1940). Vertebral neuroses. *Psychosom. Med.* **2**, 265–275.

Fleminger, J. J., McClure, G. M., and Dalton, R. (1980). Lateral response to suggestion in relation to handedness and the side of psychogenic symptoms. *Br. J. Psychiatry* **136**, 562–566.

Frankel, F. H. (1978). Hypnosis and related clinical behavior. *Am. J. Psychiatry* **135**, 644–668.

Fromm, E. (1941). "Escape from Freedom." Farrar & Rinehart, New York.

Fromm, E. (1947). "Man for Himself." Rinehart, New York.

Fromm-Reichmann, F. (1959). "Psychoanalysis and Psychotherapy: Selected Papers." Univ. of Chicago Press, Chicago, Illinois.

Frumkin, L. R., Ripley, H. S., and Cox, G. B. (1978). Changes in cerebral hemispheric lateralization with hypnosis. *Biol. Psychiatry* **13**, 741–750.

Gainotti, G. (1972). Emotional behavior and hemispheric side of lesion. *Cortex* **8**, 41–55.

Galin, D. (1974). Implications for psychiatry of left and right cerebral specialization. *Arch. Gen. Psychiatry* **31**, 572–583.

Galin, D. (1976). Hemispheric specialization: Implications for psychiatry. *In* "Biological Foundations of Psychiatry" (R. G. Grenell and S. Gabay, eds.), Vol. I, pp. 145–176. Raven Press, New York.

Galin, D. (1977). Lateralization and psychiatric issues: Speculations on development and the evolution of consciousness. *Ann. N.Y. Acad. Sci.* **299**, 397–411.

Galin, D., Diamond, R., and Braff, D. (1977). Lateralization of conversion symptoms: More frequent on the left. *Am. J. Psychiatry* **134**, 578–580.

Gazzaniga, M. S. (1970). "The Bisected Brain." Appleton, New York.

Gill, M. M., and Brenman, M. (1959). "Hypnosis and Related States." International Universities Press, New York.

Gill, M. M., and Holzman, P., eds. (1976). "Psychology vs. Metapsychology: Psychoanalytic Essays in Memory of George S. Klein," Psychol. Issues, Vol. 36. International Universities Press, New York.
Gilles de la Tourette (1981). "Traité clinique et thérapeutique de l'hystérie." Plon-Nourrit, Paris.
Goldstein, K. (1939). "The Organism: A Holistic Approach to Biology Derived from Pathological Data on Man." American Book Co., New York.
Gur, R. C., and Gur, R. E. (1974). Handedness, sex, and eyedness as moderating variables in the relation between hypnotic susceptibility and functional brain asymmetry. *J. Abnorm. Psychol.* **83**, 635–643.
Halliday, J. L. (1937). Psychological factors in rheumatism: A preliminary study. Part II. *Br. Med. J.* **1**, 264–269.
Halliday, J. L. (1941). The concept of psychosomatic rheumatism. *Ann. Intern. Med.* **15**, 666–677.
Halliday, J. L. (1949). Psychosomatic medicine: A new outlook. *Surgo.* **15**, 69–72.
Hécaen, H., and Angelergues, R. (1963). "La cécité psychique." Masson, Paris.
Henderson, D., and Batchelor, I. R. C. (1962). " A Textbook of Psychiatry," 9th ed. Oxford Univ. Press, London.
Hertz, R. (1960). "Death and the Right Hand." Free Press, Glencoe, Illinois.
Hilgard, E. R. (1977). "Divided Consciousness: Multiple Controls in Human Thought and Action." Wiley, New York.
Hilgard, E. R., Morgan, A. H., and Macdonald, H. (1975). Pain and dissociation in the cold pressor test: A study of hypnotic analgesia with "hidden reports" through automatic key pressing and automatic talking. *J. Abnorm. Psychol.* **84**, 280–289.
James, W. (1890). "The Principles of Psychology." Holt, New York.
Janet, P. (1901). "The Mental State of Hysterical: A Study of Mental Stigmata and Accidents." Putman, New York.
Janet, P. (1907). "The Major Symptoms of Hysteria." Macmillan, New York.
Jaspers, K. (1963). "General Psychopathology." Univ. of Chicago Press, Chicago, Illinois.
Kampmann, R., and Kuha, S. (1975). Hypnoanalytic case study of conversion symptoms. *Psychiatr. Fenn.* **28**, 173–176.
Kennedy, A. (1940). Recent hysterical states and their treatment. *J. Ment. Sci.* **86**, 988–1019.
Kenyon, F. E. (1964). Hypochondriasis: A clincial study. *Br. J. Psychiatry* **110**, 478–488.
Klein, G. S. (1976). "Psychoanalytic Theory: An Exploration of Essentials." International Universities Press, New York.
Kretschmer, E. (1960). "Hysteria, Reflex, and Instinct." Philosophical Library, New York.
Levenson, E. A. (1972). "The Fallacy of Understanding." Basic Books, New York.
Levenson, E. A. (1979). Language and healing. *J. Am. Acad. Psychoanal.* **7**, 271–282.
Levitt, E. E., and Chapman, R. H. (1979). Hypnosis as a research method. *In* "Hypnosis: Developments in Research and New Perspectives" (E. Fromm and R. E. Shor, eds.), 2nd ed., pp. 185–215. Aldine Publ. Co., New York.
Ley, R. G. (1980). An archival examination of an asymmetry of hysterical conversion symptoms. *J. Clin. Neuropsychol.* **2**, 61–70.
London, P., Hart, J., and Leibovitz, M. (1968). EEG alpha rhythms and hypnotic susceptibility. *Nature (London)* **219**, 71–72.
London, P., Cooper, L. M., and Engström, D. R. (1974). Increasing hypnotic susceptibility by brain wave feedback. *J. Abnorm. Psychol.* **83**, 554–560.
Luria, A. R. (1932). "The Nature of Human Conflicts." Livewright, New York.
Magee, K. R. (1962). Hysterical hemiplegia and hemianesthesia. *Postgrad. Med.* **31**, 339–345.
May, R., Angel, E., and Ellenberger, H. F., eds. (1958). "Existence." Basic Books, New York.
Merskey, H. (1965). The characteristics of persistent pain in psychological illness. *J. Psychosom. Res.* **9**, 291–298.

Merskey, H., and Buhrich, N. A. (1975). Hysteria and organic brain disease. *Br. J. Med. Psychol.* **48**, 359–366.
Merskey, H., and Spear, F. G. (1967). "Pain: Psychological and Psychiatric Aspects." Baillière, London.
Merskey, H., and Trimble, M. (1979). Personality, sexual adjustment, and brain lesions in patients with conversion symptoms. *Am. J. Psychiatry* **136**, 179–182.
Morgan, A. H., McDonald, P. J., and Macdonald, H. (1971). Differences in bilateral alpha as a function of experimental task, with a note on lateral eye movements and hypnotizability. *Neuropsychologia* **9**, 451–469.
Morgan, A. H., Macdonald, H., and Hilgard, E. R. (1974). EEG alpha: Lateral asymmetry related to task and hypnotizability. *Psychophysiology* **11**, 275–282.
Morgenstern, F. S. (1964). Effects of sensory input and concentration on post-amputation phantom limb pain. *J. Neurol., Neurosurg. Psychiatry* **27**, 58.
Morgenstern, F. S. (1970). Chronic pain: A study of some general features which play a role in maintaining a state of chronic pain after amputation. *In* "Modern Trends in Psychosomatic Medicine" (O. W. Hill, ed.), pp. 225–245. Appleton, New York.
Nowlis, D. P., and Rhead, J. C. (1968). Relation of eyes-closed resting EEG activity to hypnotic susceptibility. *Percept. Mot. Skills* **27**, 1047–1050.
Osgood, C., Suci, B. J., and Tannenbaum, P. H. (1957). "The Measurement of Meaning." Univ. of Illinois Press, Urbana.
Pitres, A. (1891). "Leçons cliniques sur l'hystérie et l'hypnotisme." Doin, Paris.
Popper, K. R., and Eccles, J. C. (1977). "The Self and Its Brain." Springer-Verlag, New York.
Purves-Stewart, J. (1924). "The Diagnosis of Nervous Diseases." Bulter & Tamner, London.
Reyher, J. (1967). Hypnosis in research on psychopathology. *In* "Handbook of Clinical and Experimental Hypnosis" (J. E. Gordon, ed.), pp. 110–147. Macmillan, New York.
Ross, E. D. (1981). The aprosodias: Functional–anatomic organization of the affective components of language in the right hemisphere. *Arch. Neurol. (Chicago)* **38**, 561–569.
Ross, E. D., and Mesulam, M. (1979). Dominant language functions of the right hemisphere? Prosody and emotional gesturing. *Arch. Neurol. (Chicago)* **36**, 144–148.
Ross, E. D., Harney, J. H., deLacoste-Utamsing, C., and Purdy, P. D. (1981). How the brain integrates affective and propositional language into a unified behavioral function: Hypothesis based on clinicoanatomic evidence. *Arch. Neurol. (Chicago)* **38**, 745–748.
Roy, A. (1977). Cerebral disease and hysteria. *Compr. Psychiatry* **18**, 607–609.
Roy, A (1979). Hysteria: A case note study. *Can. J. Psychiatry* **34**, 157–160.
Sackeim, H. A., and Gur, R. C. (1978). Lateral asymmetry in intensity of emotional expression. *Neuropsychologia* **16**, 473–481.
Sackeim, H. A., Gur, R. C., and Saucy, M. C. (1978). Emotions are expressed more intensely on the left side of the face. *Science* **202**, 434–436.
Sackeim, H. A., Nordlie, J. W., and Gur, R. C. (1979). A model of hysterical and hypnotic blindness: Cognition, motivation, and awareness. *J. Abnorm. Psychol.* **88**, 474–489.
Sandifer, P. H. (1946). Anosognosia and disorders of body scheme. *Brain* **69**, 122–137.
Schafer, R. (1976). "A New Language for Psychoanalysis." Yale Univ. Press, New Haven, Connecticut.
Schilder, P. (1950). "The Image and Appearance of the Human Body." International Universities Press, New York.
Schnall, B. S., and Smith, D. W. (1974). Nonrandom laterality of malformations in paired structures. *J. Pediatr.* **8**, 509–511.
Slater, E. (1965). Diagnosis of "hysteria." *J. Ment. Sci.* **107,** 359–381.
Slater, E., and Glithero, E. (1965). A follow-up of patients diagnosed as suffering from hysteria. *J. Psychosom. Res.* **9**, 9–13.
Sommerschield, H., and Reyher, J. (1973). Posthypnotic conflict, repression, and psychopathology. *J. Abnorm. Psychol.* **82**, 278–290.

Spear, F. G. (1964). A study of pain as a symptom in psychiatric illness. M.D. Thesis, Bristol University.

Stephánsson, J. G., Messina, J. A., and Meyerowitz, S. (1976). Hysterical neurosis, conversion type: Clinical and epidemiological considerations. *Acta Psychiatr. Scand.* **53**, 119–138.

Stern, D. B. (1977). Handedness and the lateral distribution of conversion reactions. *J. Nerv. Ment. Dis.* **164**, 122–128.

Sullivan, H. S. (1940). "Conceptions of Modern Psychiatry." Norton, New York.

Sullivan, H. S. (1953). "The Interpersonal Theory of Psychiatry." Norton, New York.

Teitelbaum, H. A. (1954). Spontaneous rhythmic ocular movements: Their possible relationship to mental activity. *Neurology* **4**, 350–354.

Thompson, C. M. (1964). *In* "Interpersonal Psychoanalysis: Selected Papers" (M. Green, ed.), Basic Books, New York.

Weinstein, E. A., and Friedland, R. P. (1977). "Hemi-inattention and Hemisphere Specialization." Raven Press, New York.

Weinstein, E. A., and Kahn, R. L. (1955). "Denial of Illness: Symbolic and Physiological Aspects." Charles C. Thomas, Springfield, Illinois.

Weinstein, E. A., Cole, M., Mitchell, M. S., and Hyerly (1964). Anosognosia and aphasia. *Arch. Neurol. (Chicago)* **10**, 76–86.

Weintraub, M. I. (1977). Hysteria: A clinical guide to diagnosis. *Ciba Found. Symp.* **29**, 1–31.

Whitlock, F. A. (1967). The aetiology of hysteria. *Acta Psychiatr. Scand.* **43**, 144–162.

Winer, D. (1978). Anger and dissociation: A case study of multiple personality. *J. Abnorm. Psychol.* **87**, 368–372.

Wolff, B. B., and Jarvik, M. E. (1964). Relationship between superficial and deep somatic thresholds of pain with a note on handedness. *Amer. J. Psychol.* **77**, 589–599.

Wolstein, B. (1981). Psychic realism and psychoanalytic inquiry. *Contemp. Psychoanal.* **17**, 595–606.

17: Pharmacopsychotherapy and Aberrant Brain Laterality

MICHAEL S. MYSLOBODSKY and MURRAY WEINER

Psychobiology Research Unit
Department of Psychology
Tel Aviv University
Ramat Aviv, Israel

Division of Clinical Pharmacology
Department of Internal Medicine
University of Cincinnati
Medical Center
Cincinnati, Ohio

I. Introduction 447
II. What, Where, and Why? 448
III. Personality and Situational Variables in Drug Response 450
IV. Psychopharmacology of the "Artistic" and "Intellectual" Brain 453
V. Components of Brain Asymmetry 456
VI. Activity and Drug Disposition 460
VII. Pharmacopsychotherapy 465
VIII. Psychotherapy and Dissociative Experience 468
IX. Epilogue 472
References 473

I. Introduction

Whatever our private opinions of the limitations of drug therapy, and they may differ a great deal, there can be little doubt about the power of psychopharmacology and some of its achievements. There exist today agents that alter physical endurance, attention, perception, mood, intellectual functions, behavior, memory, and consciousness. The effects of these agents are relatively easy to anticipate and control, and their actions are often clearly discernible in a reasonably short time. In this new atmosphere of the chemical treatment and study of the mind, clinical psychology, an ill-defined discipline devoid of the symbols of a sophisticated modern craft, with undependable, capricious methods, evokes even more suspicion than it did in the prepsychopharmacotherapeutic era, when Hebb (1949) expressed doubts as to its value in helping the mentally ill. Clinical psychologists, no doubt, have done their best to

HEMISYNDROMES:
Psychobiology, Neurology,
Psychiatry

ISBN 0-12-512460-0

summarize the achievements of human communication, but the results of their utmost zeal have been insignificant in comparison with the impact of the broad use of pharmacotherapy. Even today those who turn expectantly to "pure" psychotherapy are bound to be disappointed if they hope to find substantial clinical benefits (Tennov, 1976). Psychotherapy is lengthy and dependent on many variables, which are difficult to take into consideration; occasionally it is dangerous. In practical terms its efforts are often futile and the results infinitesimal compared with the inconveniences it imposes and the amount of time it requires. To quote May *et al.* (1981), who conducted by far the best psychotherapy–drug medication comparison:

> There was a concomitant advantage from drug therapy in terms of the clinical, social, and psychological test criteria. Patients who had received in-hospital drug treatment reached and maintained (in some but not all respects) a better level of mental health. In general, this clinical advantage could be detected for as long as three years from admission and two years from release. On the other hand, patients who had received in-hospital individual psychotherapy without concomitant drug treatment attained a poorer follow-up clinical status, spent more time in the hospital, and generally had a less adequate follow-up social adjustment [May, P. R. A, Tuma, A. H., and Dixon, W. J. (1981). Schizophrenia: A follow-up study of the results of five forms of treatment. *Arch. Gen. Psychiatry* **38,** 776–784. Copyright 1981, American Medical Association. p. 783].

That notwithstanding, the story of psychotherapy is hardly finished.

II. What, Where, and Why?

Twenty-five years of experience with psychoactive drugs have demonstrated that drug therapy by itself is not an omnipotent tool for the management of patients. Drugs help some patients a great deal, some a little, and some not at all. Some patients who remain chronically ill in spite of intensive drug therapy do better when all drugs are withdrawn (Devis, 1975). The choice of drug remains largely an empirical matter of trial and error in spite of recent efforts to classify mental illness biochemically. In many cases it is not known why a patient given an apparently appropriate drug does not improve, or why some patients on the same medication do better than others. One reason for the uncertainty of drug response is that we still target drugs to the brain in the same shotgun fashion that physicians have for many years, with little understanding of where we want them to go or how they work. It is reminiscent of the experience of Szent-Györgyi (1957), who described his medical student lessons about potassium iodide (KI) as the universal remedy.

"Nobody knew what it did, but it did something and did something good." Students used to sum up the philosophy of treatment in a little rhyme:

If ye don't know where, what, and why,
Prescribe ye then K and I.

Psychopharmacology is still challenged by the same problem.

Psychiatrically trained experts commonly attribute the unpredictability of drug action to the individual peculiarities of personality or the complexity of a disease with multiple manifestations and therefore multiple therapeutic targets (Eysenck, 1960; Rickels *et al.*, 1964; Frostad *et al.*, 1966). Many practitioners recognized a need to look for the right drug for the right patient (Klett and Moseley, 1967). However, even with the most careful selection of both patient and drug, results can vary under the management of different therapists. The nature of the response to a drug can be a *state-dependent process,* and the nature of the therapist and his approach can influence the state of the patient. To achieve an optimal and more reproducible drug effect, should one be concerned with the induction of the right state as well as the right drug for the right patient? In practice psychotherapists seldom collaborate with clinical psychopharmacologists in a conscious effort to induce the most appropriate psychological state for maximizing drug efficacy, perhaps because there is no body of knowledge to guide such an effort. In fact, there is a tendency to consider psychotherapy and pharmacotherapy mutually exclusive. Psychotherapy is "psychological treatment of psychological problems" (Corsini, 1968) conducted by clinical psychologists, in contrast to biological therapy, which is a chemical or electrophysical intervention into physiological processes commanded by physicians. Much of the conflict in this area of the interaction of psychotherapy with drug therapy has been admirably reviewed by May (1976a,b; May *et al.*, 1981) and is not repeated here.

However, there is a possibility that a psychosocial state can increase, decrease, or distort brain reactivity to a chemical substance, suggesting that psychotherapy and psychopharmacology could operate on the same therapeutic target, playing on the same neurochemical keyboard. For instance, psychotherapy and drug treatment can induce similar changes in the activity of serum enzymes (Silbergeld *et al.*, 1975). May (1976a) referred to an important statement by Paul Hock: "Psychotherapy itself is, of course, a procedure which is as organic as the introduction of a drug, but it is not applied directly to the nervous system. It has to pass through all the filtering and defense mechanisms which shield the organism against external stimulation whereas drugs are introduced directly into the organism [p. 255]." Hence, psychotherapy and pharmacotherapy could work in harmony toward the same goal. Drug action starts at a psychological base to which drug therapists ascribe the placebo effect. To the objective pharmacotherapist the placebo effect is a nuisance that complicates the evaluation of drug action. Nevertheless, pharmacotherapy must start on that base and should attempt to build on and enhance rather than eliminate the placebo effect (Weiner, 1975). Conversely, effective psychotherapy should build on the relief offered by drugs. Psychosocial therapy is likely to be more effective if successful drug treatment makes a patient more capable of accommodating a psychotherapeutic setting. Fisher *et al.* (1964) demonstrated that patients treated with drugs in an atmosphere of scientific skepticism toward drugs did not differ in response from those who received placebo, whereas in the hands of an enthusiastic physician the same substance was superior to placebo. This example suggests that the sterile and strict atmosphere of the laboratory experiment could undo the most effective aspects of the processes of pharmacotherapeutics, whereas the enthusiasm of a physician or psychologist could add to the power of a drug.

In practice psychotherapy is more often than not conducted against the background of medication. Some systems of therapy use sedatives for abreaction or recommend the inhalation of cannabis to reduce tension, increase imagery, and enhance suggestibility. In other cases psychotherapists simply do not have any choice because their patients already use neuroleptic drugs on a regular basis or obtain various kinds of medication from time to time.

Psychotherapy may affect brain reactivity to a drug by several different mechanisms. It may alter drug disposition or the state of endogenous neurohumors with which numerous drugs compete one way or another to exert their effect on the functions of the organism. How, then, ought the drug–psychotherapy "cocktail" be mixed? What should be the components? When and how should they be administered? What recommendations can be made for the recognition and induction of the "right" psychological state of the patient in order to make him more responsive to psychopharmacology? These questions are of considerable importance for both psychopharmacology and clinical psychology. A successful attack could lead not merely to the aid of one discipline by the other, but to a merging of both disciplines into *pharmacopsychotherapy*, offering a philosophy of treating mentally disturbed people that attempts to understand and control what happens, where, and why in a unified approach based on the concept of medical, biochemical, behavioral, and emotional interdependence.

III. Personality and Situational Variables in Drug Response

There are many straightforward biochemical and peripheral physiological variables that create individual differences in response to drugs (Weiner, 1975). Beyond these variables, however, there is no doubt that personality and situational differences also influence drug response; that is, there may be what are generally referred to as drug–personality interactions or situationally "channeled" response.

In reviewing factors influencing the selectivity of drug disposition and action, Myslobodsky and Weiner (1976, 1978) discussed the capacity of some drugs to release or activate a preexisting potential for some behavioral or autonomic response, a phenomenon sometimes referred to as the *prepotent hypothesis,* which was proposed by Valenstein (1969); that is, the preexisting status determines how the response to a drug or external stimulus will be channeled. Any behavior that is within the individual's repertoire and has more than zero probability of occurrence under appropriate stimulus conditions qualifies as prepotent. In this respect prepotent behavior and Pavlovian unconditioned reflexes probably belong to the same category of responses. According to Valenstein (1969), "the prepotency may reflect the differential sensitizing influence of the internal conditions associated with specific biological needs [p. 215]."

It has been demonstrated that, during electrical stimulation of the hypothalamus, animals exhibit behaviors that resemble natural drive states. It was attractive to view the hypothalamus as a complex of different systems, each controlling a specific motivational state. Valenstein reexamined some of the conclusions based on the electrical stimulation studies. He discovered that the hypothalamus elicited behaviors involving distinct learning components. Briefly, he demonstrated that stimulation of the same site of the hypothalamus can evoke various behaviors if different goal objects were paired with the stimulation. By combining electrical stimulation with motivational stimuli based on achieving a goal object, specific behavior can be elicited. For instance, the presentation of food during electrical stimulation of the hypothalamus leads subsequently to feeding behavior in response to electrical stimulation alone. Incidentally, the same sites of the brain evoke self-stimulation behavior. However, the illusion of hypothalamic specificity for this feeding behavior may be misleading, since the observation is constantly evoked in the presence of the goal object. Animals displaying this "stimulus-bound" behavior maintain it rather steadily and do not easily change from one "prepotent" response to another when the goal object is changed. Characteristically, animals that have learned to work for food do not display feeding behavior if the food is presented in a different form. Hence, this response is stimulus specific and not directed exclusively by hunger. Valenstein (1969, 1971) suggested that stimulus-bound behavior evoked by hypothalamic stimulation is a result of environmental conditions, peculiarities of the stimulus, and the generalized nondifferentiated motivational state. These factors create a "specific mode of expression" and "channel the response." The term *canalization,* or channeling, coined by Janet, was later defined as a "process by which general motives . . .

tend, upon repeated experience, to become more easily satisfied through the action of the specific satisfier than of others of the same general class . . . [Murphy, 1947, p. 162]." According to Mowrer (1960), organisms have built-in responses and what has to be learned is "wanting" to make them.

There are numerous examples of behavior in animals and man in which baseline status influences the response to drugs and external stimuli. Amphetamine enhanced side preference and rotation in rats in the direction of their natural side and direction tendency (Glick *et al.,* 1975a). A transmitter precursor, L-dopa, was demonstrated to bring out presymptomatic problems by initiating already prepotent movement (Cawein and Turney, 1971). Penfield and Perot (1963) were able to evoke dreams and memories by stimulation of the temporal lobe only in patients who had had such experience due to epileptic activities. A drug may reinforce preexisting undiagnosed or latent disease. The concept that unfavorable psychotic reactions after the administration of psychotomimetic substances occur in individuals who already have psychotic personality features is quite old (Connell, 1958). Amphetamine, which remarkably intensifies the symptoms of schizophrenia, did not have psychotic effects in persons with affective disorders or in schizophrenics in remission (Janowsky *et al.,* 1973). Also, chlorpromazine, which alters subjective experience and behavioral effects in schizophrenic patients, has reportedly unremarkable effects in healthy individuals (Frey and Winter, 1977).

Drugs that influence the general motivational state could create behaviors that are channeled by numerous situation-dependent variables. Two social psychologists (Schachter and Singer, 1962; Schachter, 1964) demonstrated that the general emotional state created by epinephrine injection to a group of normal individuals ranged from feelings of shared joy and euphoria to anger, depending on the behavior of a confederate. The confederate, who was introduced as another subject, acted according to instruction in a euphoric or angry manner. Apparently, his behavior offered a channel for the pressure of arousal experienced in response to the administered epinephrine. The experiment also demonstrated that beliefs, expectations, and environmental stimuli can markedly affect responses to drug.

Becker (1953) wrote that novice marijuana smokers have to be introduced to a new experience by a "supervisor," who reveals the desirable effects of the drug action. This sort of "initiation" may have acted as a confounding variable in some early studies with recreational drugs [see, e.g., Ames (1958), in whose study participants were kept together in an atmosphere of expectation]. Most of these studies are of historical interest because the procedures were such as to warrant no confidence in the data presented to substantiate the assertions made.

The well-established reputation of amphetamine as a stimulant and the fact that it is commonly called "speed," contribute to the response that the drug elicits. It is amazing that some subjects studied in a double-blind design were unable to differentiate between amphetamine and barbiturates (Hurst *et al.*, 1973), and the actions of amphetamine were distinguished only by an appropriate scoring system employed with sophisticated drug takers as subjects (Martin *et al.*, 1971).

Pahnke (1970) conducted a double-blind study with 20 Christian theology students. Ten of them had been given psilocybin 1.5 hr before religious services in a chapel. An effort was made to encourage positive expectations, trust, confidence, and group support and to reduce fear of drugs, that is, to create an atmosphere "comparable to that achieved by tribes who actually use psychedelic substances in religious ceremonies [p. 152]." Most of the participants who received the drug perceived unity with the surrounding environment, sacredness, joy, blessedness, love, and peace. The only person who did not respond to the psychedelic in this experiment did not believe it possible to have a mystical experience with drugs and made an effort to demonstrate that he was right. There was a high initial score of feelings of blessedness and peace, a sense of sacredness, love, and positive attitudes toward others in the group participating in this experiment. Apparently, a preexisting psychological tendency channeled the response to psilocybin. Hence, what was thought to be a drug effect was a "delicate combination of psychological set and setting in which the drug is a *necessary* but not sufficient condition [Pahnke, 1970, p. 161]." The most embarrassing and ludicrous event seldom recalled in the professional literature is the story of "bananadine" or "mellow yellow," the hoax of the novel addictive substance contained on the inside of the banana peel. Although some users of "bananadine" reported getting high or even having visual hallucinations, these proved to be the result of suggestions and expectations based on previous experience (Fort, 1969). It seems that any chemical compound given in a certain form, at certain doses, and by certain individuals to patients with certain personalities, with a certain history and expectations, and consumed in certain cultural or social setting has a fair chance of producing certain mental symptoms.

It is puzzling that the rich experience of channeled reaction in the "drug culture" has never been exploited in designing a clinical environment for drug therapy with neuroleptics. No effort so far has been made to "initiate" patients deliberately into drug treatment with behavioral strategies.

IV. Psychopharmacology of the "Artistic" and "Intellectual" Brain

If the response to drugs depends on personality and can, in addition, be channeled by various external (environmental) and internal (organismal) events, some understanding of these factors may help us to make better predictions of the effect of a specific agent given to a specific patient. Today's pharmacokineticists have made remarkable strides in describing the elements that influence the disposition of drugs within so-called body compartments (Weiner, 1964). Now, from the other end, we seek to compartmentalize personality and behavioral aspects. One result of this search has been the anatomically based concept of *hemisphericity*, a term coined by Bogen *et al.* (1972) as a tentative structural determinant of personality.

According to a German proverb, "when two do the same thing it is not the same thing." The two hemispheres of the human brain can be likened to these proverbial two. They both deal with the same problems but they deal with them differently. When a chimeric picture is flashed to the left hemisphere (right visual field) of a split-brain patient, he can correctly name the person whose image is projected, but he only points to the image when it is projected to the left visual field (Levy *et al.*, 1972). If the picture of an object is presented tachistiscopically to the right or left hemisphere, each hemisphere can find a match to the picture. However, in the search for the match the right hemisphere is guided by the similarity of shapes ("artistic" cues), whereas the left hemisphere operates analytically, identifying functionally relevant links between the objects (Levy and Trevarthen, 1976). The hemisphericity hypothesis of personality implies that operations of the normal brain may be determined by the ratio of the artistic-to-analytical style, as conjured by Pavlov long ago. Pavlov (1928) related individual behavior to the interrelations between excitatory and inhibitory processes in the central nervous system. Equilibrium between excitation and inhibition and the strength and mobility of both processes were considered to be the basic qualities that, after being mixed in different proportions, allowed for the reconstruction of the four types of human temperament of the Hippocratic scheme. This scheme was used to describe the "types of the nervous system" of dogs as well as human beings. In the final years of his life Pavlov turned to another dimension of personality characterizing human behavior in a verbal environment. He defined individuals relying predominantly on the logical, rational, verbal, analytical strategy as *thinkers*, and persons employing predominantly holistic, *gestalt*, emotional, synthetic style as *artists*. "Artists comprehend reality as a whole, as continuity, as complete living reality without any divisions, without any separations. The other group, the thinkers, pull it apart, kill it, so to speak, making out of it a temporary skeleton and then only gradually putting it together anew [Pavlov, 1941, p. 113]."

This approach to the study of personality offered a more agreeable language to those who felt that rigorous physiological vernacular was inappropriate and certainly premature as a foundation for psychology and psychiatry. However, an exploration of the differences between the two cognitive styles revealed that intellectual versus artistic strategy in the solution of everyday problems coordinated well with the two strategies of the neurochemically distinct cerebral hemisphere. Rossi and Rosadini (1967) discovered that intracarotid amobarbital injections elicited different emotional reactions depending on the side of injection in 42% of their subjects. In most cases the initial response to left side injection was a depressive reaction, whereas that to right side injections was euphoria. However, a few subjects showed the opposite effect, and in several subjects emotional reactions to right side injection contained both depression and euphoria. The authors concluded that the hemispheric specialization for mood and emotion appears to be independent of a dominance of one hemisphere over the other.

It was later demonstrated that intracarotid doses of amobarbital that were adequate to cause loss of consciousness when the injection was made into the speech-dominant hemisphere caused loss of consciousness only rarely and for short periods after injection into the nondominant hemisphere, leading to the conclusion that consciousness is generally linked with the function of the hemisphere dominant for speech [Serafetinides *et al.*, 1965]. Phenothiazines, administered orally, reduced inwardly and outwardly directed hostility (Gottschalk, 1969). In most patients phenothiazine treatment markedly improved speech and thinking, helped to relieve pressure, and allowed thoughts "to settle down" (Haase and Janssen, 1965). Myslobodsky *et al.* (Chapter 14) have interpreted their findings as suggesting that neuroleptics alter right hemisphere reactivity most significantly. It is of interest that, generally, right hemisphere functions seem to be especially vulnerable to drugs. A mean blood alcohol concentration of 0.09% selectively reduced visual evoked potentials over the right central area (Lewis *et al.*, 1969). Miglioli *et al.* (1979) and Jenkins and Parsons (1979) also provided evidence consistent with a conjecture that the right hemisphere is disproportionately sensitive to alcohol. Marijuana smoked at moderate doses caused selective slowing of responses to pictorial stimuli presented to the right hemisphere, whereas reactions to verbal stimuli were slowed equally when presented to either the right or left hemisphere (Stillman *et al.*, 1977).

The left hemisphere seems to be involved primarily in the response to the stimulant amphetamine, which increases verbal activity and performance in numerical tasks (Laties and Weiss, 1967) and produces euphoria, feelings of friendship, and cooperation (Bradley, 1950; Laties, 1961). Addicts prefer the use of amphetamine-type stimulants in groups, when the social (left) hemisphere is more active. In contrast, the color hallucinations and bright sensory illusions associated with the psychotic state produced by mescaline points to right hemisphere involvement and may be described as disphoric (Longo, 1972).

It is of interest that amphetamine, which induces elevation of mood and alertness in young normal men, caused drowsiness, annoyance, sadness, and anger when administered in a small dose (0.15 mg/kg, iv) to normal postmenopausal women (Halbreith *et al.*, 1981). This puzzling finding may be related to the inhibitory effects of estrogens on dopaminergic activity (see Chapter 5 for review) interacting with the lateralized mechanism responsible for mood. Mintz and Myslobodsky (Chapter 10) suggested that a relatively higher incidence of left-sided hemi-Parkinsonian symptoms among female patients is associated with a higher vulnerability of right hemisphere dopaminergic activity to estrogens. Since the action of estrogens is similar to that of neuroleptics, estrogens may cause dopamine (DA) receptor hypersensitivity, which is especially visible after estrogen withdrawal, that is, during menopause. It is tempting to attribute the atypical reactions to amphetamine reported by Halbreith *et al.* to supersensitive DA receptors in the mesolimbic neurons of the right ("emotional") hemisphere.

V. Components of Brain Asymmetry

At one time the asymmetric effects of "mind-altering" drugs were related to asymmetries of neurotransmitter systems (Myslobodsky and Weiner, 1976). Since Glick *et al.* (1975a) discovered an imbalance of DA in the nigrostriatal system in rats, the list of lateralized neurotransmitters has grown considerably (see Table 17.1). Oke *et al.* (1978) found that norepinephrine is strongly lateralized in the human thalamus. The pulvinar is richer in norepinephrine on the left side, whereas the somatosensory input area shows higher neurotransmitter concentration on the right. Thalamic right–left asymmetry of norepinephrine has also been noted in the rat (Oke *et al.*, 1980).

Mandell and associates found an asymmetric representation of serotonin (Knapp and Mandell, 1980). Lithium and chlorimipramine differentially altered hemispheric asymmetries of the serotonin precursor tryptophan, serotonin itself (5-HT), and 5-hydroxyindoleacetic acid, a product of 5-HT catabolism by monoamine oxidase.

Starr and Kilpatrick (1981) reported that following the inhibition of brain γ-aminobutyric acid (GABA) catabolism with either intracisternal ethanolamine *O*-sulfate or intraperitoneal aminoxyacetic acid, the elevation in brain GABA levels was asymmetric. The GABA concentration was consistently higher in the substantia nigra, superior colliculus, and nucleus accumbens on the right side and in the ventral tegmentum, ventromedial thalamus, and caudate on the left. The globus pallidus showed no lateral asymmetry. Rossor *et al.* (1980) found no evidence of neurotransmitter asymmetry in the human brain except for a small but consistent increase in nigral GABA level on the left side. A year later,

TABLE 17.1
Neurochemical Components of Brain Laterality

Component	Evidence[a]	Subjects	Reference
1. Asymmetry of enzyme activity	Larger amount of copper (DBH?) in the left hemisphere	Human	Delva (1960), cited in Petelin (1970)
	Choline acetyltransferase activity enhanced in the left temporal lobe	Human	Amaducci *et al.* (1981)
	Higher zinc concentration in left hippocampus	Long–Evans rat	Valdes *et al.* (1982)
2. Asymmetry of transmitter systems	Asymmetry of NE in the thalamus	Human; rat, strain unspecified	Oke *et al.* (1978, 1980)
	Striatal DA imbalance	Sprague–Dawley rat	Glick *et al.* (1975a), Robinson *et al.* (Chapter 5)
	5-HT asymmetry in the midbrain	Male Sprague–Dawley, rat	Knapp and Mandell (1980)
	Brain GABA asymmetry (see component 4)	Male Wistar rat	Starr and Kilpatrick (1981)
	GABA R–L differences in the substantia nigra	Human	Rossor *et al.* (1980)
	Increased uptake of NE, 5-HT, and choline into the right hippocampus in the sinistral rat	Male Long–Evans rat	Valdes *et al.* (1981)

(*Continued*)

TABLE 17.1 (*Continued*)

Component	Evidence[a]	Subjects	Reference
3. Asymmetries related to hemisphere connection	Striatal ACh asymmetry induction and increase in the striatal DA asymmetry after the section of callosal fibers	Female Sprague–Dawley rat	Glick *et al.* (1975b)
	Interdependence in the nigrostriatal DA system	Cat, both sexes	Nieoullon *et al.* (1977, 1978)
4. Regional asymmetries in different directions	NE: L > R for the pulvinar and R > L for the somatosensory input area	Human	Oke *et al.* (1978)
	Multiple metabolic asymmetries	Sprague–Dawley rat	Glick (Chapter 2)
	GABA: R > L for the nigra, superior colliculi, n. accumbens; L > R for the ventral tegmentum, ventromedial thalamus, caudate	Male Wistar rat	Starr and Kilpatrick (1981)

[a] Abbreviations: DBH, dopamine β-hydroxylase; NE, norepinephrine; DA, dopamine; GABA, γ-aminobutyric acid; 5-HT, serotonin; ACh, acetylcholine; L, left; R, right.

however, Amaducci *et al.* (1981) noted enhanced choline acetyltransferase activity in the left temporal lobe. This area was not examined by Rossor *et al.*

Data concerning the relations of various transmitter systems and their ratios in the two hemispheres are practically nonexistent. Glick *et al.* (1975b) reported that sectioning of the corpus callosum in rats unveils an asymmetry of striatal acetylcholine along with an increase in striatal DA asymmetry. Given that more than 200 putative neurotransmitters or neuromodulators (amines, amino acids, peptides, and corresponding enzymes) may theoretically participate in mediating asymmetric responses, it is clear that the complexity of lateralized transmitter systems is only beginning to show its contours.

It should be noted that rational psychotherapy would require a more profound knowledge of the excitatory and inhibitory machinery determining the "laterality balance" in normal individuals and in psychotics than is currently available. There are a number of tentative mechanisms that can lead to the overall increase in activity in the lateralized circuits: (*a*) excessive synthesis and availability of an excitatory transmitter; (*b*) increased mobilization and the number of quanta of the transmitter per nerve impulse; (*c*) prolonged neurotransmitter action due to blockade of the inactivation system (faulty uptake and/or defective destructive enzymes); (*d*) subsensitivity of autoreceptors; (*e*) enhanced sensitivity of the postsynaptic membrane (lowered membrane potential, shortened recovery cycle, etc.); and (*f*) the development of spike-generating capacity in dendrites. The inclusion of these mechanisms is justified by circumstantial evidence that can be found for most of them in the literature on rotating rodents or the neurophysiology of lateralized epileptogenic lesions. It is clear that a more detailed and fragmented list could be compiled. In addition, it could be supplemented by factors leading to inhibitory (within- and between-hemisphere) effects, mechanisms of energy generation, etc.

Whenever a new transmitter system is described, someone speculates that an imbalance of the system might be helpful in understanding the pathophysiology of aberrant behavior and effects of drug treatment. However, few reliable data on medication-related shifts of neurotransmitter balance are currently available. Two studies reporting lateralized side effects of neuroleptic treatment deserve special attention.

Rudenko and Lepakhin (1979) noted the development of an extrapyramidal hemisyndrome in 85 patients after medication with major tranquilizers. Signs of asymmetry in muscular tone were detected within 2 to 3 days of treatment in 48 right-handed patients. Forty-two of these showed left-sided motor abnormality, and in 6 extrapyramidal symptoms were seen on the right side. This peculiar result was attributed to dormant organic pathology, which supposedly was revealed by medication.

No data on treatment protocols or drug doses and no neurological or psychiatric profiles were provided.

Unlike Rudenko and Lepakhin (1979), Waziri (1980) reported greater right- than left-sided dyskinesia in patients after long-term usage of large doses of neuroleptics. This was interpreted as indicating selective vulnerability of the left hemisphere. As useful and interesting as Waziri's study may be, it does unfortunately have design errors. First, in his small sample of eight patients, four were diagnosed as manic–depressives. This subgroup, as well as one patient with a hysterical personality, are believed to have a pattern of "hemispheric balance" dissimilar to schizophrenia (Flor-Henry, 1969, 1972) and may be expected to have a different pattern of drug distribution (Myslobodsky and Weiner, 1976; see also Chapter 14). Had Waziri used a more homogeneous group of patients, a different side of dyskinetic symptoms might have been found. Second, neuroleptics of different types, including antidepressive medication, given in different combinations, can be expected to have different effects. However, there was no mention of the medication administered. Third, the patients had movement disorders at the time of admission. It is possible that lateralized neuroleptic abnormality was present before, and aggravated during, medication. Fourth, the abnormal movements were assessed during a 3-min interview and were not videotaped. Unpublished findings by L. P. Taylor (personal communication) indicate that in schizophrenic patients the left side may more often display extrapyramidal symptoms after neuroleptic medication, suggesting that the right hemisphere is more vulnerable to neuroleptic medication, contrary to the conclusion of Waziri but consistent with that of Mintz *et al.* (1982) and Myslobodsky *et al.* (Chapter 14).

VI. Activity and Drug Disposition

It is axiomatic that (*a*) the effect of a drug is dependent on the amount or concentration of drugs at the critical target sites, rather than the levels measured in the blood; (*b*) drugs rarely act on a single mechanism, area, or system; (*c*) at different doses of a drug, qualitatively different responses may be generated.

Since the safety margin of many drugs is rather narrow, it would obviously be of great value if one could increase the tissue concentration of a chemical substance to more effective levels at the desired site of action without producing a corresponding increase in its concentration at other receptor sites associated with undesirable actions. Changes in several functional systems of the organism can alter drug disposition, adding to the unpredictability of drug action. Generally, slowing metabolism or excretion unselectively enhances the likelihood of toxic effects equivalent to an increase in dose. Patients' noncompliance in taking prescribed doses of medicine may be a psychological consequence of the fear of undesired effects. Some psychiatrists attempt to reduce this fear by treating patients with a once-per-day dosage (Ayd, 1974), generally at bedtime. It is recommended that most single doses be given at night because the peripheral side effects associated with peak blood levels (dry mouth, orthostatic hypotension, blurred vision, etc.) might be prohibitive during the day but tolerated during sleep at night.

Some findings, not necessarily related to laterality, show time-dependent physiological differences in responses to drugs. The effect of a difference in the sensitivity of the two hemispheres around the clock has yet to be explored by chronopharmacologists. Weise *et al.* (1980) conducted a study comparing two dosage schedules of amitriptyline (once daily at bedtime versus three times daily) in nonpsychotic depressed outpatients. The side effects of medication were essentially the same, but improvement with a single dose was significantly superior. There is a possibility that the time of drug administration gives the right hemisphere, implicated in emotional disorders (Flor-Henry, 1979; see also Chapter 7), preferential exposure to the drug. Menon *et al.* (1980) showed that there is an inverse relationship between power of rhythms below 13 cycles per second (δ, θ, and α) and blood flow through gray matter. Since the right hemisphere lags slightly behind the left in slow-wave sleep development and therefore has a relatively reduced electroencephalographic (EEG) power (Myslobodsky, 1976; Myslobodsky *et al.*, 1977), one can predict that right hemisphere regional blood flow would be enhanced. Sakai *et al.* (1980) reported that right hemispheric regions have greater flow reduction from awake values than left regions during stage IIa and greater flow increases from sleep stage IV to stage IIb.

Unfortunately, in other studies referred to by Weise *et al.* (1980) using the same protocol favorable results were not obtained with a single bedtime dose of antidepressants. It has been reported that, in depressed patients, a single bedtime dose schedule increased the incidence of night terrors (Flemenbaum, 1976). This notwithstanding, one must consider when the single dose is given and what the hemispheric activity pattern is like at the time of exposure to the peak concentration of drug. In this way drugs can be deliberately targeted to the pathophysiologically justified region of the brain. In any event drug–local activity interaction is important to consider because psychotropic drugs themselves can significantly alter brain circulation (Sari *et al.*, 1975), thereby altering their own distribution.

Theoretically, the effect of a chemical compound at a particular target can be deliberately altered by manipulating the metabolic activity of the region in question. Indeed, the local fate of a drug is temperature and energy dependent, and the state of receptors is governed by local electrolyte and pH conditions. Thus, the excitation or inhibition of a brain area induced by a wide variety of stimuli due to a change of environment or psychotherapy could help to open or close the "gates" to the receptor sites. It has been demonstrated that sensory stimuli induce metabolic changes in the specific sensory system. McElligott and Melzack (1967) employed localized measurements of brain temperature as an indirect indicator of local metabolic activity. The thermal response is considered to be a result of local neural metabolism and concomitant change in the local cerebral microcirculation. The writers discovered that low-frequency light stimulation (2–12 Hz) produced a temperature increase, whereas high-frequency flickering light (52–62 Hz) or steady light decreased the temperature of the lateral geniculate nucleus. Auditory stimuli also produced a localized temperature increase in the inferior colliculus. Photic stimulation or auditory stimulation can lead, in accordance with theoretical expectations, to the selective accumulation of labeled (S^{35}) sulfate in the visual cortex and the lateral geniculate. Auditory stimulation produced a corresponding increase in the penetration of the material into the inferior colliculus of the cat's brain (Roth, 1965). Glassman (1974) reported that H. Rahmann kept adult carp in darkness for 10 days before injecting them intraperitoneally with [^{3}H]histidine. One eye was then exposed to light for 15 min, following which the fish were killed and autoradiograms of histological sections through optic tecti were prepared. The density of grains over the exposed (contralateral) tectum was greater than that over the nonstimulated tectum, demonstrating that the local fate of systemically injected [^{3}H]histidine was activity dependent. Manipulating the metabolic state of the brain can direct an agent more to one region than the other.

The old electrophysiological literature suggested that brain tissue can be conceived of as a complex structure with different metabolic rates in various parts of the brain under different functional states. New techniques for the measurement of regional cerebral blood flow made it possible to visualize this spatial heterogeneity of brain metabolism under different experimental and clinical states. Although the vascular system tends to distribute chemical substances randomly to various receptor sites, which may be widely represented in various brain areas serving different functions, the flow to the various sites may differ measurably with the nature of the subject's activity. Such a simple maneuver as vigorous hand exercise was shown to affect regional cerebral blood flow in the area corresponding to cortical representation of the working hand, with little or no effect in the area of the other hand (Olesen, 1971; Ingvar, 1975a). There was no associated change in systemic blood pressure, and intravenous infusion of angiotensin to increase pressure caused no local flow changes. Electrical stimulation of the thumb area also gave a moderate increase in blood flow in the corresponding area. Painful stimulation of the thumb appeared to affect cerebral metabolism markedly (Ingvar, 1975a).

An increase of blood flow in the occipital region in awake human beings was also observed by Olesen (1971) during flicker stimulation. He used several scintillation detectors spaced over the cranium and coupled to a computer to determine regional cerebral blood flow by measuring the clearance of radioactive ^{133}Xe gas from segments of cerebral tissue. Characteristic patterns of the regional blood flow ("rCBF landscape," as Ingvar calls it) were demonstrated. In awake subjects resting in a supine position, maximal flow values were found over premotor and frontal regions. In schizophrenic patients the landscape was "hypofrontal," that is, devoid of the predominance of the blood flow in the premotor and frontal areas seen in normal subjects. In older and more psychotic patients this hypofrontality was more marked (Ingvar, 1975b).

Ingvar (1975b) described the major rCBF landscapes typical for a nonpsychotic population and found that talking and reading, visual problem solving, and analytical tasks resulted in peculiar regional flow distributions. He concluded that augmentation of blood flow "reflects more or less regional functional (metabolic) accompaniment to mentation" and that "islands" of activity can be identified by techniques that are sensitive enough to measure regionally (Risberg and Ingvar, 1968).

Since there is recognized asymmetry of activity and reactivity of the cerebral hemispheres in normal waking individuals, one would anticipate that the ^{133}Xe technique, which detects differences in regional blood flow, might also detect interhemispheric differences. Indeed, such differences were observed by Risberg *et al.* (1975). A small predominance of the blood flow in the left hemisphere was apparent in the resting state. With a visual task, blood flow increased in the right hemisphere predominantly in frontal and parietal areas whereas, with a verbal task, maximal flow was noted in the parietooccipital and temporal region of the left hemisphere corresponding to the Wernicke speech area. The verbal task, unlike spatial ones, led to a more general activation of the blood flow. It has been demonstrated by Risberg *et al.* (1982) that drugs may alter the right–left asymmetry of rCBF.

Lassen *et al.* (1977) showed that, when subjects pressed a spring between finger and thumb, the corresponding primary sensory and motor areas showed increased blood flow. In the supplementary motor area blood flow increased bilaterally. When subjects were asked merely to imagine movements, bilateral response of only the supplementary motor area remained.

An *in vivo* assessment of brain metabolism has been developed by Sokoloff (1977). His method is based on a "deception" of the active transport system for glucose to carry the "inedible" compound, 2-[^{14}C] deoxyglucose across the blood–brain barrier. The metabolite of this com-

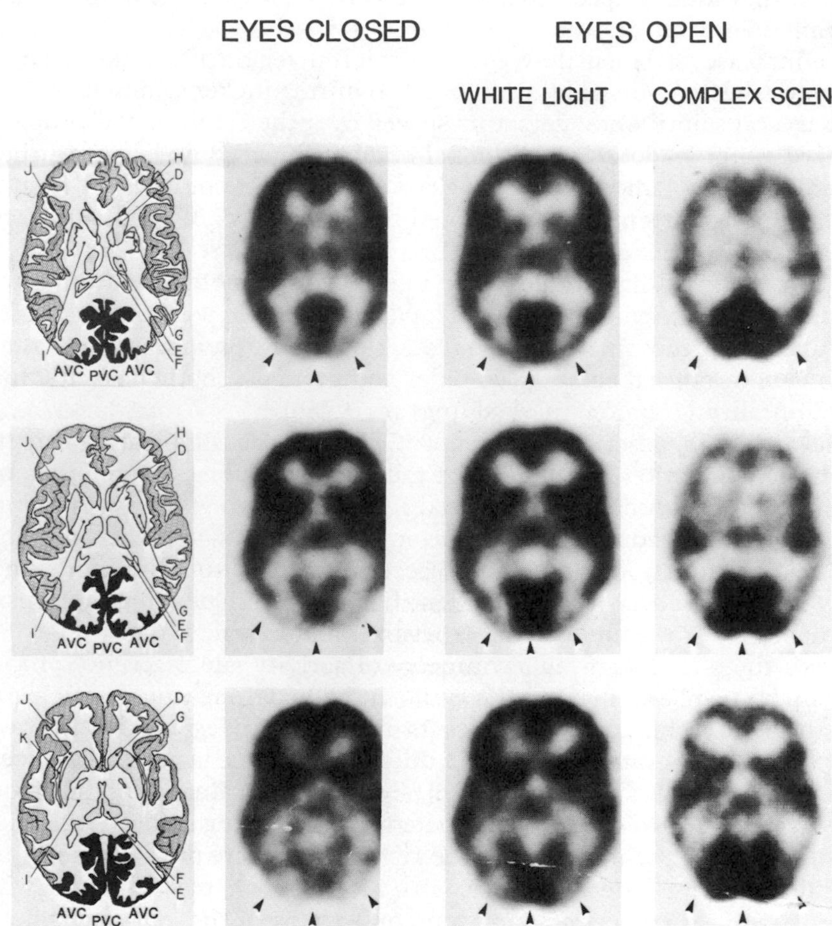

FIG. 17.1. Example of an eyes-closed control and visual stimulation with white light. Subject's left is to the reader's left, and the increasing gray scale is proportional to the glucose metabolic rate, black being the highest. Three levels containing the visual cortex at 4.4, 3.6, and 2.8 cm above the orbital–meatal plane are shown. The sketches at the left were made from actual brain slices to illustrate some of the cerebral structures at the cross-sectional levels of the tomographic study. D, Head of the caudate nucleus; E, thalamus; F, posterior horn of lateral ventricle; G, putamen and globus pallidus; H, anterior horn of lateral ventricle; I, internal capsule; J, external capsule; K, claustrum; PVC, primary visual cortex; AVC, associative visual cortex. Adapted from Phelps *et al.* (1981), with the kind permission of the authors.

pound (2-deoxyglucose-6-phosphate) accumulates at a rate reflecting activity-induced glucose utilization and remains trapped at these sites of activity. Subsequent autoradiography visualizes the tracer and indicates the local glucose asymmetries in the "metabolic landscape," including significant left–right differences of glucose utilization in the striatum, midbrain, hippocampus, and frontal cortex of the rat. This method has been adapted for use in positron-computed tomography (PCT) to assess with high precision the rate constants for 2-[^{18}F]fluoro-2-deoxyglucose. A study by the UCLA team (Phelps *et al.*, 1981) showed that it is possible to detect in the visual cortex changes of local glucose metabolism in response to simple attention tasks similar to those often employed in psychobiology. Figure 17.1, obtained through the courtesy of J. Engel, Jr., a collaborator in this project, illustrates the possibilities of the method.

VII. Pharmacopsychotherapy

The obvious objective of psychopharmacology is to administer psychotropic agents that control or alleviate symptoms of mental disease. Practitioners who use drugs developed by psycho- or neuropharmacologists are concerned with drug absorption but seldom consider influencing drug distribution after the drug passes into the bloodstream. The word *pharmacopsychology* or *pharmacopsychotherapy* as used here is to be distinguished from the generally recognized discipline of behavioral pharmacology. Pharmacopsychology is concerned with the influence of the basic psychological state of the patient and the numerous environmental variables that help to determine behavior on the efficacy of a centrally active drug. Pharmacopsychological therapy can be defined as active manipulation of environmental factors to help achieve a psychological state that will contribute to a more desirable drug distribution or response while the drug is in the body.

Today a patient commonly asks his physician if he should take a prescribed drug before or after meals. Medical research people go to great pains to evaluate the many influences that timing in relation to food intake may have on the physiological disposition and the effect of drugs, and physicians are prepared to advise their patients in this regard. However, patients rarely ask whether they should take a medicine before or after attending a concert, watching a television show, reading a book, or talking with a friend. If they did ask such a question, the most likely answer would be that it does not matter. Some day, however, a rigorous control of stimuli around the time of peak exposure to a drug could prove to be as important as dosage or duration of the treatment. Among pharmacotherapists there is a strong interest in the relationship between drug action and the state of the responding organism. One need only review the program of the Second International Symposium on Drugs as Discriminative Stimuli (Bierce, Belgium, June 30–July 3, 1982) to see the extent of this interest. The program was involved with what is called internal stimulus control of behavior and its relation to drug action, and its topics included animal and human studies on state dependency, neurochemical and neurophysiological attributes of drug and stimulation-produced discriminative stimuli, and identification of nervous system sites in drug administration.

It is unfortunate that psychotherapists are doing so little to evaluate the usefulness of controllable influences on the disposition and response to drugs. In an earlier review of mechanisms that influence drug reactivity, Myslobodsky and Weiner (1976) formulated a concept of *activity-directed drug distribution,* which postulates that the selective manipulation of functional states may be an effective means of achieving a more desirable drug disposition and reactivity. The influence of directed thought is exemplified by the Risberg *et al.* (1975) studies of regional brain–blood flow described earlier. They were conducted in two groups of subjects. One group was given no special motivation, and the results were variable and nonsignificant. The second group was offered additional money as a reward for good performance. In these motivated subjects the interhemispheric differences in blood flow were much more consistent and reached statistical significance. It is tempting to speculate that manipulation of the environment to activate one or the other hemisphere deliberately will reinforce the drug effect on either the left or the right cerebral hemisphere, as desired. When one reads that amphetamine increases feelings of friendliness (Laties, 1961), whereas others working in the same area report that it leads to aggressive, violent behavior (Lemere, 1966), it is not necessary to conclude that one report is wrong. The disagreement or paradoxical results could well be explained by the differences in the psychosocial or physical environment that existed during medication.

When a therapist treats two patients with reactive depression, provoked by a traumatic visual experience in one and associated with a verbal insult in the other, his basic therapeutic approach is very likely to be the same for both patients. However, the etiological differences suggest an opportunity for selective psychotherapy based on the hemisphere primarily involved in the processing of the traumatic situation. Will treatment be more successful if the therapist takes advantage of this opportunity? How might he do it? The ancient Galen recommended the "principle of opposites" in looking for a potential drug. When a drug caused constipation, it was thought to be a good remedy for diarrhea. Hahnemann held the opposite view. His theory of homeopathy was based on the claim, *similia similibus curantur* ("Like cures like"). He treated constipation with small ("homeopathic") doses of chemical substances that produced constipation. One might find this historical example amusing. However, it invokes a legitimate question: whether the psychotherapeutic approach to those two hypothetical patients should employ the principles of similarity or of opposites. No answer to this question is yet available. Oddly enough, we do not focus attention on the philosophy of treatment nearly as much as we do on the techniques of treatment.

We are often told, and we are inclined to agree, that theories and schools are of secondary value in psychotherapy. The personality of the therapist is thought to be more important than his techniques (Truax and Mitchell, 1971). This belief is reminiscent of Schopenhauer's dictum that the patient is the way in which the psychotherapist sees him. In fact, a theory that requires standard and rigorous treatment is seen as a handicap to the concept of individualized approach.

Although the mystery of therapist–patient interaction is an important part of the thrills of psychotherapy, it has led in practice to a bewildering variety of individual therapeutic styles, making scientific evaluation of psychotherapeutic factors virtually impossible. In 1959 Lacey proposed that some order be established in the lush overgrowth of psychotherapeutic systems using psychophysiological measurements of therapist–client interaction. Alpert *et al.* (1980) employed lateral EEG measurements to assess individual listening styles of young psychotherapists. The result, albeit highly preliminary, was promising. The therapist's sensitivity (defined as the number of concern-related clues detected in the tape-recorded patient's monologue) was significantly correlated with EEG asymmetry, suggesting relatively more right hemisphere involvement when sensitivity was greater. If replicated, this study may open the way to a reassessment of the circumstances under which current techniques address themselves to right or left hemisphere cognitive strategies, as well as the depth to which they utilize the patient's intellectual capacity, logic and linguistic ability or his imagination, emotions, or intuition. It is an interesting exercise to review some of the classical approaches to the understanding and psychological treatment of emotional disturbance in terms of the anatomical site of the problem and the therapeutic influence, bearing in mind that verbal–analytical activity is primarily of the left hemisphere, and sensory emotional imagery, of the right hemisphere. Some theories proceed from the Adlerian assumption that emotions are secondary events created by the patient's incorrect concepts. The essence of will-training procedures or the rational–emotional system of Albert Ellis, for instance, could be best summarized with a paradox of the James–Lange type: We speak wrongly not because we are mad; we are mad because we speak and think wrongly. This implies that therapists should look for ways to modify the patient's style of thinking and structure of language in order to improve his behavior and increase his ability to attain social success in our verbal culture. Verbal–analytical techniques, which have been recognized since Freud, remain to this day a dominant psychotherapeutic vehicle. However, therapies based on imagery that stimulate fantasies, encourage synthetic–*gestalt* approach, and enrich sensory–emotional content of environment are not less important for helping the mentally ill (Shorr, 1974). Psychodrama or implosive therapy also evokes patients' spontaneity, emotionality, aggression, spatial orientation, and social interaction. In fact, implosive therapy requires a patient with a poor imagination to participate in a real situation rich in anxiety-eliciting stimuli. Comparing Moreno's and Rogers's procedures, Corsini (1968) wrote that Rogers's nondirective therapy "is intended to create an Apollonian type of individual: kind, reserved, considerate. In contrast, Moreno's psychodrama is intended to create a Dionysian type of person: aggressive, spontaneous, and uninhibited [p. 1112]."

There is no single template by which to measure the degree of imagery versus analytical load in a given technique. Nor is there an understanding of when various techniques could or should be employed. Special work is needed to "translate" old techniques using the neuropsychological vernacular acceptable for the assessment of "hemisphericity."

Several examples similar to that undertaken by Stern (Chapter 16) are likely to serve as a launching pad for further trials in this area. Rossi (1977) made an attempt to neurologize some of Jung's fundamental concepts, relating them to research on hemispheric specialization. His contribution was supplemented by provocative comments by Henry (1977). Barcai (1971) found interesting differences between poor and good drug responders. The peculiarities of personality shown in clinicians' ratings of nine personality characteristics suggest different hemisphericity in good and poor responders. Louks *et al.* (1976) indicated that patients with deficits in left hemispheric functions tend to score in the psychotic range, whereas right hemispheric patients tend to score in the neurotic range of the Minnesota Multiphasic Personality Inventory (MMPI). Although the relation between lateralized deficits and MMPI neurotic versus psychotic states was moderate, these writers admitted that "the real significance of this finding is in the heuristic value it has in understanding the functions of the two hemispheres in terms of personality organization [p. 658]." Research on the roles of the right and left hemispheres in personality organization is embryonic, and this is the best time to look for new techniques. To paraphrase Sechrest (1968), these new tests are not likely to be measurably worse. They would not have to be remarkable to be better.

VIII. Psychotherapy and Dissociative Experience

The words of a therapist, like physical stimuli, can be attended to or ignored depending on the patient's state of consciousness, mood, expectations, and previous experience. Whatever the therapeutic system, all practitioners are bothered by the same questions: does the therapeutic session have an impact on the patient, and when, to what extent, and for how long?

The phenomenon of consciousness in the topographic theory of Freud is organized by attention, which, like the mythological Janus, keeps one eye on outward sensations and the other on inner experience. The pertinent portion of Webster's definition of *attention* refers to its connection with a perceptual receptivity, whereas *perception* is defined through "physical sensation as interpreted in the light of experience." In other words, attention is seen as being strongly connected to previous events. This connection not only triggers attention and alters its intensity, but provides appropriate "tags" when channeling the stimuli to storage, thereby facilitating its subsequent retrieval. Stimuli that are not attended to may also be stored in memory but unaccompanied by retrieval-relevant cues. We have not the foggiest idea as to where and how this information is "sedimented" and, for lack of a more accurate address, the residence of this stored-to-be-forgotten experience can be assigned to the realm of the "system Ucs" of Freud. This amazing trait of holding undistilled, almost untouched, all sensory and emotional experience disregarded by consciousness can lead to the accumulation of sufficient material to equip another personality with a different role but with a comparable degree of self-completeness and continuity.

There are rare cases known as syndrome de Fregoli, possession, ideas of presence, and multiple personalities, when the alter ego emerges on the stage showing different emotional, cognitive, and sensory experiences with various degrees of awareness of the parallel self. There may be more of these cases than we think. Sensations of presence or possession may be encountered in confusional states, exhaustion, the hypnagogic state, schizophrenia, epilepsy, brain lesions, etc. "The patient may be reluctant to volunteer the information; the neurologist in his ignorance may neglect to inquire for it, or to record it if mentioned. Consequently we are apt to regard it as a rare phenomenon, though perhaps unjustifiably so [Critchley, 1979, p. 3]." We must admit that in dealing with some of these isolated or uncorroborated cases there is a fair possibility of error. However, some of these cases, even if unique, may serve as a source of insight with which to analyze the enigma of the "neurochemical pentagram" with which the dissociative experience is sealed.

Since drugs are also known to alter perception, mood, and states of consciousness, experience under the influence of a drug may not necessarily be psychologically relevant or even retrievable in the nondrug state. Animals trained while under drug treatment may show little or no evidence of conditioning when in a drug-free state (see Ho *et al.*, 1977). Until recently it was not clear whether, in humans, learning and memory can be disrupted by aberrant profiles of neurotransmitter activity to the same extent as by drug experience. Weingartner and associates have collected evidence that storage and retrieval of verbal information in manic–depressive patients are mood- and treatment-dependent processes (Henry *et al.*, 1973; Weingartner *et al.*, 1977). In another study, in which alcohol was employed to alter the state during learning or retrieval of to-be-remembered low- and high-imagery words, Weingartner (1977) showed that high-imagery stimuli are less likely to be affected by state barriers. Weingartner (1977) insightfully observed that state-dependent effects may be associated with nonhomogeneous disruption of brain functions when one hemisphere is more altered by a disease or drugs than the other: "Within this [*lateralized,* M. M. & M. W.] system, input may be seen stored and retrieved not only less effectively but qualitatively differently than would be the case if the brain functioned normally [p. 375]."

Dissociative experience was reproduced by Sperry and Gazzaniga (1967), who showed that a picture of a nude flashed to the right hemisphere of a split-brain patient evoked a sneaky grin, although the patient was unable to give a reason for this response. Gazzaniga (1970) described a patient who seemed to shift to a more violent personality whenever his right hemisphere took control over behavior. According to Mesulam (1981) dissociative states more often develop in patients whose predominant EEG abnormality is in the nondominant temporal lobe. Schenk and Bear (1981) also noted that activation of the right temporal lobe is associated with ego-alien experiences, although they reported bilateral EEG abnormalities rather than clear pathology for either hemisphere. Sometimes a change from one personality to the other would result in a change not only in voice, experience, and habits but also in handedness, suggesting a real change of hemisphere dominance (Mesulam, 1981; Schenk and Bear, 1981).

Given this evidence it is likely that psychotherapeutic experience, like verbal learning, is encoded, recalled, and retrieved in a state-dependent (dissociation-prone) manner. This conjecture implies that psychotherapeutically induced strategies even leading to visible benefits may be only temporary and not necessarily reelicited or not easily accessible in a nonhospital or nondrug state, so that the efforts of the therapist may be later evaluated as futile. In experimental situations overtraining could cause learned responses to generalize across the barriers of state dependency (Bliss, 1972). Psychotherapy hardly is and should not be dependent on overtraining since we hardly understand when and under what circumstances state dependency has to be inhibited or facilitated, when it acts as a friend and when it is a foe. It is worth considering that disappointing or even negative effects of psychotherapy given alone or in a drug environment (May, 1976b; May *et al.*, 1981) have been associated with drug-induced or psychopathology-related dissociative barriers that may render psychotherapeutic intervention useless. We have to learn how to provide the medicated patient with sufficiently powerful retrieval cues of previously stored desirable behavioral strategies. Only under the assumption that all psychological factors, state dependency included, are rationally controlled could one share the optimism of Max Fink (1976) that "by using combined pharmacologic and psychological therapies it is possible to predict the type of linguistic, mood, perceptual, and attitudinal changes occasioned by specified changes in brain function, and to select appropriate psychoactive substances to enhance the adaptations regarded most useful by the therapist [p. 82]."

A current problem that extends even beyond the serious concern of drug–psychotherapy interaction is the question of drug-induced anterograde amnesia. An earlier generation of obstetricians were highly impressed with the value of "twilight sleep" induced by the combination of morphine and scopolamine in the painfully laboring woman. A major component of this treatment was the amnesia that it induced, leaving the mother with little or no recollection of the travails of childbirth. Today both the oral surgeon and his patient are grateful for rapidly acting intravenous benzodiazepines, not simply because of their relaxing and analgesic potentiating action, but also because of the patient's amnesia for the unpleasant experience of oral surgery. It is not unusual for a conscious, responsive patient undergoing a second procedure under a benzodiazepine to comment that the present procedure is lasting much longer than the first. Later, however, his memory no longer makes this distinction.

There is some concern about anterograde amnesia with potent, orally effective, short-acting benzodiazepine derivatives. A traveler who was having trouble sleeping reported the following scenario. Finding himself wide awake at 3 a.m. with an important day ahead, he swallowed a normal dose of short-acting benzodiazepine and promptly fell into a satisfying sleep. He awoke refreshed and went about his business. The following evening, when he tried to record the day's business activities, he could remember having met people but could not recall what was discussed and what conclusions were reached.

Sleep laboratory studies documented a distinct anterograde amnesia for nocturnal activities that subjects performed in an apparently fully awake status while under the influence of lorazepam (Scharf and Jacoby, 1982). How serious anterograde amnesia can be during psychotherapy, and how common and severe it is with sedatives in general and individual benzodiazepine derivatives in particular, remain to be determined. There is an intriguing possibility that asymmetric hemispheric characteristics, and particularly a disruption of hemispheric communication via the corpus callosum, might be involved in drug-induced anterograde amnesia.

IX. Epilogue

The future may teach us to exercise a direct influence, by means of particular chemical substances, on the amount of energy and their distribution in the neural apparatus.

—SIGMUND FREUD (1938)

The objective of this chapter has been to alert clinical psychologists, psychiatrists, and drug therapists to the potential of a coordinated approach to the treatment of the mentally ill. We are convinced that clinical psychologists can share responsibility and, with appropriate training, can make valuable contributions to chemotherapy. We find ourselves in full agreement with Devis (1975), who pointed out that "since patients can receive psychological therapies and drug therapies jointly . . . it is a false dichotomy to think of one versus the other [p. 1244]." In fact, clinical psychologists have always had that opportunity. The concept of psychotherapeutically channeled drug disposition simply elaborates the reality. It also reminds us that psychotherapy conducted in the chemical environment at random could be randomly salubrious or harmful. Unwittingly, the therapist could reinforce right hemispheric activity in a situation in which more emphasis should be laid on improving the activity and reactivity of the left brain. Influencing the results of drug treatment without giving another drug presents an intriguing challenge to clinical pharmacology. Clinical psychopharmacology could only benefit by combining its efforts with clinical psychology in a study of different variables affecting the disposition of chemical substances in the brain. Over two decades ago, Eysenck (1960) pointed out that "without such symbiosis both general psychology and psychopharmacology would be the poorer [p. 334]." The mission of psychotherapy is to translate into reality an old dream of physicians to develop a magic method for targeting a desirable substance into the desired site of action. A fictional situation presented with wit by Reiss (1974) illustrates this point:

> The year is 1987. . . . The scene is a dimly lit room on a research ward for study of schizophrenic patients at the Massachusetts General Hospital. Fate and science have rewarded a selfless worker as they never do in real life: Professor Emeritus has just discovered the twisted molecule that causes chronic schizophrenia (acute schizophrenia had been established as definitely of environmental origin 5 years before). Moreover, he and a large group of relative youngsters have developed a specific drug for untwisting the molecule and a set of sophisticated electronic gear for monitoring the untwisting process (to be marketed commercially as Monotwist). The Professor Emeritus is about to give the drug to the first patient, Mr. Brown. Mr. Brown is hooked up to Monotwist. A dozen colleagues crowd around the patient in the small room. The injection is given. All eyes are on Monotwist. The signals on the oscilloscope are unmistakable. The molecules

> are untwisting. Precisely on schedule, all systems indicate the molecules are completely untwisted. The colleagues are ready to burst into a loud cheer but, to a man, they catch themselves as they note that the Professor Emeritus' face still appears grim and concerned. Only he realizes that the biggest step in the entire research program has been omitted, and he sees clearly what he must do. Quietly and compassionately, he turns to the patient and says "Mr. Brown, how do you feel?"
>
> The way this question is posed and how its answer is understood will determine whether all that came before was worth the bother [p. 10].

We are sympathetic with the lesson of this story. However, if Professor Emeritus had bothered to ask this and related questions earlier, not only might he have had some answers in advance, but this conversation could have helped him to accelerate the process of untwisting schizophrenic molecules.

References

Alpert, M., Cohen, N. L., Martz, M., and Robinson, C. (1980). Electroencephalographic analysis: A methodology for evaluating psychotherapeutic process. *Psychiatry Res.* **2,** 323–329.

Amaducci, L., Sorbi, S., Albanese, A., and Gainotti, G. (1981). Choline acetyltransferase (ChAT) activity differs in right and left human temporal lobes. *Neurology* **31,** 799–805.

Ames, F. (1958). A clinical and metabolic study of acute intoxication with *Cannabis sativa* and its role in the mode psychoses. *J. Ment. Sci.* **104,** 972–999.

Ayd, F. J. (1974). Single daily dose of antidepressants. *JAMA, J. Am. Med. Assoc.* **230,** 263–264.

Barcai, A. (1971). Predicting the response of children with learning disabilities and behavior problems to dextroamphetamine sulfate. *Pediatrics* **47,** 73–80.

Becker, H. (1953). Becoming a marihuana user. *Am. J. Sociol.* **59,** 235–242.

Bliss, D. K. (1972). Dissociated learning and state-dependent retention induced by pentobarbital in rhesus monkeys. *J. Physiol. Psychol.* **84,** 149–161.

Bogen, J. E., DeZure, R., TenHouten, W., and Marsh, J. (1972). The other side of the brain. IV. The A/P ratio. *Bull. Los Angeles Neurol. Soc.* **37,** 49–61.

Bradley, C. (1950). Benzedrine and dexedrine in the treatment of children's behavior disorders. *Pediatrics* **5,** 24–36.

Cawein, M., and Turney, F. (1971). Test for incipient Huntington's chorea. *N. Engl. J. Med.* **288,** 504.

Connell, P. H. (1958). "Amphetamine Psychosis." Oxford Univ. Press, London.

Corsini, R. J. (1968). Counseling and psychotherapy. *In* "Handbook of Personality Theory and Research" (E. F. Borgatta and W. W. Lambert, eds.), pp. 1105–1129. Rand McNally, Chicago, Illinois.

Critchley, M. (1979),"The Divine Banquet of the Brain and Other Essays." Raven Press, New York.

Devis, J. M. (1975). Maintenance therapy in psychiatry. I. Schizophrenia. *Am. J. Psychiatry* **132,** 1237–1245.

Eysenck, H. J. (1960). Objective psychological tests and the assessment of drug effects. *Int. Rev. Neurobiol.* **2,** 333–384.

Fink, M. (1976). Presidential address. Brain function, verbal behavior, and psychotherapy.

In "Evaluation of Psychological Therapies" (R. L. Spitzer and D. F. Klein, eds.), pp. 74–86. Johns Hopkins Univ. Press, Baltimore, Maryland.

Fisher, S., Cole, J., Rickels, K., and Uhlenhuth, E. (1964). Drug–set interaction: The effect of expectations on drug response in out-patients. *Neuropsychopharmacology* **3,** 149–156.

Flemenbaum, A. (1976). Pavour nocturnus: A complication of single daily tricyclic or neuroleptic dosage. *Am. J. Psychiatry* **135,** 570–572.

Flor-Henry, P. (1969). Psychosis and temporal lobe epilepsy: A controlled investigation. *Epilepsia* **10,** 363–395.

Flor-Henry, P. (1972). Ictal and inter-ictal psychiatric manifestations in epilepsy, specific or non-specific. *Epilepsia* **13,** 773–783.

Flor-Henry, P. (1979). On certain aspects of the localization of the cerebral systems regulating and determining emotion. *Biol. Psychiatry* **14,** 677–698.

Fort, J. (1969). "The Pleasure Seekers: The Drug Crisis, Youth and Society." Grove Press, Inc., New York.

Freud, S. (1938). "An Outline of Psychoanalysis," pp. 172–182. Hogarth Press, London.

Frey, L. G., and Winter, J. C. (1977). Current trends in the study of drugs as discriminative stimuli. *In* "Drug Discrimination and State Dependent Learning" (B. T. Ho, D. W. Richards, III, and D. L. Chute, eds.), pp. 35–45. Academic Press, New York.

Frostad, H., Forrest, G., and Baker, C. (1966). Influence of personality type on drug response. *Am. J. Psychiatry* **22,** 1153–1158.

Gazzaniga, M. S. (1970). "The Bisected Brain." Appleton, New York.

Glassman, E. (1974). Macromolecules and behavior. *In* "Neurosciences: The Third Study Program" (F. O. Schmitt and F. G. Worden, eds.), pp. 667–677. MIT Press, Cambridge, Massachusetts.

Glick, S. D., Jerussi, T. P., and Fleisher, L. N. (1975a). Turning in circles: The neuropharmacology of rotation. *Life Sci.* **18,** 889–896.

Glick, S. D., Crane, A. M., Jerussi, T. P., Fleisher, L. N., and Green, J. P. (1975b). Functional and neurochemical correlates of potentiation of striatal asymmetry by callosal section. *Nature (London)* **254,** 616–617.

Gottschalk, L. (1969). The measurement of hostile aggression through analysis of speech: Some biological and interpersonal aspects. *In* "Aggressive Behavior" (S. Garattini and E. Sigg, eds.), pp. 299–316. Excerpta Medica, Amsterdam.

Haase, H. J., and Janssen, P. A. (1965). "The Action of Neuroleptic Drugs." North-Holland Publ., Amsterdam.

Halbreith, U., Asmis, G., Ross, D., and Endicott, J. (1981). Amphetamine-induced dysphoria in postmenopausal women. *Br. J. Psychiatry* **138,** 470–473.

Hebb, D. O. (1949). "The Organization of Behavior; A Neuropsychological Theory." Wiley, New York.

Henry, G. M., Weingartner, H., and Murphy, D. L. (1973). Influence of affective states and psychoactive drugs on verbal learning and memory. *Am. J. Psychiatry* **130,** 966–971.

Henry, J. P. (1977). Comment. *J. Anal. Psychol.* **22,** 51–53.

Ho, B. T., Richards, D. W., III, and Chute, D. L., eds. (1977). "Drug Discrimination and State Dependent Learning." Academic Press, New York.

Hurst, P. M., Weidner, M. F., Radlow, R., and Ross, S. (1973). Drugs and placebos: Drug guessing by normal volunteers. *Psychol. Rep.* **33,** 683–694.

Ingvar, D. H. (1975a). Patterns of brain activity revealed by measurements of regional cerebral blood flow. *Alfred Benzon Symp.* **8,** 397–413.

Ingvar, D. H. (1975b). Brain work in presenile dementia and in chronic schizophrenia. *Alfred Benzon Symp.* **8,** 478–497.

Janowsky, D. S., El-Yousef, M. K., Davis, J. M., and Sekerke, N. J. (1973). Provocation of schizophrenic symptoms by intravenous administration of methylphenidate. *Arch. Gen. Psychiatry* **3,** 195–211.

Jenkins, R. L., and Parsons, O. A. (1979). Lateralized patterns of tactual performance in alcoholics. *Curr. Alcohol.* **5,** 285–294.

Klett, C. J., and Moseley, E. C. (1967). The right drug for the right patient. *J. Consult. Psychol.* **29,** 546–551.

Knapp, S., and Mandell, A. J. (1980). Lithium and chlorimipramine differentially alter bilateral asymmetry in mesostriatal serotonin metabolites and kinetic conformations of midbrain tryptophan hydroxylase with respect to tetrahydrobiopterin cofactor. *Neuropharmacology* **19,** 1–7.

Lacey, J. I. (1959). Psychophysiological approach to the evaluation of psychotherapeutic process and outcome. *In* "Research in Psychotherapy" (E. A. Rubinstein and M. B. Parloff, eds.), Vol. I, pp. 160–208. Am Psychol. Assoc., Washington, D.C.

Lassen, N. A., Roland, P. E., Larsen, B. Melamed, E., and Soh, K. (1977). Mapping of human cerebral functions: A study of the regional cerebral blood flow pattern during rest, its reproducibility and the activation seen during basic sensory and motor functions. *Acta Neurol. Scand.* **56,** Suppl. 64, 25.16–25.17.

Laties, V. (1961). Modification of affect, social behavior and performance by sleep deprivation and drugs. *J. Psychiatr. Res.* **1,** 12–25.

Laties, V. G., and Weiss, B. (1967). Performance enhancement by amphetamines: A new appraisal. *In* "Neuro-psychopharmacologium" (H. Brill, ed.), pp. 800–803. Excerpta Medica, Amsterdam.

Lemere, F. (1966). The danger of amphetamine dependency. *Am. J. Psychiatry* **123,** 569–579.

Levy, J., and Trevarthen, C. B. (1976). Meta-control of hemispheric function in human split-brain patients. *J. Exp. Psychol., Hum. Percept. Performance* **2,** 299–312.

Levy, J., Trevarthen, C. B., and Sperry, R. W. (1972). Perception of bilateral chimeric figures following hemisphere deconnection. *Brain* **95,** 61–78.

Lewis, E. G., Dustman, R. E., and Beck, E. C. (1969). The effect of alcohol on sensory phenomena and cognitive and motor tasks. *Q. J. Stud. Alc.* **30,** 618–633.

Longo, V. C. (1972), "Mental Health Through Will-Training." Christopher, Boston, Massachusetts.

Louks, J., Calsyn, D., and Lindsey, F. (1976). Personality dysfunction and laterality deficits in cerebral functions as measured by the MMPI and Reitan–Halstead battery. *Percept. Mot. Skills* **43,** 655–659.

McElligott, J. C., and Melzack, R. (1967). Localized thermal charges evoked on the brain by visual and auditory stimulation. *Exp. Neurol.* **17,** 293–312.

Martin, W. R., Sloan, J. W., and Sapira, J.D. (1971). Physiologic, subjective, and behavioral effects of amphetamine, methamphetamine, ephedrine, phenmetrazine, and methylphenidate in man. *Clin. Pharmacol. Ther.* **12,** 245–258.

May, P. R. A. (1976a). Prologue: Paul Hock. *In* "Evaluation of Psychological Therapies" R. I. Spitzer and D. F. Klein, eds.), pp. 254–255. Johns Hopkins Univ. Press, Baltimore, Maryland.

May, P. R. A. (1976b). Rational treatment for irrational disorder: What does the schizophrenic patient need? *Am. J. Psychiatry* **133,** 1008–1012.

May, P. R. A., Tuma, A. H., and Dixon, W. J. (1981). Schizophrenia: A follow-up study of the results of five forms of treatment. *Arch. Gen. Psychiatry* **38,** 776–784.

Menon, D., Koles, Z., and Dobbs, A. (1980). The relationship between cerebral blood flow and the EEG in normals. *Can. J. Neurol. Sci.* **7,** 195–198.

Mesulam, M. M. (1981). Dissociative states with abnormal temporal lobe EEG: Multiple personality and the illusion of possession. *Arch. Neurol. (Chicago)* **38,** 176–181.

Miglioli, M., Buchtel, H. A., Campanini, T., and De Risio, C. (1979). Cerebral hemispheric lateralization of cognitive deficits due to alcoholism. *J. Nerv. Ment. Dis.* **167,** 212–217.

Mintz, M., Tomer, R., and Myslobodsky, M. S. (1982). Neuroleptic-induced lateral asymmetry of visual evoked potentials in schizophrenia. *Biol. Psychiatry* **17,** 673–686.
Mowrer, O. H. (1960). "Learning Theory and Behavior." Wiley, New York.
Murphy, G. (1947). "Personality: A Biosocial Approach to Origins and Structure." Harper, New York.
Myslobodsky, M. S. (1976). "Petit Mal Epilepsy: A Search for Precursors of Wave–Spike Discharges." Academic Press, New York.
Myslobodsky, M. S., and Weiner, M. (1976). Pharmacologic implications of hemispheric asymmetries. *Life Sci.* **19,** 1467–1478.
Myslobodsky, M. S., and Weiner, M. (1978). Clinical psychology in the chemical environment. *Psychol. Rep.* **43,** 247–276.
Myslobodsky, M. S., Ben-Mayor, V., Yedid-Levy, B., and Mintz, M. (1977). Hemisphere asymmetry of EEG and averaged visual evoked potentials during non-REM sleep. *In* "Sleep 1976" (W. P. Koella and P. Levin, eds.), pp. 295–297. Karger, Basel.
Nieoullon, A., Chéramy, A., and Glowinski, J. (1977). Interdependence of the nigrostriatal dopaminergic systems on the two sides of the brain in the cat. *Science* **198,** 416–417.
Nieoullon, A., Chéramy, A., and Glowinski, J. (1978). Release of dopamine evoked by electrical stimulation of the motor and visual areas of the cerebral cortex in both caudate nuclei and in the substantia nigra in the cat. *Brain Res.* **145,** 69–83.
Oke, A., Keller, R., Mefford, I., and Adams, R. N. (1978). Lateralization of norepinepherine in human thalamus. *Science* **200,** 1411–1413.
Oke, A., Lewis, R., and Adams, R. N. (1980). Hemispheric asymmetry of norepinepherine distribution in rat thalamus. *Brain Res.* **188,** 269–272.
Olesen, J. (1971). Contralateral focal increase of cerebral blood flow in man during arm work. *Brain* **94,** 635–646.
Pahnke, W. N. (1970). Drugs and mysticism. *In* "Psychedelics" (B. Aaronson and H. Osmond, eds.), pp. 145–165. Doubleday, New York.
Pavlov, I. P. (1928). "Lectures on Conditioned Reflexes." International Universities Press, New York.
Pavlov, I. P. (1941). "Conditioned Reflexes and Psychiatry." International Universities Press, New York.
Penfield, W., and Perot, P. (1963). Brain's record of auditory and visual experience. *Brain* **36,** 595–696.
Petelin, L. C. (1970). "Extrapyramidal Hyperkynesis." Medizina, Moscow.
Phelps, M. E., Mazziotta, J. C., Kuhl, D. E., Nuwer, M., Packwood, J., Metter, J., and Engel, J., Jr. (1981). Tomographic mapping of human cerebral metabolism: Visual stimulation and deprivation. *Neurology* **31,** 517–529.
Reiss, D. (1974). Competing hypotheses and warring factions: Applying knowledge of schizophrenia. *Schizophr. Bull.* **8,** 7–11.
Rickels, K., Ward, C., and Schut, L. (1964). Different populations, different drug responses. *Am. J. Med. Sci.* **247,** 328–335.
Risberg, J., and Ingvar, D. H. (1968). Regional changes in cerebral blood volume during activity. *Exp. Brain Res.* **5,** 72–78.
Risberg, J., Halsey, J. H., Wills, E. L., and Wilson, E. M. (1975). Hemispheric specialization in normal man studied by bilateral measurements of the regional cerebral blood flow. *Brain* **98,** 511–524.
Risberg, J., Hagstadius, S., Gustafson, L. (1982). rCBF-Measurements in the study of drug-effects. *rCBF Bull.* **3,** 56–57.
Rossi, E. L. (1977). The cerebral hemispheres in analytical psychology. *J. Anal. Psychol.* **22,** 32–51.
Rossi, G. F., and Rosadini, G. (1967). Experimental analysis of cerebral dominance in man. *In* "Brain Mechanisms Underlying Speech and Language" (C. H. Millikan and F. L. Darley, eds.), pp. 167–183. Grune & Stratton, New York.

Rossor, M., Garret, N., and Iversen, L. (1980). No evidence for lateral asymmetry of neurotransmitters in post-mortem human brain. *J. Neurochem.* **35,** 743–745.

Roth, L. J. (1965). Penetration of drugs into the brain. *In* "Monographs in Biology and Medicine," pp. 98–107. Grune & Stratton, New York.

Rudenko, G. M., and Lepakhin, V. K. (1979). The major tranquillizers. *Side Eff. Drugs Annu.* **3,** 39–58.

Sakai, F., Meyer, J. S., Karacan, I., Derman, S., and Yamamoto, M. (1980). Normal human sleep: Regional cerebral hemodynamics. *Ann. Neurol.* **7,** 471–478.

Sari, A., Fukuda, Y., Sakabe, T., Mackawa, T., and Ishikawa, T. (1975). Effects of psychotropic drugs on canine cerebral metabolism and circulation related to EEG-diazepam, clomipramine, and chlorpromazine. *J. Neurol., Neurosurg. Psychiatry* **38,** 838–844.

Schachter, S. (1964). The interaction of cognitive and physiological determinants of emotional state. *Adv. Exp. Soc. Psychol.* **1,** 49–80.

Schachter, S., and Singer, J. E. (1962). Cognitive, social and physiological determinants of emotional state. *Psychol. Rev.* **69,** 379–399.

Scharf, M. B., and Jacoby, J. A. (1982). Lorazepam—efficacy, side-effects and rebound phenomena. *Clin. Pharmacol. Ther.* **31,** 175–179.

Schenk, L., and Bear, D. (1981). Multiple personality and related dissociative phenomena in patients with temporal lobe epilepsy. *Am. J. Psychiatry* **138,** 1311–1316.

Sechrest, L. (1968). Testing, measuring and assessing people. *In* "Handbook of Personality Theory and Research" (E. F. Borgatta and W. W. Lambert, eds.), pp. 529–625. Rand McNally, Chicago, Illinois.

Serafetinides, E. A., Hoare, R. A., and Driver, M. V. (1965). Intracarotid sodium amylobarbitone and cerebral dominance for speech and consciousness. *Brain* **88,** 107–130.

Shorr, J. E. (1974). "Psychotherapy through Imagery." International Medical Book Corporation, New York.

Silbergeld, S., Manderscheid, R. W., O'Neill, P. H., Lamprecht, F., and Ng, L. K. Y. (1975). Changes in serum dopamine-beta-hydroxylase activity during group psychotherapy. *Psychosom. Med.* **37,** 352–367.

Sokoloff, L. (1977). Relation between psychological function and energy metabolism in the central nervous system. *J. Neurochem.* **29,** 13–26.

Sperry, R. W., and Gazzaniga, M. S. (1967). Language following surgical disconnection of the hemispheres. *In* "Brain Mechanisms Underlying Speech and Language" (C. H. Millikan and F. L. Darley, eds.), pp. 108–121. Grune & Stratton, New York.

Starr, M. S., and Kilpatrick, I. C. (1981). Bilateral asymmetry in GABA brain function? *Neurosci. Lett.* **25,** 167–172.

Stillman, R. C., Wolkowitz, O., Weingartner, H., Waldman, I., DeRenzo, E. V., and Wyatt, R. J. (1977). Marijuana: Differential effects on right and left hemisphere functions in man. *Life Sci.* **21,** 1793–1800.

Szent-Györgyi,A. (1957). "Bioenergetics." Academic Press, New York.

Tennov, D. (1976). "Psychotherapy: The Hazardous Cure." Doubleday-Anchor, New York.

Truax, C. B., and Mitchell, K. M. (1971). Rescarch on certain therapist interpersonal skills in relation to process and outcome. *In* "Handbook of Psychotherapy and Behavior Change" (A. E. Bergin and S. L. Garfield, eds.), pp. 299–344. Wiley, New York.

Valdes, J. J., Mactutus, C. F., and Cory, R. N. (1981). Lateralization of norepinephrine, serotonin and choline uptake into hippocampal synaptosomes of sinistral rats. *Physiol. Behav.* **27,** 381–383.

Valdes, J. J., Hartwell, S. W., Sato, S. M., and Frazier, J. M. (1982). Lateralization of zinc in rat brain and its relationship to a spatial behavior. *Pharmacol., Biochem. Behav.* **16,** 915–917.

Valenstein, E. S. (1969). Behavior elicited by hypothalamic stimulation. *Brain Behav. Evol.* **2,** 295–316.

Valenstein, E. S. (1971). Channelling of responses elicited by hypothalamic stimulation. *J. Psychiatr. Res.* **8**, 335–344.

Waziri, R. (1980). Lateralization of neuroleptic-induced dyskinesia indicates pharmacologic asymmetry in the brain. *Psychopharmacology* **68**, 51–53.

Weiner, M. (1964). The significance of the physiologic disposition of drugs in anticoagulant therapy. *Semin. Hematol.* **1** (4), 345–374.

Weiner, M. (1975). Conflicting concepts. *Chem. Technol.* **5**, 205–209.

Weingartner, H. (1977). Human state dependent learning. *In* "Drug Discrimination and State Dependent Learning" (B. T. Ho, D. W. Richards, III, and D. L. Chute, eds.), pp. 361–382. Academic Press, New York.

Weingartner, H., Miller, H., and Murphy, D. L. (1977). Mood–state-dependent retrieval of verbal associations. *J. Abnorm. Psychol.* **86,** 276–284.

Weise, C. C., Stein, M. K., Pereira-Ogan, J., Csanalosi, I., and Rickels, K. (1980). Amitriptyline once daily vs three times daily in depressed outpatients. *Arch. Gen. Psychiatry* **37,** 555–560.

Index

A

Acetylcholine, in Parkinson's disease, 79
Adenylate cyclase, dopamine stimulation, striatal asymmetry, 10
ADTN, *see* 2-Amino-6,7-dihydroxy-1,2,3, 4-tetrahydronaphthalene
Adversive epilepsy, *see* Gyratory epilepsy
Affect
 laterality, unilateral brain lesions (human), 175–189
 lateralization, model, 14
 nonverbal communication through facial expression, 182
 recognition and elaboration, right hemisphere, 188
Affective disorders
 and right hemisphere dysfunction, 396
Aging, 194–206; *see also* Hemiaging
 cognitive abilities, asymmetric decline, 194–195
Alcohol, right hemisphere sensitivity, 455
Alpha activity, and schizophrenia, 299–300
γ-Aminobutyric acid
 left-right asymmetries, brain structures (human), 21
 in Parkinson's disease, 78
 role, globus pallidus projections, 74–75
 systems, substantia nigra, 74
2-Amino-6,7-dihydroxy-1,2,3,4-tetrahydronaphthalene, 19
Amnesia, anterograde, drug induced, 471
Amobarbital, and emotional reactions, 455
Amphetamine, 47, 452
 effect on
  brain tetrahydrobiopterin levels, 340
  lateral hypothalamic self-stimulation asymmetries, 14–15
 left hemisphere response, 455
 rotation induction (animal), 9–10
Anatomical asymmetries, brain (animals), 95–96
Anosognosia, unilateral brain lesions, 178–180
Anterograde amnesia, drug induced, 471
Anticonvulsants
 gyratory epilepsy treatment, 136
Antiepileptic drugs
 and dyskinesias, 249
 role in gelastic epilepsy, 249–251
Anti-Parkinsonian drugs, assessment in rotating rodent model, 80–83
Aphasia, left hemisphere lesions (human), 93
Apomorphine, 47
 rotation induction (rat), 9
[^{3}H]Apomorphine, binding sites, striatum (rat), 18 19

Asymmetry, *see also* specific structure and function
behavior, sex differences, 91–121
brain
components, 456–460
dynamic process (human, rat), 22
sex differences, 91–121
endogenous, striatal dopamine content (rat), 10
functional, in different brain structures (rat), 12
hemisphere, and psychopathology, interaction, 216
human and animal, relationship, 119–121
kinds in different brain structure (rat), 12
lateral
clinical syndromes, delineation, 267–269
schizophrenia, 265–318
medication induced, 2
neuron circuits, 51
spatiotemporal, neurochemical locus, 338–342
Asymmetry index
electroencephalogram patterns during sleep in hemi-Parkinsonism, 217
lateral eye movements, schizophrenia, 349–350
Attention
arousal, in hemiaging, 205–206
connected to previous events, 469
divided, tasks, in hemiaging, 204
focused, and evoked potentials in schizophrenia, 304
induction of changes in P_{300}, 360–364
schizophrenia, 266
Attention-arousal defect
and indifference reaction, right brain damage, 186
and neglect syndrome, right brain damage, 186
Attitude, toward disability, unilateral brain damage, 179–180
Audiometry test, and schizophrenia, 285
Auditory
functions, and schizophrenia, 280–291
habituation, lateralization (bird), 97
Automatism, running, in cursive epilepsy, 142
Awareness, alteration with running, in cursive epilepsy, 142
Axon
developing, dynamic interactions, 53
regenerating terminals, replacement of sprouted synapses by, 50

B

Basal ganglia
and movement, initiation and control, 70
neurochemical laterality, 22
organization and outflows, and rotation model, 73–77, 84
Behavior
asymmetries, sex differences, 91–121
deficits, asymmetry, 51
disorders
and hemisphere dysfunction, 389–406
clinical evidence, 394–397
history, 389–390
modifications, and dendritic arborization, 59
motor, and striatal dopamine concentrations, 71–72
plasticity, after unilateral brain lesions, 27–59
product of interacting biological and environmental factors, 405
recovery from lesion-induced sensorimotor asymmetries, 28–29
temporal-spatial patterns, cooperative neural dynamics, 334
Benzidine dihydrochloride, 31
Benzodiazepines, and oral surgery, 471
Beta activity, and schizophrenia, 300–301
Binding sites, [^{3}H]apomorphine, striatum (rat), 18–19
Biogenic amine neurotransmitters, synthesis and binding by receptors, 329
Biosocial interaction, nature, 405
Blinking, in schizophrenia, effects of neuroleptics, 368–371
Brain, *see also* specific function and structure
artistic and intellectual, psychopharmacology, 453–456
asymmetry
components, 456–460
dynamic process (human, rat), 22
mechanisms (animal, human), 8
sex differences, 91–121
central measures of aging, 201–206

denervated structures, increased synapse formation, 48
dynamic states, 341
electrical activity, in hemi-Parkinsonism, 216–223
functions, effect of right and left hemisphere lesions, 1
laterality, *see* Laterality
lesions, unilateral
clinical aspects of emotional reactions, 177–181
laterality of affect (human), 175–189
multiple asymmetries, and developmental changes (rat), 12–13
neural changes, compensatory, 54
neurochemical laterality (human), 21–22
organization, lateralization, sex differences (human), 105, 115–117
pathology, and pathophysiology of epileptic laughter, 251–256
processes, dynamic patterns, 327–329
reactivity to
chemical substance, effect of psychosocial state, 449
drug, effect of psychotherapy, 450
structure damage in psychosis, 150
unilateral lesions
behavior plasticity after, 27–59
lateralization effects (rat), 11–12
neuron plasticity after, 27–59
rotation (animal), 8

C

Canalization, channeling response, 451–452
Catastrophic reaction, and left hemisphere lesions (human), 178–180
Caudate nucleus
head, horseradish peroxidase injection, 37–41
neurochemical laterality, 22
unilateral
destruction, rotation syndrome, 9
stimulation, and spatial preferences (rat), 10
Central nervous system
organization, fundamental elements: structure and function asymmetries, 164
plastic changes, 52
Cerebellum, developing axons, dynamic interactions, 53
Cerebrum
asymmetries
ontogeny, 12–13
and psychopathology, 16–17
sex differences (human), 104–105
dominance
and direction of turning, 141
and emotions, relationship, 176–177
laterality of dysfunction, and forced normalization, 157
lateralization
of mood, in epilepsy, 150
rat, extrapolations to human, 7–22
Chlorpromazine, 281
and auditory tests in schizophrenia, 290
Cholecystokinin, in Parkinson's disease, 79
Choline acetyltransferase, laterality, brain structures (human), 22
Chromic acid, 8
Circling, *see* Rotation
Clinical syndromes, and lateral asymmetries, in schizophrenia, 267–269
Clozapine, and EEG activity in schizophrenics, 157
Cluster behavior
and neuropsychobiological hemisyndromes, 337–338
in time domain, 337–338
Cognition, ideal, and intermittency, 341
Cognitive abilities, asymmetric decline with age, 193–201
Cognitive dimensions, and psychopathological dimensions, interrelation, 169
Cognitive functions
lateralization
complementary specialization (human), 93–94
sex differences (human), 103–105
Cognitive style
hemisphere differences, 328
oscillation, neurochemical locus, 338
Compulsive personality style
and dimensionality, 333
energy distribution, compact and restrained, 328
temporal and spatial dynamics, 327–342

Computed tomography
hemisphere reversals, 269–270
and schizophrenia, 270
Consciousness
state
in cursive epilepsy, 142
in gyratory epilepsy, 135–136
Coping style
hysterical mode, 342
obsessive–compulsive mode, 342
Corpus callosum
dopamine-mediated activity, effects of neuroleptics, 364
and somesthetic studies in schizophrenia, 293
transmission
deficit in schizophrenia, 371–377
and schizophrenia, 274–275
Corpus striatum, lesions, rotation (animal), 8–9
Cortex
modulation, and population bias (rat), 17–18
silent lesions, 428–430
Cortical evoked potentials, and schizophrenia, 298, 301–305
Criminal
behavior, and hemisphere dysfunction, 390
left hemisphere dysfunction, 393–394
Criminology
psychobiological theories, 390
psychopathy and behavior disorders in, 389
Crying, and left-sided lesions, 161
Cursive epilepsy, 130, 141–146
clinical features, 141–143
differential diagnosis, 144–145
electroencephalography, 143
psychiatric aspects, 143–144

D

Dendrite, arborization, and behavior modifications, 59
Dentate gyrus, neuron plasticity, 56–57
2-Deoxy-D-glucose technique, brain multiple asymmetries, and developmental changes (rat), 12–13
Deprenyl, anti-Parkinsonian drug, 82
Depression, psychiatric disorder associated with age, 206
Depressive syndrome, and right hemisphere damage, 160
Diagnosis
based on results of treatment, and schizophrenia, 377–379
controversies, schizophrenia, 269
Dichotic listening
and hemiaging, 199–201
and schizophrenia, 286
L-3,4-Dihydroxyphenylalanine, *see* L-Dopa
Dimensionality
and compulsive personality style, 333
and hysterical personality style, 333
and neuropsychobiological hemisyndromes, 331–335
and stability, concept, 331–335
Dimethyltryptamine, abnormal neurological signs on left side, normal subjects, 164
Dissociative experience, and psychotherapy, 468–471
Divided attention tasks, in hemiaging, 204
Divided-field technique, and visual tests in schizophrenia, 294–297
Domperidone, 19
L-Dopa, 452
effect on
attention-related visual evoked potentials asymmetry reduction, 223–225
electroencephalogram patterns over Parkinsonian and non-Parkinsonian hemispheres during sleep, 217
visual evoked potential from Parkinsonian and non-Parkinsonian hemispheres, 219–221
and motor function restoration, 71–72
rotation induction (rat), 9
Dopamine
deficit
and electrodermal activity in hemi-Parkinsonism, 230–233
in hemi-Parkinsonism, 77–78
extrastriatal sites, 80
laterality, brain structures (human), 22
nigrostriatum content, endogenous asymmetry (rat), 10
striatum
asymmetry, and side preferences (rat), 10–11
concentrations, and unilateral motor behavior, 71–72
Dopamine agonists, direct and indirect, 80–81
Dopamine receptor
presynaptic, 83

striatum, asymmetries and sex differences (rat), 18–20
D3 Dopamine receptor
striatum, asymmetry, sex differences (rat), 19–20
Dopaminergic system
brain, locus for
disconnections of hemisyndromes, 338
oscillation in cognitive style, 338
spatiotemporal asymmetries, 338
Dreams, loss or reduction, right hemisphere lesions, 165–166
Drug
action starts at psychological base, placebo effect, 449–450
alteration of perception, mood, and states of consciousness, 469
brain reactivity to, effect of psychotherapy, 450
commonly abused, mechanisms of action, 16
disposition
and activity, 460–465
effect of
blood flow, 461–463
metabolism and excretion, 460
distribution, activity directed, 466
euphoria, and lateralization of reward mechanisms, 13–17
induction of anterograde amnesia, 471
response
effects of beliefs, expectations, and environmental stimuli, 452
influence of
personality, 450
situational variables, 450
state-dependent process, 449
rotation induction (animal), 9
Drug-personality interactions, 451
Dynamic process model, hemisphere functions, 265–267, 311–314

E

Earedness, sex differences (human), 106
Electrical activity, brain, in hemi-Parkinsonism, 216–223
Electroconvulsive therapy, unilateral, emotional response pattern, 162
Electrodermal activity
asymmetries
in hemi-Parkinsonism, 229–234
in schizophrenia, 267–269
syndrome differentiation, 268
in schizophrenia, effects of neuroleptics, 364–368
Electroencephalography
in cursive epilepsy, 143
in gelastic epilepsy, 244–246
in gyratory epilepsy, 136–137
and schizophrenia, 298–301
sleep abnormalities, symmetry in hemi-Parkinsonism, 216–219
Electromyography, face, asymmetries after questions about positive or negative emotions, 185
Electrooculogram, recording eye movements, in schizophrenia, 308
Electrophysiology, and hemiaging, 201–202
Emotion
and cerebral dominance, relationship, 176–177
and right hemisphere, 432
Emotional appropriateness, unilateral brain lesions, 181–184
Emotional behavior
patterns, unilateral brain lesions (human), 177–180
and right hemisphere lesions (human), 176–177
unilateral brain lesions
clinical aspects, 177–181
human, 175–189
meaning, 184–188
Emotional comprehension, unilateral brain lesions, 181–184
Emotional control, mechanisms, left hemisphere, 188
Emotional expression, unilateral brain lesions, 181–184
Emotional outbursts, positive and negative, hemispheric asymmetry, 189
Emotional reactions, effect of right and left hemisphere lesions, 1
Endogenous psychoses, *see* Psychosis
Energy
distribution
compact, compulsive personality style, 328
diffuse, hysterical personality style, 328
Entorhinal lesions, unilateral, neuron sprouting induction, 48

Enzymes, brain, intermittent catalytic and binding actions, 334
Epilepsy, 1–2, 129–146
brain lesions and psychiatric disorders, 1
convulsions, whole body, 130
history, 129–131
laterality and psychopathology, 150, 156
lateralized pathology, 2
loss of consciousness, 130
partial, 130
right- and left-sided, relation to psychopathological manifestations, 149–169
Epileptic laughter, 239–258; *see also* Gelastic epilepsy
pathophysiology, and brain pathology, 251–256
Erotic arousal, and right brain processes, 166
Euphoria
function of left brain systems, 162
Experience, dissociative, and psychotherapy, 468–471
Extrapyramidal system
activation, and turning behavior (human), 139
lateralization, gyratory epilepsy, 146
Eye
lateral movements
index of abnormal hemisphere balance in schizophrenia, 348–350
neuroleptic effects, 348–350, 371
in schizophrenia, 307–310
pursuit movements, in hemiaging, 204
tracking,
in hemiaging, 203–204
in schizophrenia, 309–310
Eyedness, sex differences (human), 105–106

F

Face, left side, expression of positive and negative emotions, 186
Fiber connections, lesion-induced asymmetry, 52
Fixed structure, model of hemisphere functions, 265–267, 315
Fluorescent tracers, injection, caudate nucleus head, 37–41
Focal slowing, and electrophysiology, in hemiaging, 201
Footedness, sex differences (human), 105–106
Forced normalization, 156–159
and laterality of cerebral dysfunction, interaction in psychosis, 157
parameter of psychosis, 150
in psychosis, 157
Function
asymmetries
after accident, stroke, or surgery (human), 93
animals, 96–103

G

GABA, *see* γ-Aminobutyric acid
Galin's hypothesis, 423–424
right hemisphere, locus for unconscious mental contents, 423
Galvanic skin response, painful stimuli, and unilateral brain damage (human), 183–184
Gelastic epilepsy, 240–251; *see also* Epileptic laughter
and antiepileptic medication, 249, 251
electroencephalography and laterality, 244–246
psychopathology, 242–244
role of pleasure, 240–242
symptoms, 240–251
Globus pallidus
neurochemical laterality, 22
projections, 74–75
Glutamate decarboxylase, left-right asymmetries, brain structures (human), 21–22
Gyratory epilepsy, 130–141, 146
clinical features, 131–137
electroencephalography, 136
experimental data, extrapolation to, 139–141
and laughter, 246–249
treatment, 136

H

Haloperidol, and EEG activity in schizophrenics, 157
Halstead–Reitan battery, and schizophrenia, 276–278
Handedness
and schizophrenia, 275–276
sex differences (human), 105–106
in study of hemiaging, 207
and symptom lateralization, 427–428

Happiness, leads to movement, skipping, hopping, 165
Hatred, toward paralyzed limbs, unilateral brain damage, 179–180
Health status, in testing for hemiaging, 207
Hearing, loss, and aging, 200
Hebb's Recurring Digits Test, and schizophrenia, 283
Hemiaging, 193–208
  cognitive abilities, 194–201
    dichotic listening, 199–201
    intelligence, 194–195
    visuospatial abilities, 195–199
  electrophysiology, 201–202
  neurotransmitters, 202–203, 206
  time sharing, 203–206
Hemi-Parkinsonism
  brain electrical activity, 216–223
  electrodermal activity, asymmetries, 229–234
  failing dopamine system, 214
  hemisphere
    imbalance, two types, 213–234
    interdependence, 223–229
  model
    experimental, 69–84
    hemidecline with age (human), 203
    laterality research in schizophrenia and depression, 214–215
    rotating rodent, 77, 80
  patient distribution by sex and side of symptoms, 216
  sleep electroencephalogram abnormalities, symmetry, 216–219
  visual evoked potentials, 219–222
Hemisphere
  abnormal balance in schizophrenia, 348–350
    and lateral eye movements, 348–350
  asymmetries, and psychopathology, interaction, 216
  balance, personality determinant, 156
  cognitive style differences, 328
  disconnection, neurochemical locus, 338–342
  dominant, and temporal lobe epilepsy psychosis, 149–150
  dysfunction
    in behavior disorders, 389–406
      clinical evidence, 394–397
    in psychopathy, 389–406
  functions
    model
      dynamic process, 265–267, 311–314
      fixed structure, 265–267, 315
    and personality organization, 468
  imbalance
    in hemi-Parkinsonism, two types, 213–234
    in psychoses, 2
  interdependence, 4, 406
    in hemi-Parkinsonism, 223–229
  left
    activation, right-sided machinery requirement, 355–357
    deficit, in schizophrenia, 371–377
    discrete organization, 168
  reversals
    and computed tomography, 269–270
    and schizophrenia, 270
  right
    decompensation by schizophrenic process, 355
    deficit, in schizophrenia, 371-377
    diffuse organization, 168
    dominant for emotions and affects, 186–187
    and emotion, 432–433
    in hemiaging, 193–208
    and hypnotism, 433–436
    influences on vegetative functions, 416
    silent cortical lesions, and symptom lateralization, 428–430
Hemisphere disconnection syndrome, from neuroleptic treatment, 357–360
Hemisphericity, structural determinant of personality, 454
Hemisyndromes, 3–4
  clinical, and aberrant laterality, 3–4
  disconnections, locus, brain dopaminergic systems, 338
  experimental, roles of age, gender, and activity in organization, 4
  in laterality research, 4–5
  neuropsychobiological, 327–342
  temporal lobe epilepsy, 149–169
Hippocampus
  morphological asymmetry, sex differences 108
  neuron plasticity, 56–57
  and schizophrenia, 316–317

Hippocampus (*cont.*)
self-stimulation asymmetries (rat), 15–16
Hoffman reflex, *see* Neuromuscular reflexes
Hormone control systems, sex differences (human), 103
Horseradish peroxidase
injection
caudate nucleus head, 37–41
thalamus, 28–37
6-Hydroxydopamine
nigrostriatum lesion induction, 72–73
substantia nigra unilateral lesion, 35–42
Hydroxylase cofactor, *see* Tetrahydrobiopterin
5-Hydroxytryptamine, in Parkinson's disease, 78
Hypnotism, and right hemisphere, 433–436
Hypothalamopituitary system, organization, sex differences (human), 103
Hypothalamus
lateral, self-stimulation threshold asymmetries (rat), 13–14
in laughter system, 251
organization, sex differences (human), 103
Hysterical personality style
and dimensionality, 333
energy distribution, diffuse, 328
temporal and spatial dynamics, 327–342

I

Imagery
and hemiaging, 196, 198
in therapy, 467
Imipramine
EEG changes, normal subjects, 163
effect on cognitive styles, 341–342
Index of dimensionality, 339–340
Index of sensory processing, P_{300}, 362
Indifference reaction
and right hemisphere lesions (human), 178–179
and attention-arousal defect, 186
Information processing
additive and multiplicative, 335–337
and neuropsychobiological hemisyndromes, 335–337
Intelligence
crystallized and fluid abilities, in hemiaging, 194–195
and hemiaging, 194–195
verbal and performance subtests, in hemiaging, 194–195
Interhemisphere
communication, corticotectal, 56
fiber connections
plasticity, 51–59
projection systems, 51
projections
and function recovery
after lesion, 59
from lesion-induced behavior asymmetries, 46
substantia nigra neurons, 28–51
Intermittency
cluster behavior in time domain, 337–338
and ideal cognition, 341
and neuropsychobiological hemisyndromes, 337–338
mechanisms, 337–338

K

Kainic acid, substantia nigra unilateral lesion, 35–37

L

Language
abilities, effect of left hemisphere lesions (human), 93
affective components, and right hemisphere lesions, 182
structure, modification, 467
Laterality
affect, unilateral brain lesions (human), 175–189
brain
functions, 2
and pharmacopsychotherapy, 447–473
changes, in psychopathological syndromes, 2
and endogenous psychoses, 159–164
in gelastic epilepsy, 244–246
neurochemistry, brain (human), 21–22
patterns, assessment, 348
and psychopathology, in epilepsy, 150–156
Laterality index, auditory studies, and schizophrenia, 288, 290
Lateralization, *see also* specific structure and function

affect, model, 14
cerebrum, function (animal, human), 8
cognitive
functions, complementary specialization (human), 93–94
symptoms, left hemisphere, 271
effects of unilateral brain lesions (rat), 11–12
patterns
for optimal function in specific neural systems, 121
in population, 108
reward mechanisms (rat), 13–17
sex differences
animal, 117–119
human, 115–117
and understanding of function of neural systems, 121
Laughter
and adversive epilepsy, 246–249
affective syndromes, 251
automatic, reflectoral reaction, 251
clinical, mechanisms, 251
epileptic, *see* Epileptic laughter
inappropriate, in epileptic laughter, 258
medication side effect, 257
reaction to pain cessation, 255
and right-sided lesions, 161
Learning
experience, and terminal arborization, 59
lateralization (bird), 97
tasks, compensation for lesion-induced sensorimotor asymmetry, 49
Limbic epilepsy, laterality and psychopathology, 152, 154
Lithium
EEG changes, normal subjects, 164
effect on cognitive styles, 342
Locus of dysfunction, schizophrenia, 315–318
Lorazepam, and anterograde amnesia, 471
D-Lysergic acid diethylamide
effects on hippocampus self-stimulation asymmetries (rat), 15–16
rotation induction (rat), 9

M

Manic-depressive states
and bilateral involvement, 272
mood alterations, 271
Marijuana, smoke, effect on hemisphere responses, 455
Mathematical theory, in temporal and spatial dynamics of neuropsychobiological hemisyndromes, 329–331
Meaning, of emotional behavior after unilateral brain damage, 184–188
Memory, 195–198; *see also* specific type of memory
for faces, in hemiaging, 195–196
Mental manipulation, visual information, in hemiaging, 196–197
Mood
cerebral lateralization, 150
disturbance, and lesions of dominant hemisphere, 161
and movement, interdependence, 165
states
and visuospatial processes, 165
and volitional motility, 165
systems, and lateralization, 165
Morphine
effects on lateral hypothalamic self-stimulation asymmetries, 14–15
rotation induction (rat), 9
Motivational defect, and right brain damage, 181
Motor
asymmetries
animal, 98
sex differences
animal, 108–115
human 105–106
laterality, right (human), 167
system, activation by temporal discharges, cursive epilepsy, 146
Movement
initiation and control, and basal ganglia, 70
and mood, interdependence, 165
Multiple personality, and temporal lobe epilepsy, 156
Muscimol, 75

N

Nardil, EEG changes, depressed patients, 164
Neglect syndrome, and attention-arousal defect, right brain damage, 186
Nerve cell, *see* Neuron
Neural asymmetries, sex differences (animal), 107–108

Neural dynamics, cooperative, 334
Neuroanatomical indices, and neural asymmetries, sex differences (animal), 108
Neurobiology
  data, vertically integrated phenomena, 334
  states
    dimensionality and amplitude of fluctuations, 332
    invariant geometries, 332
  systems, intermittent pattern of activity, 337
Neurochemical indices, and neural asymmetries, sex differences (animal), 107–108
Neurochemical locus
  for hemispheric disconnection, 338–342
  for spatiotemporal asymmetries, 338–342
Neurochemistry
  asymmetries
    brain regions (rat), 96
    and cerebral dominance (rat), 20
  brain, laterality (human), 21–22
Neuroleptic drug
  alteration of right hemisphere reactivity, 455
  effects
    on lateral eye movements, 348–350, 371
    and site of abnormality, schizophrenia, 347–379
  induction of visual evoked potential asymmetry, 350–360
  multiple sites of action, 378
  treatment
    and hemisphere disconnection syndrome, 357–360
    lateralized side effects, 459–460
Neuromuscular reflexes, and schizophrenia, 305–307
Neuron
  circuits, lesion-induced asymmetry, 51
  connections, plastic changes, 52
  plastic changes in terminal arborization, 59
  plasticity
    dentate gyrus, 56–57
    red nucleus, 52–54
    superior colliculus, 55–56
    after unilateral brain lesions, 27–59
    reorganization, compensatory, 51
    sprouting, 48
      forebrain, 52
Neuropsychiatry, 270–272, 275–280
  handedness, 275–276
  neuropsychological tests, 276–280
  organic lesions, 276
  and schizophrenia, 270–272, 275–280
Neuropsychobiological hemisyndromes
  hysterical and compulsive personality styles, 327–342
  temporal and spatial dynamics, 327–342
    dimensionality and stability, concept, 331–335
    information processing, 335–337
    intermittency, 337–338
    mathematical theory, 329–331
Neuropsychological tests, and schizophrenia, 276–280
Neurotransmitter
  biogenic amines, synthesis and binding by receptors, 329
  central systems, motor behavior modification, 73
  lateral asymmetry, brain (human), 21–22
  in Parkinson's disease, 78–79
  systems, asymmetric organization
    in hemiaging, 202–203, 206
    brain, 164
Nigral afferents, to ventromedial thalamus, 41–42
Nigrocaudate projections, 39–41
Nigrostriatum
  dopamine
    concentrations, and unilateral motor behavior, 71
    content, endogenous asymmetry (rat), 10
    metabolites, asymmetry, 10
  lesions
    induction by 6-hydroxydopamine, 72–73
    partial, 79–80
Nigrothalamic projections, 32
  reorganization, 42–44
Nondirective therapy, 468
Nonpiperazine drugs, and lateral eye movements in schizophrenia, 350
Nonverbal expressiveness, and unilateral brain damage, 183

Nonverbal tasks, deficits, right hemisphere lesions, 93
Norepinephrine, in Parkinson's disease, 78
Nucleus accumbens
  dopamine receptors, 80
  and posture deviation, 80
Nucleus ruber, *see* Red nucleus
Nucleus tegmentum pedunculopontinus, 74–77

O

Organic bias hypothesis, and symptom lateralization, 430–431
Organization
  diffuse, right hemisphere, 168
  discrete, left hemisphere, 168
Orgasmic epilepsy, and right hemisphere systems, 166
Orofacial dyskinesia, and antiepileptic treatment, 250

P

P_{300}, *see* Surface positive potential
Pain, lateralized, usually on left side, 422
Paralysis, unilateral, nigrothalamic projection reorganization after (rat), 42–44
Paralyzed limbs, hatred toward, unilateral brain damage, 179–180
Parkinsonism
  basal ganglion disease, 70
  failure of dopamine neurotransmission in nigrostriatal tract, 215
  model, rotating rodent, 70–73
  neurotransmitter involvement, 78–79
Parkinson's disease, *see* Parkinsonism
Pathology, brain, and pathophysiology of epileptic laughter, 251, 256
Pathophysiology, epileptic laughter, 251–256
Pawedness, *see also* Handedness
  brain asymmetry 97–98
  lateralization, sex differences (mouse), 114–115
Peptide
  role in neurological disorders, 79
  transmitters, assessment, 84
Periaqueductal gray, and basal ganglion outflow site, 77
Personality
  in drug response, 450
  organization, roles of right and left hemispheres, 468
Perspective-taking, mental manipulation task, in hemiaging, 196–197
Pharmacopsychotherapy, 447–473
  and aberrant brain laterality, 447–473
  and desirable drug response, 465
Pharmacotherapy, and differentiation of pathological conditions, 378
Phencyclidine
  effects on hippocampus self-stimulation asymmetries (rat), 15–16
  rotation induction (rat), 9
Phenothiazines, hostility reduction, 455
Pindolol, 281
Piperazine derivatives
  effect on visual evoked potentials, 352
  and lateral eye movements in schizophrenia, 350
Placebo effect, psychological base of drug action, 449–450
Planum temporale, size, asymmetry (human), 92
Plasticity
  interhemispheric fiber connections, 51–59
  interhemispherically projecting neurons, 57–58
  neuron
    dentate gyrus, 56–57
    red nucleus, 52–54
    superior colliculus, 55–56
  redirected growth of axons, 58
  sprouting of projecting neurons, 58
Pleasure, role in gelastic epilepsy, 240–242
Population bias, cortex modulation (rat), 17–18
Posture
  asymmetries
    animal, 98
    sex differences
      animal, 108–115
      human, 105–106
  deviation, and nucleus accumbens, 80
Prepotent hypothesis, response to drug, 451
Problem-solving mode
  compulsive personality style, 328
  hysterical personality style, 328
Processing strategies, auditory studies, and schizophrenia, 287

Projections
globus pallidus, 74–75
interhemispheric, 28–51
nigrocaudate, 39–41
nigrothalamic, 32
sites, dentate gyrus, 56
substantia nigra, 75–77
systems, interhemispheric fiber connections, 51
Psychiatry, and hemispheric asymmetry of function, 423–424
Psychodrama, in therapy, 468
Psychogenic hemisensory disturbances, on left side, 416
Psychogenic somatic symptoms, on left side, 415–441
Psychology
experimental, 280–298
auditory studies, 280–291
hemisphere equivalence and acute symptoms, 288–290
lateralized drug influences, 290–291
left hemisphere overactivation in paranoid schizophrenia, 286–288
left hemisphere temporal variation and limbic locus, 281–286
and schizophrenia, 280–298
somesthetic studies, 291–293
and callosal hypothesis, 291–293
visual studies, 293–298
Psychopathology
gelastic epilepsy, 242–244
and hemisphere asymmetries, interaction, 216
and laterality, in epilepsy, 150–156
manifestations, relation to right- and left-sided epilepsy, 149–169
states, and lateralization of reward mechanisms, 13–17
Psychopathy
and hemisphere dysfunction, 389–406
experimental evidence, 397–399
electrodermal responsivity, 397–399
lateral preferences, 399–403
visual field differences, 399
history, 389–390
Psychopharmacology
artistic and intellectual brain, 453–456
clinical, and clinical psychology, 472
Psychophysiology, 272–273, 298–310
conjugate lateral eye movements, 307–310
cortical evoked potentials, 298, 301–305
electroencephalogram, 298–301
neuromuscular reflexes, 305–307
and schizophrenia, 272–273, 298–310
Psychosis, 1–3
association with disorders of cerebral laterality, 16
bilateral involvement, 272
bipartite laterality model, 273–274
endogenous, and laterality, 159–164
laterality of cerebral dysfunction and forced normalization, interaction, 157
relation to hemisphere imbalance, 2
temporal lobe epilepsy, and dominant hemisphere, 149–150
Psychosocial state, effect on brain reactivity to chemical substance, 449
Psychotherapy
and dissociative experience, 468–471
effect on brain reactivity to drug, 450
Putamen, neurochemical laterality, 22

R

Receptors, brain, intermittent catalytic and binding actions, 334
Red nucleus
lesion-induced reorganization, 53
neuron plasticity, 52–54
Reward mechanisms, lateralization (rat), 13–17
Right versus left, neurochemical asymmetries and cerebral dominance (rat, human), 20
Rotating rodent model
anti-Parkinsonian drug assessment, 80–83
and basal ganglion organization and outflows, 73–77
hemi-Parkinsonism, 77–80
Parkinson's disease, 70–73
Rotation
asymmetries, sex differences (animal), 110–111
and epileptic laughter, 247–248
in gyratory epilepsy, 131–137
history, 8–10
and corpus striatum, 8–9
and dopaminergic nigrostriatal system, 9
and interhemispheric projections, 28–51

mental, of visual information, in hemiaging, 196
sustained, experimental data, 137–139
Rotatory epilepsy, *see* Gyratory epilepsy
Running
in cursive epilepsy, 141–145
experimental data, relation to cursive epilepsy, 145

S

Sadness
function of right brain systems, 162
linked to immobility or agitation, 165
Schizophrenia, 1
abnormal hemisphere balance, 348–350
and lateral eye movements, 348–350
and auditory functions, 280–291
and bilateral involvement, 272, 280
and blinking, effects of neuroleptics, 368–371
and callosal transmission, 274–275
and cerebral asymmetries, 16–17
and conjugate lateral eye movements, 307–310
and diagnosis based on results of treatment, 377–379
electrodermal activity, effects of neuroleptics, 364–368
and electroencephalogram, 298–301
and experimental psychology, 280–298
hallucinations, mechanisms, 17
and handedness, 275–276
hemisphere functions, model
dynamic process, 265–267, 311–314
fixed structure, 265–267, 315
and hemisphere reversals, 270
heterogeneous character, 159
and interhemispheric transfer problems, 274
lateral asymmetries, 265–318
neuroleptic effects, 348–350
and neuromuscular reflexes, 305–307
and neuropsychiatry, 270–272, 275–280
and neuropsychological tests, 276–280
psychophysiology, 272–273, 298–301
site of abnormality, and neuroleptic effects, 347–379
symptoms, diminished or reduced with age, 203
and temporal lobe epilepsy, 153
Scopolamine, rotation induction (rat), 9
Self-stimulation
lateral hypothalamus, asymmetries (rat), 13–15
Sensorimotor
asymmetries, behavior recovery from, 28–29
deprivation, after unilateral substantia nigra lesion, 41–42
Sensory
data
conceptual elaboration, left hemisphere, 187
immediateness and rich affective value, right hemisphere, 187
deprivation, unilateral, nigrothalamic projection reorganization after (rat), 42–44
Sex
differences
[^{3}H]apomorphine binding to D3 dopamine receptor, 19–20
behavioral and brain asymmetries, 91–121
and symptom lateralization, 427
Sexuality
normal, and intact interhemispheric connections, 167
Side preferences
and lateralized dopamine function, 10–11
pinched tail, asymmetries, sex differences (rat), 112–113
two-lever operant situation, asymmetries, sex differences (rat), 113–114
Silent cortical lesions, right hemisphere, and symptom lateralization, 428–430
Situational variables, in drug response, 450
Sleep, electroencephalogram abnormalities, symmetry in hemi-Parkinsonism, 216–219
Social judgement, and right brain damage, 181
Somatic symptoms, *see* Psychogenic somatic symptoms
Song, neural control, asymmetry (bird), 96–97
Spatial
abilities, lateralization, sex differences (human), 104–105
dynamics, and neuropsychobiological hemisyndromes, 327–342

Spatial (*cont.*)
memory, in hemiaging, 195, 198
neglect, and right brain damage, 181
tasks, impairment, right hemisphere lesions (human), 93
Spatiotemporal asymmetry, neurochemical locus, 338–342
Speech, affective components, and right hemisphere, 182
Spike-wave discharge
bilateral synchronous, 136
in cursive epilepsy, 143
Sprouting
dentate gyrus, 56
initiation stimulus, 51
neuron, 48
forebrain, 52
postoperative, behavior concomitants, 51
Stability
and dimensionality, concept, 331–335
and neuropsychobiological hemisyndromes, 331–335
Striatum, dopamine receptor asymmetries and sex differences (rat), 18–20
Substantia nigra
anatomical connections, 138
efferent site in basal ganglion outflow systems, 74
locus of brain excitability modulation, 138
neuron interhemispheric projections, 28–51
projections, 75–77
and turning behavior, 137–139
unilateral lesion, 35–37
sensorimotor deprivation after, 41–42
Superior colliculus
neuron plasticity, 55–56
projections, and visual field mapping, 56
in substantia nigra projections, 75–76
Surface positive potential, component P_{300}, attention-induced changes 360–364
Symbolism hypothesis, and symptom lateralization, 431–432
Symptom
lateralization, 415–441
clinical observations, 416–417
Galin's (1974) hypothesis, 423–424
and handedness, 427–428
research findings, 417–426
and sex, 427
lateralization, explanations
alternatives to hemispheric specialization, 428–432
organic bias hypothesis, 430–431
silent cortical lesions in right hemisphere, 428–430
symbolism hypothesis, 431–432
hemispheric specialization, 432–441
emotion and right hemisphere, 432–433
emotional influence on somatic input from left side, 438–441
hypnosis and right hemisphere, 433–436
right hemisphere mechanism 436–438
psychogenic somatic, on left side, 415–441
Synapse
contacts, hippocampus, 57
formation, increased in denervated brain structures, 48
sprouted, replacement by regenerating axon terminals, 50
Synthetic Sentence Identification Test, and schizophrenia, 283

T

Tactual memory, in hemiaging, 197
Tail deviation, newborn, asymmetries, sex differences (rat), 114
Task, complexity, in hemiaging, 204–205
Telencephalon
unilateral removal
adult (rat), 29–33
newborn (rat), 33–35
Temporal dynamics, and neuropsychobiological hemisyndromes, 327–342
Temporal lobe epilepsy
hemisyndromes, 149–169
left, schizophrenic symptoms, 150
right, manic-depressive symptoms, 150
Tetrahydrobiopterin, hydroxylase cofactor, 339–340
Tetramethylbenzidine, 31
Thalamus
horseradish peroxidase injection, 28–37
in substantia nigra projections, 75–76
ventromedial, nigral afferents to, 41–42
Therapist–patient, interaction, 467
Thinking, style, modification to improve behavior, 467

Thought
modes
holistic or gestalt processing capacity, right hemisphere, 187
verbal-analytical-logical, left hemisphere, 187
Time
domain
cluster behavior in, 337–338
and neuropsychobiological hemisyndromes, 337–338
sharing, and hemiaging, 203–206
Tomography, *see* Computed tomography
Touch, localization tests, and schizophrenia, 291–292
Tracking, in schizophrenia, 309–310
Trait factor, and schizophrenia, 286–288
Trimetadione, gyratory epilepsy treatment, 136
Turning, *see* Rotation
Turn preferences
in open field
asymmetries, sex differences (animal), 111–112
effects of handling, 112
in T maze, asymmetries, sex differences (rat), 113
Tyrosine hydroxylase, brain homogenates (rat), 339

U

Unilateral paralysis agitans, *see* Hemi-Parkinsonism
Uptake blockers, anti-Parkinsonian drugs, 81–82

V

Verbal abilities, lateralization, sex differences (human), 104–105
Verbal–performance difference, and hemiaging, 194–195
Violent behavior, psychopathic, associated with left hemisphere dysfunctions, 396
Visual discrimination, lateralization (bird), 97
Visual evoked potentials
attention-related, asymmetry reduction, 222–223
in hemi-Parkinsonism, 219–226
neuroleptic-induced asymmetry, 350–360
Visual processing, and schizophrenia, 293–294
Visual system, neuron changes, compensatory, 55
Visuospatial
abilities, and hemiaging, 195–199
processing, and hemiaging, 194–199
systems, and mood states, 164–165

W

Wechsler Adult Intelligence Scale
performance > verbal pattern, 390–394
criminals, 393–394
delinquents, 392–393
learning difficulties, 392–393
left hemisphere dysfunction, 391–394
psychopaths, 392–393
and schizophrenia, 277–278
verbal > performance pattern
alcoholics, 394
depresive patients, 393
right hemisphere dysfunction, 391–394